IMAGING OF CARDIAC DISORDERS

VOLUME 1: CONGENITAL DISORDERS

IMAGING OF CARDIAC DISORDERS

VOLUME 1: CONGENITAL DISORDERS

Benigno Soto, M.D.
Professor of Radiology
Director of Cardiopulmonary Radiology
University of Alabama at Birmingham School of Medicine
Birmingham, AL

E. George Kassner, M.D.
Director of Diagnostic Radiology
Kings County Hospital Center
Professor of Radiology
State University of New York
Health Science Center at Brooklyn
Brooklyn, NY

William A. Baxley, M.D.
Professor of Medicine
Division of Cardiovascular Disease
University of Alabama at Birmingham School of Medicine
Birmingham, AL

JB Lippincott • Philadelphia
Gower Medical Publishing • New York • London

LIBRARY OF CONGRESS CATALOGING-IN-PUBLICATION DATA
Soto, Benigno, 1929–
Imaging of cardiac disorders / Benigno Soto, E. George Kassner,
William A. Baxley.
p. cm.
Includes bibliographical references and index.
Contents: v. 1. Congenital disorders — v. 2. Acquired disorders.
ISBN 1-56375-093-7 (v. 1). — ISBN 1-56375-094-5 (v. 2)
1. Heart—Imaging—Atlases. 2. Pediatric cardiology—Diagnosis—
-Atlases. 3. Heart—Interventional radiology—Atlases.
I. Kassner, E. George. II. Baxley, W. A. (Williams A.) III. Title.
[DNLM: 1. Cardiovascular Diseases—diagnosis—atlases.
2. Diagnostic Imaging—atlases. 3. Heart Defects, Congenital—
-diagnosis—atlases. WG 17 S7181]
RC683.5.I42S67 1991
616. 1'20754—dc20
91-22715

BRITISH LIBRARY CATALOGUING IN PUBLICATION DATA
Imaging of cardiac disorders.
Vol. 1 : Congenital disorders.
I. Benigno, Soto II. Kassner, E. George, 1937-
III. Baxley, William A.
616.120757

ISBN 1563750937

DISTRIBUTED IN USA AND CANADA BY:
JB Lippincott Company
East Washington Square
Philadelphia, PA 19105, USA

DISTRIBUTED IN THE REST OF THE WORLD
(EXCEPT JAPAN) BY:
Gower Medical Publishing Ltd.
Middlesex House
34-42 Cleveland Street
London W1P 5FB, UK

DISTRIBUTED IN JAPAN BY:
Nankodo Co., Ltd.
42-6, Hongo 3-Chome
Bunkyo-Ku
Tokyo 113, Japan

ISBN 0-397-44678-0 (Set)
ISBN 1-56375-093-7 (Volume 1)
ISBN 1-56375-094-5 (Volume 2)

10 9 8 7 6 5 4 3 2 1

ILLUSTRATORS: Wendy Jackelow, Patricia Gast (line tracings)
ART DIRECTOR: Jill Feltham
INTERIOR DESIGN AND LAYOUT: Jeff Brown
COVER DESIGN AND LAYOUT: Selina Waxman

Printed in the United States by Arcata Graphics/Kingsport

Dedicated to the patients who suffer from the cardiac diseases described in this book, and to their families.

CONTRIBUTORS

William A. Baxley, M.D.
Professor of Medicine
Division of Cardiovascular Disease
University of Alabama at Birmingham School of Medicine

Vera A. Bittner, M.D.
Assistant Professor of Medicine
Division of Cardiovascular Disease
University of Alabama at Birmingham School of Medicine

Robert C. Bourge, M.D., F.A.C.C.
Associate Professor of Medicine and Radiology
Division of Cardiovascular Disease
University of Alabama at Birmingham School of Medicine

Edward C. Colvin, M.D.
Associate Professor of Pediatrics
Division of Pediatric Cardiology
University of Alabama at Birmingham School of Medicine

Gregory B. Cranney, M.D.
Assistant Professor of Medicine
Division of Cardiovascular Disease
Clinical Director, Cardiovascular NMR Laboratory
University of Alabama at Birmingham School of Medicine
Clinical Director, Cardiovascular NMR Laboratory
University of Alabama Hospitals
Birmingham, Alabama

Milena J. Henzlova, M.D., F.A.C.C.
Assistant Professor of Medicine
Division of Cardiovascular Disease
University of Alabama at Birmingham School of Medicine

E. George Kassner, M.D., F.A.C.P.
Professor of Radiology
State University of New York Health Science Center at Brooklyn
Director of Diagnostic Radiology, Kings County Hospital Center
Head of Section of Pediatric Radiology, University Hospital
Brooklyn, New York

William R. Morrow, M.D.
Assistant Professor of Pediatrics
Division of Pediatric Cardiology
University of Alabama at Birmingham School of Medicine

Navin C. Nanda, M.D.
Professor of Medicine
Division of Cardiovascular Disease
University of Alabama at Birmingham School of Medicine
Director, Heart Station and Echocardiography-Graphics Laboratories
University of Alabama Hospitals
Birmingham, Alabama

Benigno Soto, M.D.
Professor of Radiology
University of Alabama at Birmingham School of Medicine
Director of Cardiopulmonary Radiology, University of Alabama Hospitals
Birmingham, Alabama

Isidre Vilaicosta, M.D.
Associate
Division of Cardiovascular Disease
University of Alabama at Birmingham School of Medicine
Assistant Professor
Division of Cardiology
University Hospital "San Carlos"
Madrid, Spain

PREFACE

Before the twentieth century, cardiovascular diagnosis was based on clinical observation and physical diagnosis. In the early years of this century, this limited armamentarium was augmented by plain radiography and fluoroscopy of the chest and by electrocardiography. Objective evaluation of cardiovascular physiology in vivo became possible in 1941 when Cournand demonstrated that intravascular exploration, using percutaneously introduced catheters, was both feasible and safe. Cardiac catheterization was soon followed by the advent of angiocardiography, which made it possible to identify morphologic abnormalities of the heart and great vessels in the living patient. The precise physiologic and anatomic data provided by cardiac catheterization and angiocardiography led to rapid advances in the field of cardiac surgery.

The past two decades have seen revolutionary advances in diagnostic imaging. The introduction of noninvasive (or minimally invasive) modalities such as echocardiography, nuclear cardiology, computed tomography, and magnetic resonance imaging has dramatically altered the diagnostic approach to the patient with cardiovascular disease. In some instances, sophisticated noninvasive techniques have decreased (or eliminated) the need for invasive diagnosis. In others, noninvasive techniques have provided new insights into the pathophysiology and natural history of cardiovascular disease. The ability of these modalities to detect cardiac disease in its earliest stages (e.g., silent ischemia, subclinical diastolic dysfunction) has important implications for the clinician. Rapid advances in interventional cardiology—coronary balloon angioplasty in particular—have stimulated major advances in imaging technology. Digital subtraction and other image enhancement techniques that provide high-resolution instant replay images are now available in all state-of-the-art interventional laboratories.

Imaging of Cardiac Disorders represents an effort to bridge the gap between introductory texts and more encyclopedic and highly specialized works on cardiology and specific imaging modalities. The emphasis is on plain radiography and angiocardiography, which continue to be the pillars of cardiac diagnosis; however, the newer modalities are extensively discussed and illustrated.

As the scope of the book widened, and production costs increased, the publisher suggested publishing it as a two-volume set. The authors agreed, since the two-volume format would make the book available to a wider audience (each volume can be purchased separately). Volume I discusses congenital heart disease in the child and adult. [A chapter on fetal cardiac diagnosis ("Imaging the Fetal Heart"), added because of the importance of sophisticated fetal cardiac diagnosis for pediatricians and pediatric cardiologists, appears as Chapter 15A.] Acquired heart disease in the child and adult, including ischemic heart disease resulting from congenital anomalies of the coronary arteries, is discussed in Volume II. A series of introductory chapters on imaging techniques and electrocardiography appears in both volumes. (Not included in the initial numbering scheme, a chapter on nuclear cardiology has been added as Chapter 4A.) Invasive catheter techniques employed in the treatment of congenital and acquired heart disease are discussed in Volume I and Volume II, respectively. Embolization techniques used in the treatment of congenital heart disease are discussed in Volume II.

The authors are indebted to their colleagues at the University of Alabama Medical Center and elsewhere who contributed chapters in their areas of expertise and provided images that appear throughout the book. We also wish to thank Abe Krieger and his team at Gower, who have captured our highly visual discipline in this beautifully produced book.

E. George Kassner, M.D.

Contents

VOLUME I: CONGENITAL DISORDERS

Chapter 10 140
Abnormal Atrioventricular Connections

Chapter 11 156
Abnormal Ventriculoarterial Connections

Chapter 12 178
Congenital Obstructing Lesions

Chapter 13 204
Valvular Insufficiency

Chapter 14 220
Extracardiac Shunts

Chapter 15 228
Anomalies of the Aortic Arch and Pulmonary Arteries

CHAPTER 1

Noninvasive Radiologic Techniques and Electrocardiography

CHEST RADIOGRAPHY AND FLUOROSCOPY

The initial radiologic examination in any patient with suspected heart disease consists of frontal and lateral radiographs of the chest. This simple, inexpensive technique provides important information about the size and configuration of the heart, atrial and visceral situs, the great arteries, and the pulmonary vasculature. The high-kilovoltage (140–160 kVp) technique normally used in adults usually provides excellent visualization of the trachea, bronchi, mediastinal structures, and pulmonary vasculature (Fig. 1.1). The ultra-high kilovoltage/magnification technique may be helpful when atrial situs is uncertain or when compression or displacement of the trachea is suspected (Fig. 1.2). Although no longer employed routinely, the four-film "cardiac series" is useful for evaluating the size of the cardiac

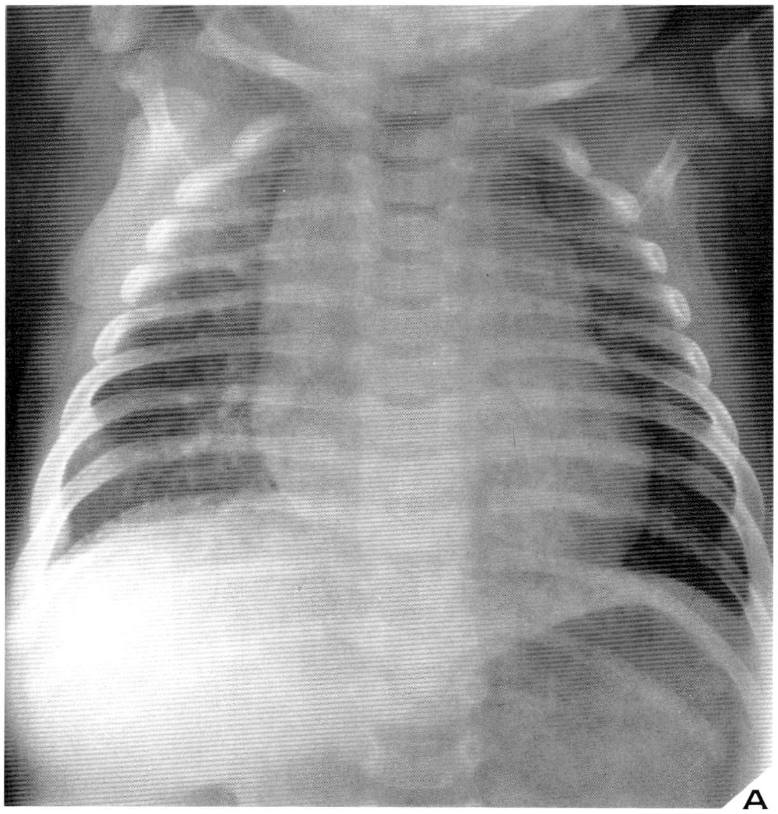

Fig. 1.1 High-kilovoltage chest films. (A) Frontal and (B) lateral chest films of an infant with transposition of the great arteries, obtained with 160 KVp using a very short exposure, clearly demonstrate the trachea, bronchi, mediastinal structures, and cardiovascular silhouette. The plethoric pulmonary vasculature is well demonstrated.

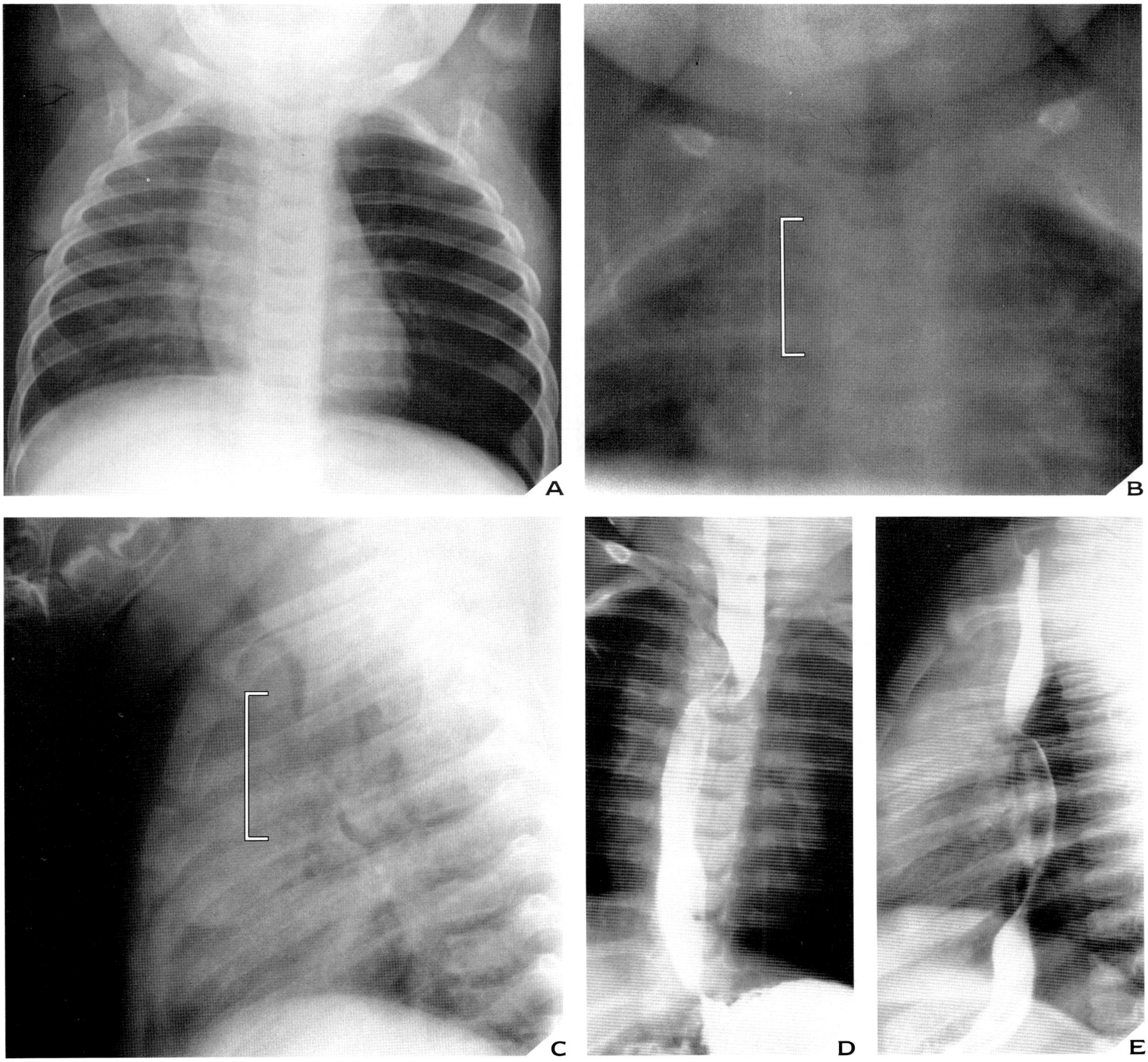

Fig. 1.2 Ultra-high kilovoltage/magnification technique and barium esophagram in investigation of vascular ring. Infant with stridor and feeding difficulty associated with a vascular ring (right aortic arch and left descending thoracic aorta). (A) Frontal chest film shows hyperlucency of the left lung. The tracheal air column cannot be identified. (B) Ultra-high kilovoltage magnification film shows absence of the tracheal air column ("empty segment sign") between the carina and the thoracic inlet (*brace*). (C) Conventional lateral chest film shows anterior displacement of the thoracic segment of the trachea, with complete effacement of its lumen. (D) Frontal and (E) lateral projections of esophagram show characteristic indentations of the right and posterior aspects of the esophagus produced by the vascular ring.

In the ultra-high kilovoltage/magnification technique illustrated in B, a Thoreus (tin–copper–aluminum) filter is placed in the X-ray beam to "harden" the radiation to an effective peak kilovoltage of about 300 kVp. At this energy, Compton scattering predominates and photoelectric interactions are relatively insignificant. The probability of photoelectric interactions between X-rays and the inner orbital electrons of the calcium atom is greatest on the low-kilovoltage films; consequently, the trachea and main bronchi are often obscured by overlying bony structures in infants' chest films. Because Compton scattering is related to electron density (which is approximately the same in bone and soft tissue), the ultra-high kilovoltage technique largely negates the "hiding" power of the thoracic and cervical vertebrae. Because electron density of soft tissue is much greater than that of air, there is excellent contrast between the tracheal air column and the surrounding soft tissues. The presence of an "empty" segment implies narrowing of the trachea by intrinsic or extrinsic pathology (in this instance, a tight vascular ring).

chambers (particularly the left atrium) and great arteries (Fig. 1.3). The barium esophagram is invaluable in patients with suspected vascular rings or aortopulmonary collaterals, which produce characteristic impressions on the barium-filled esophagus (see Fig. 1.2). With the advent of echocardiography, cardiac fluoroscopy is no longer performed routinely; however, it remains the most sensitive means of detecting calcifications of the cardiac valves and coronary arteries. Certain classical findings (eg, the "hilar dance" of pulmonary vavular insufficiency) can be detected only by fluoroscopy.

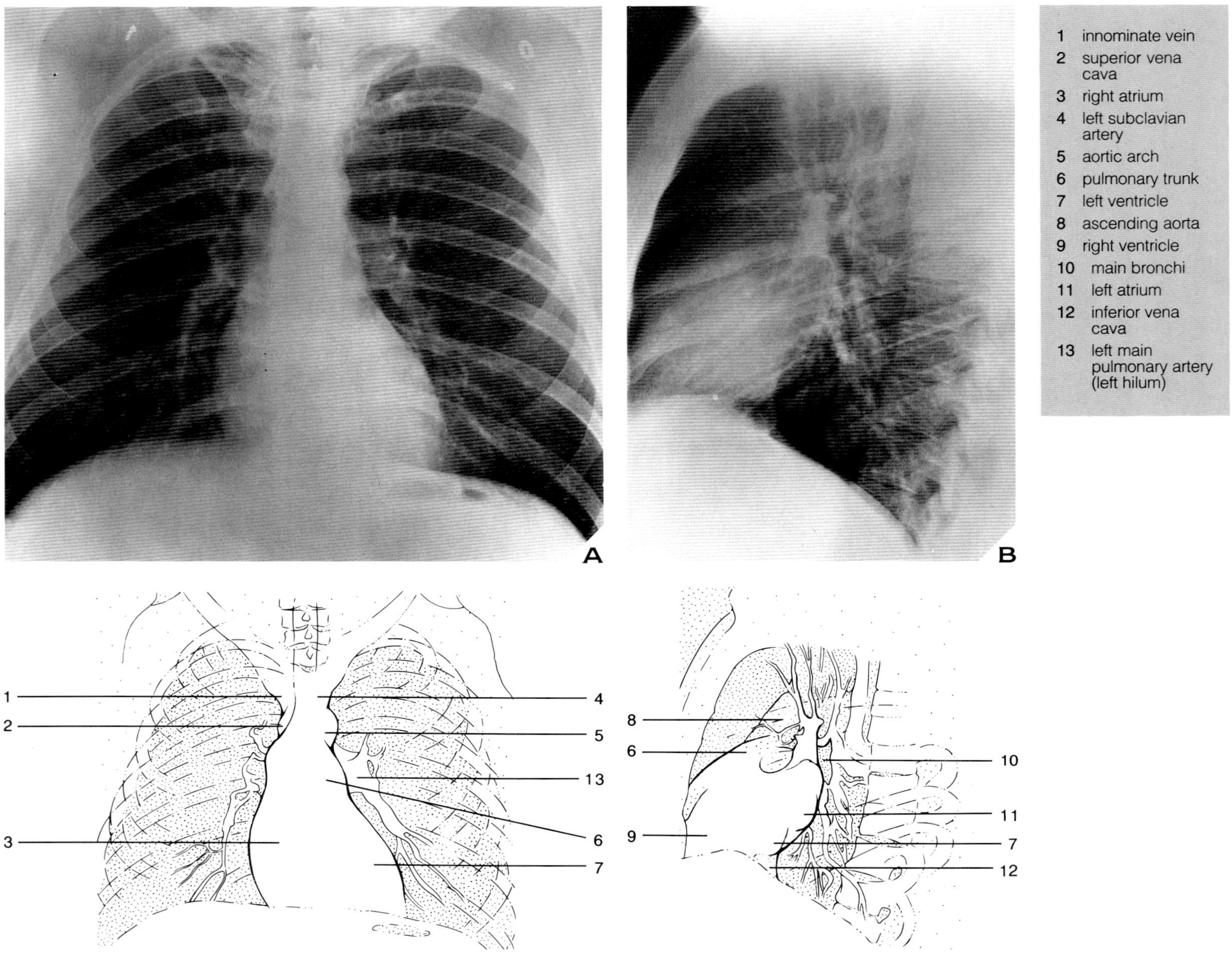

Fig. 1.3 Normal cardiac series. The standard cardiac series consists of four projections: posterior (PA), lateral, 60° left anterior oblique (LAO), and 45° right anterior oblique (RAO). (A) Posteroanterior (PA) projection. The right border of the cardiovascular silhouette is formed (from above downward) by the innominate vein, superior vena cava, and right atrium The border-forming structures on the left are (from above downward) the left subclavian artery, left aortic arch, pulmonary trunk, and left ventricle. The left atrial appendage normally does not contribute to the left heart border; in patients with an enlarged left atrium the left atrial appendage appears as a discrete bulge between the pulmonary trunk and the left ventricle. The left pulmonary artery, which forms the central portion of the left hilum, lies posterior to the pulmonary trunk and is distinctly separate from it. (B) Lateral projection. The anterior border of the cardiovascular silhouette is formed (from above downward) by the ascending aorta, pulmonary trunk, and right ventricle. Normally, the ascending aorta and pulmonary trunk are not well visualized in the lateral projection. The lower one third of the right ventricle normally makes contact with the anterior chest wall. The posterior border of the cardiovascular silhouette extends from the inferior margin of the mainstem bronchi and extends to the diaphragm; the border-forming structures are (from above downward) the left atrium, left ventricle, and inferior vena cava. (C) 60° left anterior oblique (LAO) projection. In this projection the anterior border of the cardiovascular silhouette is formed (from above downward) by the right innominate vein, superior vena cava, right atrium, and right ventricle.

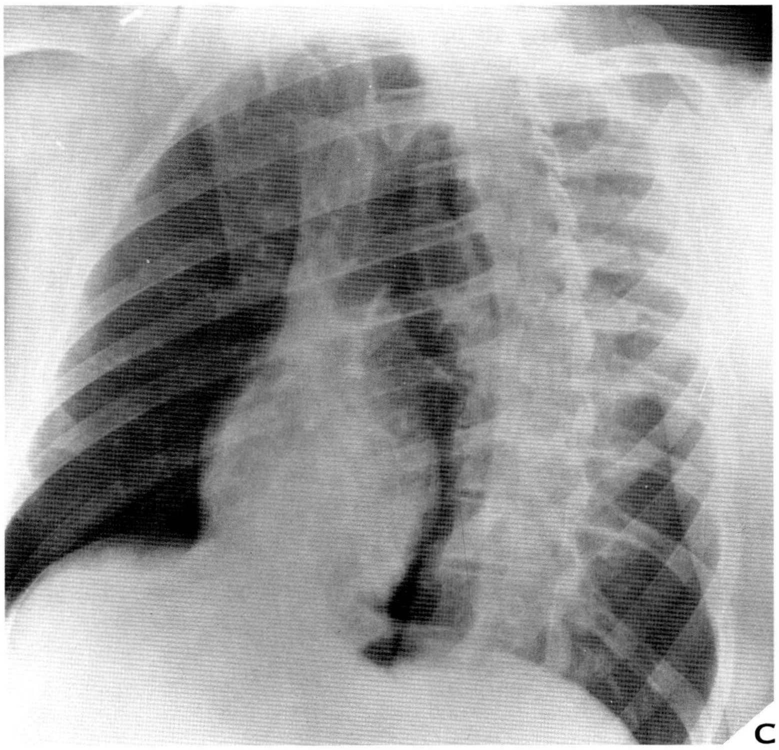

C

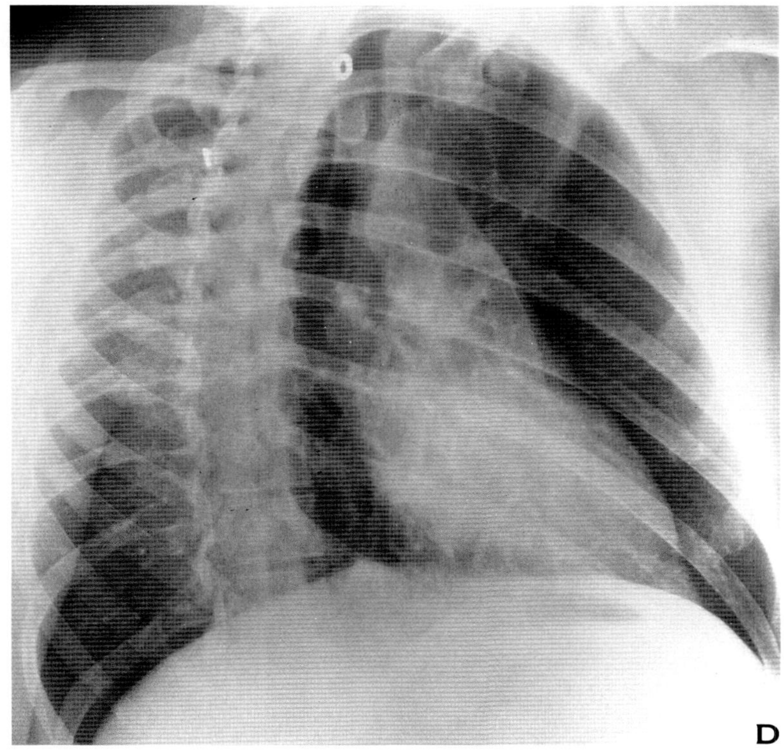

D

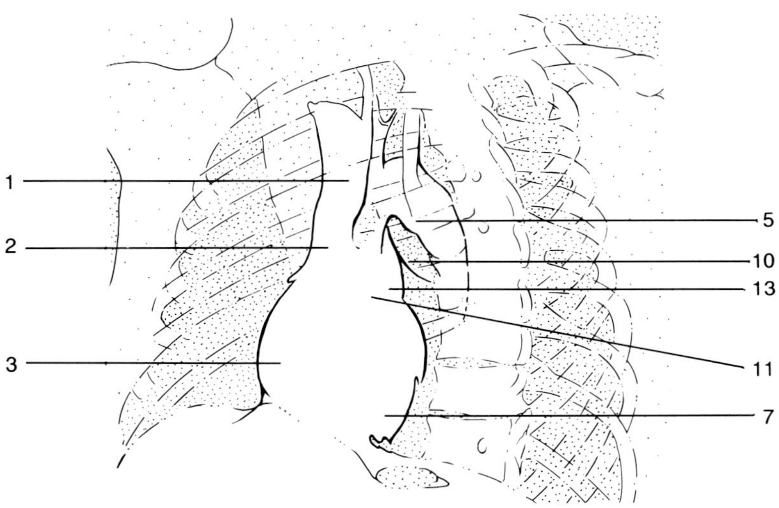

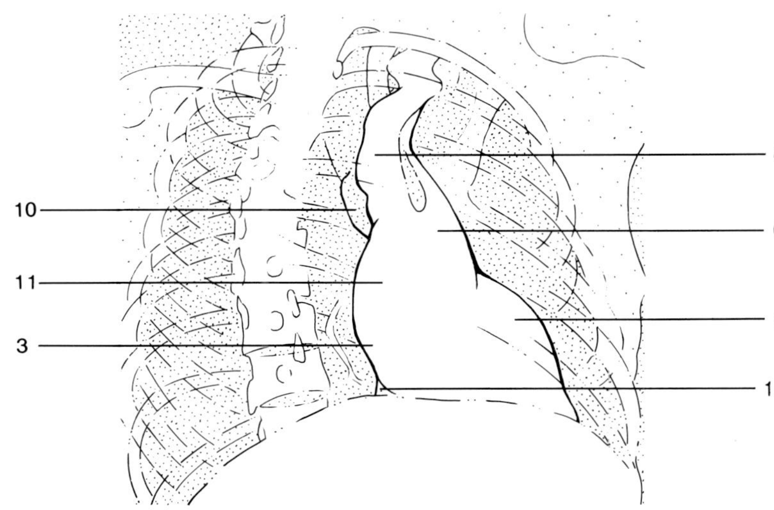

Depending on its size, the ascending aorta may or may not contribute to the contour anterior contour in this projection. An enlarged or tortuous ascending aorta appears as a discrete structure between the superior vena cava and the right atrium. The right ventricle is usually not visualized in this projection; however, in some individuals the inlet portion of the right ventricle is border forming. On the left, the border-forming structures are the left atrium, the upper margin of which lies just below the left main bronchus, and the left ventricle, which extends to the level of the diaphragm. The inferior aspect of the aortic arch and the upper aspect of the left pulmonary artery are separated by a clear space, the aortopulmonary window. (In this example, the left main bronchus is projected over the aortopulmonary window.) Enlargement or displacement of either (or both) of these structures may narrow or obliterate the aortopulmonary window. (D) 45° right anterior oblique (RAO) projection. The anterior border of the cardiovascular silhouette is formed (from above downward) by the ascending aorta, the pulmonary trunk, and the right ventricle. The posterior border is formed by the left atrium (just beneath the main bronchi) and the right atrium.

Administering barium paste to opacify the esophagus facilitates identification of an enlarged left atrium (in the RAO and lateral projections) or dilated descending aorta (in the PA and lateral projections).

COMPUTED TOMOGRAPHY

Unlike plain films and angiography, CT is capable of displaying anatomic structures without overlapping. The standard study consists of a set of contiguous transverse slices. To evaluate the heart and great vessels, rapid-sequence images are obtained after an intravenous bolus injection of contrast material (Fig. 1.4). By adjusting window and level settings, it is possible to create images with a wide range of contrast.

Whereas most thoracic structures, including the great vessels, are adequately visualized on conventional contrast-enhanced CT scans, motion artifacts often severely degrade images of the

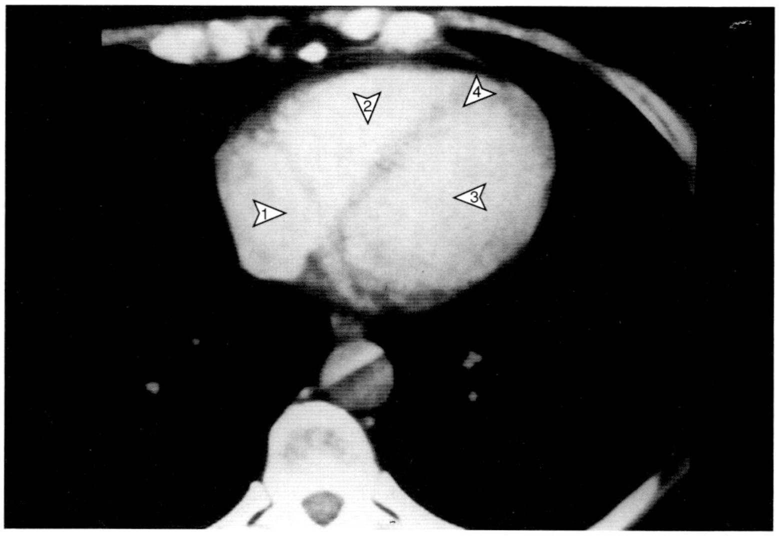

Fig. 1.4 Conventional CT of the heart. Nongated axial image at the level of the ventricles. The right ventricle is anterior and to the right of the left ventricle. The left atrium is not included in this section.

1 right atrium
2 right ventricle
3 left ventricle
4 ventricular septum

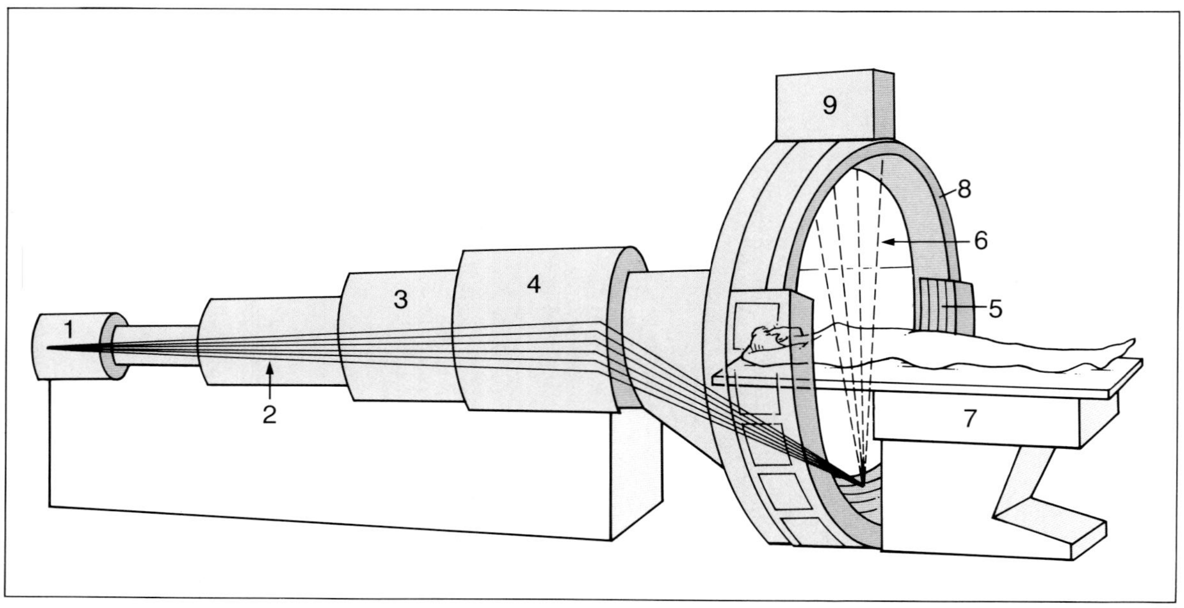

1 electron gun (cathode)
2 electron beam
3 focusing coil
4 deflector coil
5 tungsten target ring (anodes)
6 fan-shaped X-ray beam
7 patient couch
8 detectors
9 data acquisition system (computer)

Fig. 1.5 Cine CT scanner. Schematic cross-section of the Imatron C-100 cine CT scanner. In this device a focused beam of electrons originating in the cathode ("electron gun") is accelerated by electromagnetic fields and directed to four fixed tungsten targets (anodes), which are arrayed in a semicircle beneath the patient. The fan-shaped beam of radiation emitted by the tungsten targets passes upward through the patient and is collimated by the detector array, which comprises two rows of stationary detectors located above the patient. The detectors, which consist of scintillation crystals coupled to photodiode arrays, feed the data into an acquisition system which digitizes and stores information at the rate of eight million 16-bit words per second. The reconstructed images are similar to those of a conventional CT scan. Unlike a conventional CT scanner, which depends on the mechanical motion of a motorized gantry, the cine CT scanner has no moving parts. By minimizing the constraints imposed by heat loading in a conventional CT scanner, the cine CT scanner allows a rapid scanning speed (short exposure time), multiplanar images, and continuous multilevel scanning.

heart. Therefore, conventional CT is largely limited to the evaluation of pericardial disease and mediastinal masses contiguous with the heart and great vessels.

A "cine" CT scanner, which produces very short (millisecond) exposures, overcomes most of the problems associated with conventional CT. Unlike conventional CT scanners, which employ X-ray tubes, the cine CT scanner employs an electron gun and accelerator to generate a beam of electrons, which is steered magnetically to four tungsten cathode rings (targets) located beneath the patient. Each target generates a fan beam of photons which pass through the patient and activate a double ring of stationary detectors arranged in a semicircle overhead (Fig. 1.5). Because cine CT does not employ moving parts or X-ray tubes, it is not limited by mechanical inertia or tube heating capacity.

Three modes of cardiac cine CT are currently available. In the *cine mode*, electrocardiographically triggered images are created at a rate of 17 images per second on each target ring. Such images clearly depict changes in the ventricular chamber and wall thickness throughout the cardiac cycle (Fig. 1.6). In the *flow mode*, electrocardiographically gated images are acquired at each of two to eight levels; at each level the data are acquired at precisely the same point in the cardiac cycle. A computer-generated time-density curve, which correlates with cardiac output, is used to measure blood flow in a region of interest (cardiac chamber, vessel, or myocardium). In the *volume mode*, rapid scanning on two target rings is combined with automated movement of the patient couch at 17 cm/sec, generating 80 contiguous slices covering an area of 64 cm². The images are reformatted to display the entire ventricular cavity in systole and diastole. Using these images, it is possible to measure end diastolic volume, ejection fraction, and ventricular wall motion. The quantitative assessment of ventricular function provided by cine CT correlates well with data obtained from combined cardiac catheterization and angiocardiography, which remains the "gold standard."

Although cine CT provides valuable structural and functional data, it may be superseded by advances in echocardiography and magnetic resonance imaging (MRI) (see Chapters 2 and 4). At present, cine CT is available in only a few centers; whether it will assume a major role in cardiac diagnosis remains to be seen.

ELECTROCARDIOGRAPHY

The electrocardiogram (ECG) detects the electrical activity of the heart. It is an essential part of the work-up of patients with both congenital and acquired heart disease.

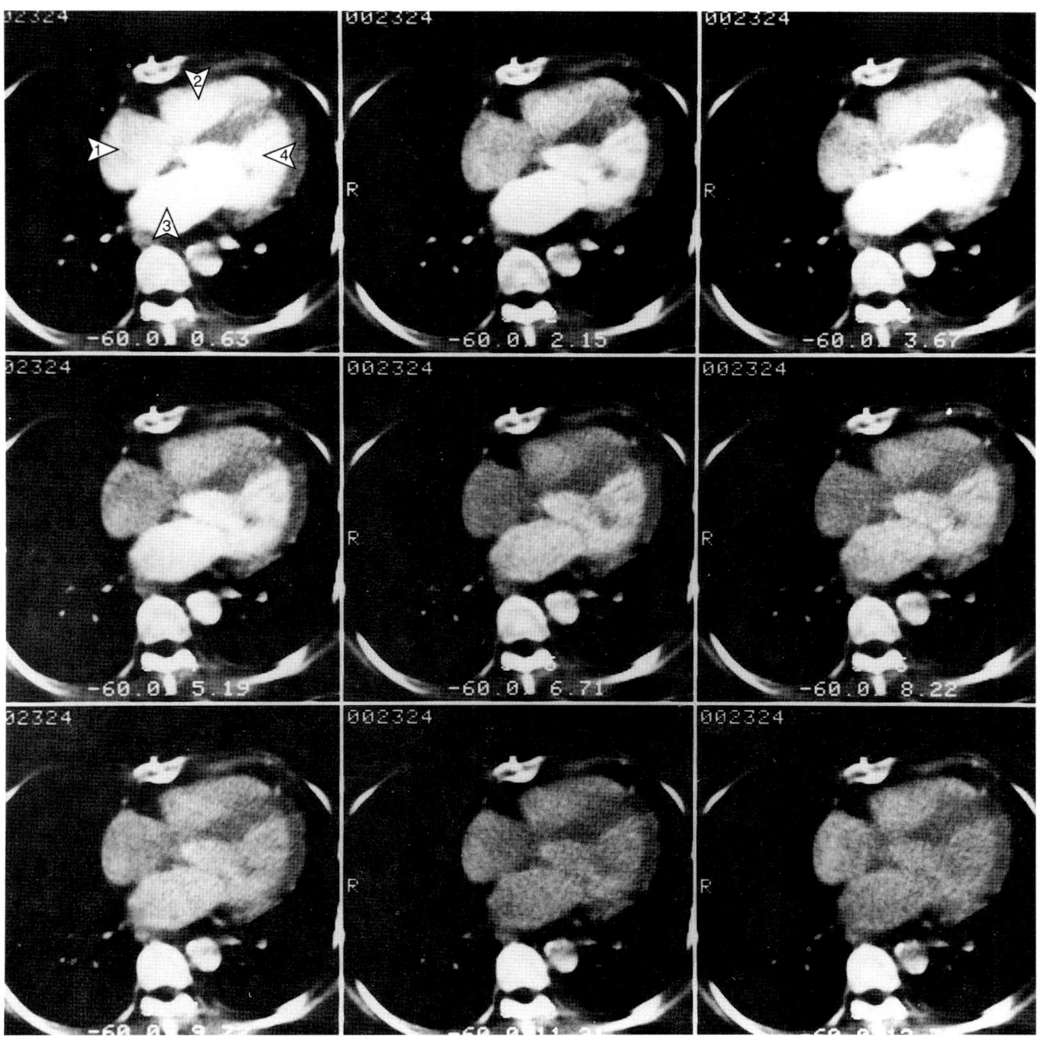

Fig. 1.6 Cardiac cine CT. Rapid-sequence images through midportion of the heart. The first frame is at the top left, the last is at the bottom right.

1	right atrium	3	left atrium
2	right ventricle	4	left ventricle

EXTERNAL ELECTROCARDIOGRAPHY

The normal external ECG consists of a series of waves which represent cardiac electrical activity (Figs. 1.7 and 1.8). The P-wave reflects electrical activity during atrial depolarization. The T-wave is produced by repolarization of the atria. The Q-wave (negative deflection), R-wave (positive deflection), and S-wave (negative deflection) result from ventricular depolarization. The time needed for atrial depolarization and subsequent atrial repolarization, as well as for conduction through the atrioventricular node, is indicated by the PR-interval (the inter-

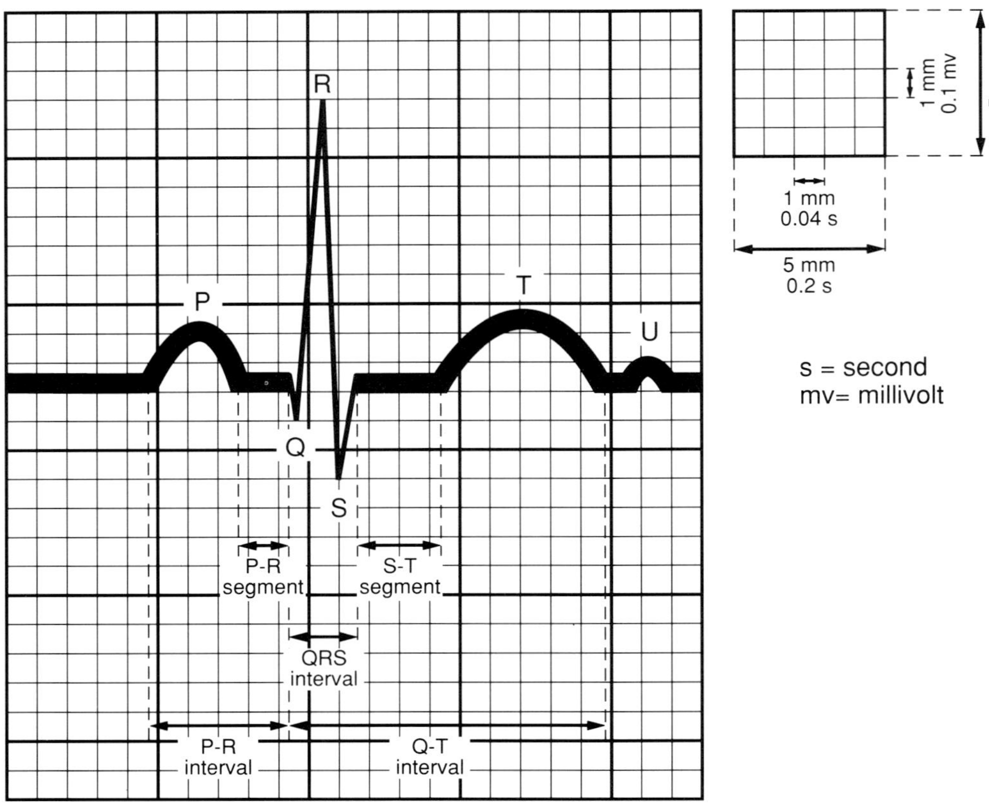

NORMAL RANGES

	P-R Interval (seconds)	QRS Interval (seconds)	Rate	Q-T Interval (seconds)
ADULTS	0.12-0.20	0.07-0.10	60	< 0.42
			70	< 0.40
			80	< 0.37
			90	< 0.35
			100	< 0.34
			120	< 0.31

Fig. 1.7 Normal electrocardiogram (schematic).

val between the P-wave and the initial deflection of the QRS complex). Ventricular repolarization occurs during the ST-segment and T-wave. (The junction between the end of ventricular depolarization and the ST-segment is known as the J-point.) The fetal ECG normally exhibits considerable variation in voltage and duration of electrical activity. This normal variability persists throughout infancy, childhood, and adolescence.

INTERNAL ELECTROCARDIOGRAPHY

Electrophysiological abnormalities that are not apparent on the external ECG can be quantitated by mapping the endocardium electrophysiologically with an intracardiac electrode ("electrophysiologic study"). Such abnormalities include aberrant con-

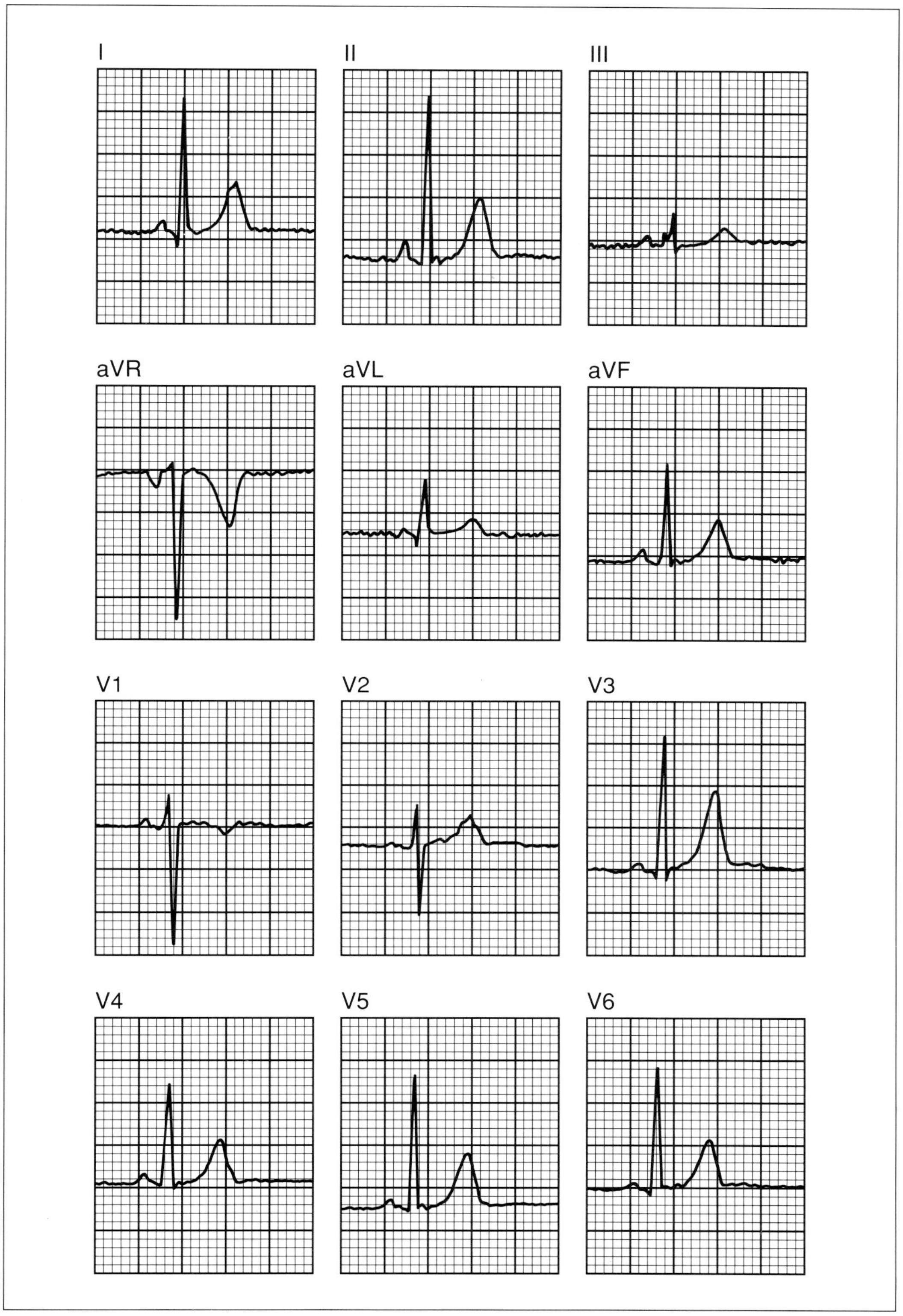

Fig. 1.8 Normal electrocardiogram. In this normal subject the ventricular rate is 75 beats/minute; the PR-interval is 112 milliseconds; the QRS duration is 68 milliseconds; and the P, R, and T axes are 57, 38, and 39, respectively.

duction pathways, ectopic foci, and gaps in the intraventricular conduction system (Fig. 1.9). Intracardiac electrodes can also be used therapeutically. For example, by applying a strong electrical pulse it is possible to excise ectopic foci, which can lead to dramatic improvement in patients with severe arrhythmias caused by an ectopic focus or an aberrant conduction pathway.

CONTINUOUS MONITORING

The Holter system, which enables the cardiologist to monitor electrical activity for prolonged periods, is commonly used in the diagnosis and management of intractable arrhythmias (Fig. 1.10). Continuous monitoring is also used to diagnose ar-

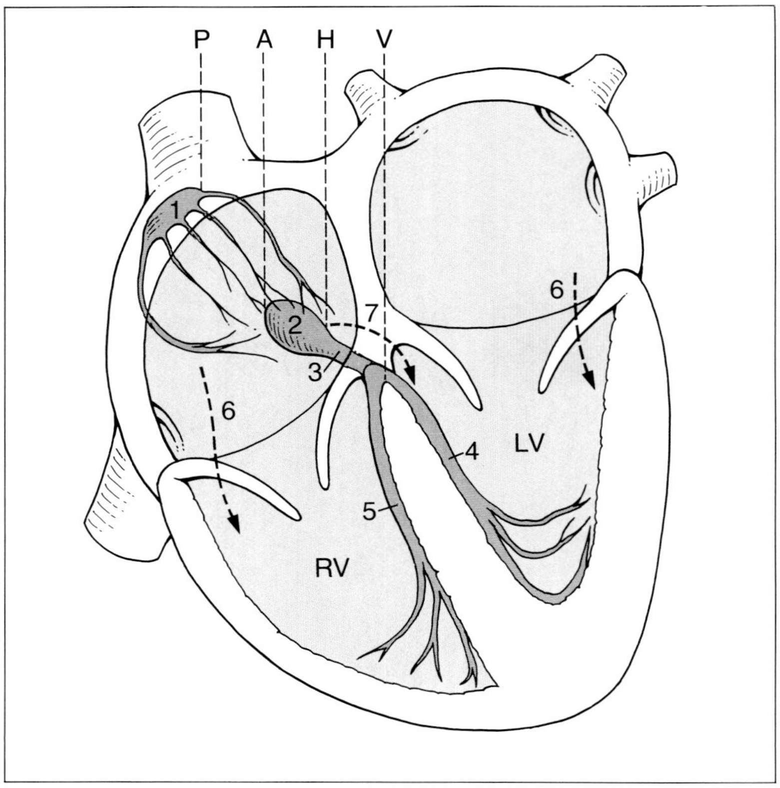

Fig. 1.9 Electrophysiological mapping of the endocardium. Tracings obtained at the superior vena cava–right atrial junction reflect the electrical activity of the sinus node. The electrical activity of the atrioventricular node, the bundle of His, and bundle branches is monitored by moving the electrode to the appropriate position. The P-A interval indicates the intraatrial conduction time (normal, 5–40 milliseconds). The A-H interval indicates the transit time between the atrioventricular node and the bundle of His (normal, 50–150 milliseconds). The His–ventricular (H-V) interval is a parameter of ventricular depolarization (normal, 30–55 milliseconds). By recording and stimulating different segments of the endocardium, it is possible to detect aberrant connections such as Kent's fascicle or the bundle of Mahaim.

1	sinus node	**LA**	left atrium
2	atrioventricular node	**RA**	right atrium
3	bundle of his	**LV**	left ventricle
4	left bundle branch	**RV**	right ventricle
5	right bundle branch	**P-A**	interval intra-atrial conduction
6	Kent's fascicle	**A-H**	atrioventricular node transit
7	bundle of Mahaim	**H-V**	ventricular depolarization

Strip #	Time	Date	Marker	Arrhythmia	Symptoms/Activities
1	09:46:40	07-SEP-90		Couplet	
2	10:19:50	07-SEP-90		Couplet	
3	11:30:00	07-SEP-90	*	Isolated PVC	Palpitations
4	11:30:16	07-SEP-90		Couplet	
5	12:00:00	07-SEP-90	*	Isolated PVC	Palpitations
6	12:49:34	07-SEP-90		Isolated PVC	
7	15:00:00	07-SEP-90	*	Bigeminy	Palpitations
8	15:49:56	07-SEP-90		VTACH, 7 bts, 168 BPM	
9	16:43:17	07-SEP-90		VTACH, 4 bts, 103 BPM	
10	17:00:00	07-SEP-90	*	Isolated PVC	Palpitations
11	18:14:10	07-SEP-90		VITACH, 4 bts. 106 BPM	
12	18:14:13	07-SEP-90		VTACH, 4 bts, 106 BPM	
13	18:54:48	07-SEP-90		HR 109	
14	19:30:00	07-SEP-90	*	Isolated PVC	Palpitations
15	21:00:00	07-SEP-90	*	Couplet	Palpitations
	21:00:00	07-SEP-90	*	Couplet	Palpitations
16	22:12:41	07-SEP-90		VTACH, 4 bts, 128 BPM	
17	23:13:59	07-SEP-90		VTACH, 4 bts, 126 BPM	
18	02:31:40	08-SEP-90		HR 51	
19	03:49:20	08-SEP-90		HR 51	
20	05:39:14	08-SEP-90		Isolated PVC	
21	06:00:00	08-SEP-90	*	Couplet	Palpitations
22	06:06:03	08-SEP-90		Isolated PVC	
23	06:06:07	08-SEP-90		Couplet	
24	07:48:43	08-SEP-90		VRHY, 3 bts, 53 BPM	

A

Fig. 1.10 Holter monitoring system. This system enables one to obtain a continuous record of the electrical activity of the heart over a prolonged period. The example shown is from a 60-year-old patient with dilated cardiomyopathy. (A) The time of abnormal electrical activity (arrhythmia) is indicated.

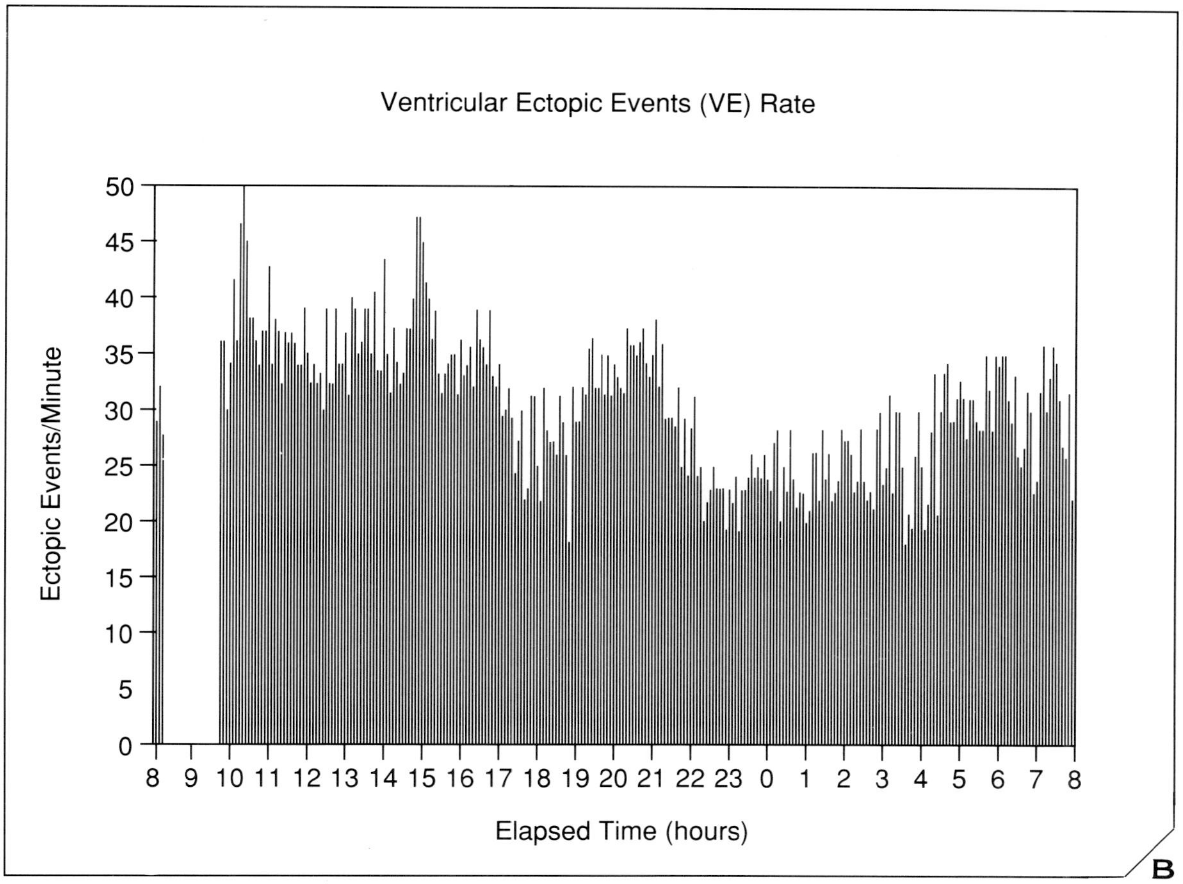

B

Fig. 1.10 (continued) (B) The frequency of ventricular ectopic events is displayed graphically. The vertical axis indicates the number of ectopic events per minute and the horizontal axis indicates elapsed time in hours. (C) The summary indicates that this patient has a severe arrhythmia characterized by couplets, premature ventricular contractions (PVCs), isolated PVCs, bigeminy, ventricular tachycardia, and bradycardia. Altogether, ventricular ectopic events account for 31 percent of the QRS complexes. These detailed data are very helpful in assessing the severity of the arrhythmias in a given patient.

104085 QRS complexes

32641	Ventricular	ectopics which represent	31% of total QRS complexes
194	Supraventricular	ectopics which represent	1% of total QRS complexes
	Paced QRS complexes	which represent	% of total QRS complexes

Ventricular Ectopy

16157 Isolated
1805 Bigeminal Cycles
7974 Couplets
174 Runs
536 Beats in Runs
7 Beats LONGEST at 168 BPM at
15:49:55 07-SEP-90
7 Beats FASTEST at 168 BPT at
15:49:55 07-SEP-90

Supraventricular Ectopy

165 Isolated
5 Couplets
4 Runs
19 Beats in Runs
7 Beats LONGEST at 80 BPM at
06:06:03 08-SEP-90
7 Beats FASTEST at 80 BPM at
06:06:03 08-SEP-90

Heart Rates

49 MIN at 07:48:43 08-SEP-90
76 AVG
109 MAX at 18:54:48 07-SEP-90

S-T Levels Channel

mm at
mm at

C

rhythmias that are intermittent or occur during physical activity or emotional stress, and to monitor the response to medical therapy.

ELECTROCARDIOGRAPHY IN CONGENITAL HEART DISEASE

The external ECG provides information about heart rate, rhythm, abnormalities of the conduction system, and chamber enlargement in patients with suspected or documented congenital heart disease; it can also be used to monitor ventricular function over time. Hypertrophy of one or both ventricles is a feature of many congenital defects (Fig. 1.11). Certain cardiac malformations [eg, atrioventricular septal defect (endocardial cushion defect), corrected transposition of the great arteries, univentricular atrioventricular connection] are associated with abnormal patterns of depolarization and repolarization. The atrioventricular node and penetrating bundle (of His), which are abnormally positioned in these malformations, are likely to be injured during corrective surgery. Certain malformations (eg, Ebstein's malformation, right ventricular dysplasia) are associated with accessory conduction pathways (Fig. 1.12).

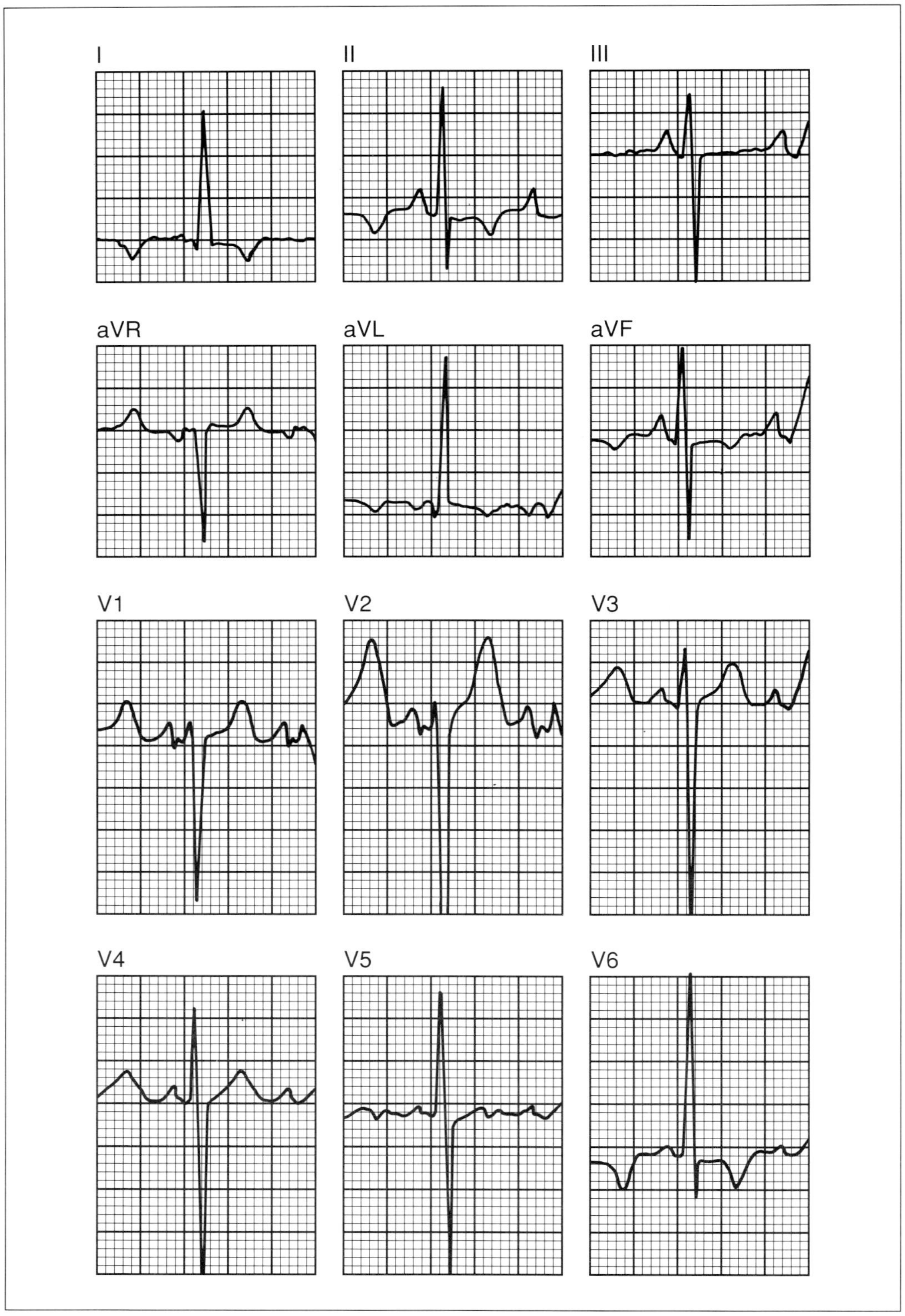

Fig. 1.11 Electrocardiographic findings in left ventricular hypertrophy. Note the small R-wave in V1 and V2, the tall R-wave in V5 and V6, and the absence of S-wave in V5 and V6.

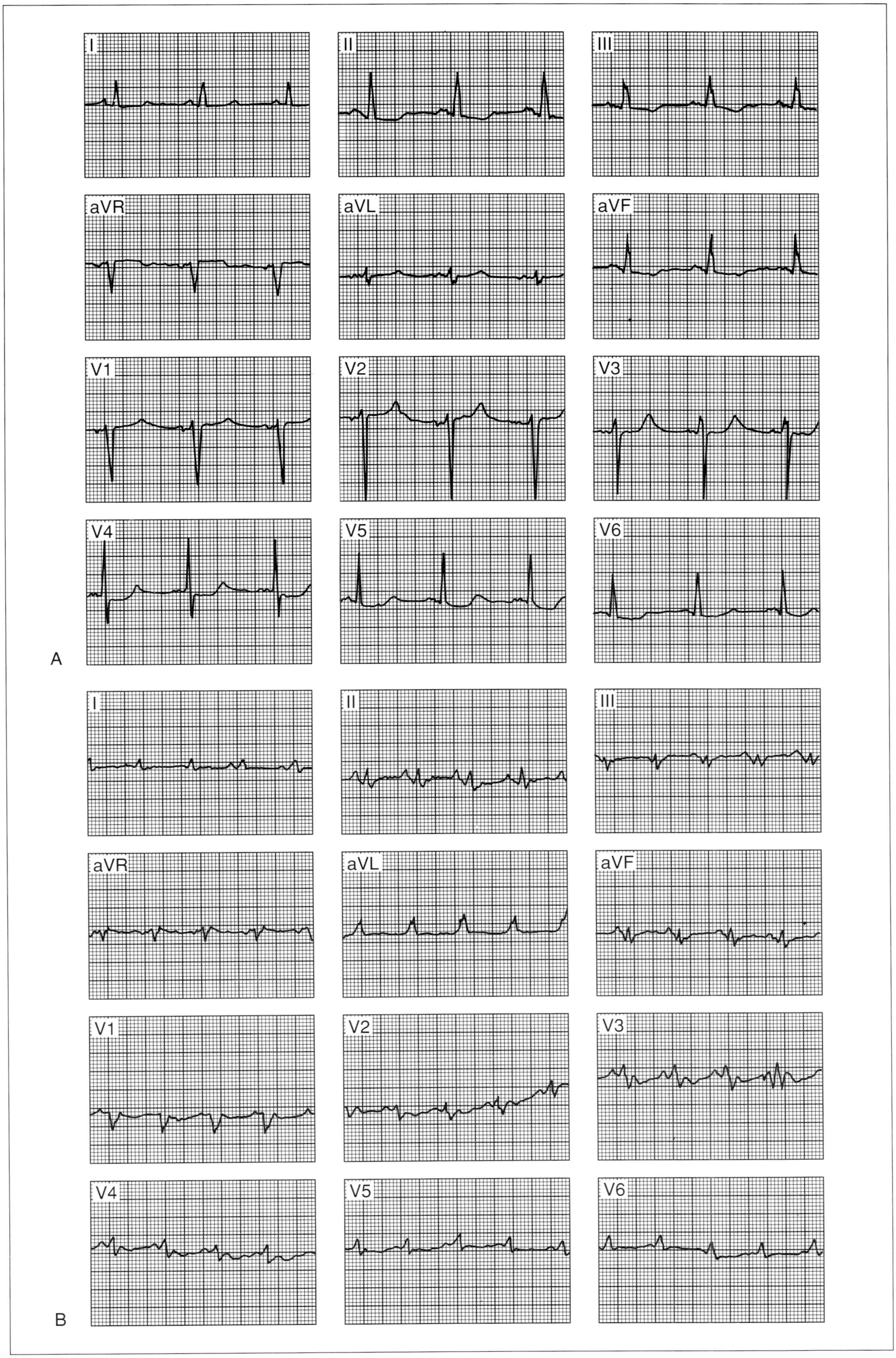

Fig. 1.12 Arrythmia due to congenital heart disease. This man with Ebstein's malformation of the tricuspid valve had experienced repeated episodes of supraventricular tachycardia. (A) ECG demonstrates typical features of the Wolff–Parkinson–White syndrome (type B): a short P-R interval and slurring of the initial inscription of the QRS complex, producing a delta wave that is directed superiorly, posteriorly, and to the left. (B) A subsequent tracing in the same patient demonstrates peaked P-waves (indicating right atrial overload) and low-voltage "splintered" QRS complexes (indicating right ventricular conduction delay). This pattern is typical of Ebstein's malformation (see Chapter 12).

Patients with these anomalies tend to develop ectopic foci of electrical activity, which can lead to an intractable arrhythmia. Such pathways can usually be detected with an electrophysiologic study.

ELECTROCARDIOGRAPHY IN ACQUIRED HEART DISEASE

The electrocardiographic findings in patients with acquired heart disease are quite variable and depend on the portion of the heart affected. Valvular disease is usually associated with pressure or volume overload, which may affect one or more chambers. Abnormal myocardial perfusion secondary to ischemic heart disease is manifested electrocardiographically by altered depolarization and repolarization.

Increased right atrial pressure and right atrial volume overload are manifested on the ECG by tall, peaked, and narrow P-waves ("P-pulmonale"), which are best seen in leads II, III, and aVf.

Left atrial enlargement secondary to mitral stenosis or mitral insufficiency is manifested electrocardiographically by wide, notched P-waves ("P-mitrale") in leads II and V6. The abnormal P-waves are typically 0.11 seconds or longer in lead II.

Right ventricular hypertrophy is manifested electrocardiographically by QR forces that are directed to the right. The R-waves are abnormally tall in leads V1 and V2, and there are deep S-waves in leads V4 and V5. Characteristically, the direction of the ST-segments and T-waves is opposite to that of the widest portion of the QRS complex.

Left ventricular hypertrophy causes distortion of the QRS loop in the direction of the left scapula. This is manifested on the ECG by small R-waves and deep S-waves in leads V1 and V2, and tall R-waves and small or absent S-waves in leads V5 and V6. The ST-segment and T-wave are positive in V1 and negative in V6 (see Fig. 1.10).

The transmission of electrical activity through the heart is altered in many types of acquired heart disease (Figs. 1.13 to 1.15). Conduction defects (eg, complete atrioventricular disso-

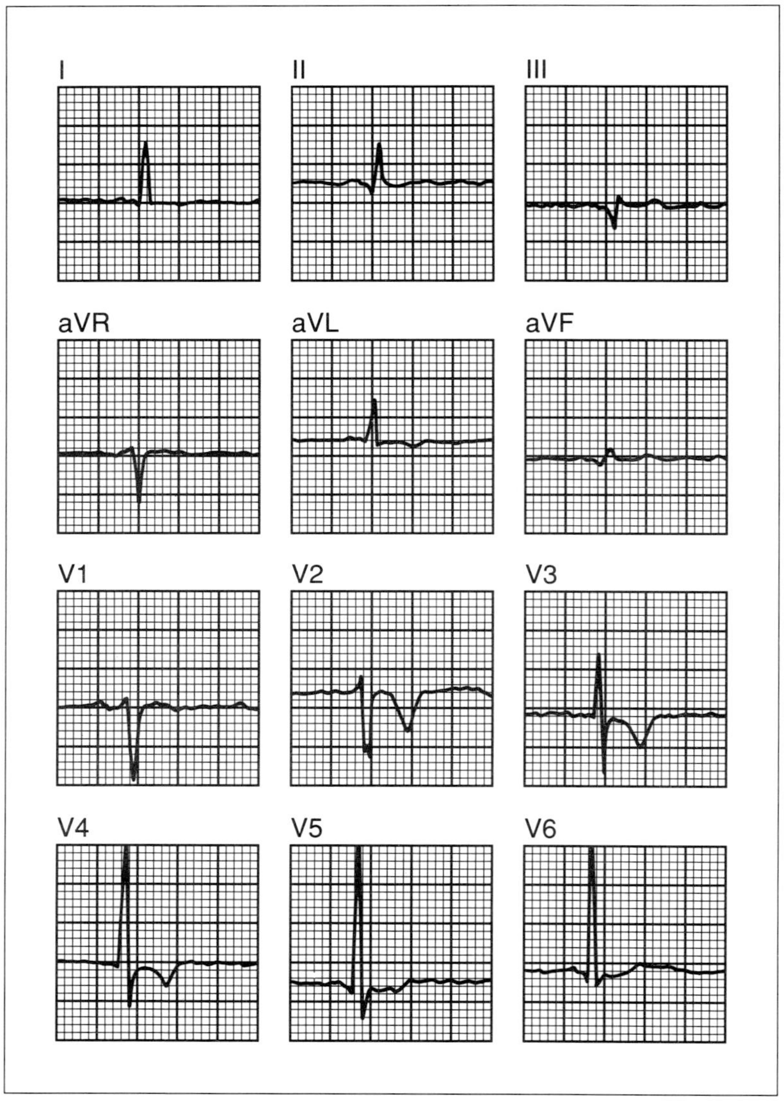

Fig. 1.13 Anterior myocardial infarction. ECG of a 72-year-old patient demonstrates inverted T-waves in leads I, aVl, V5, and V6; poor progression of the R-wave; and Q-waves in V1, V3, and V4. The QRS is prolonged (128 milliseconds). These ECG findings are typical of an anterior wall infarction of the left ventricle.

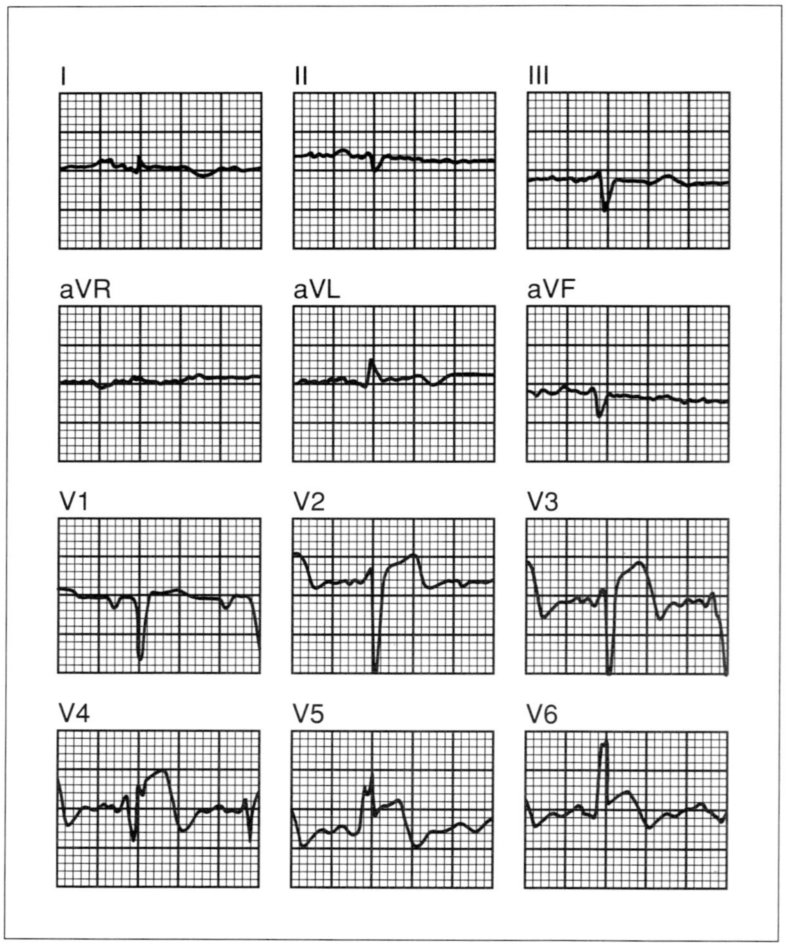

Fig. 1.14 Anteroseptal myocardial infarction. ECG of a 50-year-old man shows absence of the R-wave in V1 through V4 and T-wave inversion in I, aVl, V5, and V6. This pattern is typical for an anteroseptal infarction of the left ventricle.

ciation, bundle branch block) are quite common in patients with ischemic heart disease.

Altered transmission through branches of the conduction system (bundle branch block) is common in patients with acquired heart disease. It can affect the left ventricle, right ventricle, or both. When the duration of the QRS complex is moderately prolonged (0.1–0.12 seconds) the conduction disturbance is called an incomplete bundle branch block; when the QRS complex is longer than 0.12 seconds, it is called a complete bundle branch block (Fig. 1.16). In patients with a right bundle branch block, the first 0.04 seconds of the QRS complex are normal in configuration but the last part is abnormal. In patients with a left bundle branch block the entire QRS complex is "written" by an abnormal depolarization wave, resulting in a markedly abnormal tracing.

Some individuals have accessory conduction pathways between the right atrium and the ventricles. One anomaly, which is manifested electrocardiographically by a short PR-interval and an abnormally wide QRS complex, is known as the *Wolf–Parkinson–White complex* (see Fig. 1.12). Clinical manifestations include atrial tachycardia and other arrhythmias.

Acquired heart disease is associated with a wide variety of arrhythmias. One of the most common is atrial fibrillation, which is typically associated with mitral stenosis (Fig. 1.16).

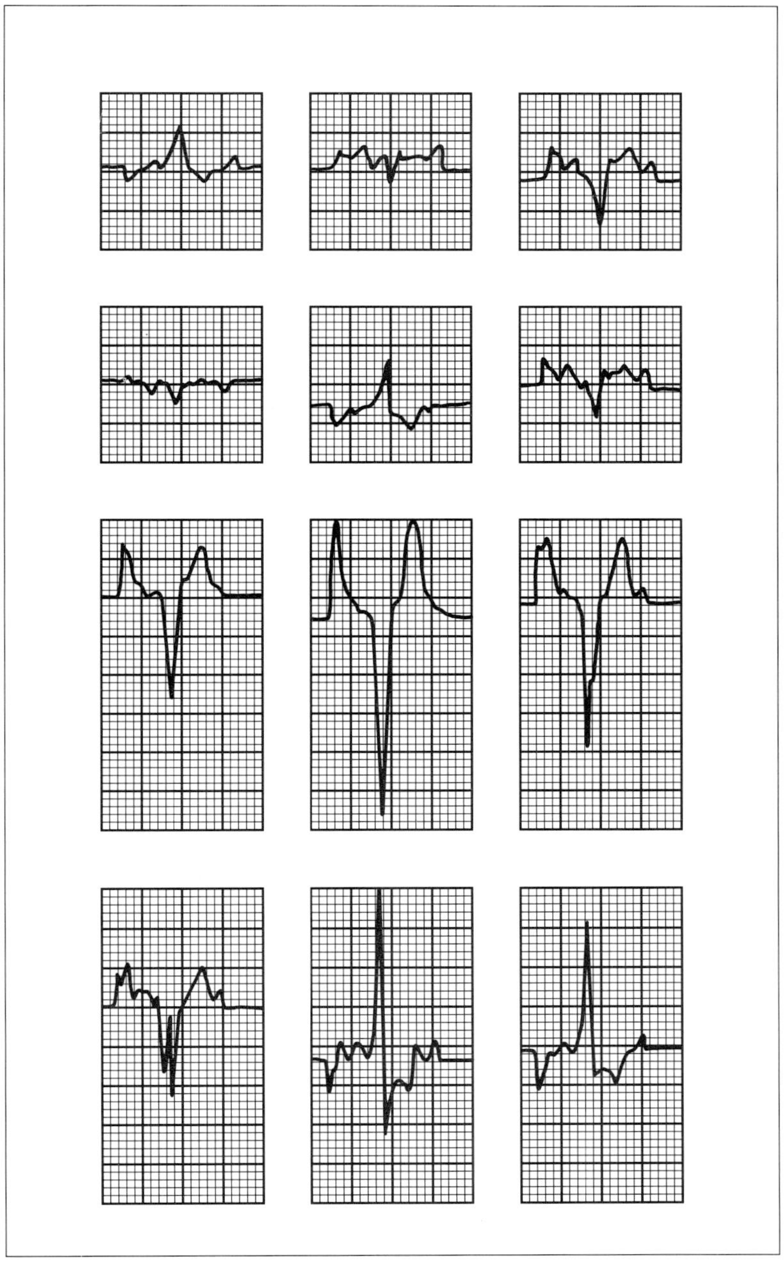

Fig. 1.15 Inferoseptal myocardial infarction. ECG of a 72-year-old patient shows a sinus tachycardia (154 beats/minute) and an abnormally short P-Q interval (104 milliseconds). Abnormal repolarization is seen in leads V5, V6, I, and aVI. This pattern meets the criteria for an inferoseptal infarction of the left ventricle.

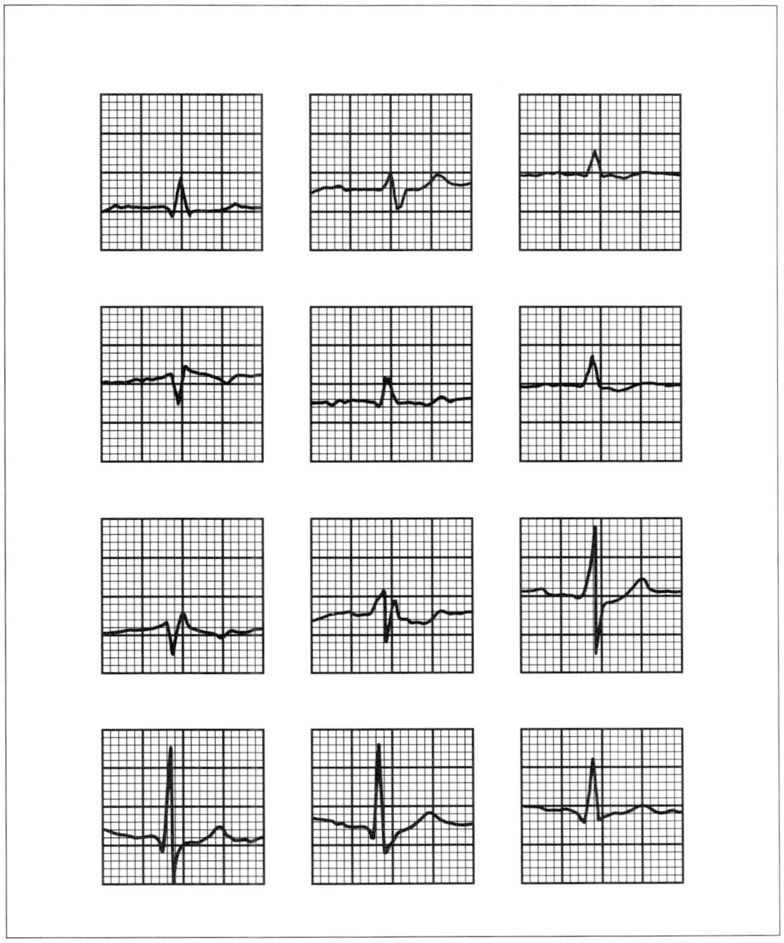

Fig. 1.16 Atrial fibrillation and right bundle branch block. ECG of a 72-year-old patient shows an irregular rhythm with a ventricular rate of 102 beats/minute. P-waves are absent. There is left axis deviation of 30°, as well as a right bundle branch block.

CHAPTER 2

Echocardiography

ISIDRE VILAICOSTA, M.D.
NAVIN C. NANDA, M.D.

The piezoelectric effect was first described by Curie. Rhythmic changes in the shape of a piezoelectric crystal are induced

modality has been improved dramatically with ongoing new developments in technology

decubitus position. This creates tomographic sections that transect the heart parallel to its long axis (Figs. 2.3 and 2.4). The same parasternal window also yields tomographic sections perpendicular to the long axis of the heart (short-axis tomographic views), transecting the heart at several levels from the apex (Figs. 2.5 and 2.6) to the base (Figs. 2.7 and 2.8).

The apical planes are obtained by placing the transducer near (usually inferior to) the palpable cardiac apex while the patient is in the left lateral decubitus position. The apical

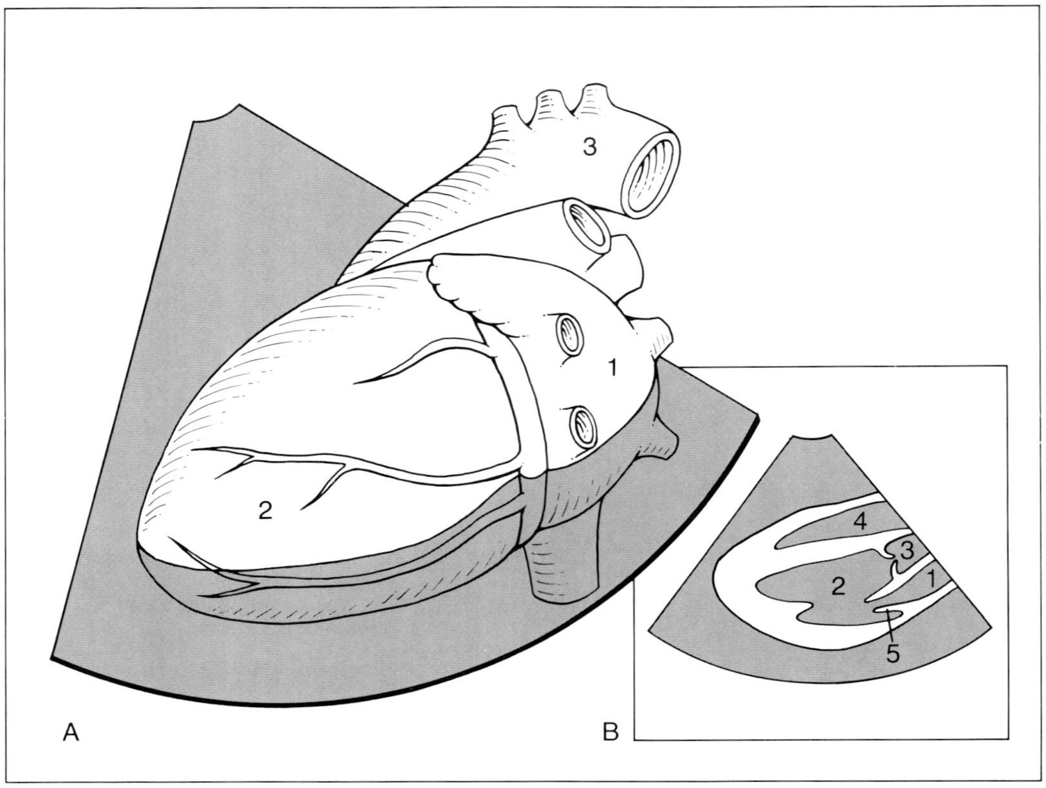

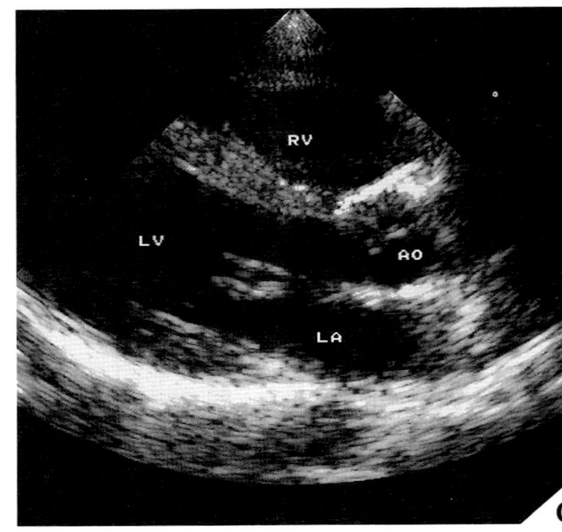

1 left atrium
2 left ventricle
3 aorta
4 right ventricle
5 mitral valve

Fig. 2.3 Normal heart in parasternal long axial plane. (A) Schematic representation shows the parasternal long-axis plane, which passes through the heart, including the two ventricular chambers, arteries, and part of the septum. (B) Schematic representation shows the heart through this view. (C) Parasternal long-axis echocardiogram, in which the echocardiographic section passes through the heart such that it exposes the posterior aspect of the right and left ventricles, left atrium, and aorta.

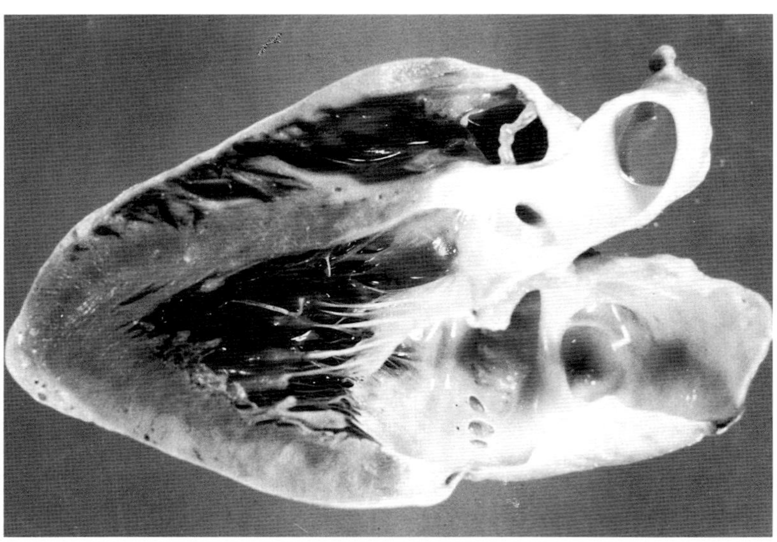

Fig. 2.4 Section of the heart using the same plane as in echocardiography long-axis view.

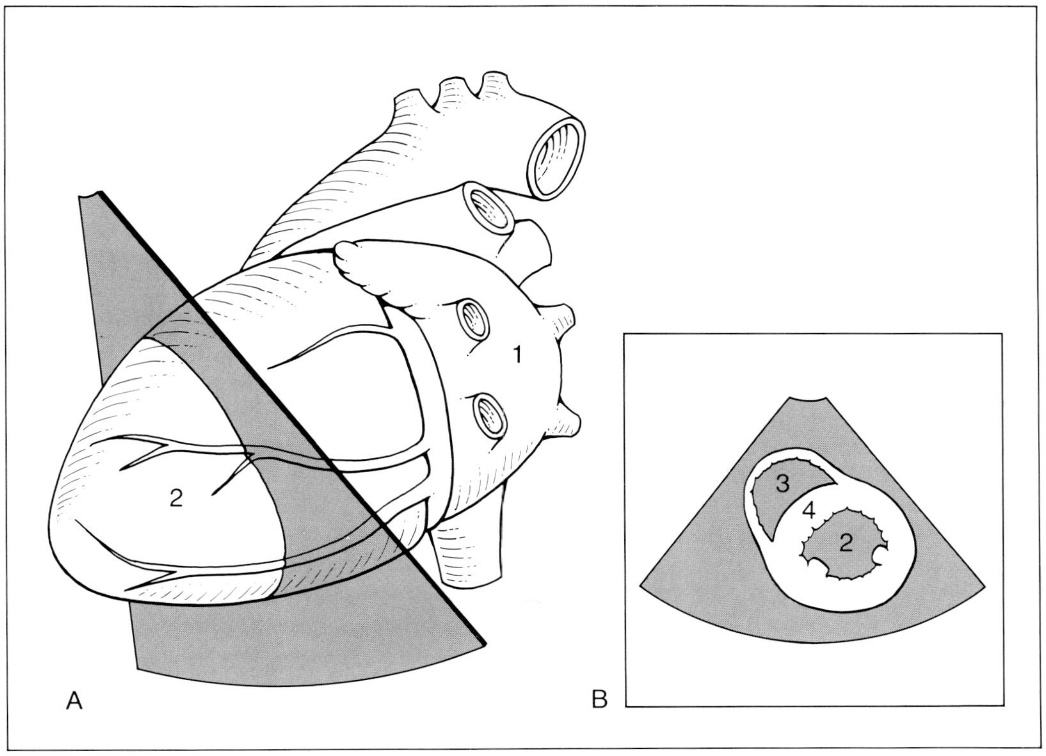

Fig. 2.5 Schematic representation of the plane used for short-axis view at the middle portion of the ventricular chambers; parasternal window. (A) Diagram of the approximate plane, as seen from outside of the heart, is shown. (B) Representation of the ventricular chamber morphology is shown, as seen from this view. (C) An echocardiogram through the base of the left ventricle is shown.

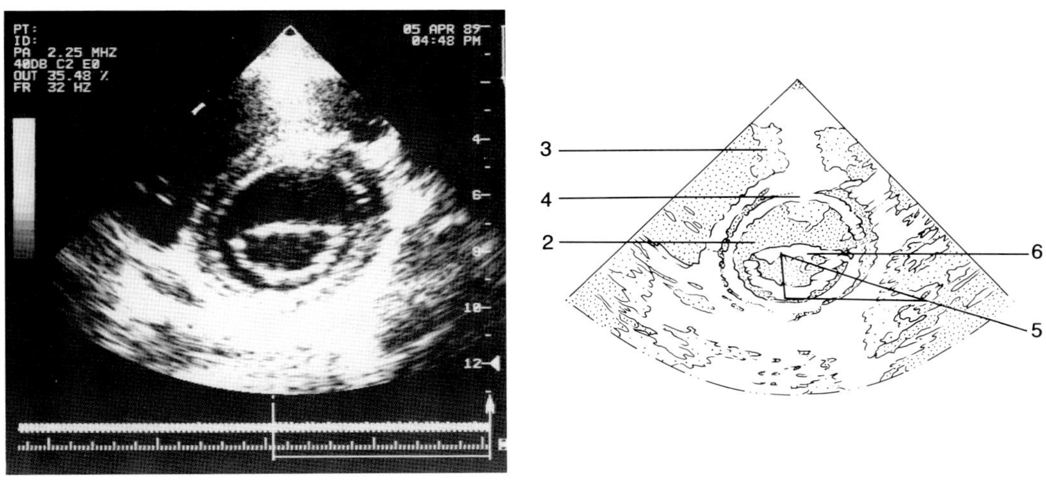

1	left atrium	4	ventricular septum
2	left ventricle	5	mitral valve
3	right ventricle	6	anterior mitral leaflet

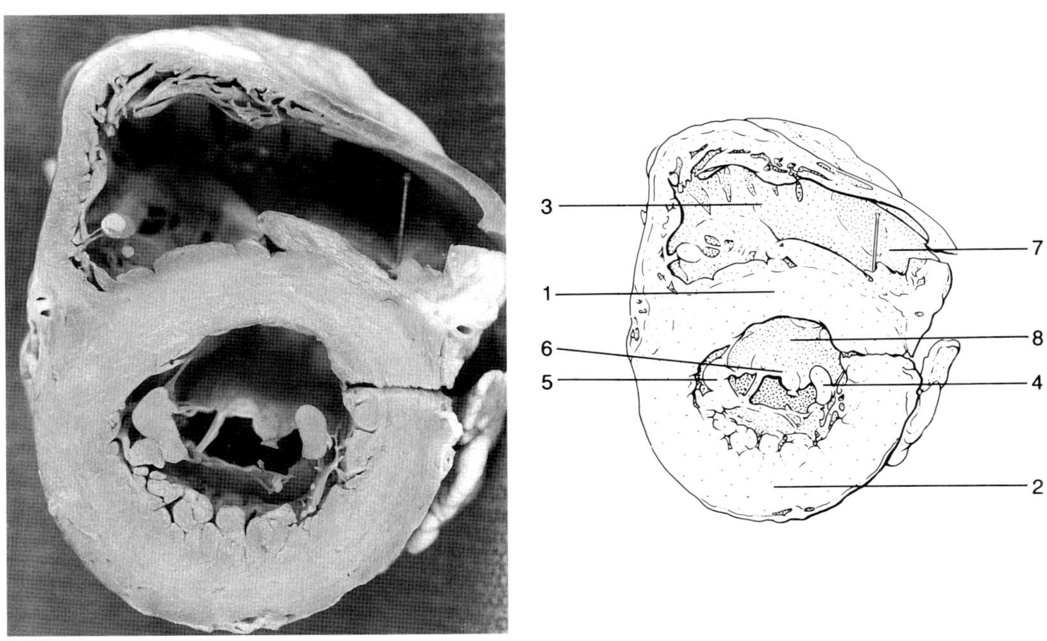

Fig. 2.6 Section of the ventricular chamber as seen through a short axis at the level of the atrioventricular valves. Left ventricle has a circular appearance; the right ventricle makes a semicircle around the left ventricle in its upper and right aspects.

1	ventricular septum	5	posterior papillary muscle
2	free wall of the left ventricle	6	anterior mitral leaflet
3	right ventricle	7	right ventricular outflow tract
4	anterior papillary muscle	8	left ventricular outflow tract

window enables one to obtain four-chamber tomographic sections (Figs. 2.9 and 2.10), apical long-axis views, two-chamber views of both sides of the heart, and a variety of short-axis views of the ventricles.

In the subcostal window, the transducer is placed just under the subxiphoid process, allowing visualization of the four chambers of the heart, the interatrial septum along its entire length, and a variety of short-axis planes, as well as depiction of the systemic venous drainage.

For the suprasternal window, the patient should be supine with a pillow under the shoulders so that the head and neck are slightly hyperextended. This position gives the operator

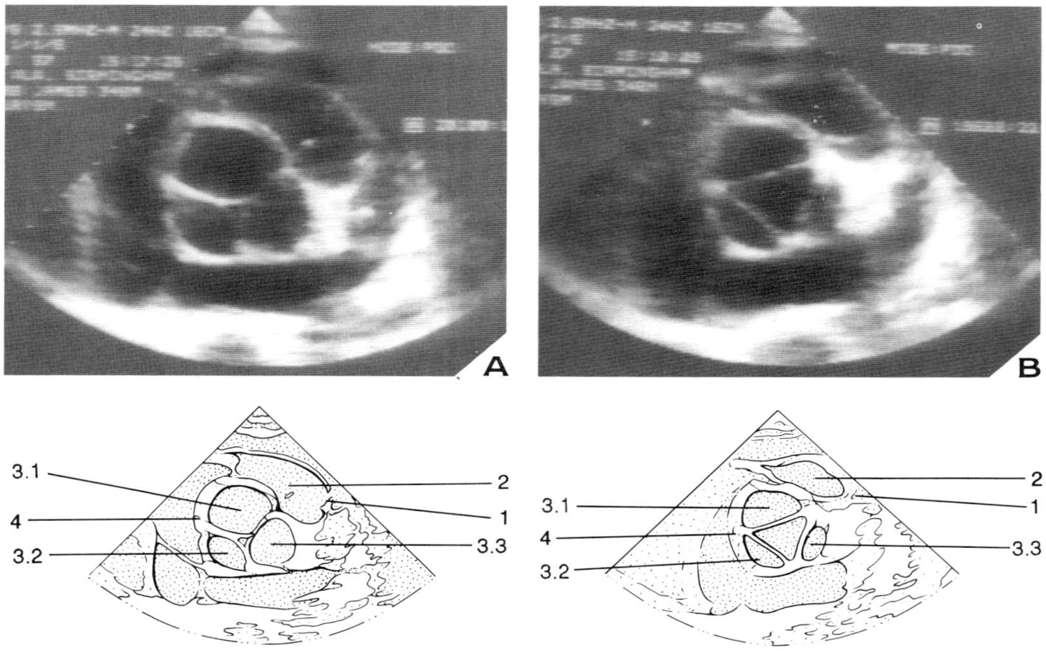

Fig. 2.7 Short-axis 2-D echocardiographic plane of the heart at the level of the aortic valve obtained through transesophageal approach. (A) Diastolic frame and (B) systolic frame are shown. The aorta lies between the right ventricular outflow tract and the left atrium.

1 pulmonic valve
2 right ventricular outflow tract
3 aortic valve with:
3.1 right coronary cusp
3.2 noncoronary cusp
3.3 left coronary cusp
4 position of membranous septum

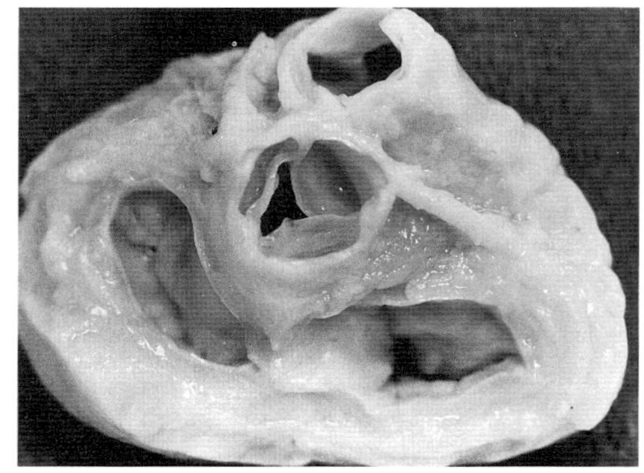

Fig. 2.8 Short-axis, section of the heart, 2-D echocardiographic plane, at the aortic level. The aortic valve lies between the right ventricular outflow tract and the left atrium.

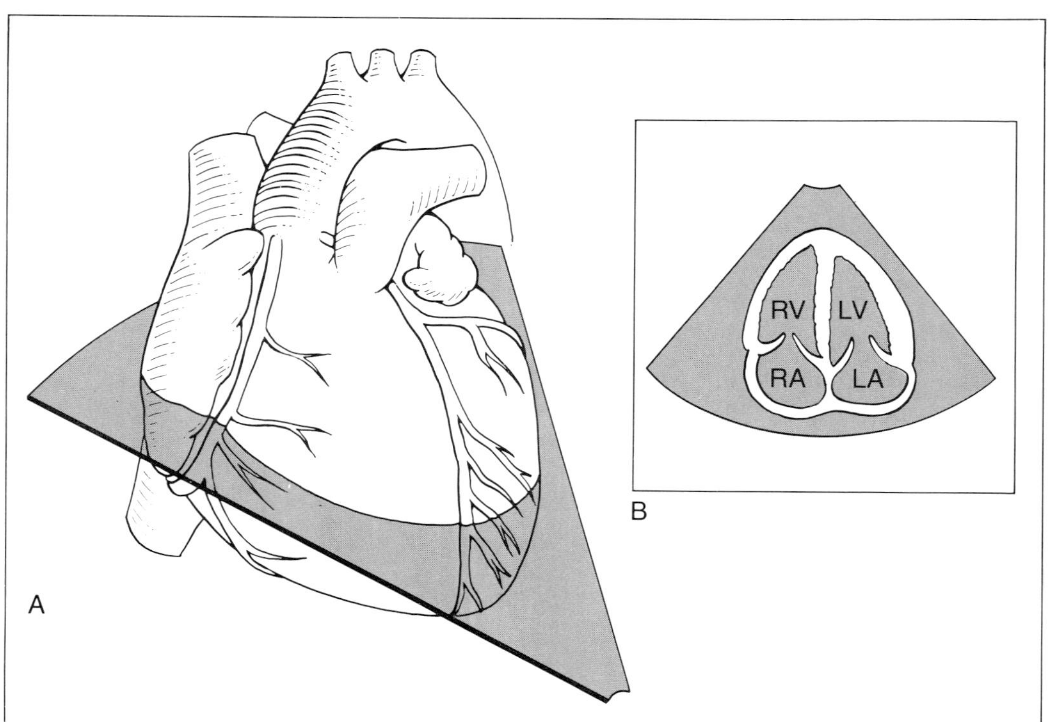

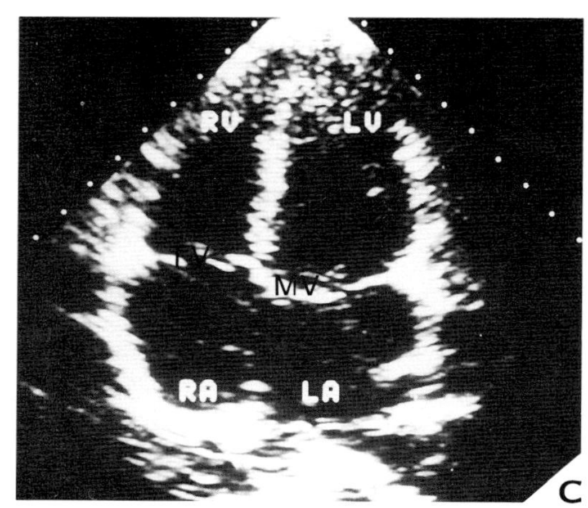

TV tricuspid valve MV mitral valve

Fig. 2.9 Schematic representation of 2-D echocardiography obtained in four-chamber view. (A) Apical approach is shown. (B) Schematic represents the cardiac chambers in this view. (C) Normal echocardiogram of a normal heart is shown. The echocardiographic section is through the atria and ventricles separated by septal structures. The four cardiac chambers are well demonstrated; the septal mitral leaflet is higher than the septal tricuspid leaflet, delineating a portion of the septum between them, the so-called "atrioventricular septum".

better access to the suprasternal and/or supraclavicular spaces and can provide tomographic sections of the ascending aorta, aortic arch, descending aorta, superior vena cava, pulmonary trunk, and main pulmonary arteries. A properly performed two-dimensional echocardiographic study permits a comprehensive and precise three-dimensional anatomic study of the heart (Fig. 2.11).

DOPPLER ECHOCARDIOGRAPHY

Doppler echocardiography uses ultrasound to evaluate the direction, velocity, and character of blood flow within the cardiovascular system. All Doppler instruments work on the *Doppler principle,* which states that the frequencies received from an energy source differ from those sent according to the

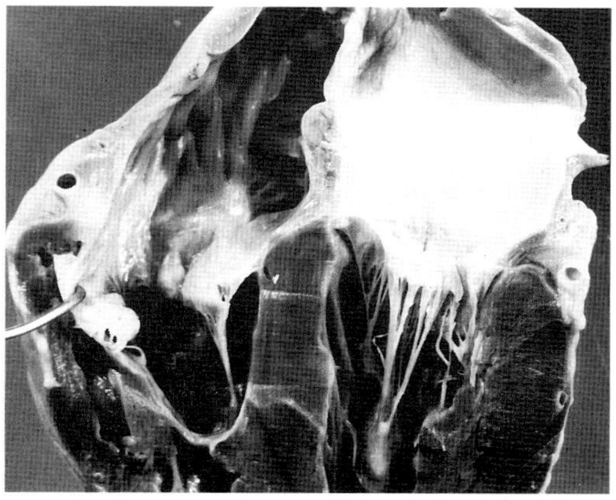

Fig. 2.10 Section of normal heart as seen on four-chamber view, similar to that observed in Fig. 2.9. Note the different level of implantation of the septal leaflets of the tricuspid and mitral valves.

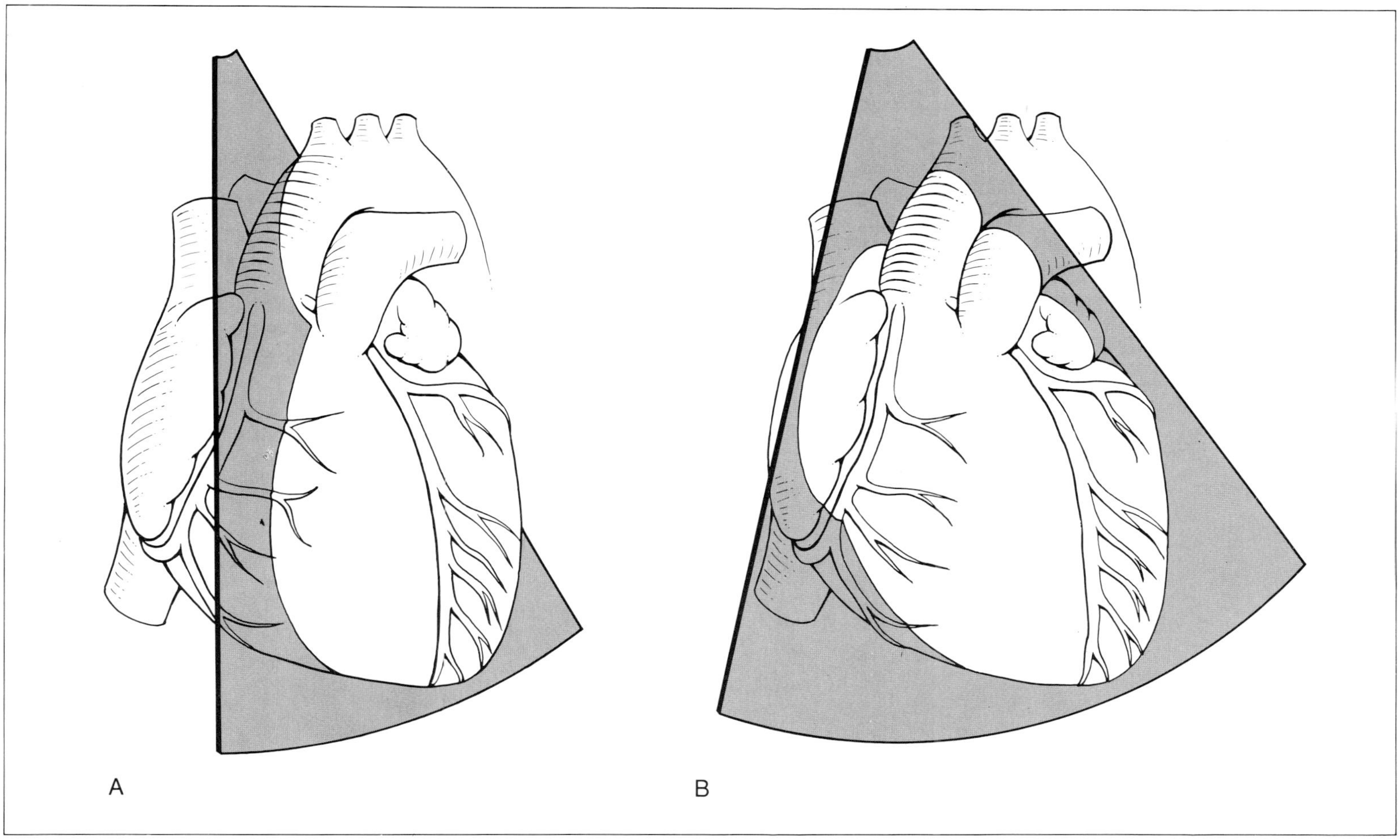

Fig. 2.11 Schematic representation of orientation of the sections when the transducer is in a suprasternal location. (A) Suprasternal long axial view. (B) Suprasternal short-axis view.

direction and velocity of motion relative to the receiver. If an ultrasonic beam is reflected by a stationary object, the transmitted frequency (F_0) and the received frequency (F_1) are equal. However, if the target reflecting the ultrasonic energy is moving towards the transducer, the received frequency is greater than the transmitted frequency. When the target is moving away from the transducer, the received frequency is less than the transmitted frequency. The difference between the reflected and transmitted frequency represents the *Doppler frequency shift.* By knowing the degree of shift, it is possible to calculate the velocity of the moving target, which is the red blood cells. The Doppler equation can be summarized by

$$V = \frac{C}{2F_o} \cdot \frac{f}{(\mathrm{Cos}\ \phi)}$$

where Doppler blood flow velocity is f ($F_1 - F_0$), the velocity of sound in tissue (c), the frequency of transmitted sound is (F_0), and the cosine of the ultrasound beam is the angle of incidence. The velocity of the sound in soft tissue and blood is assumed to be 1540 cm/sec. From this equation, for clinical evaluation the ultrasonic beam must be almost parallel to the direction of blood flow to obtain an accurate determination of the blood flow. The cosine functions, however, allow variations between the Doppler beam and the velocity axis to result in minor changes in the calculated velocity.

There are two basic modes of Doppler interrogation: continuous-wave Doppler and pulsed Doppler. The former mode was the first mode of Doppler interrogation; it requires separate transmission and reception elements so that one piezoelectric element continuously transmits ultrasonic energy and the other continuously and passively receives the reflected sound. The continuous-wave Doppler technique is capable of resolving very high velocities. In this mode, the sound energy is processed for the Doppler frequency shift along the course of the beam; however, this technique is limited by its inability to interrogate and characterize flow in specific regions.

The pulsed Doppler mode employs only one crystal. Crystal deactivation between pulses for specific periods of time enables a temporal gate to be established so that reflections from blood flow at a specific distance from the transducer can be analyzed for Doppler shift. Changes in duration of the reactivation period prior to the next pulse allow selection of the size of the specific region to be interrogated (the *sample volume*). Because the *Nyquist limit* (the highest frequency shift that can be unambiguously resolved) is equal to one half the pulse repetition frequency, the long interval necessary between pulses with the pulsed Doppler mode interferes with velocity determination. However, pulsed Doppler's primary utility is to locate and characterize blood flow; continuous-wave Doppler, with its extremely high pulse repetition frequency but poor range gating capability, can be used for high-velocity determination.

A third mode of pulsed Doppler ultrasound, called *high pulse repetition frequency* Doppler, uses multiple range gates. By sacrificing unambiguous range gating, this system allows the resolution of higher velocities than is usually possible with conventional pulsed Doppler.

Conventional Doppler visual display is in the form of an analog trace or a Fast Fourier Transform (FFT) spectral trace, both of which are graphic, with time along the X-axis and frequency shift (or velocity) along the Y-axis. FFT spectral trace is the more common mode of display presently in use. This mode displays, insofar as possible, all frequency shifts present over time. The analog trace displays the modular (mean) frequency shift over time linearly (Fig. 2.12, Appendix). Because the Doppler frequency shifts fall within the range of human hearing, an audio signal is usually available as an adjunct to the visible graphic trace, and represents an important aspect of the Doppler examination.

COLOR DOPPLER IMAGING

A standard echocardiographic transducer is used and the returning signals are split after being received. One part of the signal is used to create a standard black and white two-dimensional echocardiographic tomogram and the other part is evaluated for Doppler phase shift information analogous to conventional Doppler frequency shift, which is subsequently encoded in color and superimposed on the black portions of the two-dimensional echocardiographic image. Because color Doppler imaging is analogous to conventional pulsed Doppler, it is susceptible to all the constraints of pulsed Doppler. However, the velocity display modes are somewhat different. Conventional pulsed Doppler provides a display of the full spectrum of velocities within a single sample region, whereas color Doppler provides an estimate of the mean velocity for multiple sample volume sites. In addition, pulsed Doppler provides information for one sample volume site along one beam path, and Doppler flow mapping provides information regarding multiple sample sites along multiple beam paths, allowing a semblance of real-time two-dimensional display of the signals (Fig. 2.13, Appendix).

The velocity data are depicted for each site in terms of two characteristics: direction and relative velocity of blood flow. These parameters are displayed in color: flow towards the transducer is depicted in red, and flow away from the transducer in blue (Fig. 2.14, Appendix). Color brightness is increased in proportion to flow velocity. This is done using standard television technology; green is added to the primary direction color in proportion to the degree of phase shift. The more green, the lighter the shade of the color. Most instruments also add green as a distinct color when there is evidence of disturbed blood flow. In contrast to Doppler spectral recordings, flow mapping provides measurements only of the mean velocity within a sample volume site, and also allows excellent two-dimensional orientation, as the flows are displayed directly within the chambers and vessels.

TRANSESOPHAGEAL ECHOCARDIOGRAPHY

Although advances in two-dimensional echocardiography, pulsed and continuous-wave Doppler, and color Doppler imaging have revolutionized noninvasive assessment of cardiac disorders, a major limitation of transthoracic echocardiography is its inability to obtain consistently high-quality imaging of the heart and aorta in all patients. Transesophageal echocardiography overcomes this limitation and opens up "a new window to the heart." This new and rapidly expanding technique allows ultrasonic imaging of the cardiac structures and great vessels via the esophagus. The transesophageal approach uses a 3.5 or 5.0 mHZ transducer fixed to the tip of a modified flexible gastroscope without fiberoptics. The probe is passed into the esophagus and manipulated in a manner similar to that in gastrointestinal endoscopy. A transverse view can be obtained at any given level with the conventional uniplanar transesophageal probe. Recently, a transesophageal biplanar probe has been developed; transverse and longitudinal transducers are mounted side by side, 1.5 mm apart on the same transesophageal shaft. This arrangement enables transverse and longitudinal views to be obtained. This new technique provides ultrasonic access to the heart and thoracic aorta from the esophagus without being restricted by lung tissue or bone, and the proximity of both structures allows the use of high-frequency, near-focused transducers, resulting in better image quality (Fig. 2.7). Transesophageal echocardiography can be performed in an outpatient setting for ambulatory patients, intraoperatively for patients undergoing cardiac or noncardiac surgery, or at the bedside for those in intensive care units.

ASSESSMENT OF VENTRICULAR PERFORMANCE

One of the most valuable clinical applications of two-dimensional and Doppler echocardiography is the evaluation of left ventricular performance by assessment of both systolic and diastolic function. M-mode echocardiography permits an accurate measurement of left ventricular dimension and wall thickness. Precise endocardial definition and correct orientation of imaging planes with regard to internal landmarks is required. The rapid sampling rate provides a continuous record of the motion of the ventricular septum and the left ventricular free wall, allowing determination of chamber dimension, wall thickness, and rate of change of these variables over the course of the cardiac cycle. The most commonly used echocardiographic indexes of left ventricular performance are dimensional fractional shortening, fractional area change, and ejection fraction.

$$\text{fractional shortening} = \frac{\text{end diastolic dimension} - \text{end systolic dimension}}{\text{end diastolic dimension}}$$

$$\text{fractional area change} = \frac{\text{end diastolic area} - \text{end systolic area}}{\text{end diastolic area}}$$

$$\text{ejection fraction} = \frac{\text{end diastolic volume} - \text{end systolic volume}}{\text{end diastolic volume}}$$

Under certain conditions, these indexes provide a reliable and reproducible estimate of ventricular performance. Determination of left ventricular muscle mass is the accepted standard for identifying the presence or absence of left ventricular hypertrophy. M-mode and two-dimensional echocardiography have been shown to be reliable noninvasive methods for determining left ventricular mass (LVM).

$$\text{Anatomic LVM} = 1.04\,[(\text{LVID} + \text{PWT} + \text{IVST})^3 - (\text{LVID})^3] - 13.6 \text{ gm}$$

Altered geometry of the cavity due to an aneurysm, localized thinning from myocardial infarction, and asymmetrical or segmental hypertrophy limit the accurate determination of left ventricular volume and mass. The American Society of Echocardiography recommends that left ventricular volume be computed from the dimensions and area measurements obtained from four-chamber and two-chamber views using the modified Simpson's rule or "method of discs," which treats the ventricle as a stack of discs or slices. This algorithm is recommended because it is independent of preconceived ventricular shape (Fig. 2.15). The noninvasive determination

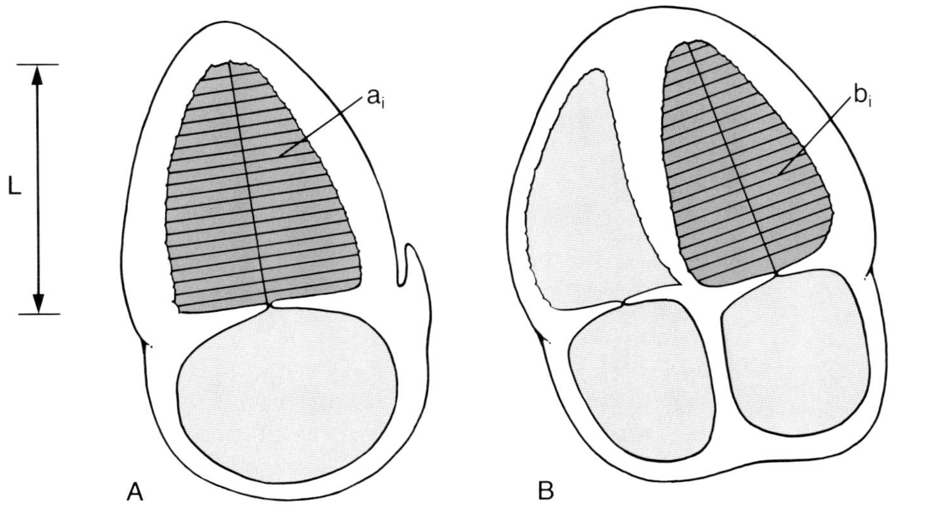

$$V = \frac{\pi}{4} \sum_{i=1}^{20} a_i b_i \frac{L}{20}$$

Fig. 2.15 Biplanar method of discs (modified Simpson's rule) from apical two- and four-chamber views. Calculation of volume (formula) results from summation of areas from diameters a_i and b_i of 20 cylinders of discs of equal height.

of left ventricular wall stress has been validated. The force per unit area, or "stress," acting along the circumference of the left ventricle at its minor axis is directly dependent on intracavitary pressure and radius of curvature, and is inversely dependent on wall thickness.

As a real-time tomographic technique, two-dimensional echocardiography is especially suitable for study of regional wall motion. The American Society of Echocardiography recommends a 16-segment model (Fig. 2.16) based on the following considerations: anatomic logic, easy identification of the segments using internal anatomic landmarks, relationship of the segments to known coronary arterial supply, and a uniform scoring system for grading the severity of segmental wall motion abnormalities.

Doppler echocardiography has been used in many clinical studies to assess left ventricular diastolic function by evaluating the ventricle's diastolic filling characteristics. Diastolic time intervals, peak flow velocities, and the proportion of flow during the various phases of diastole can be accurately measured from the Doppler recording with the pulsed-wave sample volume positioned properly in the left ventricular inflow tract. Abnormal patterns of diastolic filling include: delayed onset of flow, with resultant decreased total duration of diastolic filling; decreased velocity and total volumetric flow during the early rapid filling phase; prolonged time to early peak filling; decreased rates of left ventricular relaxation; increased velocity and total volumetric flow during late diastolic (atrial) filling (A wave); abnormal E/A flow ratios; and decreased or absent atrial filling despite sinus rhythm. Diastolic filling of the heart is a complex sequence of interrelated events. Therefore, attempts to interpret these Doppler findings should take into consideration the complex nature of the subject.

ECHO DOPPLER IN MANAGEMENT OF PATIENTS WITH VALVULAR HEART DISEASE

Echocardiographic visualization of each of the four cardiac valves can identify specific anatomic abnormalities characteristic of each type of valvular heart disease. Optimal echocardiographic evaluation of a patient with valvular heart disease requires determination of the following issues: detection of the particular valve lesion, its etiology and severity; valve morphology; complications of disease such as left atrial

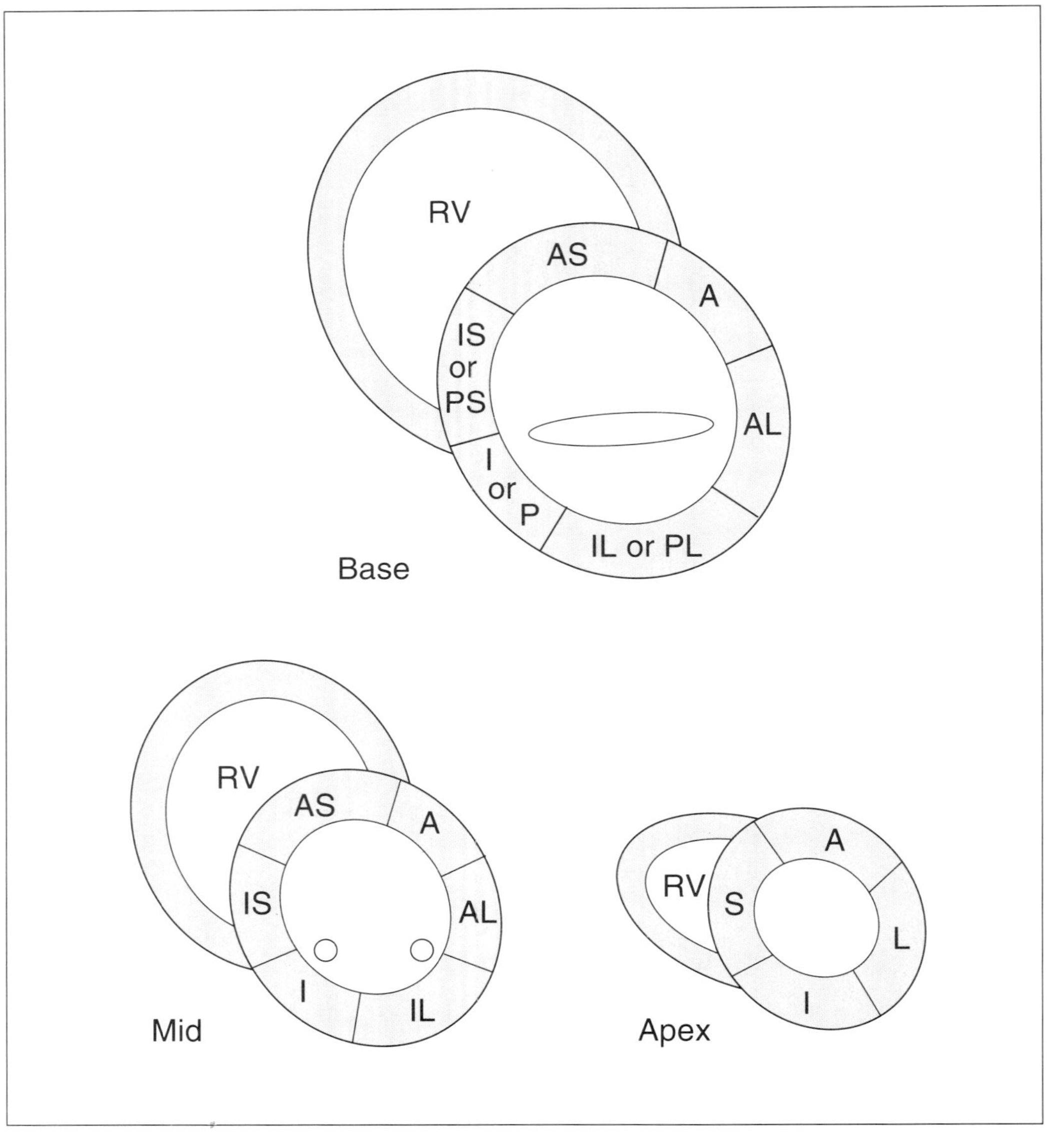

Fig. 2.16 Proposed 16-segment model for wall motion analysis.

A	anterior	IS	inferior septum
I	inferior	PL	posterior lateral
P	posterior	PS	posterior septum
AL	anterior lateral	S	septum
AS	anterior septum	L	lateral
IL	inferior lateral		

thrombus and endocarditis; presence of pulmonary hypertension; presence of other congenital or acquired heart lesions; and assessment of ventricular function.

One of the most important contributions to the usefulness of Doppler ultrasonography for the quantitative assessment of pressure gradients across stenotic valves has been the application of the modified Bernoulli equation. This equation is based on the Bernoulli principle for short segment stenosis and states

$$P = P/2 \times (V_2^2 - V_1^2)$$

where P is the pressure drop in mm Hg, P is the mass density of blood, V_2 is the velocity distal to an area of obstruction, and V_1 is the velocity proximal to it, both measured in meters per second. The equation has generally been further modified to yield the pressure drop: $P = 4 \times V_2^2$. If the proximal velocity rises to values of 2 meters per second or more, it must also be considered in the equation as $P = 4 \times (V_2^2 - V_1^2)$. When the Doppler velocity is defining a pressure difference from a jet, the pressure differences are assessed instantaneously. These are referred to as *peak instantaneous gradients.* The measurement of all the pressure drops during the ejection phase of the cardiac cycle divided by the ejection times yields the mean gradient. Mean pressure gradients calculated by Doppler ultrasonography appear to correlate better with those measured at cardiac catheterization than do peak pressure gradients. The examination of peak jet velocity must be performed from many transducer locations. Obtaining the highest velocity indicates that the jet and transducer are closely aligned.

A combination of two-dimensional and Doppler parameters is used to calculate the valvular area with the simplified continuity equation. The continuity equation states that because flow (Q) is a product of mean velocity and cross-sectional area, the product of the proximal mean velocity (V_1) and the proximal area (A_1) equals the product of the distal velocity (V_2) and the distal area (A_2), which is the valve area. Therefore, the valve area can be calculated from $A_2 = (V_1 \times A_1)/V_2$. In atrioventricular valve stenosis, the concept of *pressure half-time* has been applied to calculate the valvular area on the basis of hemodynamic studies in patients with mitral stenosis. Pressure half-time is the time taken for the initial maximum diastolic gradient to drop to one half; it is prolonged in atrioventricular valve stenosis, and the degree of prolongation is proportional to the severity of stenosis. Hatle et al. noted that mitral valve area was 1 cm^2 at a pressure half-time of 220 msec; therefore, mitral valve area can be calculated by the formula MVA = 220/pressure half-time in msec. Valvular regurgitation is mainly assessed either by pulsed Doppler echocardiography or color Doppler mapping; both are equally able to detect the regurgitant flow (Fig. 2.17, Appendix). The size of the regurgitant jet can be determined more easily and accurately with color Doppler mapping.

Doppler echocardiography has also been useful for noninvasive estimation of pulmonary artery pressure. Tricuspid regurgitation is fairly common in adults (Fig. 2.18, Appendix). The difference between right ventricular and right atrial pressure can be calculated from the transtricuspid velocity using the modified Bernoulli equation. Right ventricular systolic pressure is then approximated by adding the right atrial mean pressure to the pressure drop across the tricuspid valve. In the absence of pulmonary stenosis, this is a very reliable method for calculating the systolic pulmonary artery pressure.

In the past decade, echocardiography has been used increasingly in patients with bacterial endocarditis, as this technique can detect vegetations, delineate valvular lesions, and document progression of the disease. The presence of vegetations is of prognostic importance in patients with subacute bacterial endocarditis, as it is correlated with a higher rate of complications. Ultrasonographic detection of vegetations, in general, is limited by the size of the vegetation (lesions as small as 2 mm in diameter can be resolved) the relative echogenicity of the lesion, the presence of preexisting valvular disease, the timing of the examination in relation to the course of the illness, the sensitivity of the instrument used, and the skill of the operator. Transesophageal echocardiography can be performed in patients with suspected SBE but may yield equivocal results as compared with transthoracic echocardiography. In addition, prosthetic valve endocarditis, often difficult to evaluate by precordial echocardiography, may be more reliably assessed with transesophageal echocardiography.

ASSESSMENT OF PROSTHETIC HEART VALVE FUNCTION

All prosthetic valves are mildly stenotic as well as insufficient. Likewise, all are subject to such complications as thrombosis, infection, degeneration, dehiscence, fibrous ingrowth, and embolization, all of which may lead to hemodynamically significant insufficiency or obstruction (Fig. 2.19). Doppler

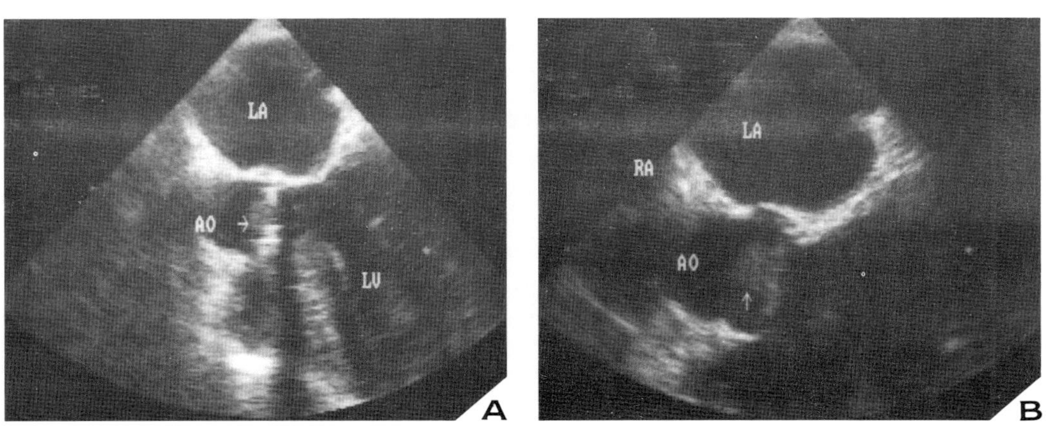

Fig. 2.19 Short axis of the heart at the level of the aorta in a patient with prosthetic Bjork–Shirley valve. The support of the valve is positioned in anterior–posterior direction. The disk is in open position in A and in closed position in B. (AO = aorta)

echocardiography is the procedure of choice for evaluation of the patient with suspected prosthetic heart valve dysfunction. An excellent correlation has been demonstrated between Doppler and catheterization techniques for both peak instantaneous and mean pressure gradients. In evaluation of patients with suspected prosthetic valve stenosis, if the interrogating Doppler beam is carefully aligned parallel to flow, the peak and mean transvalvular pressure gradients can be accurately measured by applying the modified Bernoulli equation. Physiologic insufficiency is detected in a higher percentage of patients with prosthetic heart valves. The regurgitant jet has a relatively small area, usually confined to within a centimeter of the valve plane, and a weak Doppler signal. Paravalvular leaks are much more readily identified using color Doppler mapping techniques. Several studies have demonstrated the high sensitivity and specificity of Doppler echocardiographic diagnosis of significant prosthetic valve insufficiency, particularly in the presence of an aortic prosthesis. Demonstration of mitral prosthetic insufficiency has been slightly more difficult, mainly owing to technical factors such as increased distance of the left atrium from the transducer and masking of the regurgitant signal by the prosthetic valve. Transesophageal echocardiography has been shown to be very helpful in this regard.

ECHOCARDIOGRAPHY AND DOPPLER TECHNIQUES IN EVALUATION OF PERICARDIAL DISEASES

Echocardiography has proved to be an important diagnostic tool for assessment of pericardial disease. As a semiquantitative technique, two-dimensional echocardiography has become the procedure of choice for detection and serial follow-up studies of pericardial effusion. A small amount of pericardial fluid (ie, 30 to 50 mL) can be accurately detected. The echocardiographic hallmark of pericardial effusion is the presence of an echo-free space posterior to the heart. M-mode echocardiography is usually adequate for the diagnosis of pericardial effusion in most patients; however, two-dimensional echocardiography provides valuable additional information. Precise quantitation of pericardial fluid is not extremely accurate, and most laboratories roughly estimate the size of an effusion as minimal, small, medium, or large. In large pericardial effusions the heart tends to move freely within the pericardial cavity; this type of motion has been called *swinging heart sign.* Using multiple tomographic sections, one can obtain a precise idea of the distribution of pericardial fluid and thereby determine the safest approach for pericardiocentesis.

Cardiac tamponade is an abnormal hemodynamic state resulting from impaired diastolic filling of the heart, usually due to a large collection of pericardial fluid under pressure. Cardiac tamponade should probably be defined in hemodynamic and clinical terms. A variety of M-mode, two-dimensional, and Doppler echocardiographic findings have been reported; among them, right atrial collapse and right ventricular collapse are very sensitive indicators. Pericardial constriction is accompanied by thickening, fibrosis, and calcification of the pericardium, with fusion of the epicardium and parietal pericardium and ensuing visceral constriction. A high index of suspicion is required to diagnose pericardial thickening. Among the echocardiographic features of constrictive pericarditis are rapid early and flat mid-diastolic motion of the posterior wall of the left ventricle, abnormal early diastolic ventricular septal motion, atrial systolic notch on the interventricular septum, a dense, rigid shell of pericardium, enlarged atria, ventricular septal bulging towards the left ventricle during inspiration (septal bounce), dilated inferior vena cava and hepatic veins, and marked inspiratory decrease in mitral "E" velocity. Characteristic echo Doppler features differentiate constrictive pericarditis from restrictive cardiomyopathy. The echocardiographer should have a high index of suspicion and should utilize the various M-mode, two-dimensional, and Doppler echocardiographic features to make the diagnosis of constrictive pericarditis. Total or partial absence of the pericardium is a rare congenital anomaly and is usually asymptomatic; M-mode and two-dimensional echocardiography may show features of right ventricular volume overload. Pericardial cysts, usually asymptomatic and typically located at the right costophrenic angle, can be accurately diagnosed by two-dimensional echocardiography.

ECHOCARDIOGRAPHY FOR ASSESSMENT OF INTRACAVITARY MASSES

Adequate identification of the nature of an intracavitary mass (eg, ventricular thrombus, primary cardiac tumor, metastatic tumor, hydatid cyst, vegetations) is mandatory before appropriate therapy can be undertaken. Two-dimensional echocardiography, the procedure of choice for detection of cardiac masses, yields precise anatomic information regarding the morphology of the mass, its attachment, mobility, location, and its relation to cardiac structures. The procedure can be repeated as often as necessary. With this technique, previously unrecognized intracavitary lesions can now be diagnosed, the natural history of vegetative endocarditis can be better defined, and the incidence of left ventricular thrombi accompanying myocardial infarctions can be ascertained. Transesophageal echocardiography yields images of cardiac structures that are superior in quality and structural resolution to two-dimensional echocardiography; the detailed anatomic visualization of the atrial chambers, interatrial septum, and atrial appendages makes this technique a superb tool for evaluation of atrial masses.

ECHOCARDIOGRAPHY FOR ASSESSMENT OF CONGENITAL HEART DISEASE

The instrumentation used in infants and children includes either phased-array or mechanical sector scanners and high-resolution, medium-focused 3.5 and 5.0 mHZ transducers. In addition to the standard parasternal long- and short-axis, apical, and suprasternal notch windows, infants and young children have an excellent subxiphoid window that enables intracardiac anatomy to be assessed. Ultrasonographic techniques now allow examination of human fetal cardiac development and function in utero. Diagnostic quality images of the fetal heart in utero can be obtained as early as 16 weeks of gestation, thus delineating congenital heart defects.

Analysis of the morphology and function of the fetal heart during the second and third trimesters of pregnancy enables cardiologists to counsel prospective parents and to formulate management plans for pregnancy, delivery, and the immediate postnatal period. It appears clear, for example, that nonimmune fetal hydrops often represents end-stage fetal cardiac decompensation. Pulsed Doppler examination of the fetus supplements the echocardiographic findings in identifying the responsible defects. Fetal cardiac echocardiography is of particular importance in analyzing disturbances of fetal cardiac rhythm.

To assess intracardiac anatomy and to obtain detailed morphologic information, a segmental approach to echocardiographic examination should be employed. The three cardiac segments are the atria, ventricles, and great arteries. *Atrial situs* describes the arrangement of the atrial chambers within the chest. The atria are identified by defining the morphology of the atrial appendages. A transverse cross-section of the abdomen displaying the liver, inferior vena cava, and aorta is useful to define the situs. To define ventricular position, ventricular morphology must be assessed. The morphologic characteristics of the right ventricle include a coarse trabecular pattern, a pyramidal shape with a moderator band and a crista supraventricularis, and a discrete outlet portion (ie, the arterial and atrioventricular valves are not in continuity). In contrast, the morphologic left ventricle has a prolate elliptical shape, a thin trabecular pattern, and no discrete outlet portion (ie, arterial valve is in fibrous continuity with the atrioventricular valve). There are two distinct papillary muscle masses, one in the anterior lateral position and one in the posterior medial position. Finally, it is important to note that the tricuspid valve rests in a slightly more apical position than the anatomic mitral valve. The great arteries are considered to be normally connected with the ventricles when the aorta exits the morphologic left ventricle and the pulmonary trunk exits the morphologic right ventricle. These arteries are normally related when the pulmonary artery lies anterior and to the left of the aorta.

Echocardiographic diagnoses that can often be made with certainty include: aortic valvular, subvalvular, and supravalvular stenosis; aortic coarctation; hypoplastic left heart syndrome; atrial, ventricular, and atrioventricular septal defects; cor triatriatum; tricuspid atresia; Ebstein's anomaly; valvular and subvalvular pulmonic stenosis; univentricular–atrioventricular connection; double-outlet right ventricle; transposition of the great arteries; patent ductus arteriosus; tetralogy of Fallot; truncus arteriosus; anomalous pulmonary venous connection; and pulmonary atresia. Color Doppler imaging is extremely useful for detection and assessment of cardiac shunts. Using Doppler echocardiography it is possible to measure gradients across stenotic valves, to calculate cardiac output, to identify blood flow patterns in the cardiac chambers and great arteries, and to estimate the size of a shunt. Many methods use Doppler echocardiography to quantitate pulmonary to systemic flow ratios (Q_p/Q_s). This requires sampling of a Doppler flow velocity profile in the pulmonary artery and the aorta, and calculation of mean flow velocity. In these methods, the area beneath the flow velocity curve is measured by planimetry. The cross-sectional area of the vessel is calculated according to the following formula: vessel area $= \pi r^2$, where r = radius of the vessel. Pulmonary flow can be calculated from the equation: flow = mean pulmonary artery velocity × pulmonary artery vessel area × right ventricular ejection time × heart rate. Systemic flow can be calculated by the equation: flow = mean aortic velocity × aortic root area × left ventricular ejection time × heart rate. The ratio between pulmonary and systemic flow (Q_p/Q_s) can then be calculated.

The interventricular systolic pressure drop across ventricular septal defects can also be evaluated using the modified Bernoulli equation (Fig. 2.14). Correct alignment of the transducer with the jet is quite critical. The transducer must be axial to the direction of the jet across the ventricular septal defect to obtain an accurate velocity signal (this can be best achieved by color Doppler mapping). In many circumstances, a fair estimate of the interventricular pressure difference can be assessed. A peak velocity across a ventricular septal defect of 3.5 meters per second or more suggests that the defect is restrictive in nature.

DISEASES OF THE AORTA

A portion of the ascending aorta is imaged in the parasternal and the apical long-axis views; however, right parasternal, supraclavicular, and suprasternal notch imaging is required to image the entire ascending aorta, transverse aortic arch, and part of the descending aorta. With routine parasternal imaging, the descending aorta is visualized posterior to the left atrium and left ventricle (it should not be mistaken for the echo-free space in the atrioventricular groove region produced by the coronary sinus). Dilatation and aneurysms of the ascending aorta can usually be diagnosed from the parasternal long-axis position.

Aneurysms of the sinuses of Valsalva are well depicted on parasternal and apical views. Color Doppler imaging is valuable for identifying any rupture site and blood flow into the recipient chamber. Although the diagnosis of dissecting aortic aneurysm can be made by M-mode echocardiography, it is more clearly defined with two-dimensional imaging. The echocardiographic hallmark of aortic dissection is the demonstration of an abnormal linear echo in the lumen of the aorta in more than one scan plane. Color Doppler imaging provides comprehensive evaluation of flow dynamics in aortic dissection. Transesophageal echocardiography yields accurate anatomic information in patients with aortic dissection, and is becoming the diagnostic technique of choice in this disease.

CHAPTER 3

Invasive Cardiac Diagnosis

THE CARDIAC CATHETERIZATION LABORATORY

IMAGING EQUIPMENT

Sophisticated imaging equipment is essential for proper performance of cardiac catheterization and angiography. Most invasive cardiologists prefer 35-mm techniques for angiocardiography and coronary arteriography. (Large-format roll- or cut-film is usually preferred for studies of the aortic arch and great vessels.) Both biplane and single-plane systems are available in a variety of designs, most of which employ movable floor mounts or cantilever tables (Fig. 3.1). Useful enhancements include a video recording system and a digital subtraction system that allows selective magnification and computerized image enhancement and image analysis. A power injector and film processing equipment complete the imaging component of the cardiac catheterization suite.

Modern angiocardiographic systems, which operate at low peak kilovoltage (kVp) and high milliamperage (mA), have high photon flux (photons/frame). The resulting cine images have high resolution with wide contrast latitude (long gray scale), which enhances slight differences in radiographic density.

Cardiac catheterization and angiocardiography often entail extensive, time-consuming catheter manipulations; therefore, they may expose the patient, as well as the operating personnel, to a significant radiation hazard. The danger is greatest for children, owing to their longer life expectancy and relatively greater sensitivity to radiation (the risk of radiation-induced leukemia is approximately twice as great in children as in adults). Because of their small body size, which results in increased exposure from internal scatter, the thyroid and gonadal doses are higher in children than in adults. The average entrance (skin) dose from a combined cardiac catheterization/angiocardiographic procedure is about 10 rad in a 5-year-old child and 30 rad in a 15-year-old adolescent. Although dose levels do not exceed permissible limits, every effort should be made to reduce radiation exposure, particularly in infants and young children.

Modern angiocardiographic suites incorporate "low-dose" fluoroscopy systems which significantly decrease radiation exposure to patient and staff when compared with conventional fluoroscopic equipment. It is possible to substantially decrease patient dose, with little if any loss of information, by using low pulse-rate fluoroscopy systems mated to videodisc recorders that can store a single image or dynamic sequence. Thyroid and gonadal exposure can be further reduced by placing the image intensifier as close as possible to the patient, by carefully collimating the beam, and by accurately calibrating the equipment. By using protective eyeglasses and lead shields, it is possible to reduce scattered radiation to the operator's eyes (lens) and thyroid to negligible levels.

PHYSIOLOGIC MONITORING AND RECORDING EQUIPMENT

In addition to imaging apparatus, the catheterization laboratory is equipped with a basic physiologic recording system, which is used to monitor, display, and record the patient's ECG and heart rate, intravascular and intracardiac pressures, and related hemodynamic data (Fig. 3.2). Transducers connected to fluid-filled catheters near the vascular access site are used to record intravascular and intracardiac pressures. Cardiac output is measured by the thermodilution method or, in certain situations, by the Fick method (see below). The availability of an oximeter in the catheterization laboratory permits more accurate measurements of cardiac output by the Fick method and facilitates the

CHAPTER LABELING KEY

RA	right atrium	LV	left ventricle
LA	left atrium	Ao	aorta
RV	right ventricle		

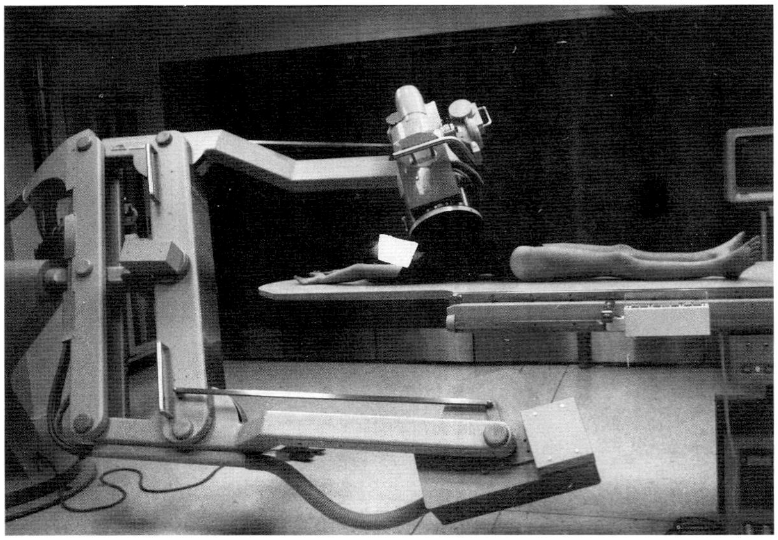

Fig. 3.1 X-ray equipment used for angiocardiography. Rotation and angulation of the X-ray tube and image intensifier system is simplified by this type of support. When combined with an additional X-ray tube and image intensifier for the horizontal plane, it is possible to perform biplane 35-mm cine angiography in multiple projections.

evaluation of shunts; by using fluoroscopy and transcatheter pressure monitoring to ascertain the position of the catheter tip, one can ascertain the location and magnitude (volume) of the shunt.

Recently, computerized systems for processing physiologic data have become popular. These sophisticated systems tabulate the catheterization data and generate a computerized report which includes automated wave-form and heart rate analysis and various calculated parameters (eg, transvalvular pressure gradients, calculated valve area of stenotic valves). On many of the more popular systems, left ventricular volume can be calculated by using a light pen or similar digitizing device to trace the outline of the chamber on the ventriculogram. (Applying the concept of quantitative ventriculography entails three-dimensional mathematical modeling. For accurate results, it is necessary to correct for magnification and "pincushion" distortion of the image. The correction factor is obtained by making an exposure with a grid or metal ball of known dimensions in the position of the left ventricle after the patient has been removed from the table.) Although these sophisticated systems have many useful features they are not necessary in small-volume laboratories that specialize in routine coronary arteriography.

EMERGENCY EQUIPMENT

In addition to systems for imaging and recording physiologic data, equipment and drugs needed to deal with medical emergencies should be available in the catheterization laboratory. Basic equipment and supplies consist of a defibrillator, oxygen, suction, ventilation devices, pacemakers, pericardiocentesis instruments, and appropriate medications. Many laboratories also stock an intra-aortic balloon assist device. Some laboratories with high patient volumes have ready access to an anesthesia machine and portable cardiopulmonary bypass equipment. Although the sophistication of the equipment may vary, it is

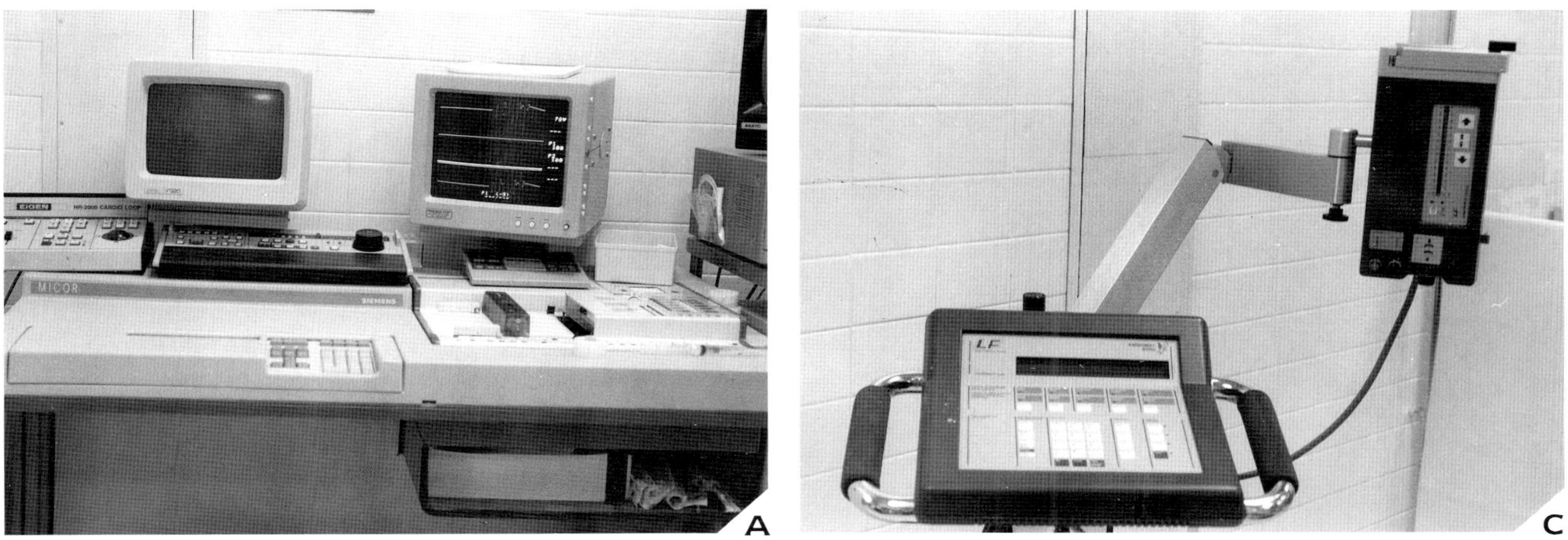

A

C

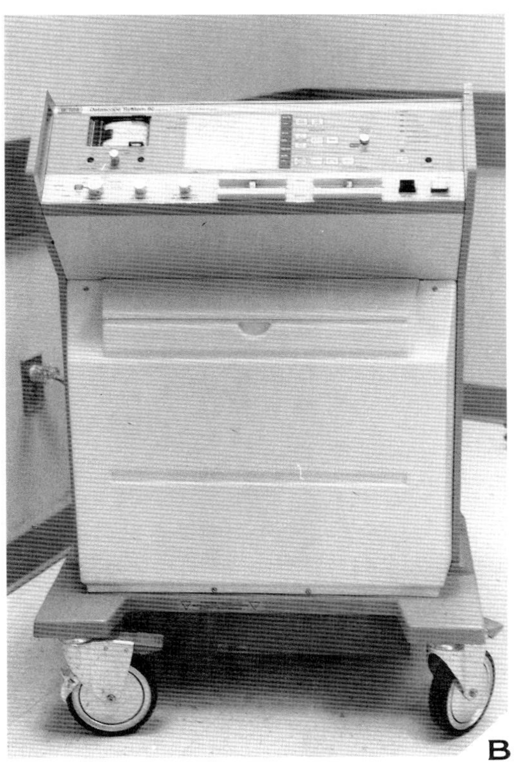

B

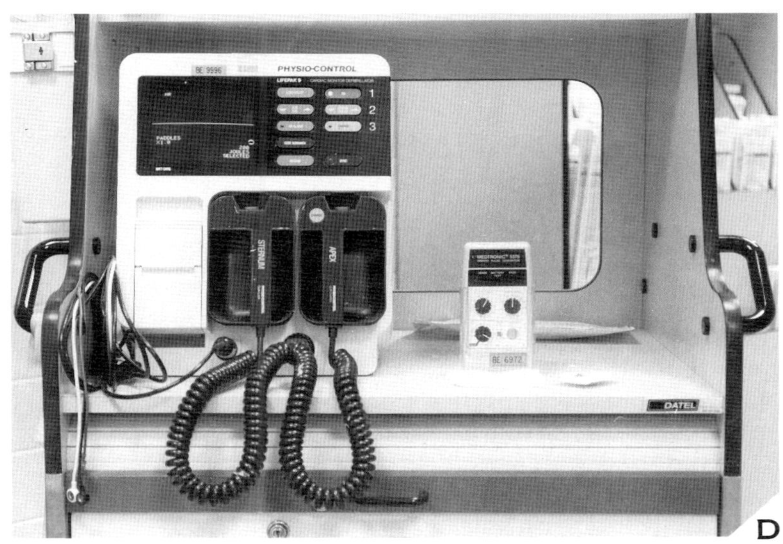

D

Fig. 3.2 Equipment used for cardiac catheterization and angiocardiography. (A) Equipment for recording pressures during catheterization; (B) intra-aortic balloon monitor; (C) power injector for contrast media; (D) ECG monitor and defibrillator.

axiomatic that laboratory personnel must be proficient in its use, so that emergency measures can be carried out quickly and effectively.

STAFF

The composition of the catheterization laboratory team has evolved over the years; in many respects it resembles its surgical counterpart. In addition to the cardiologist and assistant (if there is one), who may be a cardiology fellow or resident, the team commonly includes a scrub technician, a circulating nurse, a radiology technologist, and a technologist to record the physiologic data. Some laboratories utilize one person for more than one function.

PRINCIPLES OF CARDIAC CATHETERIZATION

In this technique, one or more catheters are introduced through a peripheral vein or artery and positioned under fluoroscopic guidance in the cardiac chambers and/or great vessels. (An abnormal course taken by the catheter is often a clue to the presence of cardiac malformation.) Pressures and oxygen content (saturation) are measured at various sites. By carefully analyzing the data, the cardiologist can obtain a wealth of anatomic, physiologic, and functional data (Fig. 3.3).

To catheterize the right side of the heart, the catheter is introduced into a systemic vein and advanced successively into the right atrium, right ventricle, and pulmonary trunk (Fig. 3.4). Left heart catheterization can be performed by either a retrograde or an antegrade approach. Retrograde catheterization is accomplished by introducing the catheter into a systemic artery and passing it retrogradely into the aorta and left ventricle; if necessary, the catheter can be passed retrogradely through the mitral valve into the left atrium (Fig. 3.5). In the antegrade approach, the catheter is introduced into a systemic vein and advanced into the right atrium; it is then passed into the left atrium via the foramen ovale (which generally remains "probe patent" throughout life) or an existing atrial septal defect. Once the catheter has entered the left atrium it can be manipulated across the aortic valve into the left ventricle and aorta. An alternative method of antegrade left heart catheterization is to perforate the atrial septum (transseptal catheterization) (Fig. 3.6).

The design of the catheter varies according to the use for which it is intended. Catheters employed exclusively for pressure measurements usually have an end hole. (This is always the case for catheters introduced into peripheral branches of the pulmonary arteries to measure wedge pressure.) Catheters used for angiocardiography, which is usually performed after the physiologic data have been collected, have an end hole and multiple side holes. A variety of specialized catheters have been developed for coronary arteriography (see Chapter 21). Swan–Ganz catheters, which are used to measure pressure in pulmonary arteries, have an inflatable balloon at the tip. When the catheter tip is positioned in a main pulmonary artery, the balloon is swept by the flowing blood into a peripheral branch. Specially designed balloon angioplasty catheters are used to treat congenital and acquired valvular stenoses, aortic coarctation, and coronary artery stenoses (see Chapters 16, 30 and 31).

Pressures are recorded by means of a transducer, a device that transforms mechanical into electrical energy. The data are displayed on a video monitor and inscribed on a continuous roll

FIG. 3.3 ANATOMIC, PHYSIOLOGIC, AND FUNCTIONAL DATA PROVIDED BY CARDIAC CATHETERIZATION

- Anatomic Data
  - Catheter position
    - Septal defects
    - Patent ductus arteriosus
    - Anomalies of great veins
    - Anomalies of great arteries

- Physiologic Data*
  - Pressures
    - Cardiac chambers
    - Aorta
    - Pulmonary arterial tree
    - Pulmonary capillary bed (wedge pressure)
    - Gradient across a stenotic valve or coarctation
  - Oxygen saturation
    - Cardiac chambers
    - Great arteries
    - Great veins
    - Pulmonary arterial tree
  - Calculated parameters
    - Pulmonary resistance
    - Systemic resistance
    - Ratio between pulmonary and systemic resistance

- Functional data*
  - Calculated parameters
    - Cardiac output
    - Cardiac index
    - Left ventricular end diastolic volume
    - Cardiac ejection fraction
    - Left ventricular mass
    - Right ventricular mass
    - Oxygen consumption

**At rest and in response to exercise or administration of drugs or oxygen.*

Fig. 3.3 Anatomic, physiologic, and functional data provided by cardiac catheterization.

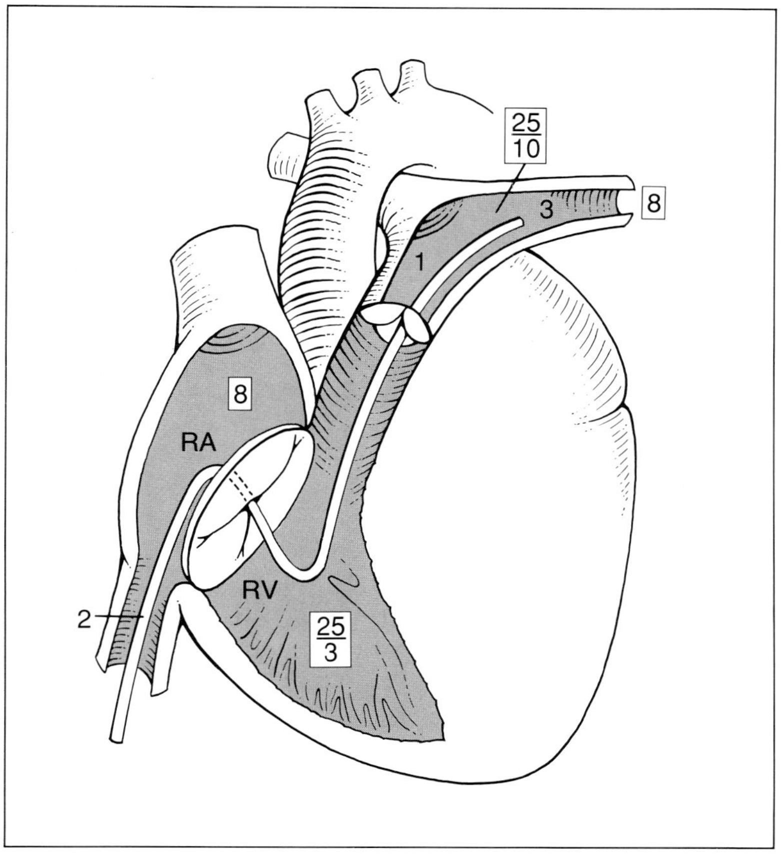

RA right atrium
RV right ventricle
1 pulmonary trunk
2 catheter (in inferior vena cava)
3 catheter position for pulmonary wedge pressure

Fig. 3.4 Right-sided catheterization via the inferior vena cava. Right ventricular pressure normally increases with exercise.

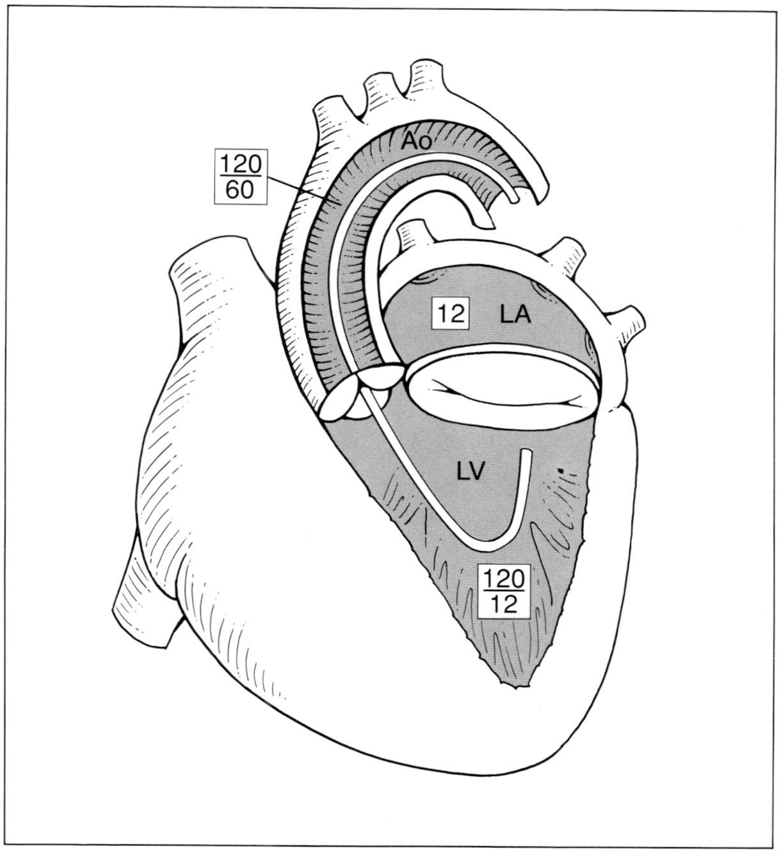

LA left atrium
LV left ventricle
Ao aorta

Fig. 3.5 Antegrade catheterization of left side of heart in the evaluation of congenital heart disease. The left heart can also be approached from the right atrium via the foramen ovale, which generally remains "probe patent" throughout life, or via a natural or surgically created atrial septal defect [eg, following a Rashkind procedure (balloon atrial septosomy)].

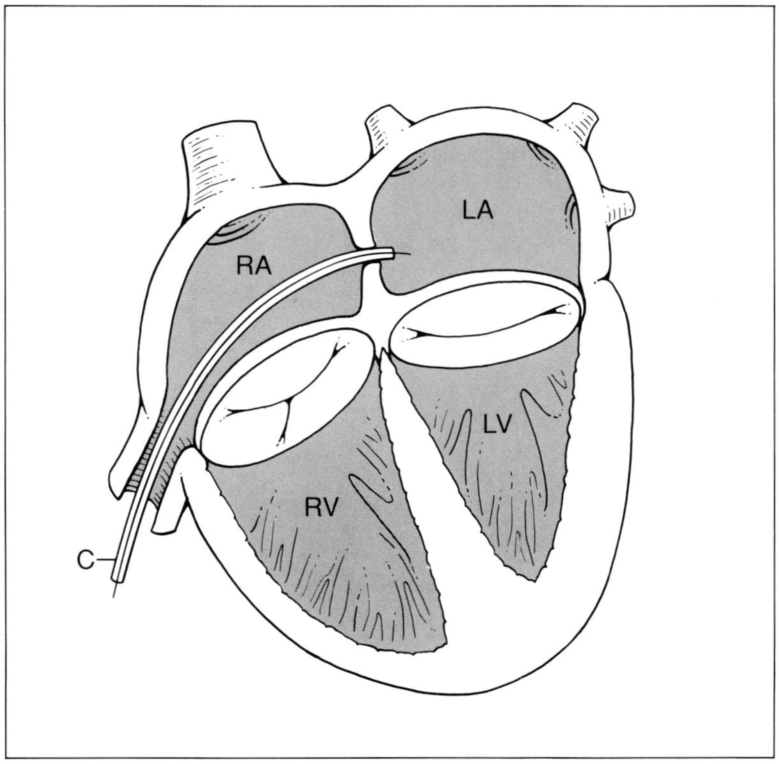

Fig. 3.6 Transseptal catheterization. The catheter (C) has been advanced from the inferior vena cava into the right atrium, and via the iatrogenic septal perforation into the left atrium. The catheter tip is positioned in the midportion of the left atrium. The catheter can be exchanged for larger catheters or a balloon catheter to create an atrial septal defect, or it can be advanced into the left ventricle. Applications include balloon valvotomy for mitral stenosis, left ventriculography following aortic valve replacement, percutaneous insertion of left ventricular assist devices, and left heart catheterization in patients with aortic stenosis when retrograde catheterization is not feasible.

of paper. Blood oxygen content at various sites is measured by oximetry; the data are used to calculate the magnitude of intra- and extracardiac shunts and other functional parameters.

The normal pressures on the left and right sides of the heart are shown in Figs. 3.4 and 3.5; (see also Fig. 3.9). By wedging an end-hole catheter into a peripheral pulmonary arterial branch, it is possible to measure the pulmonary wedge (capillary) pressure; the latter value, which reflects the pulmonary venous pressure, serves as an indirect measurement of left atrial pressure. The normal left atrial pressure is 12 mm Hg or less. The left ventricular diastolic pressure is normally equal to the main left atrial pressure (ie, 12 mm Hg or less). The normal left ventricular systolic pressure is 110 to 120 mm Hg. The normal aortic systolic pressure is the same as left ventricular systolic pressure. Aortic diastolic pressure is normally 80 mm Hg or less.

The catheterization data can be used to calculate the volume of blood in the systemic and pulmonary circulations, as well as the magnitude (volume) of any left to right or right to left shunt that may be present. The amount of blood pumped per minute equals the *cardiac output;* by normalizing this value to body surface, it is possible to calculate the *cardiac index* (blood flow per minute per square meter of body surface). The *ejection fraction,* the percentage of the ventricular content ejected during systole, is a useful parameter of ventricular function; it equals the end diastolic volume minus end systolic volume, divided by the end diastolic volume × 100). The normal left ventricular ejection fraction is above 50 percent. The left ventricular ejection fraction can also be estimated by echocardiography or MRI.

Cardiac output is most commonly measured by the thermodilution method, with computer analysis of the temperature curve; data analysis can be performed by a computer incorporated into the physiologic recording system or by a free-standing microcomputer. In the thermodilution technique, cold saline solution is injected through the proximal (right atrial) port of a balloon-tipped right heart catheter which has a thermistor at the distal (pulmonary artery) end. Although useful for routine studies, the thermodilution technique is inaccurate in a number of situations (eg, intra- and extracardiac shunts, tricuspid insufficiency, extremely low cardiac output). In such cases, cardiac output is usually measured by techniques based on the Fick principle (cardiac output equals oxygen consumption divided by the arterial–venous oxygen difference). If a metabolic analyzer is available, oxygen consumption can be measured directly; otherwise, a normal value (90 to 120 mL/min/M^2 body surface area) must be assumed.

To evaluate intra- or extracardiac shunts, O_2 saturation is measured at appropriate sites (determined by fluoroscopy or transcatheter pressure monitoring). Using the Fick principle, it is possible to calculate the magnitude (volume) of the shunt by measuring the difference between the arterial and venous oxygen content in each circuit. Using the Fick principle, it is also possible to estimate the pulmonary blood flow per unit time. [The volume of blood traversing the pulmonary circulation per minute is proportional to the amount of oxygen consumed during a given period of time; the latter value is calculated by subtracting the oxygen content of expired air from the oxygen content of room air (21 percent).] In a normal subject, the ratio of pulmonary to systemic blood flow is 1:1. If a shunt is present, the volume of blood flowing from the systemic circuit to the pulmonary circuit, or vice versa, can be calculated. The magnitude (volume) of the shunt, expressed in liters/minute, is expressed as the ratio between pulmonary and systemic blood flow; it may be 3:1 or greater in a patient with a large ventricular septal defect.

Blood flowing through the pulmonary vascular bed must overcome a certain resistance. Pulmonary vascular resistance, expressed mathematically as the pressure drop across the pulmonary vascular bed divided by the pulmonary blood flow, is another important parameter that can be determined from the catheterization data (Fig. 3.7). In both children and adults, pulmonary resistance is normally 1 to 6 units/M^2 (that is, corrected for body surface area). (To express pulmonary resistance as dyne–sec/cm^2, multiply units by 80.) In an infant with a large left to right shunt, pulmonary resistance typically begins to rise immediately after birth, progressively increasing until it reaches systemic or suprasystemic levels. A value greater than 8 units/M^2 suggests fixed, increased pulmonary resistance. Pa-

FIG. 3.7 FORMULA FOR CALCULATING PULMONARY VASCULAR RESISTANCE*

$$\text{Pulmonary resistance} = \frac{P_{PA}\,(\text{mean}) - P_{PV}\,(\text{mean})}{Q_P}$$

*P_{PA} (mean) = mean pulmonary arterial pressure (mm Hg);
PPV (mean) = mean pulmonary venous pressure (mm Hg);
QP = pulmonary blood flow (L/min).

Fig. 3.7 Formula for calculating pulmonary vascular resistance.

FIG. 3.8 FORMULA FOR CALCULATING SYSTEMIC VASULAR RESISTANCE*

$$\text{Systemic resistance} = \frac{P_{AO}\,(\text{mean}) - P_{RA}\,(\text{mean})}{S_f}$$

*For example, in a patient with a (normal) mean aortic pressure of 83 mm Hg, a (normal) mean right atrial pressure of 4 mm Hg, and a body surface of 4.4 square meters, the calculated systemic resistance is 18 units/square meter of body surface.
P_{AO} (mean) = mean aortic pressure (mm Hg);
P_{PV} (mean) = mean right atrial pressure (mm Hg);
S_F = systemic blood flow (liters/min).

Fig. 3.8 Formula for calculating systemic vascular resistance.

tients with levels above 40 units/M^2 have a very poor prognosis. Pulmonary resistance is decreased in patients with pulmonary arteriovenous fistulas, an anomaly in which a portion of the pulmonary blood flow bypasses the pulmonary capillary bed.

Systemic (peripheral) vascular resistance is calculated in the same manner as pulmonary vascular resistance (Fig. 3.8). Systemic resistance is normally 15 to 40 units/M^2 (to express resistance as dyne-sec/cm^2, multiply by 80). Increased peripheral resistance is characteristic of systemic hypertension, whereas decreased peripheral resistance is seen in patients with systemic arteriovenous fistulas (see Chapter 14), severe aortic insufficiency, and other disorders with similar hemodynamic features.

To sum up, cardiac catheterization accurately depicts the pathophysiology as well as the functional status of the heart in patients with congenital or acquired heart disease. In some instances the position of the catheter may also provide important anatomic information (see Fig. 3.3). Normal cardiac catheterization values are shown in Fig. 3.9.

PERFORMING THE STUDY

INDICATIONS AND RISKS

Invasive diagnostic procedures are performed to precisely define the pathophysiology and pathologic anatomy in patients whose clinical findings suggest a cardiac abnormality. In general, an invasive study is indicated when quantitative data needed to guide therapy or indicate prognosis cannot be obtained by noninvasive techniques such as echocardiography or MRI. Examples include symptomatic structural defects (congenital or acquired) and angina with a positive exercise stress test. Many physicians believe that any clinical findings compatible with coronary artery disease warrant coronary arteriography, even when the symptoms and/or objective evidence are minimal. This concept is based on data suggesting that the pathologic anatomy is a more accurate predictor of prognosis than the patient's symptoms.

Other candidates for invasive diagnostic studies include patients with a known diagnosis in whom it necessary to quantify the results of an intervention or to assess changes occurring over a period of time. Examples include patients with recurrent angina after coronary angioplasty for single-vessel disease and patients with recurrent symptoms after valve surgery.

Invasive diagnostic procedures are not always necessary or appropriate. For example, catheterization and angiocardiography can be omitted in an elderly patient with well-tolerated aortic incompetence which appears mild on echocardiography, or in a symptomatic patient with echocardiographically demonstrated mitral valve prolapse and a normal exercise stress test. In other words, an invasive diagnostic procedure is indicated only when it is clearly justified by the benefit-to-risk ratio. In each instance, the clinician must weigh both the medical risk and the cost and inconvenience to the patient, and then ask, "How will these data affect the management of this patient?"

In a relatively healthy patient, routine catheterization/angiography is associated with a relatively small risk. Advanced age, heart failure, peripheral vascular disease, renal or pulmonary insufficiency, and a history of asthma or severe allergy are

FIG. 3.9 NORMAL HEMODYNAMIC PARAMETERS OBTAINED FROM CARDIAC CATHETERIZATION

Normal values and pressures	
O_2 consumption (VO_2)	110–150/ml/min/M^2
Pulmonary A-V O_2 difference	3.5–4.7 vol.%
Systemic A-V O_2 difference	3.5–4.7 vol.%
Systemic O_2 saturation	>94%
Cardiac index (C.I.)	2.5–4.0 L/min/M^2
Systemic vascular resistance (SVR)	8.0–15.0 units
Pulmonary vascular resistance (PVR)	0.2–1.2 units
Total pulmonary resistance (TPR)	1.0–3.0 units
Aortic valve area (AVA)	2.6–3.5 cm^2
Mitral valve area (MVA)	4.0–6.0 cm^2
LV end diastolic volume	<90 ml/M^2
Ejection fraction	55–70%

Normal pressures (mm Hg)	
Right atrium (RA), mean	1–8
Right ventricle (RV), systolic	15–28
End diastolic (RVEDP)	0–8
Pulmonary artery (PA)	
Systolic	15–28
Diastolic	5–16
Mean	10–22
Pulmonary artery wedge (PAW)	
Mean	4–12
Left atrium (LA)	
Mean	4–12
Left ventricle (LV)	
Systolic	85–150
End diastolic (LVEDP)	4–12
Aortic (AO)	
Systolic	85–150
Diastolic	60–90
Mean	70–105

Fig. 3.9 Normal hemodynamic parameters obtained from cardiac catheterization.

LV apex should be considered (Figs. 3.16 and 3.17). This demanding technique is best employed in centers with considerable experience with complex interventions.

In general, standard techniques can be used in patients with mechanical mitral valve prostheses, provided that the catheter is kept clear of the valve to minimize the risk of dislodging a thrombus or entrapment of the catheter. Rarely, it is necessary to pass a catheter across a mechanical tricuspid or pulmonic valve prosthesis. A small balloon catheter can be used in such cases; although ball-cage prostheses usually present no problem, entrapment of the catheter is a potential risk in patients with flap valves. Whereas valvular incompetence secondary to catheter entrapment on the left side of the heart may have serious consequences, temporary valvular incompetence on the right side of the heart is usually well tolerated, even in patients who are quite ill.

AORTIC STENOSIS

Most invasive cardiologists have developed their own repertory of "tricks" for passing catheters retrogradely through stenotic aortic valves. The small valve orifice, dilated aortic root, turbulent blood flow, and the often ragged surface of the cusps contribute to the difficulty of the procedure. Nevertheless, it is necessary to persevere, since in many clinical settings (eg, elderly patients, poor ventricular function, associated coronary artery or noncardiac disease) the surgeon relies heavily on the pressure gradient and the calculated valve area in assessing the need for corrective surgery.

One technique that we have found to be reliable employs an Amplatz-configuration (S-shaped) coronary artery catheter containing a straight guidewire (Fig. 3.18). Using biplane or multiview fluoroscopy for guidance, the catheter tip is "aimed" at the valve from a distance of 1 or 2 cm, and repeated attempts are made to pass the guidewire across the valve. Once the guidewire has crossed the valve, it is usually possible to feed the catheter into the left ventricle. If this results in an excessive number of ventricular ectopic beats, or if a ventriculogram is desired, the Amplatz catheter can be replaced with a pigtail catheter (Fig. 3.19). The catheter exchange is done cautiously over a long J-shaped guidewire to minimize the risk of perforating the ventricular wall.

An alternative approach that can be employed when the retrograde technique is unsuccessful is to enter the left atrium via the transseptal approach, after which the catheter is passed through the mitral valve into the left ventricle (Fig. 3.20).

PROBLEMS OF VASCULAR ACCESS AND CATHETER PLACEMENT

Because of its ease and the low radiation dose to the operator, most angiographers prefer the femoral approach for aortography and coronary arteriography. Occasionally it may be very difficult—rarely, impossible—to position the catheter tip in the aortic root for these procedures. A number of special maneuvers can be employed in such cases. (The side with the strongest femoral pulse should be used.) A J-tip guidewire (or one with a soft tip and "torqueable" curve) can be employed if the iliac vessels or aorta are tortuous or stenotic, or both. Another frequently successful technique is to use a Judkins-shape right coronary artery catheter, making frequent test injections of contrast material to find a passage through which the catheter

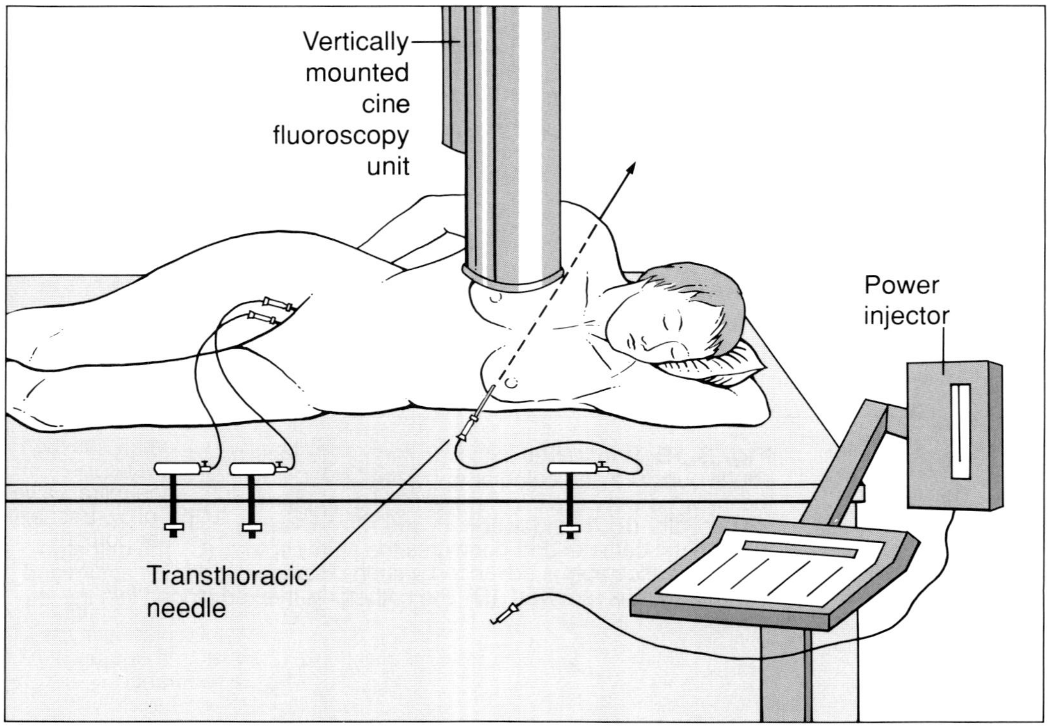

Fig. 3.16 Direct transthoracic transapical needle puncture of the left ventricle. The patient lies comfortably with his or her left side down. The patient's right side is slightly elevated so that the mitral prosthesis is in profile when viewed through the vertically mounted cine fluoroscopy unit. The shortest route between the skin surface and the cardiac apex is identified and the puncture site is prepared and anethetized. Under fluoroscopic control, the transthoracic needle is introduced and advanced in the direction of the right scapula until it enters the left ventricle. Contrast is then injected through a power injector (shown at patient's left). Systemic and pulmonary arterial "wedge" pressures are continuosly monitored during the procedure.

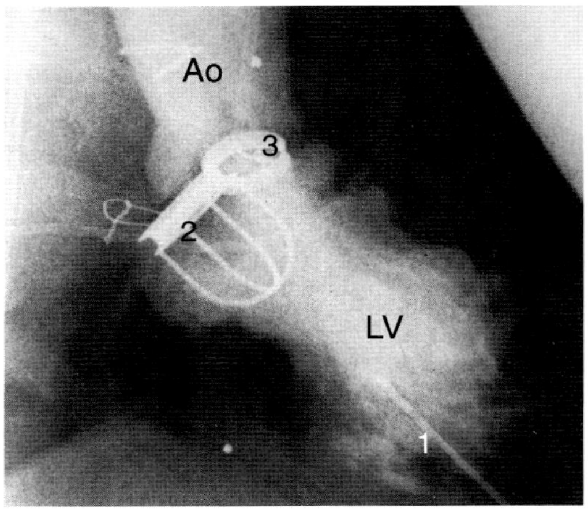

1 transapical catheter
LV left ventricle
2 prosthetic mitral valve
3 prosthetic aortic valve
Ao aorta

Fig. 3.17 Left ventriculography after transthoracic needle puncture of the left ventricle. Right anterior oblique projection of left ventriculogram in a patient with aortic and mitral valve prostheses. The tip of the catheter has been positioned in the midportion of the left ventricular cavity (the absence of contrast material in the left atrium rules out mitral incompetence). To complete the evaluation of a patient with mitral and aortic valve prostheses, the transthoracic transapical study is followed with a conventional thoracic aortogram to rule out aortic valvular incompetence.

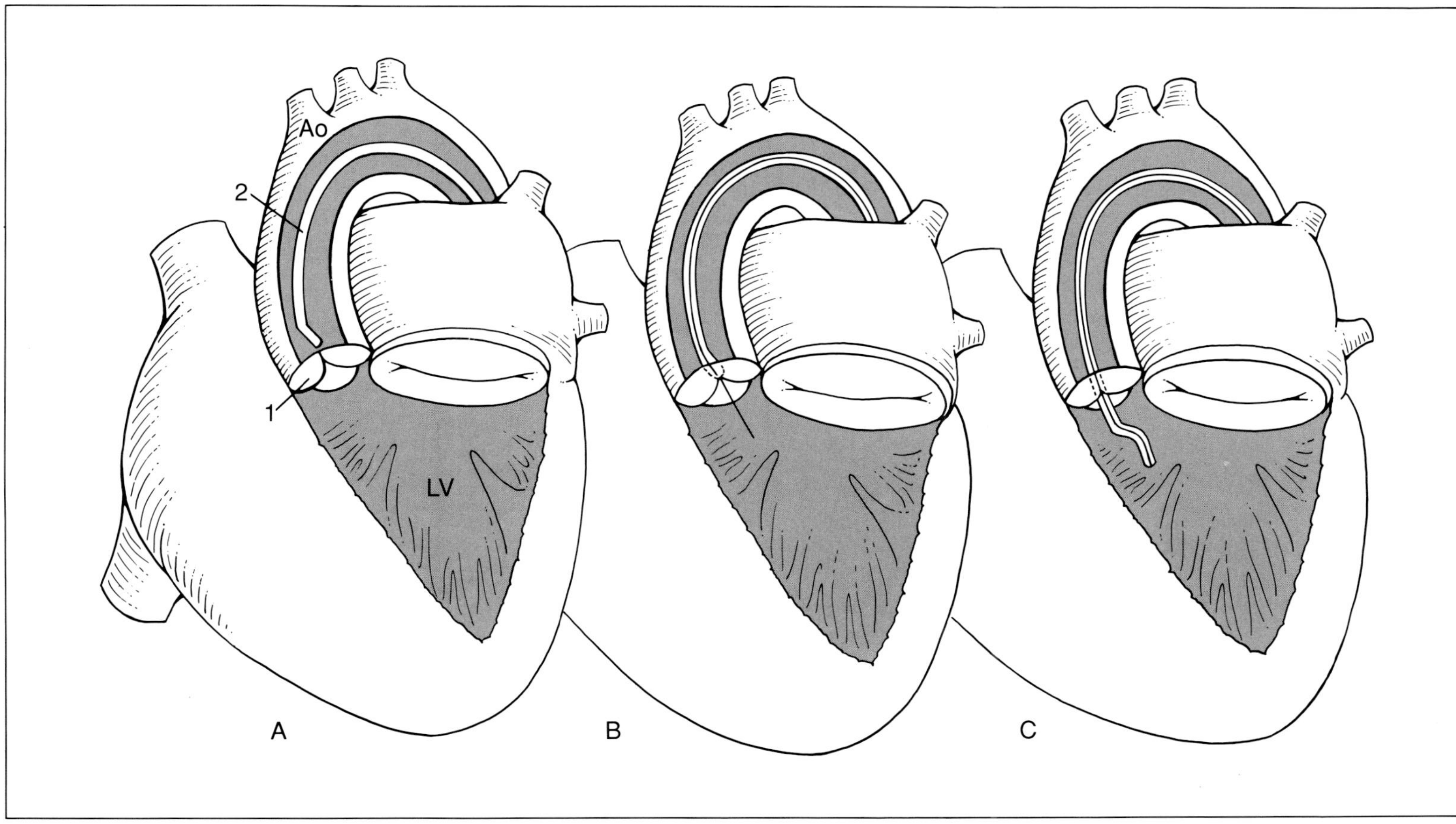

1	aortic valve	Ao	aorta
2	Amplatz catheter	LV	left ventricle

Fig. 3.18 Retrograde catheterization of left ventricle in patient with aortic stenosis using an Amplatz coronary artery catheter. (A) The Amplatz catheter, which has an angulated tip, is positioned with the end hole just above the aperture of the aortic valve. (B) The guidewire is advanced through the catheter tip, passing easily through the aortic valve into the left ventricle. (C) The catheter–guidewire assembly is then passed into the left ventricular cavity and the guidewire is withdrawn.

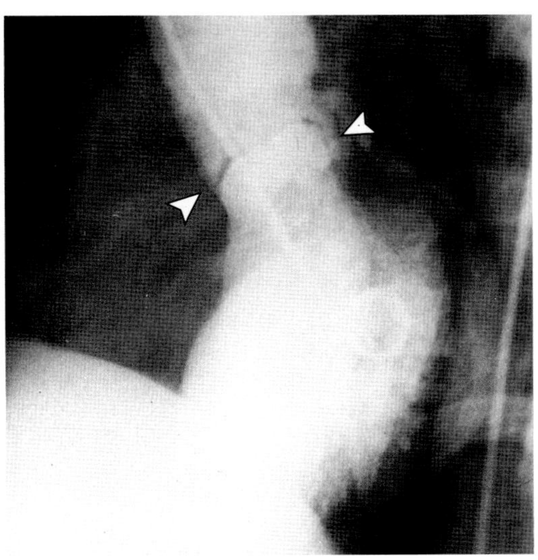

Fig. 3.19 Left ventriculogram in a patient with severe aortic stenosis (retrograde technique). The angiographic catheter has been passed from the aortic root across the stenotic aortic valve into the left ventricle. Note the domed appearance (*arrows*) of the aortic valve, indicating severe aortic stenosis.

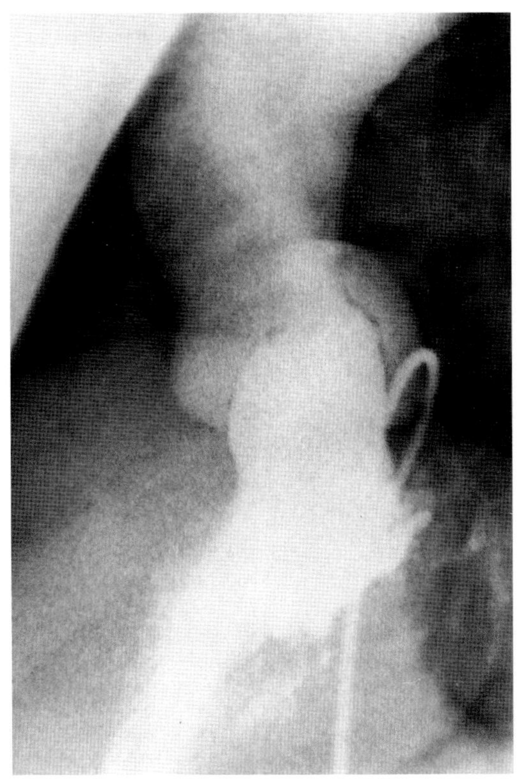

Fig. 3.20 Left ventriculogram in patient with aortic stenosis (transseptal technique). Left anterior oblique projection of left ventriculogram. The catheter has been passed from the inferior vena cava into the right atrum, through the atrial septum, and into the left atrium. It has then been advanced across the mitral valve into the inflow tract or trabecular portion of the left ventricle. Contrast material outlines the entire left ventricular cavity. Note the domed appearance of the severely stenotic aortic valve. The transseptal technique is employed in patients with severe aortic stenosis in whom it is not possible to pass a guidewire retrogradely through the valve orifice.

can be guided. The use of an extra-long (15 cm) sheath improves torque control in patients with very tortuous iliac arteries. Extreme care should be taken in patients with abdominal aortic aneurysms, particularly symptomatic ones, to avoid traumatizing the aorta during passage of the guidewire or catheter.

Femoral puncture is contraindicated in patients with a graft or scar from previous vascular surgery; entry into the vessel is likely to be difficult owing to the hard, noncompliant tissue, and hemostasis may be difficult or impossible to achieve when the catheter is removed. Alternatives include percutaneous puncture of the brachial or axillary artery or a brachial artery cutdown. (Heparin should be administered intra-arterially in such cases.) In patients undergoing coronary arteriography, the right arm is preferred for multipurpose and Sones catheters, whereas Judkins catheters can be used in either arm (Fig. 3.21). Percutaneously placed 6F sheaths are commonly used when Judkins catheters are employed. Excessive radiation exposure to the operator is a potential problem when the upper extremities are used for access. Technical aspects of coronary arteriography are discussed further in Chapter 21.

STUDY OF PATIENTS WITH COMPLEX CONGENITAL HEART DISEASE

These investigations, which may be technically very difficult, are best performed in larger centers. As much detailed information as possible should be available to help the invasive cardiologist plan the procedure. In planning the study of an adult patient with a complex defect, consultation with the pediatric cardiologist, radiologist, and surgeon may be helpful. Because many teenagers and adult patients are emotionally labile, general anesthesia may be necessary if the study is to progress in satisfactory fashion.

Polycythemia is a common problem in cyanotic patients. It predisposes to clotting of catheters and yet, paradoxically, impedes hemostasis after the catheter is removed. However, a preliminary phlebotomy is likely to have adverse hemodynamic effects and should be avoided. Great care should be taken to avoid air bubbles in the venous circulation in patients with right to left shunts. Arrthymias are common and usually transient. The most frequently encountered arrhythmias are transient ectopic beats of atrial or ventricular origin. Patients with Ebstein's malformation and congenital defects associated

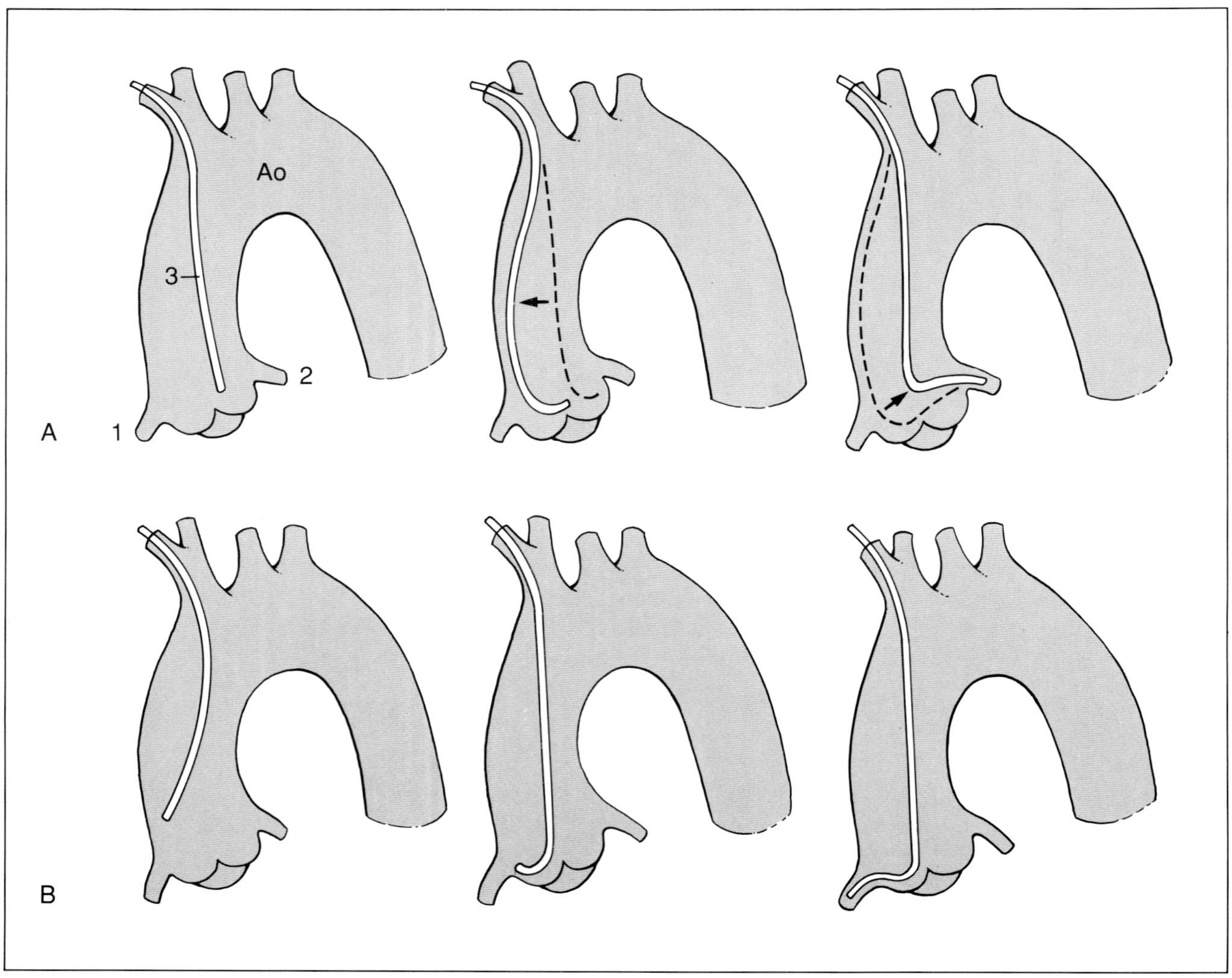

Fig. 3.21 Catheter course for coronary arteriography performed via right brachial artery. (A) Selective catheterization of left coronary artery. (B) Selective catheterization of right coronary artery.

Ao aorta
1 right coronary artery
2 left coronary artery
3 catheter

with left axis deviation or right bundle branch block (eg, atrioventricular septal defect, discordant atrioventricular connection) are prone to develop arrhythmias during catheterization. Although most arrhythmias resolve spontaneously, a DC countershock may sometimes be necessary to restore a sinus rhythm.

When dealing with a complex defect, it may be necessary to deviate from the "physiological data first, angiography last" rule, since it is sometimes desirable to perform angiography early in the procedure to guide the operator in catheterizing a markedly disordered cardiovascular system (Fig. 3.22).

POSTPROCEDURAL HEMOSTASIS

Hemostasis at the entry site is seldom a problem after routine studies performed with the Seldinger technique via a femoral arterial puncture; manual compression just proximal to the entry site, maintained for 15 minutes and followed by 6 to 18 hours of bed rest, usually results in an uneventful recovery with minimal scarring. The steady increase in the number of interventional procedures which take longer than diagnostic procedures and entail a greater number of catheter and guidewire exchanges has led to increased concern about postprocedural bleeding.

Complications associated with inadequate hemostasis, which may occasionally require surgical intervention, include perivascular hematoma, arteriovenous fistula, arterial occlusion, and false aneurysm. Complications of this type can usually be avoided by making the arterial puncture well below the groin crease, so that when the catheter is withdrawn sufficient compressive force can be applied proximal to the puncture site to transiently occlude the artery. This is especially important in formerly obese patients who have recently lost a great deal of weight, resulting in an abnormally low interstitial tissue pressure.

Patients on anticoagulant therapy present a special problem. Simple compression may be insufficient in these patients, in which case it may be necessary to use a vascular clamp or pressure girdle to stop the bleeding. Hypertensive patients also present a special problem; lowering the blood pressure to normal with nitrates or sublingual liquid nifedipine may be effective in preventing or controlling bleeding at the entry site. The risk of postprocedural bleeding is particularly great in patients with aortic incompetence, owing to the elevated systolic pressure.

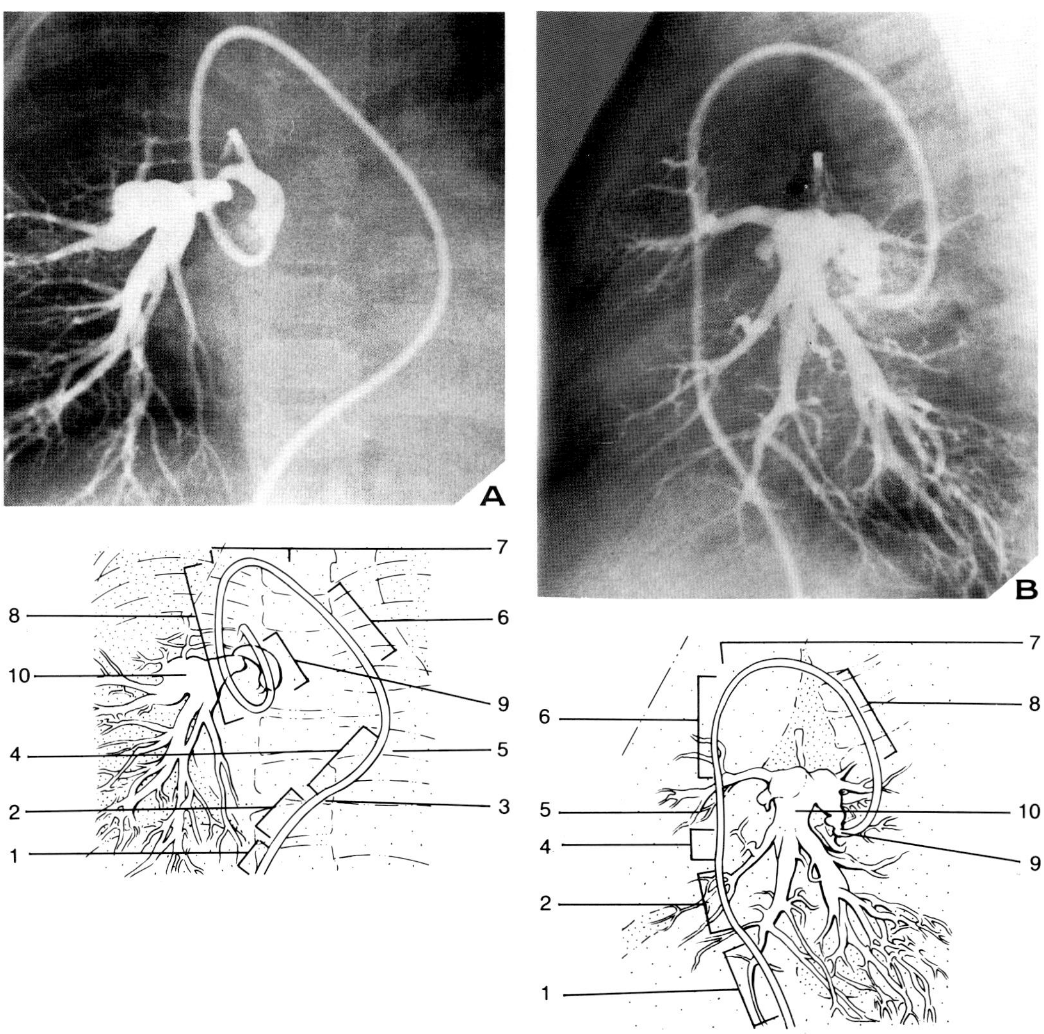

Fig. 3.22 Course of catheter in patient with complex congenital heart disease. (A) Frontal and (B) lateral projections of subselective right pulmonary arteriogram in a patient with pulmonary atresia with ventricular septal defect. The catheter was introduced into a femoral vein, advanced into the inferior vena cava, and passed into the right atrium. It then passed through the tricuspid valve to enter the right ventricle, crossed the ventriclar septal defect, and passed throgh the aortic valve into the ascending aorta. The upward course of the catheter indicates that it is in a right aortic arch. The catheter then courses downward to the right of the spine, indicating that the descending thoracic aorta is on the right. The catheter tip is in an aortopulmonary collateral that arises from the descending thoracic aorta and connects with lobar arteries supplying the right lower lobe. A preliminary arteriogram may be helpful when the course of the catheter is confusing.

1	inferior vena cava right atrium	7	right aortic arch
2	tricuspid valve	8	descending thoracic aorta
3	ventricular septal defect	9	aortopulmonary collateral (catheter tip)
4	right ventricle	10	lower lobe pulmonary artery
6	ascending aorta		

CHAPTER 4

Nuclear Magnetic Resonance Imaging

VERA A. BITTNER, M.D.
GEORGE B. CRANNEY, M.D.

Proton nuclear magnetic resonance (NMR) imaging, also known as magnetic resonance imaging (MRI), has been applied clinically to many areas of the body. It is noninvasive, yields excellent anatomic resolution, is intrinsically three dimensional, provides inherent contrast between tissues and flowing blood, and can often distinguish between normal and abnormal tissue on the basis of tissue relaxation properties. This chapter reviews basic principles of NMR physics and spectroscopy, discusses some common imaging sequences, and briefly outlines present and potential cardiovascular applications. The role of MRI in specific disease states will be addressed in later chapters.

BASIC PRINCIPLES

NMR PHYSICS

Certain atomic nuclei (usually those possessing odd numbers of nucleons) possess a net spin and an electric charge, and thus generate a small magnetic field. They can be thought of as small bar magnets. These nuclei exhibit nuclear magnetic resonance. Those with actual or potential medical relevance include ^{1}H (proton), ^{31}P (phosphorus), ^{23}Na (sodium), ^{13}C (carbon), and ^{19}F (fluorine).

In the absence of an external magnetic field, the magnetic fields associated with these nuclei are randomly oriented, and there is no net magnetic moment. When placed in a magnetic field, the nuclei become aligned parallel or antiparallel to the extrinsic field and precess around its axis. Individual magnetic fields generated by the spinning charges no longer cancel each other, and a net magnetic moment in the direction of the external magnetic field is generated. The strength of this magnetic moment depends on the external field strength and on the concentration and the intrinsic magnetic sensitivity of the nuclei.

Nuclear magnetic resonance is exhibited because sensitive nuclei can absorb radiofrequency (RF) energy at a characteristic resonance frequency (or Larmor frequency). Absorption of the RF energy causes the nuclei to be tipped away from their alignment with the external magnetic field (Fig. 4.1). The degree of displacement is proportional to the duration and the power of the RF pulse. RF pulses strong enough to rotate the vector by 90 degrees ("90-degree pulses") and 180 degrees ("180-degree pulses") are frequently used in standard MRI (see below).

After cessation of the RF pulse, the nuclei realign with the external magnetic field through a process called relaxation (Fig. 4.2). During relaxation, a characteristic RF signal is released from these nuclei and can be measured as the so-called *free in-*

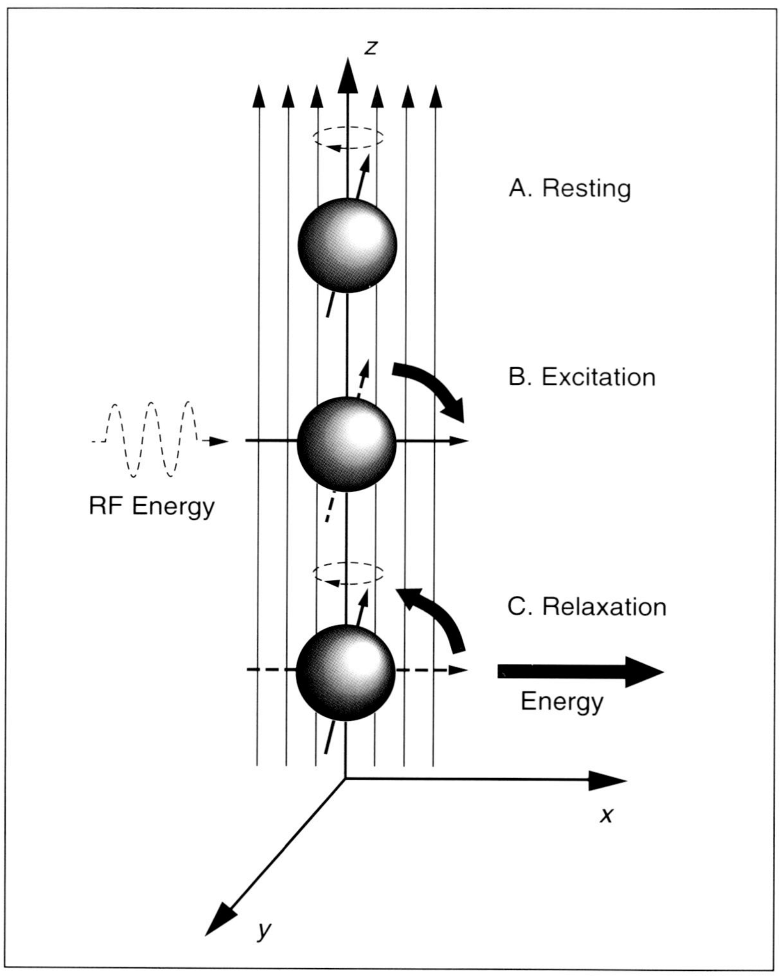

Fig. 4.1 Behavior of spins in a magnetic field. (A) Nuclei are aligned with the external magnetic field (vertical arrows) and precess around its axis (z-axis). (B) Radiofrequency (RF) energy at the Larmor frequency tips the nuclei away from the z-axis into the xy-plane, a process called excitation. (C) The nuclei gradually realign with the external magnetic field. During this process of relaxation, energy is released and a signal (the so-called FID or free induction decay) can be measured.

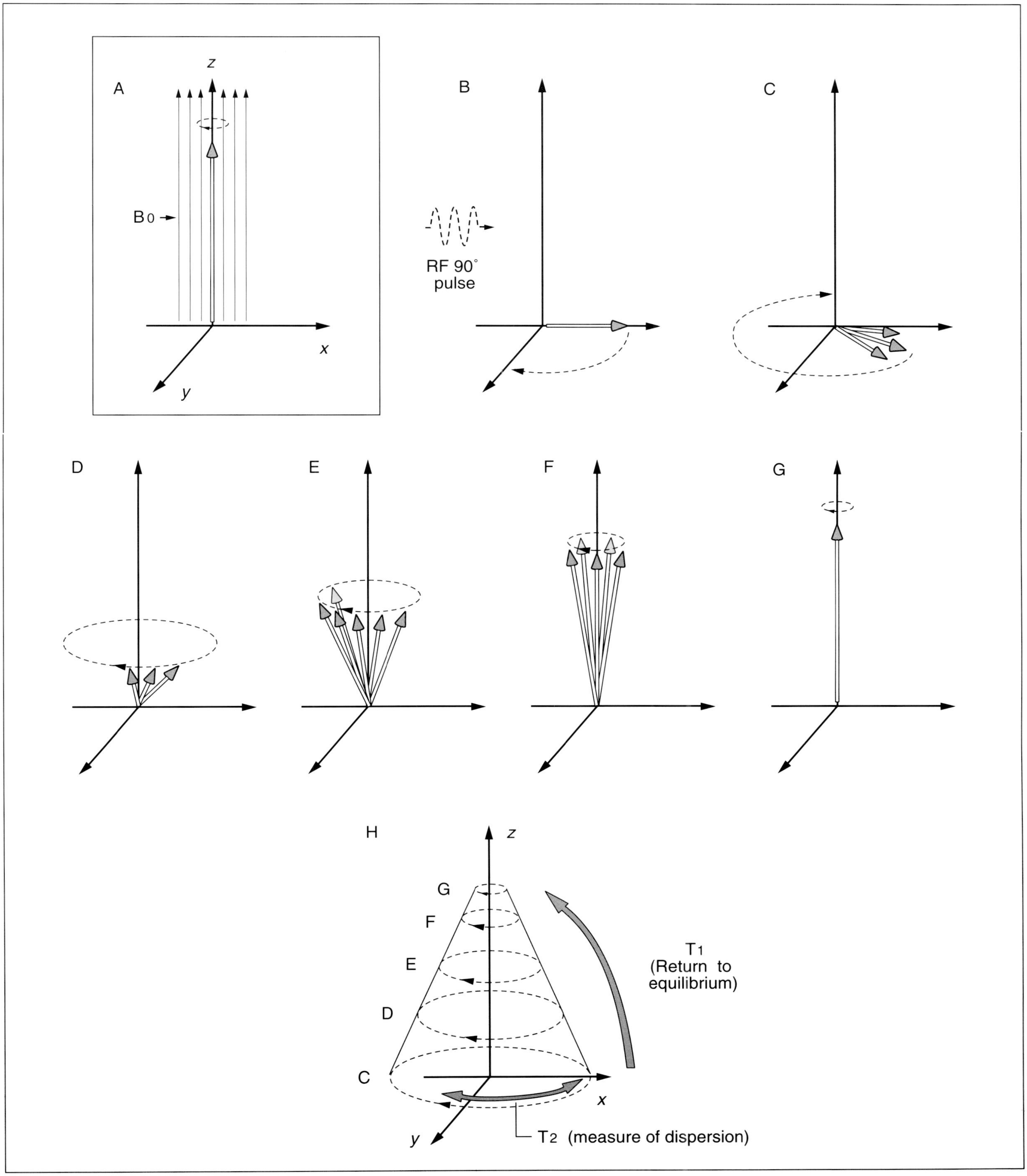

Fig. 4.2 Relaxation. (A) Spin magnetization (vertical arrow) is aligned with the external magnetic field (B_0) along the z-axis. (B) After experiencing a 90-degree RF pulse spins are now precessing around B_0 in the xy-plane. (C) Spins rotate around B_0 with slightly different speeds, resulting in dispersion of spins. The time constant of this relaxation process is called T2 (see H). (D–G) Nuclei gradually realign along the z-axis until spin magnetization is again aligned with B_0. The time constant of this portion of relaxation is called T1 (see H). (H) Summary diagram. T1 is the time constant that describes regrowth of magnetization along the z-axis. T2 describes the dispersion of spins in the xy-plane.

duction decay (FID). The relaxation process is characterized by two time constants, the *longitudinal* or spin–lattice relaxation time (T1) and the *transverse* or spin–spin relaxation time (T2). T1 relaxation is determined by the rate of growth of the magnetization vector along the direction of the extrinsic magnetic field (the "z-axis") from zero immediately after the RF pulse to a maximum value. After an RF pulse, all nuclei initially precess in phase. T2 describes the rate of dephasing of these nuclei that results in cancellation of the magnetization vector in the "xy-plane" perpendicular to the z-axis. The factors that influence proton T1 and T2 in tissue are complex; they include temperature, concentration, and compartmentalization of tissue water, intercompartmental exchange, the presence of macromolecules and paramagnetic metal ions, and the concentration and distribution of lipid. Relaxation times greatly influence NMR signal intensities during spectroscopy and imaging.

As indicated above, each nucleus has a characteristic resonance or Larmor frequency, which is dependent on magnetic field strength. Nuclei are subject to the external magnetic field modified by the magnetic microenvironment of the lattice surrounding the nucleus. Thus, nuclei of a given species at different positions within a molecule or in different molecules are exposed to a slightly different magnetic field, and therefore precess at slightly different frequencies. Corresponding differences in the resonance frequencies are referred to as "chemical shift." On the basis of this chemical shift, molecular structures can be determined in high-resolution NMR spectroscopy, and the signals from water protons and lipid protons can be distinguished in proton NMR spectroscopy as well as in chemical shift imaging. The field dependence of the Larmor frequency can also be exploited for spatial encoding in imaging. Instead of a homogeneous magnetic field, a magnetic field gradient is applied to the tissue, causing the magnetic field to differ from point to point within the sample. Accordingly, resonance frequency differs from point to point, and the particular location of a nucleus within the sample can thus be determined.

SPECTROSCOPY

NMR spectroscopy is based on the chemical shift phenomenon described above. Because chemical shift increases with increasing field strength, high field magnet systems provide better spectral resolution than systems operating at lower field strengths. Clinical spectroscopy is feasible at 1.5 Tesla and above.

In a basic spectroscopic experiment, an RF pulse tailored to the Larmor frequency of the nuclear species under investigation is delivered to the tissue sample and the FID is recorded. Multiple scans are averaged to achieve a better signal-to-noise ratio. Fourier transformation converts the averaged FIDs (signal in the time domain) to a spectrum (signal in the frequency domain). The chemical microenvironments of the nuclear species under investigation generate separate peaks at distinct locations. The area underneath the peaks is proportional to the concentration of the nuclei in the respective environment. Figure 4.3 shows a sample ^{31}P spectrum from a perfused rat heart. Distinct peaks of inorganic phosphate, phosphocreatine, and the three phosphates of ATP are visible.

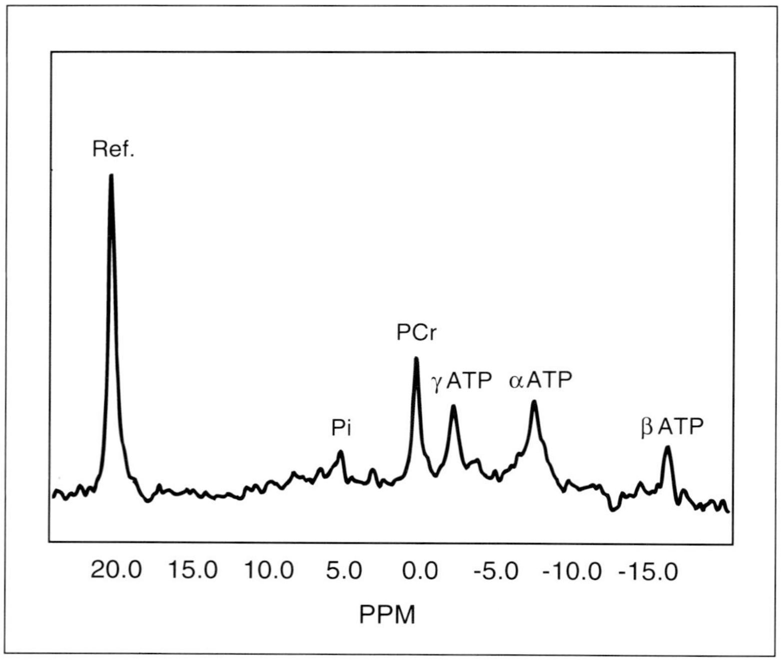

Fig. 4.3 ^{31}P spectrum of a perfused rat heart. The peaks for phosphocreatine (PCr) and ATP (gamma, alpha, and beta for the three phosphate groups) are well resolved. The inorganic phosphate peak is also visible upfield from phosphocreatine. Metabolite concentrations can be determined by normalizing peak areas to the MDP reference peak at 20 ppm (parts per million).

Proton, phosphorus, sodium, and carbon NMR spectroscopy have been widely applied to the study of myocardial metabolism in vitro, in perfused heart models, and in in vivo animal models of hypoxia, ischemia, and infarction, cardiomyopathy, and cardiac allograft rejection. In humans, ^{31}P spectroscopy has been successfully used to study skeletal muscle metabolism in normal volunteers, patients with myopathies, and those with peripheral vascular disease. Human cardiac ^{31}P spectroscopy is still in its infancy, although several recent reports describing localized spectroscopy in normal volunteers with surface coils at 1.5 T are encouraging. Further improvement in spectral quality can be expected at higher field strengths.

PRINCIPLES OF MRI IMAGING

As discussed above, the intensity of the signal generated during imaging of biological tissue depends on the species of nucleus being imaged, its concentration, the relaxation times (T1 and T2), and its motion. Protons have the highest NMR sensitivity and are the most abundant nuclei in biological tissue. Therefore, clinical applications of MRI have mainly utilized the proton. The appearance of tissue in MRI and the contrasts among various tissues in the same image can be manipulated to predominantly reflect proton concentration, T1, or T2, by varying the strength, duration, and timing of the perturbing RF pulses and the time at which the emitted RF signal is measured. Flowing blood provides natural contrast, appearing as either increased or decreased signal intensity depending on the flow velocity and the pulse sequence used. The RF signal emitted by the relaxing nuclei is detected by a receiver coil (analogous to an antenna). The coil is oriented such that only magnetization in the transverse plane (orthogonal to the axis of the external magnetic field) can be detected. To overcome motion artifact in cardiovascular imaging, imaging pulse sequences are triggered by successive R-waves of the electrocardiogram (''cardiac gating''). Respiratory gating may enhance image quality, but it markedly prolongs imaging time.

The pulse sequence most commonly used in imaging is the *spin–echo* sequence (Fig. 4.4A). An initial 90-degree pulse is followed after a short period by a 180-degree pulse. This 180-degree pulse rephases spins that had undergone transverse re-

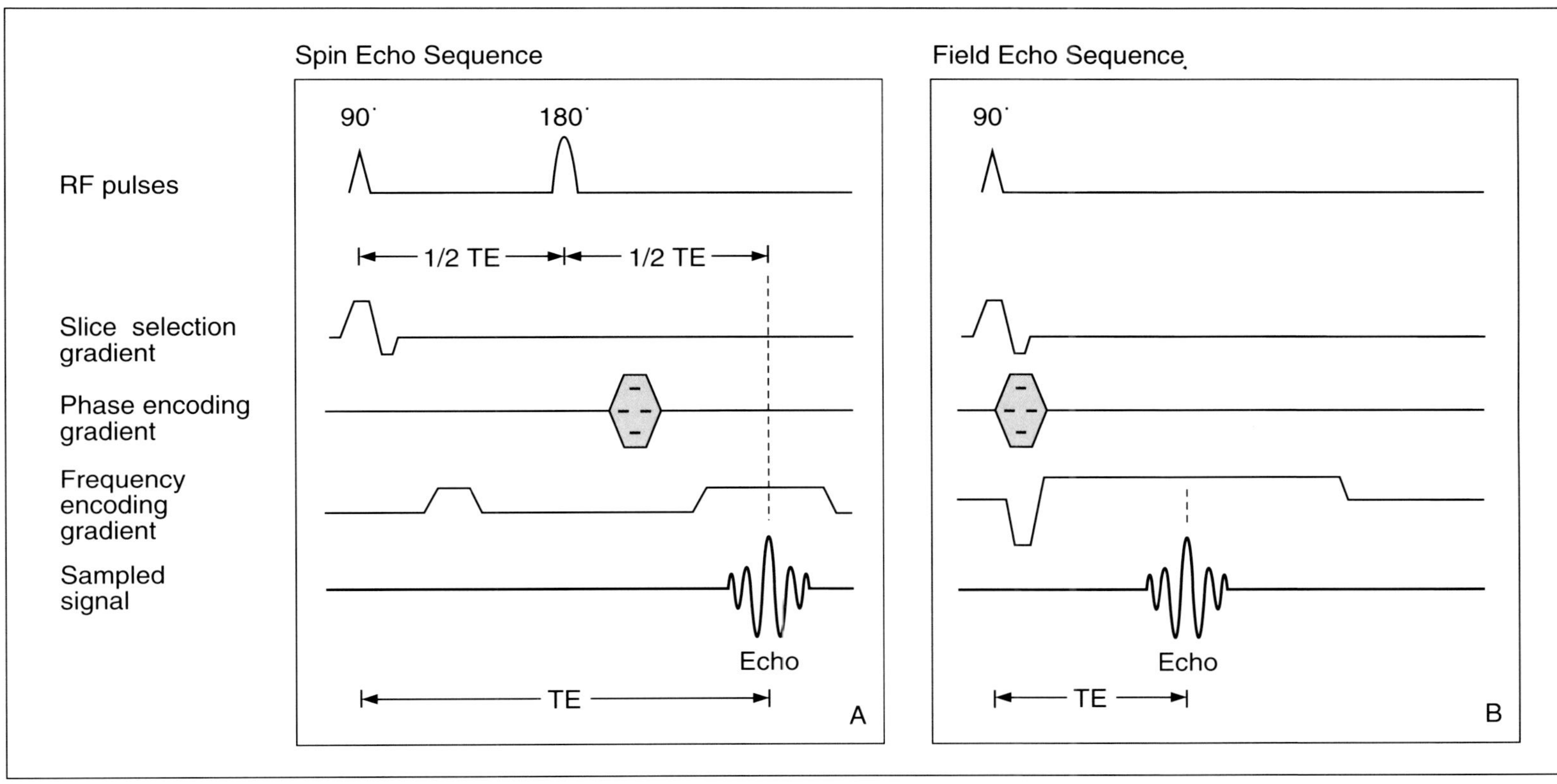

Fig. 4.4 Basic imaging sequences. (A) Spin–echo sequence. The basic spin–echo sequence consists of a 90-degree radiofrequency (RF) pulse followed after a time period of 1/2 TE (time to echo) by a 180-degree RF pulse. At time TE a free induction decay called an "echo" is generated and can be recorded. Slice selection, phase encoding, and frequency encoding gradients are applied for spin localization. During imaging this basic sequence is repeated many times to achieve an adequate signal-to-noise ratio. (B) Field echo sequence. This sequence forms the basis for gradient echo imaging sequences. Again a 90-degree pulse is applied at the beginning. In contrast to the spin– echo sequence, the echo is now generated by reversal of the frequency encoding gradient rather than by an additional RF pulse. Echo times are much shorter than with the spin–echo sequence and allow faster image acquisition.

laxation during the interpulse delay. When rephasing is complete after an echo time (TE), magnetization in the transverse plane is measured. The sequence can then be repeated. The repetition time between successive 90-degree pulses is called TR. This spin–echo sequence can be T2 weighted by using long TR and TE, or can be tailored to reflect primarily spin density (by using long TR and short TE) or to reflect T1 and spin density (by using short TR and TE). If T1 weighting is desired, a different sequence called "inversion recovery" (180-degree pulse followed by 90-degree pulse and a second 180-degree pulse) can be utilized. T1 and T2 are altered in many disease states, and MRI imaging can therefore be used to characterize tissue pathology. Paramagnetic substances, such as gadolinium, can be used to selectively alter intrinsic T1 and T2, and therefore have potential usefulness as contrast and perfusion agents.

During imaging, magnetic field gradients are superimposed on the homogeneous static magnetic field. Magnetic field strength therefore varies with position. As mentioned earlier, because the resonance frequency of a nucleus is proportional to the strength of the extrinsic magnetic field, protons at different locations in a graded magnetic field have unique resonance frequencies and can be selectively excited by tailored RF pulses. One or more parallel slices or a volume of tissue can thus be defined and imaged. Many systems not only allow imaging in the standard orthogonal planes (coronal, sagittal, transverse) but also allow definition of oblique imaging planes. Slice thickness can be varied by the operator. Images can be acquired either one slice at a time or by multi-slice imaging sequences. Slices may be contiguous, with or without a small interslice gap, or spatially remote. In traditional multi-slice imaging, each slice is imaged during a different phase of the cardiac cycle. Multi-slice, multi-phase spin–echo imaging is also feasible but very time consuming. Faster imaging techniques (see below) have made the latter technique more practical.

Several modifications of the spin–echo technique have been developed. A basic sequence called "field echo" is shown in Fig. 4.4B. After an initial 90-degree pulse, spins are rephased by application of a magnetic gradient. As in the spin–echo sequence, a signal can be recorded after an echo time TE. Faster imaging methods that generate echoes by application of magnetic field gradients, and which utilize excitation angles of less than 90 degrees and faster repetition times, are now widely applied in clinical imaging. These imaging methods are known as "gradient echo" MRI. Acquisition times are markedly reduced. With these methods, the flowing blood has a higher image intensity than the surrounding tissue. Up to 32 phases per slice can be obtained during a single acquisition, and the resultant images can be displayed in an endless-loop movie which resembles a conventional angiogram (thus the designation "cine MRI"). Echoplanar imaging and other rapid acquisition methods require specialized hardware and have only recently become available on whole-body imaging systems. These techniques generate single "shot" or multiple-shot images in 30 to 200 milliseconds. Image resolution is not yet equivalent to that of standard imaging methods, but is steadily improving.

ANGIOGRAPHY AND FLOW QUANTITATION

MRI has inherent flow sensitivity. In spin–echo MRI, flowing blood has lower signal intensity than stationary tissue because excited spins in flowing blood move out of the tissue slice selected for imaging before the spins can be refocused by the 180-degree pulse. In gradient–echo MRI, tissue signal intensity is lower owing to partial saturation of spins with rapid pulsing, whereas blood flowing into the slice being imaged contains fully magnetized spins and therefore appears bright. Flow not only affects signal amplitude by these wash-in/wash-out phenomena but also affects spin phase. Movement of spins along a magnetic gradient results in accumulation of a phase that is proportional to the spin velocity. Stationary spins do not acquire any phase shift. Images based on phase shift information can be reconstructed and used to differentiate flow from stationary tissue ("phase display imaging"). Quantitation of flow velocity based on phase shift information is also possible and, when combined with standard anatomic imaging to measure vessel cross-sectional area, allows determination of flow volume.

INSTRUMENTATION AND SAFETY

The external magnetic field of an MRI unit can be supplied by a permanent, a resistive, or a superconductive magnet. Only the latter is suitable for operation at the higher field strengths necessary to optimize in vivo NMR spectroscopy and imaging of nuclei other than protons. Most imaging units operate at a magnetic field strength of 0.15 to 2 Tesla; newer systems utilize 4 Tesla magnets. In comparison, the earth's magnetic field ranges from 0.0003 Tesla (3 gauss) at the equator to 0.0007 Tesla (7 gauss) at the north pole. Software for data acquisition and processing is continuously evolving. Even though MRI at current field strengths is believed to be safe, certain precautions must be taken (Fig. 4.5). A patient's predisposition to claustro-

FIGURE 5. CONTRAINDICATIONS TO MRI

- Unstable, acutely ill patient
- Claustrophobia
- Ferromagnetic intracerebral surgical clips
- Temporary or permanent pacemaker
- Automatic internal defibrillator
- Other implanted electronic devices
- Ocular foreign bodies

Fig. 4.5 Contraindications to MRI.

phobia is at least a relative contraindication to MRI, because the internal diameter of current imaging systems is frequently reduced to approximately 60 cm when gradient and receiver coils are in place and the limited space may trigger a panic response. Imaging is contraindicated in patients with pacemakers or other implanted electronic devices because the magnetic field can interfere with the operation of these devices. Change to asynchronous mode, reed switch inhibition, and rapid pacing during RF pulsing have all been reported. MRI is similarly contraindicated in patients with ferromagnetic intracerebral surgical clips, although selected nonferromagnetic clips may be safe for imaging. Imaging of patients with weight-bearing prostheses or with prosthetic valves is safe, but image quality in the vicinity of the prosthetic material may be significantly degraded.

Loose ferromagnetic objects in the imaging room are attracted to the magnet and can become high-speed flying projectiles. Patients and employees must be carefully screened before entering the imaging room. Patient monitoring ability is limited during MRI, and access to the patient is cumbersome. MRI should therefore not be performed in clinically unstable patients. Even in patients considered to be stable, medical emergencies can arise. Procedures for patient evacuation from the immediate vicinity of the magnet and transport to an adjacent area where resuscitation can proceed without endangering the patient or members of the resuscitation team must be clearly defined and rehearsed at regular intervals.

CLINICAL APPLICATIONS

CARDIOVASCULAR ANATOMY

Spin–echo MRI provides high-resolution images of cardiovascular anatomy (Figs. 4.6 and 4.7). Cardiac chamber sizes, orientations, and wall thicknesses are well seen. Atrioventricular and ventriculoarterial connections are easily identified. Valve

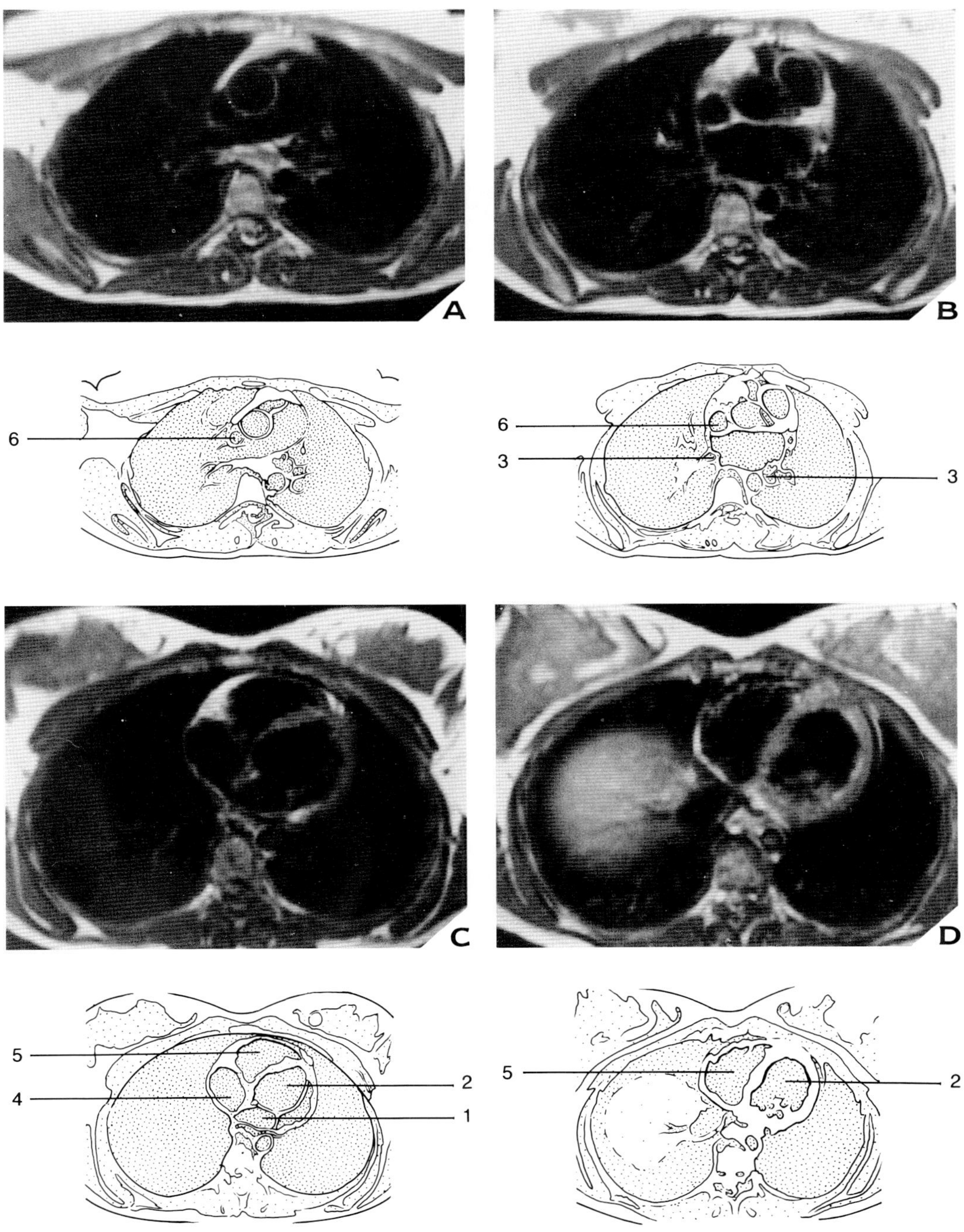

Fig. 4.6 Spin–echo imaging in the transverse plane in a normal volunteer. Four slices at different levels are shown. (A) Slice at the level of the pulmonary arteries. Ascending and descending thoracic aorta are also depicted. (B) Slice at the level of the left atrium and origin of the great vessels. Superior vena cava, ascending and descending aorta are easily distinguished. Pulmonary veins are seen to enter the left atrium. (C) Slightly lower than slice B. Right and left ventricles and portions of the left and right atrium are seen. (D) Slice just above the diaphragm. Both ventricles are again visualized.

1	left atrium;	4	right atrium;
2	left ventricle;	5	right ventricle;
3	pulmonary veins;	6	right superior vena cava.

leaflets, however, are not reliably imaged. The ventricular septum is well seen, and frequently the thinner atrial septum is also visualized. The pericardium appears as a thin, low signal intensity line between the bright signals originating from epicardial and pericardial fat. Systemic and pulmonary venous return can usually be seen. The central pulmonary arteries and the ascending and descending thoracic aorta are clearly depicted. Although most of the anatomic information can be derived from standard axial imaging planes, right and left ventricular wall thicknesses and chamber dimensions are more appropriately depicted with oblique imaging planes corresponding to the axes of the heart.

Clinically, cardiovascular spin–echo MRI has been applied in a variety of settings, including depiction of intra- and paracardiac masses, assessment of patients with congenital cardiac anomalies, demonstration of congenital and acquired anomalies of the great vessels (such as hypoplasia or dilatation of the central pulmonary arteries, aortic coarctation, aortic dissection, and aneurysmal dilatation of the thoracic and abdominal aorta), depiction of sequelae of myocardial infarction (such as wall thinning, ventricular aneurysm, and mural thrombus), and demonstration of the extent and distribution of hypertrophy in hypertensive heart disease and hypertrophic cardiomyopathy. Qualitative and quantitative diagnostic information derived from these MR images appears to correlate well with similar data obtained by traditional invasive and noninvasive imaging modalities.

GLOBAL AND REGIONAL VENTRICULAR FUNCTION

As discussed above, angulated spin–echo MRI can accurately assess ventricular wall thickness and chamber sizes. However, imaging times for multi-slice, multi-phase acquisitions with

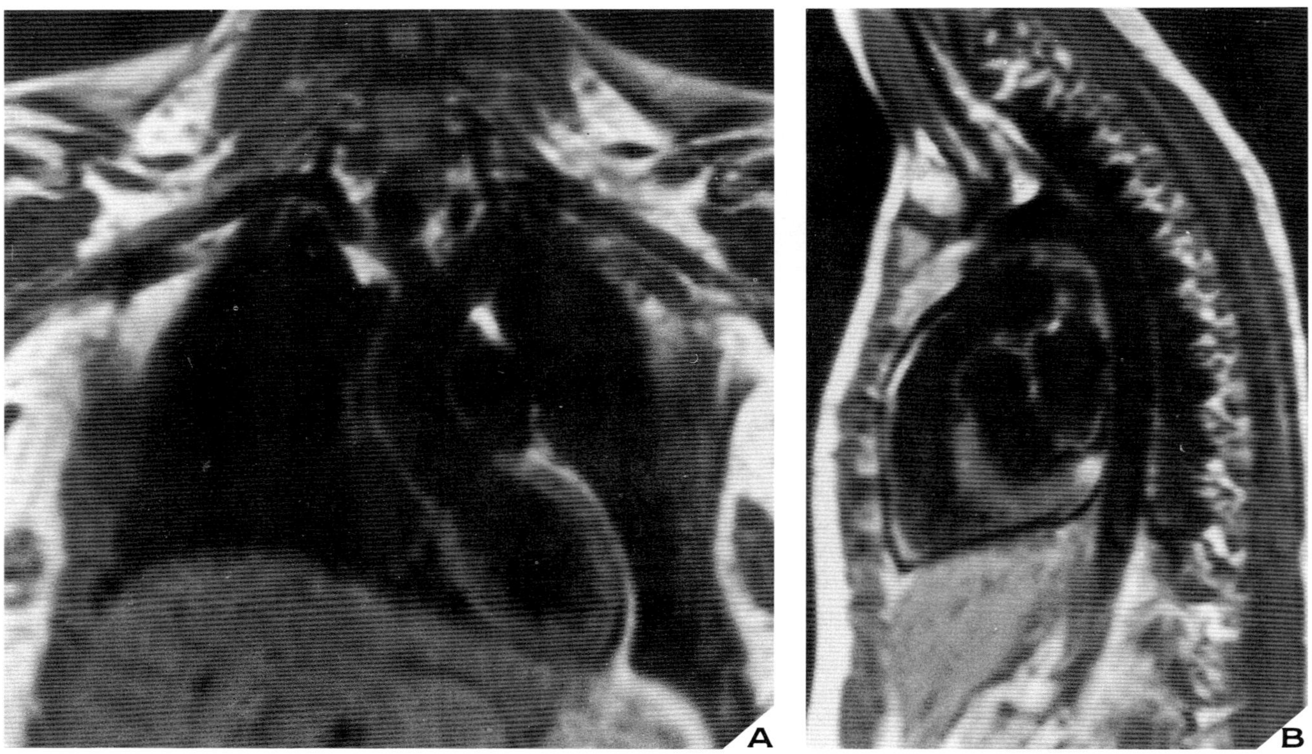

Fig. 4.7 Spin-echo imaging in the coronal and sagittal planes. (A) Coronal image at the level of the left ventricular outflow tract. The right atrium, the left ventricle, the ascending aorta, and the pulmonary trunk are clearly shown. (B) Sagittal image showing the right ventricular outflow tract. The aortic arch and descending aorta are well seen. A portion of the left ventricle and the left atrium are also depicted.

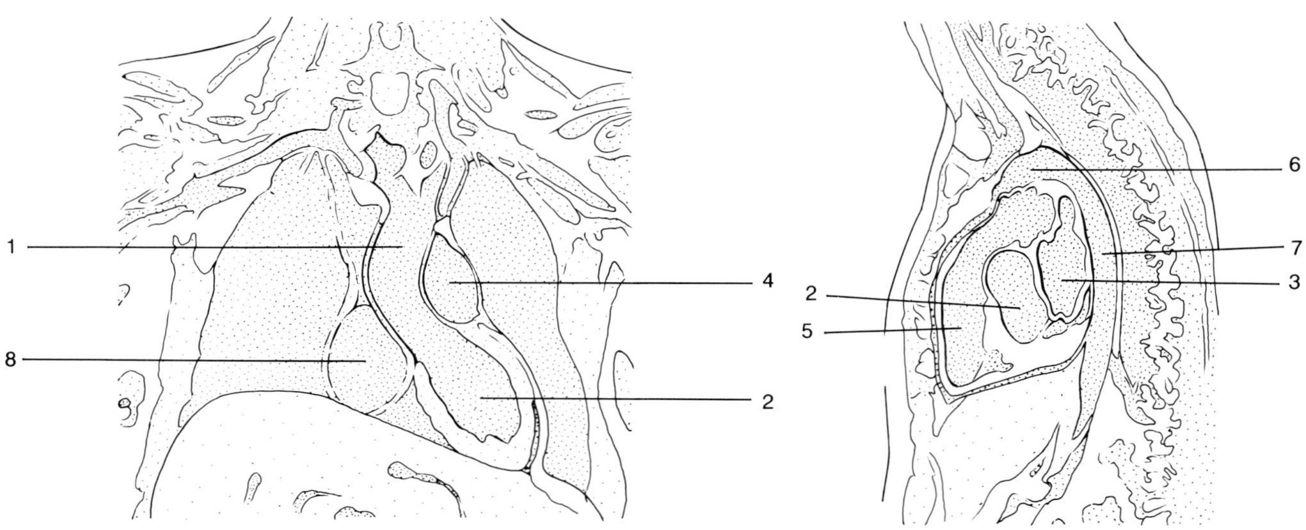

1 aorta
2 left ventricle
3 left atrium
4 pulmonary trunk
5 right ventricle
6 aortic arch
7 descending aorta
8 right atrium

standard spin–echo sequences are prohibitively long. Gradient–echo imaging allows clear depiction of anatomic detail and is considerably faster than spin–echo imaging. By applying standard formulas validated in the cardiac catheterization laboratory (Simpson's rule, Dodge–Sandler area length method, and others), parameters such as right and left ventricular end diastolic and end systolic volumes, ejection fraction, stroke volumes, cardiac output, and ventricular mass can be quantitated. Comparison of right and left ventricular stroke volumes allows calculation of shunts or regurgitant volumes in selected patients with congenital or acquired septal defects or univalvular regurgitation, respectively. Regional wall motion can be qualitatively assessed by cine loop display of multi-phase gradient echo images or quantitated by measuring regional shortening and wall thickening. Gradient–echo imaging is therefore the imaging sequence of choice at present for the evaluation of ventricular function by MRI (Figure 4.8). Even more precise analysis of regional wall motion may be possible in the future by radiofrequency tagging of selected myocardial segments. Off-line analysis of images with most current MRI processing software requires manual tracing of chamber outlines and is therefore cumbersome and time consuming. More sophisticated software for semiautomatic or automatic edge detection is under development and should markedly facilitate data analysis. The value of MRI for evaluation of ventricular function should improve even further when three-dimensional acquisition and processing strategies become available.

VISUALIZATION AND QUANTITATION OF FLOW

Cine MR images show laminar blood as a bright signal that contrasts well with the lower signal intensity of myocardium and vascular walls. Turbulent blood flow is seen as intraluminal loss of signal and has been observed distal to stenotic valves or vessels, at sites of intracardiac shunting, and proximal to regurgitant valves. Aortic regurgitation, for example, is seen as a low signal area in the left ventricle during diastole, and mitral regurgitation as a low signal area in the left atrium during systole. Sensitivity for the detection of regurgitation appears to be excellent, and qualitative estimates of its severity can be obtained by measuring the area of signal loss. Visualization of flow by cine MRI has also been used to identify coronary artery bypass graft patency. Because stenoses of grafts can not be assessed with this method, MRI is at best a screening device for graft patency and does not replace angiography at this time.

Imaging methods specifically geared towards detection of flow and depiction of vessel anatomy are based either on wash-

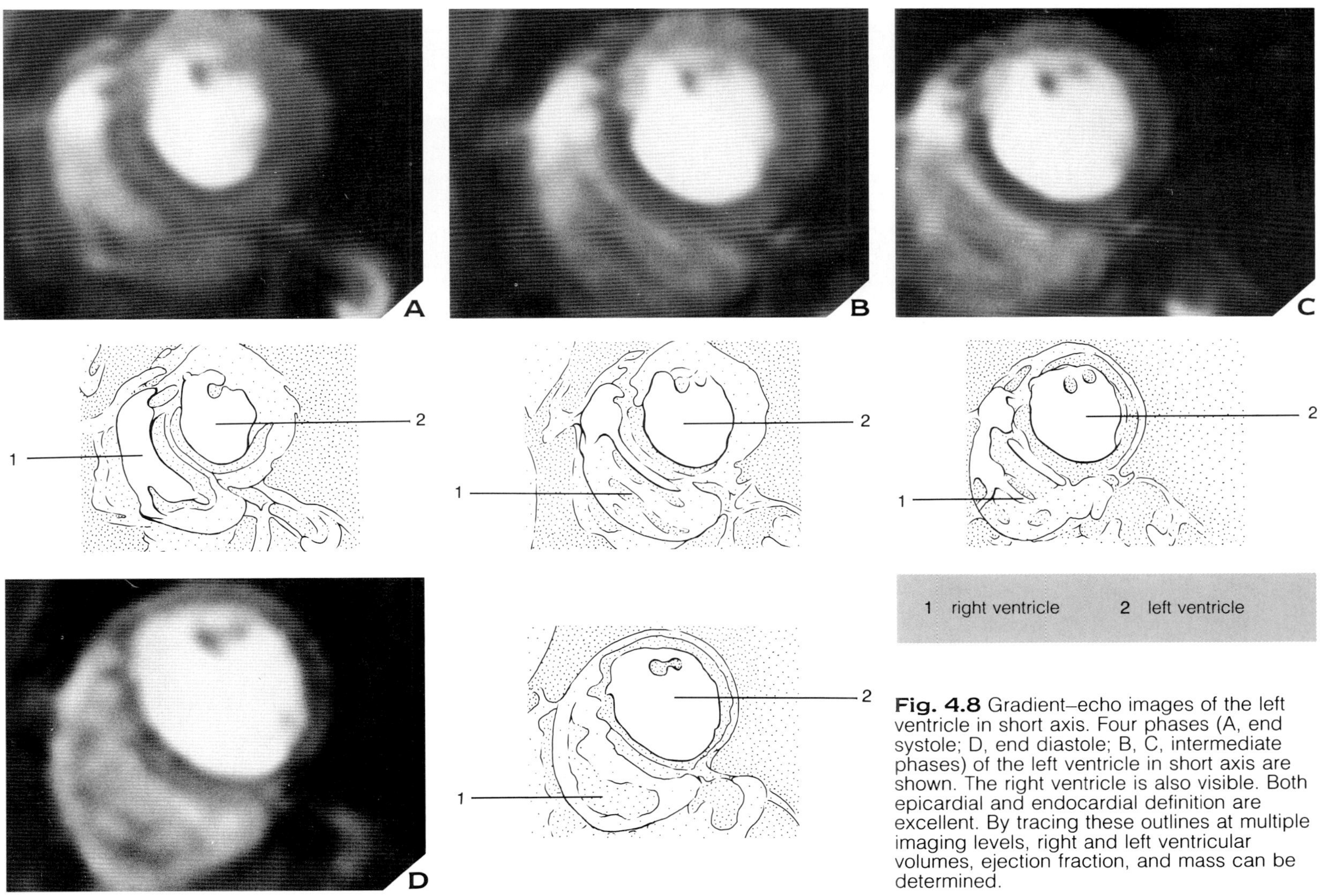

Fig. 4.8 Gradient–echo images of the left ventricle in short axis. Four phases (A, end systole; D, end diastole; B, C, intermediate phases) of the left ventricle in short axis are shown. The right ventricle is also visible. Both epicardial and endocardial definition are excellent. By tracing these outlines at multiple imaging levels, right and left ventricular volumes, ejection fraction, and mass can be determined.

in/wash-out phenomena or on velocity induced phase shifts. Excellent quality images of peripheral vessels have been obtained in healthy volunteers by either approach (Figure 4.9), and preliminary data in patients are encouraging. Coronary vessels cannot be reliably imaged with current technology. Bulk flows in the main pulmonary artery and in the ascending aorta have been quantitated and used to estimate shunt volume in patients with congenital heart disease. Pixel-by-pixel flow velocities can be determined in cross-sections of large vessels and have, for example, been used to construct detailed three-dimensional velocity profiles across the aorta throughout the cardiac cycle. Angiography and flow quantitation remain research tools at present but show great promise for future clinical application.

MYOCARDIAL TISSUE CHARACTERIZATION

Myocardial tissue characterization based on the relaxation parameters T1 and T2 has been applied to the evaluation of myocardial ischemia and infarction. Some investigators have seen increased signal intensity on T2 weighted images in areas of myocardial infarction (Figure 4.10), but the sensitivity and specificity of this signal enhancement appear to be limited. Paramagnetic contrast agents are compounds that possess unpaired electrons and can therefore alter T1 and T2 of surrounding protons by changing the local magnetic field. After intravenous infusion, these contrast agents are distributed in the myocardium according to regional blood flow, regional differences in cellular uptake by the myocardium, and diffusion of the contrast agent into and out of the interstitium. Differences in regional concentration of the contrast agent have been shown to induce differences in relaxation parameters between normal myocardium and infarcted tissue, and may thus allow detection of infarcts and quantitation of infarct size. Although these preliminary studies are encouraging, a clinical role for MRI contrast agents has not yet been defined.

Tissue characterization has also been suggested as a method to detect cardiac allograft rejection by MRI, but the results obtained by different investigators have been highly variable. Detection of abnormal metabolism by in vivo ^{31}P spectroscopy has greater potential as an eventual replacement for the more hazardous technique of serial endomyocardial biopsy as a means for diagnosing rejection.

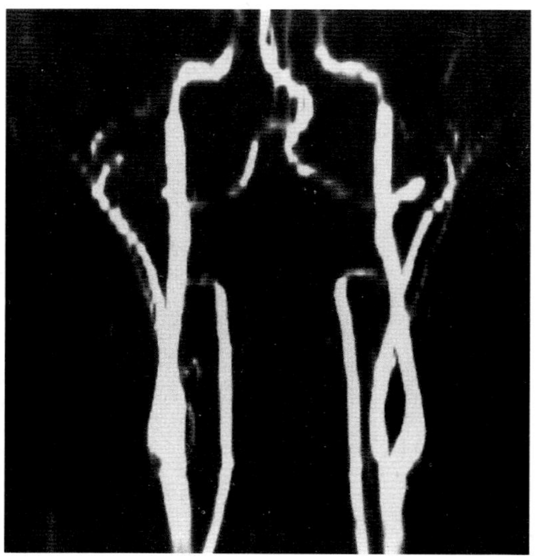

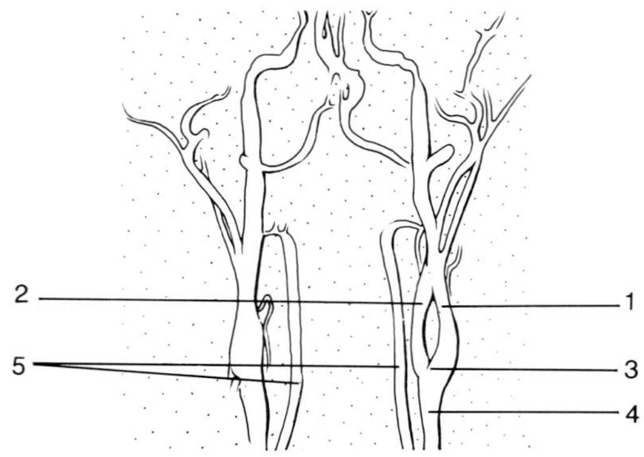

1	internal carotid artery	3	carotid bifurcation
2	external carotid artery	4	common carotid artery
		5	vertebral arteries

Fig. 4.9 MRI angiogram of the carotid circulation in a normal volunteer. Both common carotids and both internal and external carotids are well outlined. The carotid bifurcation, a frequent site of stenosis, is well visualized. The vertebral arteries are seen medial to the carotid vessels.

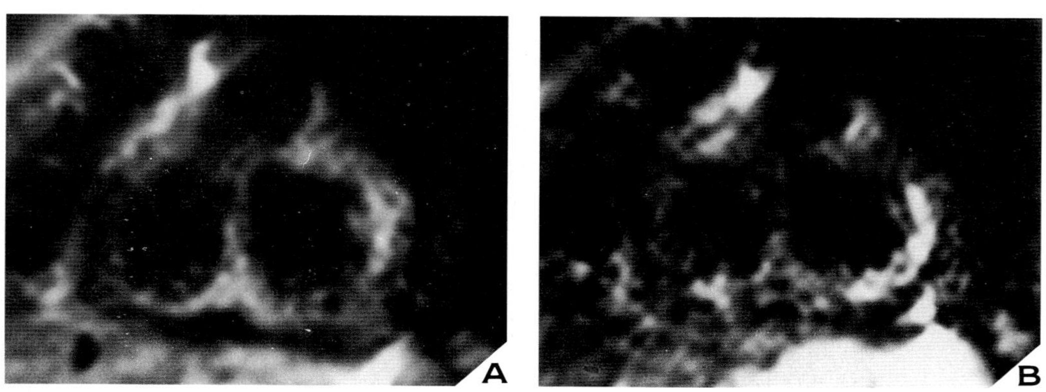

Fig. 4.10 T2 signal enhancement of myocardial infarction. (A) Spin–echo image of the left ventricle with TE of 30 msec and repetition time TR of 1 sec. There is some signal inhomogeneity but the area of myocardial infarction is not clearly visible. (B) Spin–echo image of the left ventricle in the same projection and with the same TR as in A but obtained with a longer TE of 100 msec. Increased signal is seen in the region of infarction.

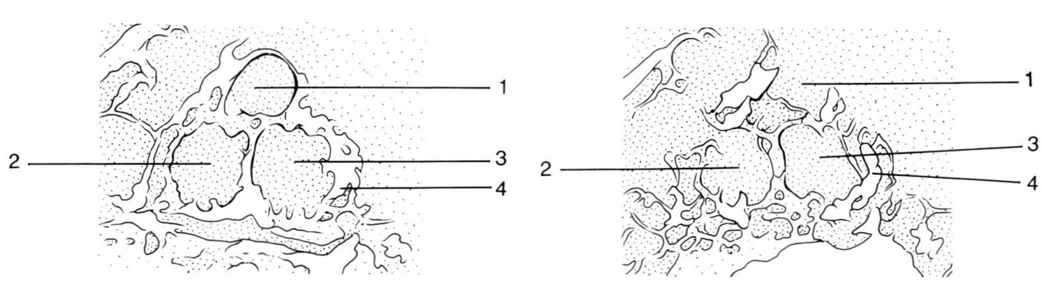

1	pulmonary trunk	4	increased signal in area of infarction
2	right ventricle		
3	left ventricle		

CHAPTER 4A

Nuclear Cardiology

MILENA HENZLOVA, M.D.
ROBERT C. BOURGE, M.D.

All radionuclide methods have in common the use of intravascularly introduced radiopharmaceuticals, which decay with the emission of gamma rays (originating from the nucleus), characteristic X-rays (originating from the orbital electrons), and/or positrons. Emitted radiation interacts with matter; the most important interactions include the Compton effect and the photoelectric effect. Before the emitted energy is detected externally, usually in a thin sodium iodine (NaI) crystal, some attenuation and scatter of the electromagnetic energy occurs owing to the interaction with the surrounding tissue. In addition, absorption of a small amount of the emitted energy represents the radiation exposure of the body, estimated to be equivalent to a standard chest X-ray for some nuclear medicine procedures.

RADIOACTIVE DECAY

The nucleus of an atom is composed of positively charged protons and neutral neutrons. Nonradioactive atoms have a stable neutron-to-proton ratio. Radioisotopes or radionuclides can achieve stability by emission of particles, which is usually accompanied by emission of electromagnetic energy. The nucleus is surrounded by negatively charged electrons arranged in orbits or shells. Electrons belonging to the same shell have the same energy. Movement of the electrons from one shell to another (caused by forces within or outside of the atom) is also accompanied by emission of electromagnetic energy.

The types of decay of the radionuclides utilized for cardiac imaging include beta (β-) decay, electron capture, internal conversion, and positron (β+) decay. *Beta (β-) decay* (examples: ^{3}H, ^{14}C, ^{32}P, ^{131}I) is characterized by the transformation of a neutron into a proton and an electron, accompanied by gamma ray emission. *Electron capture* (examples: ^{67}Ga, ^{111}In, ^{123}I, ^{125}I) is characterized by the "capture" of an orbital electron by the nucleus. The captured electron combines with a proton to form a neutron, and the process is accompanied by the emission of a characteristic X-ray. *Internal conversion* (example: ^{99m}Tc) is characterized by the transfer of the nuclear energy of an unstable radionuclide to an orbital electron; gamma rays are emitted. *Positron decay* (examples: ^{11}C, ^{13}N, ^{15}O) is characterized by the emission of a positively charged electron (e+) from the nucleus. The ejected positron ultimately comes to rest and interacts with an electron (e-). Both particles are annihilated in the process and mass is converted into energy. During the interaction, a pair of equally energetic photons (0.511 MeV) is released, traveling in opposite directions. Two opposing detectors, connected in coincidence to record simultaneous events, make positron emission tomography (PET) imaging possible.

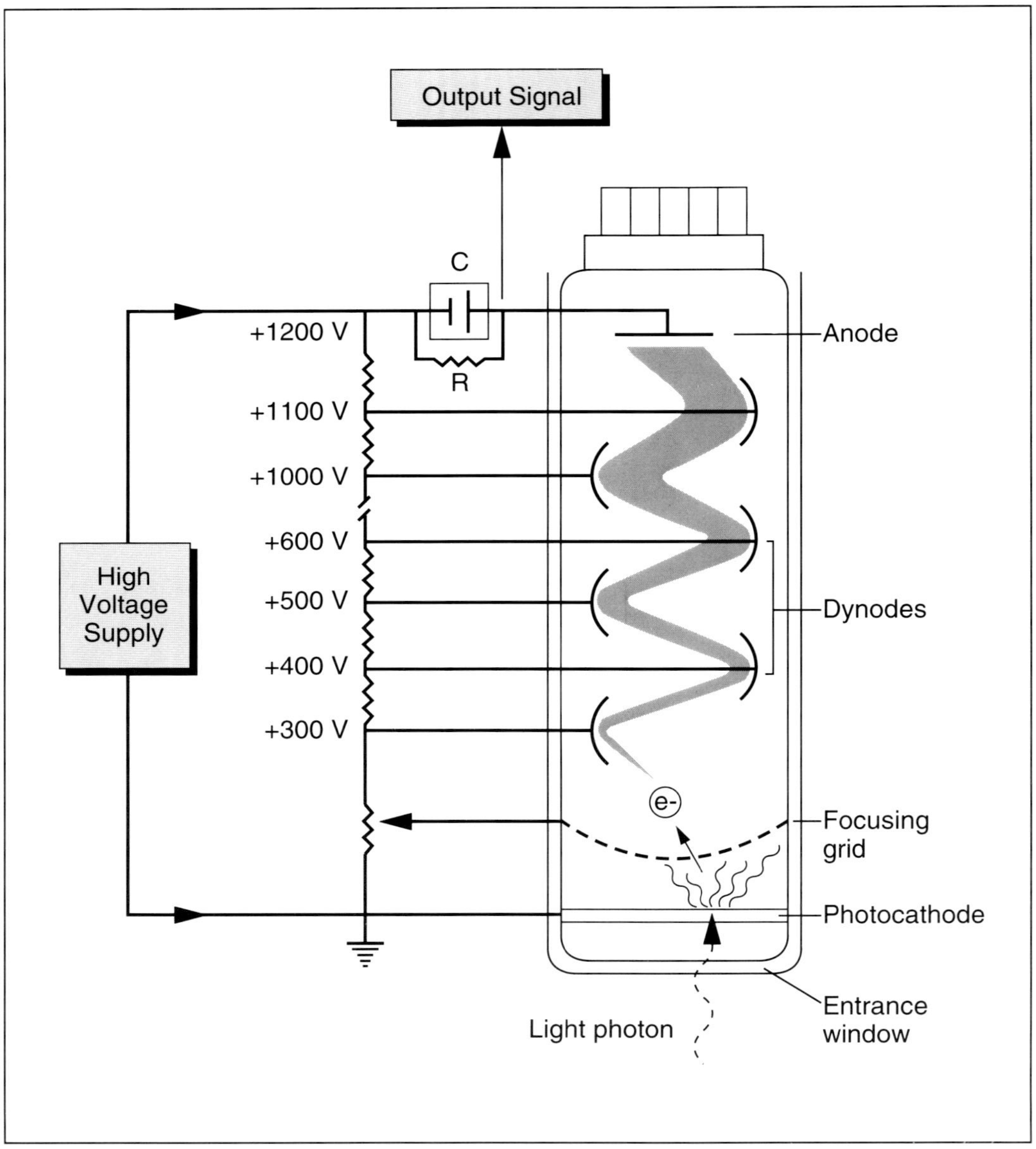

Fig. 4A.1 Components and principles of a photomultiplier tube.

Gamma and/or X-ray photons of different energies interact with the surrounding matter. A medium-energy photon can dislodge an outer (orbital) shell electron and continue to travel in a different direction and with lower energy (Compton scatter). A low-energy photon transfers all its energy to an inner shell electron and dislodges it from its orbital shell.

RADIATION DETECTION AND DETECTION DEVICES

When the described interactions occur in a sodium crystal, a flow of high-speed electrons is created. This leads to formation of ion pairs, which are subsequently trapped in the detection crystal by intentionally introduced impurities (such as thallium) and give rise to a visible light or scintillation (photoelectric effect). Visible light is converted to an electrical impulse, which is augmented in a photomultiplier tube (Fig. 4A.1). The signal is then analyzed by a pulse height analyzer to discriminate the radionuclides of different energies and to eliminate scattered gama rays, which degrade the nuclear images.

Since the late 1950s, the *Anger camera* (Fig. 4A.2) has been the instrument used most often for nuclear imaging. Components of this device include a collimator (to select desirable photons and "focus" the image information on the crystal), a sodium iodine crystal (0.25–0.5 inch thick, 300–500 mm in diameter), an array of photomultiplier tubes to detect and strengthen the energy detected in the crystal, position logic

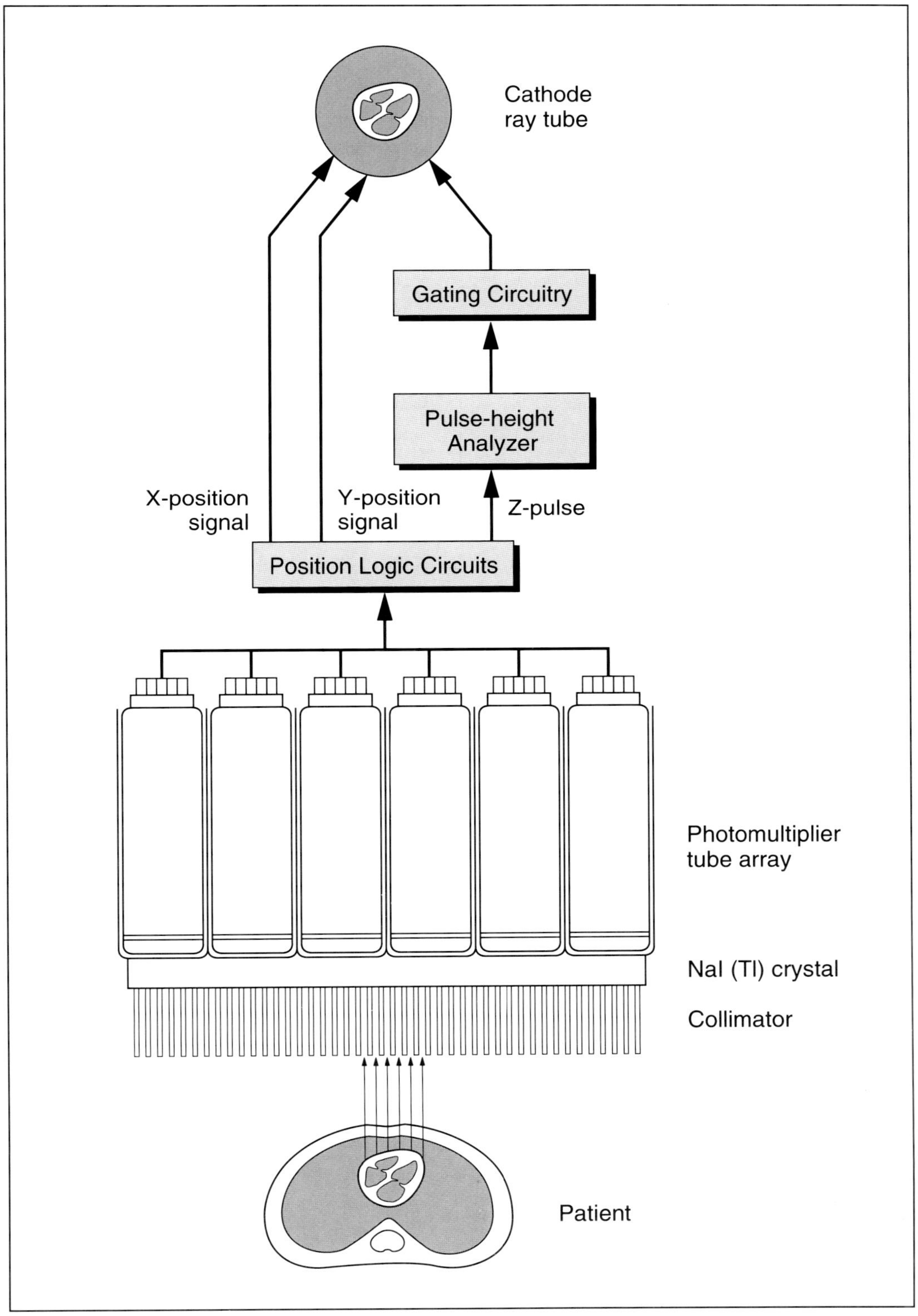

Fig. 4A.2 Components of the Anger camera.

circuits (for spatial orientation of the received signals), a pulse height analyzer (to analyze the energy of the individual detected photons), and a cathode ray tube (to display the localization and intensity of the energy detected in the crystal). Anger cameras can be stationary or mobile, and planar or rotational (Fig. 4A.3, Appendix).

The *multicrystal camera* consists of an array of up to 294 NaI crystals (1 cm × 1 cm × 1 inch), each coupled to two photomultiplier tubes. Fast counting is possible (>400,000 counts/sec), and dead time (time to process occurring events before responding to a new event) is shortened with these cameras. This device is particularly suitable for first-pass studies (see below).

The *PET camera* consists of two opposing crystals with appropriate electronics so that only simultaneously occurring events (release of a pair of equi-energetic annihilation photons traveling in opposite directions) are recorded and spatially oriented.

CARDIOPULMONARY RADIONUCLIDE IMAGING

Despite some limitations, radionuclide pulmonary arterial perfusion imaging (with or without ventilation imaging) remains the screening test of choice for most patients with suspected pulmonary thromboembolism. The radiopharmaceuticals most often used for perfusion imaging are ^{99m}Tc-labeled macroaggregated albumin or human albumin microspheres. Planar imaging is usually done with a single crystal gamma camera. Ventilation studies are optimally performed utilizing ^{133}Xe or ^{127}Xe gas techniques. Recently, ^{99m}Tc DTPA aerosol ventilation studies have become more widely used owing to the lack of need for very specialized equipment used in gas ventilation studies and lower cost. The clinical applications of pulmonary scanning techniques are outlined in Chapter 24.

CLINICAL APPLICATION OF CARDIAC RADIONUCLIDE IMAGING

Radionuclide imaging is unique in its ability to provide quantitative physiologic information. It can not compete with other invasive and noninvasive imaging methods in morphologic assessment, because radionuclide image resolution is low.

Clinically used cardiac radionuclide imaging methods include:

1. Assessment of global and regional ventricular function.
2. Imaging of myocardial perfusion.
3. Detection of myocardial viability, myocardial necrosis, and myocardial substrate utilization.

ASSESSMENT OF GLOBAL AND REGIONAL VENTRICULAR FUNCTION

Radionuclide angiography has been used for more than a decade to evaluate ventricular function. Left and right ventricular function can be assessed using the first-pass (or initial transit) technique or multigated equilibrium radionuclide angiography.

The *first-pass technique* follows the passage of the bolus of the tracer through the cardiac chambers during rapid serial imaging. A single-crystal Anger camera or, preferably, a multicrystal camera, is employed to acquire 400,000 to one million counts per second. Images are acquired at 25-millisecond intervals. Cardiac chambers are visualized in one view per injection of 25–30 mCi of ^{99m}Tc pertechnate, ^{99m}Tc sulfur colloid, or ^{99m}Tc DTPA. After the acquisition, a time–activity curve of the region of interest is generated. Three to six cycles are usually available for analysis. Good separation of the right and left ventricle in the 30° right anterior oblique (RAO) position allows evaluation of right and left ventricular function and visualization of intracardiac shunts. After injection of another bolus of the isotope, usually minutes after the previous bolus, a different projection of the heart or function during a different physiologic state (exercise, drug effect) can be imaged. However, repeated imaging is limited by increased background radiation after each injection.

Red blood cells labeled with ^{99m}Tc make *blood pool imaging* possible. Three methods are available for labeling: the in vivo method, the modified in vivo method, and the in vitro method. All three methods employ stannous pyrophosphate, a bone-scanning agent that sensitizes the red blood cell membrane and makes it permeable to ^{99m}Tc pertechnate, which binds irreversibly to the globin portion of the hemoglobin molecule.

For the *in vivo method*, the patient receives 50 mg of pyrophosphate intravenously; 20 minutes later 15–30 mCi of ^{99m}Tc pertechnate are injected intravenously. Labeling efficiency is approximately 85 percent.

The *in vitro method*, which is used least often, requires withdrawal of 20 mL of the patient's blood, which is incubated for 20 minutes with pyrophosphate, is then mixed with 30 mCi of ^{99m}Tc pertechnate, and is reinjected into the patient. Tagging efficiency approaches 95 percent. The *modified in vitro method* combines features of the other two methods. The patient is injected with pyrophosphate to sensitize the red blood cells. However, the ^{99m}Tc erythrocyte labeling is done in vitro, in a syringe of withdrawn blood, which is reinjected after 15 minutes of equilibration. Tagging efficiency is again close to 95 percent. Some pharmaceuticals, such as heparin and sulfa drugs, may interfere with erythrocyte labeling.

The labeled blood pool can be imaged a number of times over a 6-hr period. When the scintillation Anger camera is used, image acquisition requires 2 to 10 minutes. The left anterior oblique (LAO) view, which best delineates the intraventricular septum, is usually obtained first. Subsequent views are standardized in relation to the optimal LAO angulation. Data acquisition is computerized. Electronic gating permits accumulation of data from specified portions of multiple cardiac cycles. The R-R interval is usually divided into 16–24 sections, and image frames are acquired for a preselected number of cycles or a desired number of counts. Most cameras are equipped with an arrhythmia beat rejection system. Frame-mode acquisition rejects all abnormally long or abnormally short cycles. When too many cycles are rejected, a longer acquisition time is needed to compensate. List-mode acquisition, which requires more computer memory, stores all data for each cycle.

An R-R histogram is plotted after completion of the acquisition. To create the histogram, the operator selects the acceptable cycle length for image reconstruction. For each part of the cardiac cycle, a sufficient number of frames are summated to create a cycle of sufficient length to permit computerized calculation of the ejection fraction and an image adequate for visual analysis (Fig. 4A.4). Processed data are displayed in a cine loop mode for qualitative analysis. Ventricular size, motion, and shape can be assessed by observing the endless loop movie on a computer console or on a videotape. Global ventricular function, expressed most often as an ejection fraction value, can be derived from end diastolic and end systolic counts, independent of ventricular geometry. Regional ventricular function can be assessed semiquantitatively by dividing each left ventricular projection into three to five segments and grading the wall motion as normal, hypokinetic, akinetic, or dyskinetic. Quantitative analysis of wall motion is also possible. Right ventricular ejection fraction can also be calculated from both the first-pass and the blood pool study. However, the accuracy and validation of right ventricular ejection fraction remain elusive owing to variability of right ventricular shape and the overlay with other cardiac structures.

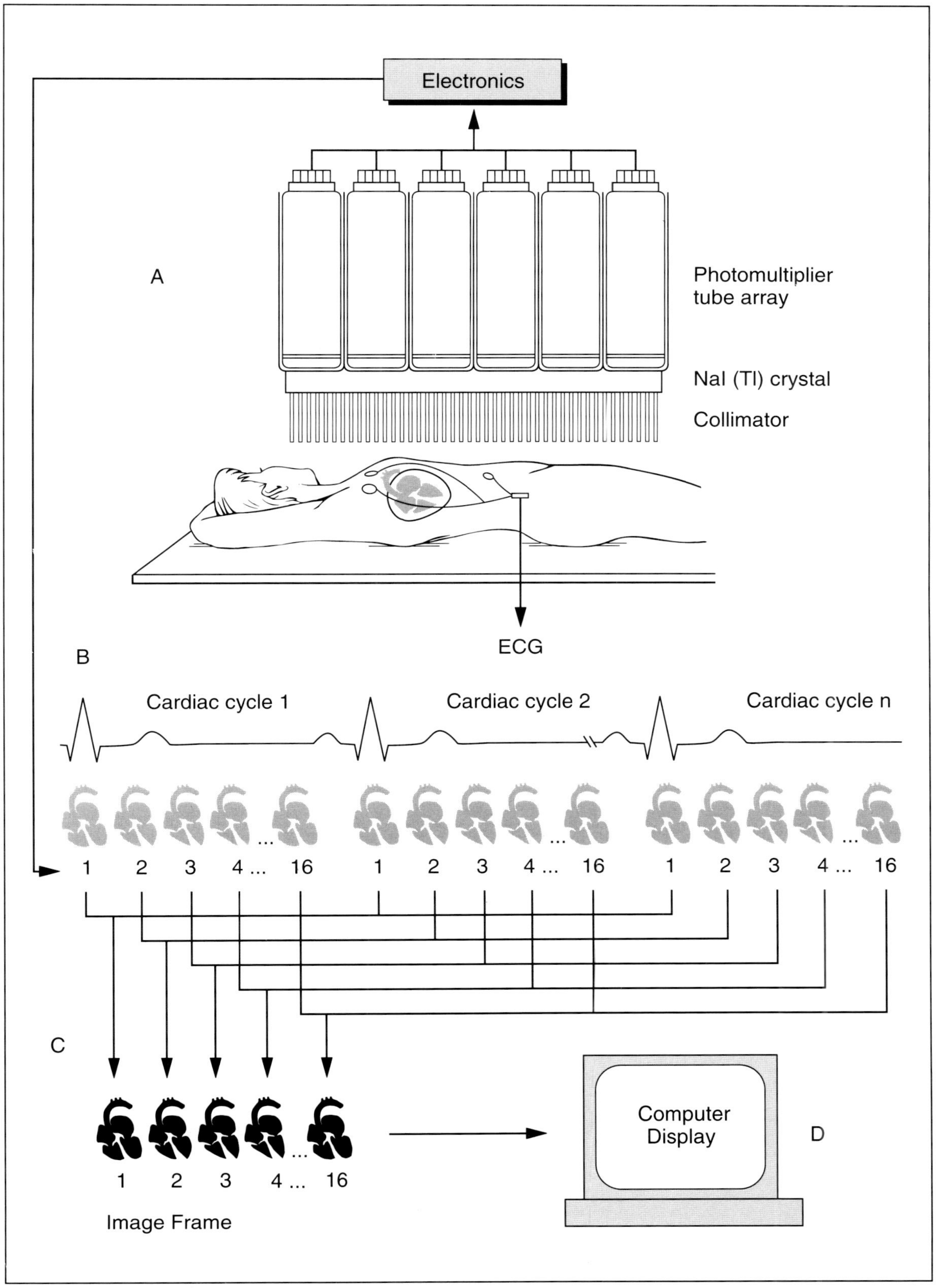

Fig. 4A.4 Principles of gated radionuclide angiography. After labeling of the blood pool (see text): (A) the patient is positioned under an Anger camera with ECG signal from the patient routed to the computer controlling acquisition of data. (B) Each cardiac cycle is divided into 16 or more frames, which represent specific portions of the cardiac cycle referenced to the R-wave of the ECG. Individual frames are stored in the computer memory. (C) The frames are then summed to allow enough image information representing each portion of the cardiac cycle to be used for ejection fraction processing and display. (D) The computer allows display of the cardiac cycle via an "endless loop" display of the summed frames for visual analysis.

MYOCARDIAL PERFUSION TECHNIQUES

THALLIUM (^{201}Tl)

^{201}Tl is a cyclotron-produced isotope with a physical half-life of 73.5 hours. The most abundant photon emission has an energy of 69–83 keV, which is somewhat less than the optimal energy for Anger camera imaging (greater than 100 keV). ^{201}Tl is a monovalent cation with biologic characteristics similar to potassium. After intravenous injection of 2–3 mCi of ^{201}Tl, distribution of the tracer in the myocardium is proportional to the regional blood flow, with a first-pass extraction of 80 percent. Myocyte uptake of ^{201}Tl is an active process, requiring energy to activate the sodium–potassium ATPase mechanism. Therefore, only viable myocytes can accumulate ^{201}Tl. After initial uptake, ^{201}Tl clears from the myocardium with a biologic half-life of 4 to 6 hours. The clearance rate is known to depend on the extent of regional ischemia (washout is slower in ischemic segments), level of exercise (washout is faster after a higher level of exercise), and plasma insulin level (washout is faster with a higher insulin level).

Initial ^{201}Tl images, usually obtained after exercise minutes after radionuclide injection, depict initial myocardial perfusion distribution. Areas with decreased flow (eg, supplied by stenosed coronary arteries) appear as defects on the initial image. Late images are obtained 3 to 4 hours after tracer injection. The phenomenon of ^{201}Tl "redistribution" enables one to distinguish between a "fixed" defect, usually representing nonviable myocardium, and a "reversible" defect, probably representing hypoperfused but viable myocardium. Two mechanisms contribute to the "redistribution" or "fill-in" of the initial defect. First, tracer clearance from the ischemic segments is slow. Therefore, the initial activity persists longer in the hypoperfused segments, decreasing the regional disparity on late images. In addition, ^{201}Tl continues to be taken up from the circulating blood, making the initial disparity less pronounced on late images. The utility of thallium imaging in patients with chronic coronary artery disease is described in Chapter 20. Imaging can be done in planar or tomographic modes (see Figs. 20.13–20.16).

Intraobserver variability is a significant factor in the interpretation of ^{201}Tl scans. For this reason, computerized programs have been devised to quantify initial and delayed abnormalities, thus decreasing the subjectivity of the interpretation. A program developed at our institution realigns early and late images, subtracts left ventricular background activity, and generates circumferential activity profiles for each view acquired. Early and delayed ventricular activity profiles are then superimposed, and the ratio between early and delayed activity is expressed as a percentage. The hottest myocardial pixel, which is considered to represent normal myocardium, is assigned a value of 100 percent. With the data displayed in this fashion it is easy to appreciate both segmental activity differences and temporal changes (Fig. 4A.5).

Additional information which can be derived from the planar images includes: assessment of left ventricular cavity size and of stress-induced changes in cavity size; demonstration of exercise-induced increase in lung ^{201}Tl activity, expressed as a "heart: lung ratio," which has been observed in patients with exercise-induced left ventricular dysfunction (seen most often in patients with diffuse three-vessel coronary artery disease) and transient pulmonary hypertension; and delayed segmental ^{201}Tl clearance, which corresponds to regional hypoperfusion and ischemia.

Like the planar images, the tomographic slices are arranged side by side to facilitate qualitative assessment. Circumferential profiles can be generated for quantitative analysis. Another type of display uses short-axis circumferential profiles to construct a myocardial map (see Chapter 20).

TECHNETIUM-99m (^{99m}Tc) IMAGING

The use of ^{99m}Tc radiopharmaceuticals for myocardial perfusion studies results in improved image resolution and decreased soft-tissue attenuation. ^{99m}Tc, which is usually produced on site from a molybdenum generator, emits photons with an energy of 140 keV—optimal for Anger camera imaging—and has a physical half-life of 6 hours. Two classes of ^{99m}Tc-labeled agents are being clinically tested for myocardial perfusion studies: ^{99m}Tc-labeled isonitriles (MIBI agents; Sestamibi or Cardiolite), and ^{99m}Tc-labeled boronic acid derivatives (BATO agents; Teboroxime or Cardiotec). Isonitriles are efficiently extracted by the myocardium by passive diffusion; because they bind to intracellular protein, they do not significantly redistribute. Therefore, stress imaging requires a separate study. However, since no significant redistribution occurs, initial imaging can be delayed by several hours.

Teboroxime is extracted by the myocardium at slightly higher rate than isonitriles; however, myocardial retention is much shorter, lasting only minutes. Initial imaging must therefore be done immediately after injection; repeat studies or stress studies can be done shortly afterward.

POSITRON EMISSION IMAGING

The positron-emitting nuclide most often used for cardiac perfusion studies is rubidium-82 (^{82}Rb), produced in a strontium-82 (^{82}Sr) generator. ^{82}Rb distributes in the myocardium in a manner similar to potassium and ^{201}Tl. Because it has a half-life of 75 seconds it must be continuously infused for imaging studies. N-13 (^{13}N) ammonia, which is cyclotron produced, is also taken up by the myocardium proportionally to the regional blood flow; it has a half-life of 10 minutes. Both ^{82}Rb and ^{13}N-ammonia are used to assess myocardial blood flow distribution at rest or with stress (dipyridamole infusion or hand-grip exercise.)

DETECTION OF VIABILITY, MYOCARDIAL NECROSIS, AND SUBSTRATE UTILIZATION

Many patients with persistent thallium defects on 3- or 4-hour scans have no history or other evidence of previous myocardial infarction. Up to 40 percent of these persistent defects do not represent "scar." Three methods are presently available to study persistent defects, which were until recently considered to represent nonviable myocardium. The first technique uses late imaging: a third set of scans is obtained 18 to 72 hours after the ^{201}Tl injection. The disadvantages of this approach are that it requires a second visit by the patient to the nuclear cardiology laboratory and that late images are of poor quality owing to a decreased concentration of the tracer in the myocardium.

Another recently described technique uses ^{201}Tl "reinjection." A second smaller dose of ^{201}Tl (1–2 mCi) is injected 2 to 4 hours after the initial scan; the scan is then repeated 15 to 20 minutes later. The third method uses dual positron-emitting isotope imaging (PET). ^{13}N-labeled ammonia is used as a perfusion agent and F-18 fluorodextrose is used as a tracer of glucose metabolism. Ischemic myocardium preferentially utilizes glucose as opposed to preferential lipid utilization in nonischemic myocardium (see also Chapter 20). PET perfusion defects that accumulate labeled glucose are considered to be underperfused but viable.

Infarct-avid tracers (eg, the bone imaging agent ^{99}Tc-labeled stannous pyrophosphate) bind to the intracellular calcium, which crystallizes within the necrotic myocyte. Delivery of the tracer depends on residual regional coronary blood flow. Planar or gated SPECT images are acquired 1 to 2 hours after administration of the tracer. Pyrophosphate uptake in necrotic myocardium begins 6 to 12 hours after the onset of injury, peaks at 24 to 72 hours, and often becomes undetectable in 10 to 14 days. Qualitative interpretation is based on a relative scale (0–4+) which relates myocardial activity to the adjacent bone activity. Pyrophosphate imaging is useful in patients with difficult to interpret ECG and enzyme changes, eg, patients who present late (>18 to 24 hours after symptom onset) or patients who have recently undergone cardiac surgery. An obvious drawback of the technique is the long interval before the scan becomes positive. In addition, the specificity of a positive scan is low. Recent chest contusion, cardioversion, myocarditis, amyloidosis, radiation therapy, chemotherapy, and remote myocardial infarction are known causes of a false-positive pyrophosphate scan.

The newest method of myocardial necrosis imaging uses labeled antimyosin antibodies. Antimyosin (Myoscint) is an F(ab) fragment of a monoclonal antibody which binds to the exposed myosin of an irreversibly damaged myocyte. The antibody, which is tagged with indium-111 (^{111}In) and injected intravenously, is taken up by the necrotic myocardium; images are obtained 24 to 48 hours later. Antimyosin imaging has also been used for detection of necrosis in patients with chest trauma or cardiomyopathy, and for detection of rejection in patients who have undergone cardiac transplantation.

PERSPECTIVES IN NUCLEAR CARDIOLOGY

The first-pass and blood pool studies provide both an accurate assessment of the global and regional ventricular function and an estimate of ventricular volumes. Particularly in patients with chronic coronary artery disease, data obtained at rest and during exercise have been proven to be of significant prognostic value and of use for patient risk stratification. The ejection fraction at peak exercise, rather than the difference between the resting and the exercise value, appears to be the most powerful predictor of future cardiac mortality and is comparable to cardiac catheterization data in its predictive power.

The newest technetium-labeled myocardial perfusion agents permit simultaneous assessment of ventricular function and of myocardial perfusion. With these agents, radionuclide ventriculography can be performed, using the first-pass technique, at the time of bolus injection of the radiopharmaceutical agent.

After almost a decade in which only a single radiopharmaceutical agent was available for myocardial perfusion studies, three agents will soon be available: ^{201}Tl, ^{99m}Tc Sestamibi, and ^{99m}Tc Teboroxime. The choice of the perfusion agent will

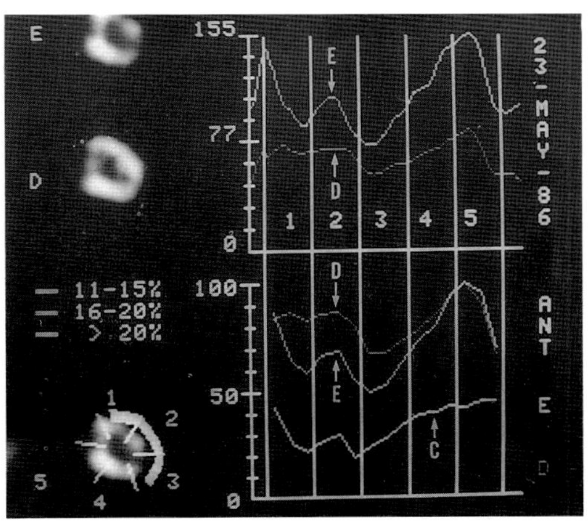

Fig. 4A.5 Quantitative computerized analysis of a ^{201}Tl myocardial perfusion image in the anterior view, depicting anterolateral wall redistribution (ischemia). The background-corrected images (early and delayed) are on the left (left upper panel). Circumferential myocardial activity in 5 myocardial segments (depicted in the left lower panel) is expressed in absolute counts (right upper panel) and in percent, normalized to the hottest pixel (right lower panel). Early images have higher absolute counts (upper line in the right upper panel) than the delayed images (lower line).

depend on the indication for the test performance and on the clinical circumstances. Some of the similarities and differences of the three agents are summarized in Fig. 4A.6.

In patients who are unable to exercise adequately (eg, because of orthopedic disability, leg claudication, pulmonary disease, or poor motivation), pharmacologic alternatives to exercise can be used for perfusion imaging. Two vasodilating agents will soon be available for intravenous infusion: dipyridamole (0.14 mg/kg/min for 4 minutes) and adenosine (140 μg/kg/min for 6 minutes). Dipyridamole induces coronary vasodilatation by inhibition of endogenous adenosine breakdown. Adenosine has a direct vasodilating effect on the precapillary arterioles. Because the hyperemic response to the increased adenosine concentration is reduced or absent in significantly stenosed coronary arteries, regional perfusion inhomogeneities are accentuated. Compared with adequate exercise, which increases resting coronary blood flow 2–2.5 times, intravenous dipyridamole or adenosine increases resting coronary blood flow four to five times. The diagnostic and prognostic agreement, as well as the safety of the pharmacological stress tests, has been confirmed in several recent comparative studies.

^{201}Tl and PET glucose imaging are used for detection of myocardial viability. Dual isotope imaging with ^{112}In-labeled antimyosin and ^{201}Tl has emerged as another method for assessing viability. Antimyosin, a "cold spot" agent, images necrotic myocardium with high sensitivity and specificity; ^{201}Tl a "hot spot" agent, is taken up only by viable myocardium. Antimyosin-thallium "match" (no overlap) indicates absence of viability in a hypoperfused myocardial segment; a "mismatch" (overlap of the territory avid for both agents) indicates the presence of viable myocardium in the hypoperfused segment.

Fig. 4A.7 depicts the spectrum of different states of the myocardium and imaging options. "Stunned" myocardium represents myocardial function altered by a recent insult. "Hibernating" myocardium represents myocardial function altered by chronic hypoperfusion.

Fig. 4A.6 Some comparisons of myocardial perfusion imaging agents

	201 Thallium	Isonitriles (MIBI)	BATO Agents (Teboroxine)
Radiopharmaceutical	201 Thallium Chloride	99m Technetium	99m Technetium
Charge	Cation	Cation	Neutral
Dose	2-3 mCi	15-30 mCi	15-30 mCi
Energy for imaging	68-83 keV	140 keV	140 keV
Myocardial extraction fraction	0.80	0.65	0.71
Myocardial T-½	3-4 hrs	6-7 hrs	10-15 minutes
Optimal time for imaging after injection	5-10 minutes	1-2 hours	1-2 minutes
First-pass imaging	No	Yes	Yes
Redistribution	Yes	No	Yes
Myocardial counts	Low	High	High
SPECT imaging	Yes	Yes	Possibly
Duration of the test	3-4 hours	3-4 hours	60-90 minutes

Fig. 4A.7 Imaging options for different states of myocardial function

Myocardium	Contractility	Viability	Tl-201 Stress	Tl-201 Delayed (up to 72 hrs)	Antimyosin Uptake	PET Viability
Normal	Normal	+	No defect	No change	No	+
"Stunned"	↓ - ↓ ↓	+	Defect	No change/Redist.	No	+
"Hibernating"	↓ - ↓ ↓	+	Defect	No change/Redist.	No	+
Acutely infarcted	↓ ↓ ↓	+/−	NA	NA	Yes	−
Chronically infarcted	↓ ↓ ↓	−	Defect +/−	No Change	No	−

NA = Nonapplicable, Redist. = Redistribution

CHAPTER 5

The Child with Congenital Heart Disease

Cardiac disease is common in infants and children. The great majority of these patients have congenital malformations, which occur at a frequency of 3 to 8 per 1000 births. Thus, cardiac malformations account for 10 percent of all major congenital defects.

ETIOLOGY AND RISK FACTORS

Although the etiology of most congenital cardiac malformations is unknown, a number of endogenous and exogenous risk factors have been identified. For example, children born to

CHAPTER LABELING KEY			
RA	right atrium	LV	left ventricle
LA	left atrium	Ao	aorta
RV	right ventricle	PT	pulmonary trunk

FIG. 5.1. CONGENITAL HEART DISEASES (CHD) IN SELECTED CHROMOSOMAL ABERRATIONS

Population Studied	Incidence of CHD	Most Common Lesions 1	2	3
General population	1%	VSD	PDA	ASD
Trisomy 21	50%	VSD or AV canal	ASD	PDA
Trisomy 18	99+%	VSD	PDA	PS
Trisomy 13	90%	VSD	PDA	Dex
Trisomy 22	67%	ASD complex	VSD	PDA
Partial trisomy 22 (cat-eye)	40%	TAPVR	VSD	ASD
4p−	≈40%	ASD	VSD	PDA
5p−(Cri-du-chat)	≈20%	VSD	PDA	ASD
Trisomy 8 (mosaic)	≈50%	VSD	ASD	PDA
Trisomy 9 (mosaic)	>50%	VSD	Coarc	DORV
13q−	≈25%	VSD		
+14q−	>50%	PDA	ASD	Tet
18q−	<50%	VSD		
XO Turner	35%	Coarc	AS	ASD
XXXXY("superfemale")	14%	PDA	ASD	ARCA

Abbreviations: ARCA, anomalous right coronary artery origination from pulmonary artery; ASD, atrial septal defect; AV canal, atrioventricular canal; Coarc, coarctation of the aorta; Dex, dextroversion (right-sided heart with situs solitus of abdominal viscera and atria); DORV, double outlet right ventricle; PDA, patent ductus arteriosus; PS, pulmonary stenosis; TAPVR, total anomalous pulmonary venous return; Tet, tetralogy of Fallot; 4p−, deletion of short arm of chromosome 4; 5p−, deletion of short arm of chromosome 5; 13q−, deletion of long arm of chromosome 13; +14q−, additional chromosome 14 with deletion of long arm; 18q−, deletion of long arm of chromosome 18. (Reproduced from Nora JJ, Nora AH: The evolution of specific genetic and environmental counseling in congenital heart diseases. Circulation *1978; 57:205. By permission of the American Heart Association, Inc.)*

Fig. 5.1 Frequency of congenital heart disease in selected chromosomal aberrations.

women over 40 years of age are at increased risk for trisomy 21 and trisomy 18, both of which are associated with a variety of cardiac malformations (see Fig. 5.1). Infants of insulin-dependent diabetic mothers are at increased risk for transposition of the great arteries, coarctation of the aorta, and ventricular septal defect (VSD). Certain environmental agents have been clearly implicated as having teratogenic effects on the developing cardiovascular system. For example, transplacental infection with the rubella virus early in gestation leads to cardiovascular malformations [peripheral pulmonary artery stenosis, VSD, patent ductus arteriosus (PDA), atrial septal defect (ASD)] in about one third of affected fetuses. Fetal exposure to ethanol has been associated with congenital cardiac defects (VSD, PDA, ASD) in about one quarter of the affected offspring. Ebstein's malformation, tricuspid atresia, and ASD occur in about 10 percent of children exposed to lithium carbonate during early gestation, and conotruncal anormalities (eg, transposition of the great arteries) occur two to four times as often as expected in infants whose mothers were treated with certain sex hormones during the first trimester. Severe cardiovascular malformations are common in the infants of mothers treated with isotretinoin (Accutane). This agent, a vitamin A congener, is used in the treatment of severe cystic acne and carries a warning against use during pregnancy.

Congenital cardiac malformations occur with relative frequency in children with chromosomal aberrations (Fig. 5.1). For example, major cardiac defects are present in about 50 percent of children with trisomy 21 (Down syndrome) and in more than 99 percent of those with trisomy 18.

The risk of cardiac malformations is significantly increased in the offspring of parents with congenital heart disease (Fig. 5.2). The malformations tend to be similar in each generation of an affected family. In general, such familial patterns are best explained by multifactorial inheritance (ie, a genetic predisposition interacting with an environmental trigger to produce cardiovascular maldevelopment). In such cases the genetic predisposition is usually presumed to be polygenic, based on the small additive effects of many genes (in some instances a single locus or a small number of loci may interact with environmental influences).

FIG. 5.2. AFFECTED OFFSPRING (ONE PARENT WITH CONGENITAL HEART DISEASE)

	Affected Offspring	
Anomaly	Number	Percent
VSD	7/174	4
PDA	6/139	4.3
ASD	5/199	2.5
Tetralogy	6/141	4.2
PS	4/111	3.6
Coarctation	7/253	2.7
AS	4/103	3.9

*Abbreviations: VSD, ventricular septal defect; PDA, patent ductus arteriosus; ASD, atrial septal defect; PS, pulmonic stenosis; AS, aortic stenosis. (Adapted from Nora JJ, Nora AH: The evolution of specific genetic and environmental counseling in congenital heart diseases.*Circulation *1978; 57:205. By permission of the American Heart Association, Inc.)*

Fig. 5.2 Frequency of affected offspring (given one parent with congenital heart disease).

Classical Mendelian inheritance accounts for a small but important subset of congenital cardiovascular diseases (Fig. 5.3). Congenital cardiac defects produced by a single mutant gene are usually part of a syndrome or anomalad (association) of multiple phenotypic features. Some inherited syndromes or anomalads are characterized by congenital cardiac defects (eg, Holt–Oram syndrome, Noonan syndrome), whereas others are characterized by a predilection for degenerative valvular disease (eg, Marfan syndrome, osteogenesis imperfecta, Ehlers–Danlos syndrome) or cardiac tumors (eg, tuberous sclerosis).

FIG. 5.3 RISK OF CARDIOVASCULAR ABNORMALITIES IN INHERITED SYNDROMES AND ANOMALADS (ASSOCIATIONS).*

Abnormality	Type of Cardiovascular Abnormality	Risk of Penetrance of Cardiovascular Disease
	AUTOSOMAL DOMINANT	
Apert	VSD, TOF, coarctation of the aorta	10%
Crouzon	Coarctation of the aorta, PDA	Low
Ehlers–Danlos	Atrioventricular valve regurgitation, rupture of large blood vessels, aortic dissection	50%
Forney	Mitral insufficiency	? moderate
Holt–Oram	ASD, VSD	50%
Idiopathic hypertrophic subaortic stenosis	Obstructive myocardial disease	100%
Leopard	PS, prolonged PR interval	50%
Marfan	Mitral and aortic disease	60 to 80%
Mitral click/murmur	Mitral insufficiency, dysrhythmias	100% in certain families
Myocardial disease (nonobstructive)	Cardiomegaly, CHF	High
Myotonic dystrophy (Steinert)	Conduction defects, myocardial disease	65%
Neurofibromatosis	PS, pheochromocytoma with hypertension, coarctation of the aorta, renal artery stenosis	4–10%
Noonan	PS, ASD, left ventricular disease	50%
Osteogenesis imperfecta	Aortic insufficiency	5–10%
Primary pulmonary hypertension	Primary pulmonary hypertension	Moderate
Supravalvular aortic stenosis (with and without elfin facies)	Supravalvular aortic and pulmonic stenosis, peripheral pulmonary artery stenosis	100%
Treacher–Collins	VSD, PDA, AS	10%
Tuberous sclerosis	Myocardial rhabdomyoma and angioma	Moderate
Waardenburg	VSD	Low

Fig. 5.3 Risk of cardiovascular abnormalities in inherited syndromes and anomalads.

FIG. 5.3 RISK OF CARDIOVASCULAR ABNORMALITIES IN INHERITED SYNDROMES AND ANOMALADS (ASSOCIATIONS).* CONTINUED

Abnormality	Type of Cardiovascular Abnormality	Risk or Penetrance of Cardiovascular Disease
	AUTOSOMAL RECESSIVE	
Alkaptonuria	Aortic and mitral disease, ? premature arteriosclerosis	Moderate to high
Carpenter syndrome	PDA, VSD, PS, TGA	20%
Cutix laxa	ASD (usually single atrium), peripheral pulmonary artery stenosis	Moderate
Friedreich ataxia	Myocardiopathy, conduction defects	75–90%
Glycogenosis IIa (Pompe)	Myocardiopathy	100%
Glycogenosis III (Cori) and IV (Andersen)	Myocardiopathy	Moderate
Ivemark	Asplenia with cardiovascular abnormalities	100%
Laurence–Moon–Bardet–Biedl	VSD, other structural defects	moderate
Meckel–Gruber	Simple and complex defects	>25%
Mucolipidosis II and III	Valvular disease	>50%
MPS, IH, IS, IV, VI	Coronary artery and valvular disease	50–85%
Muscular dystrophy I, II	Myocardiopathy	Low
Pseudoxanthoma elasticum	Generalized vascular disease, coronary insufficiency, mitral insufficiency, hypertension	100%
Seckel ("bird-headed dwarf")	VSD, PDA	Low
Sickle cell disease	Myocardipathy, mitral insufficiency	85%
Smith–Lemli–Opitz	VSD, PSA, other congenital defects	15%
Thrombocytopenia–absent radius (TAR)	ASD, TOF, dextrocardia	30%
Weill–Marchesani	PS, VSD, ?PDA	15%
Zellweger	PSA, VSD, ASD	Low
	X-LINKED DOMINANT	
Focal dermal hypoplasia	Various cardiovascular defects	3–10%
Incontinentia pigmenti	PDA, primary pulmonary hypertension	Low
	X-LINKED RECESSIVE	
MPS II (Hunter)	Coronary artery and valvular disease	100%
Muscular dystrophy (Duchenne, Dreifuss)	Myocardiopathy	67%

Abbreviations: MPS, mucopolysaccharidosis; PDA, patent ductus arteriosus; VSD, ventricular septal defect; PS, pulmonic stenosis; TGA, transposition of the great arteries; TOF, tetralogy of Fallot; CHF, congestive heart failure.

**Only conditions associated with structural cardiovascular disease are listed. Some cardiovascular abnormalities are not manifest during childhood. (Adapted with permission from data in Nora JJ, Norah AH: The evolution of specific genetic and environmental counseling in congenital heart diseases.* Circulation *1978; 57:205. By permission of the American Heart Association, Inc.)*

Skeletal abnormalities serve as a useful marker for several chromosomal and genetic disorders associated with cardiac malformations (Figs. 5.4 to 5.7; see also Chapter 17).

Certain chromosomal and genetic disorders associated with congenital heart defects (eg, trisomy 13, 18, 21; Turner syndrome; Holt–Oram syndrome; Meckel–Gruber syndrome) are reliably detected by prenatal ultrasound. Careful echocardiographic evaluation of the affected fetus may demonstrate a cardiac malformation that warrants prompt intervention after birth. A similar approach is warranted when the fetus has been exposed to nongenetic factors (eg, uncontrolled maternal diabetes, lithium) associated with a significant risk of congenital heart disease.

Genetic factors are becoming increasingly important in cardiovascular disease because of the growing number of children with congenital defects who survive corrective surgery and grow up to have children of their own.

PATHOGENESIS

Cardiac malformations may be caused by a variety of errors in organogenesis, including persistence of fetal structures that normally disappear, resorption of structures that normally persist, malalignment of normal cardiac components, and abnormal connection of the cardiovascular segments. Complex mal-

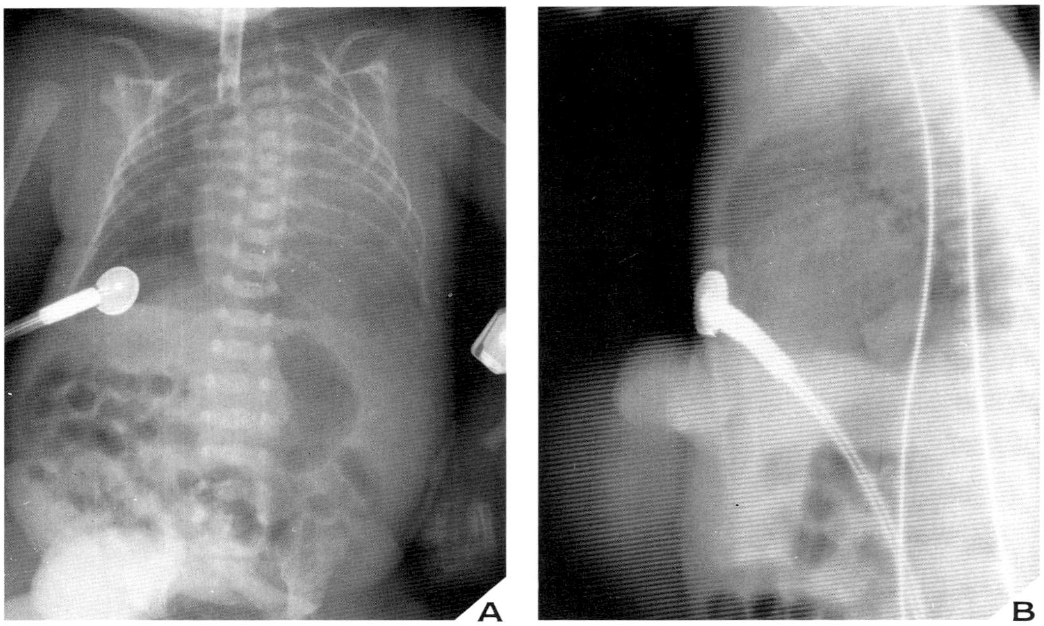

Fig. 5.4 Trisomy 18. (A) Frontal and (B) lateral radiographs of a neonate with trisomy 18 show many features characteristic of this disorder: gracile ribs, "handlebar" clavicles, absence of normal flaring of the iliac wings, and a large omphalocele. The cardiac enlargement is secondary to a ventricular septal defect, the most common cardiac defect in this chromosomal disorder. The left lung is atelectatic.

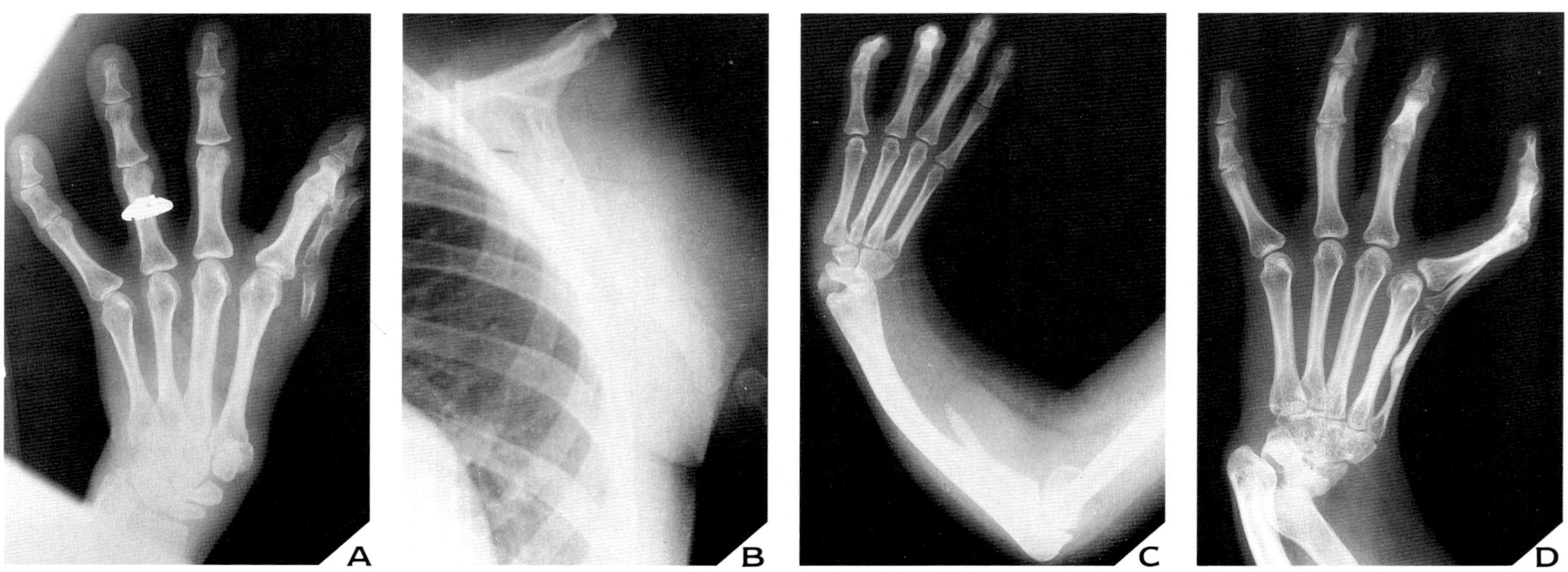

Fig. 5.5 Holt–Oram syndrome. Radiographs of three members of a family show abnormalities of the uppper extremities characteristic of this autosomal dominant disorder. The mother and both daughters have ostium secundum atrial septal defects, and both daughters have cardiac arrhythmias (heart block). (A) Mother. Radiograph of the left hand shows a hypoplastic first ray. The right thumb (not illustrated) was also hypoplastic. (B) Older daughter. Detail of the left upper extremity shows hypoplasia of the scapula, humerus, and forearm bones. A similar abnormality was present on the right. (C, D) Younger daughter. Radiograph of the right forearm and hand (C) shows absence of all but the proximal portion of the right radius and absence of the first metatarsal and thumb. Radiograph of the left hand (D) shows hypoplasia of the first ray, soft tissue syndactyly between the second and third digits, abnormal alignment of the carpal bones, and malalignment at the radiocarpal and ulnocarpal joints. (Courtesy of Jack G. Rabinowitz, MD, New York, NY, and Anthony Camera, MD, Brooklyn, NY)

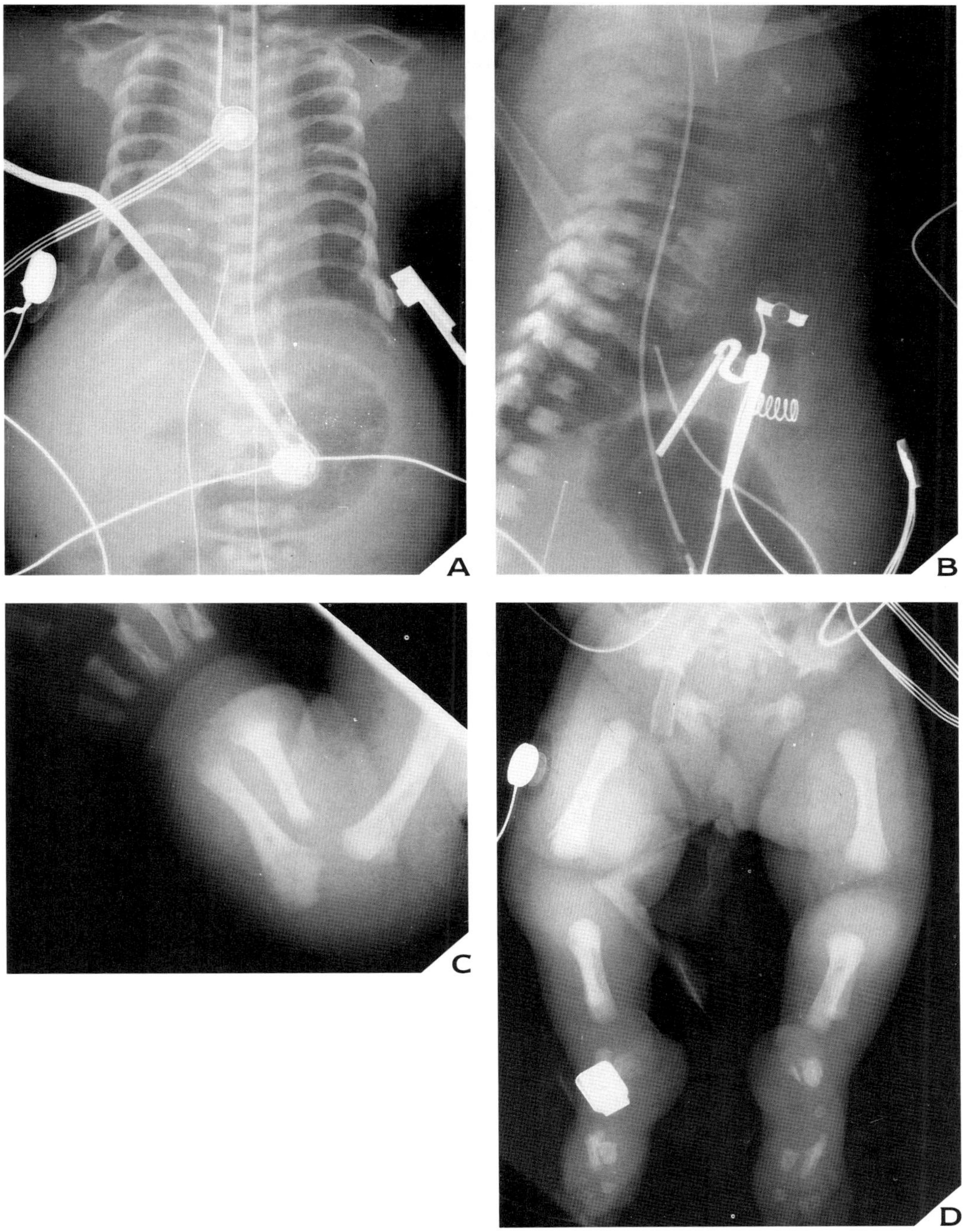

Fig. 5.6 Ellis–van Creveld syndrome. A newborn girl exhibits the characteristic skeletal features of this autosomal recessive disorder. (A) Frontal and (B) lateral chest films show a small thorax and short ribs. (The relative smallness of the thorax in this infant is exaggerated by the presence of marked hepatomegaly secondary to coexisting sepsis.) (C) Right arm. Note the short ulna, bulbous enlargement of the proximal ulna and distal radius, dislocation of the radial head, and postaxial polydactyly (extra digit on ulnar aspect of hand). (D) Pelvis and lower extremities. Note the small, squared-off iliac wings with narrowing of the sciatic notch and flattening of acetabular roof, shortening of the long bones, fibular hypoplasia, and clubfeet. The patient died at 2 weeks of age of complications of sepsis; autopsy revealed a single atrium and a cleft mitral valve.

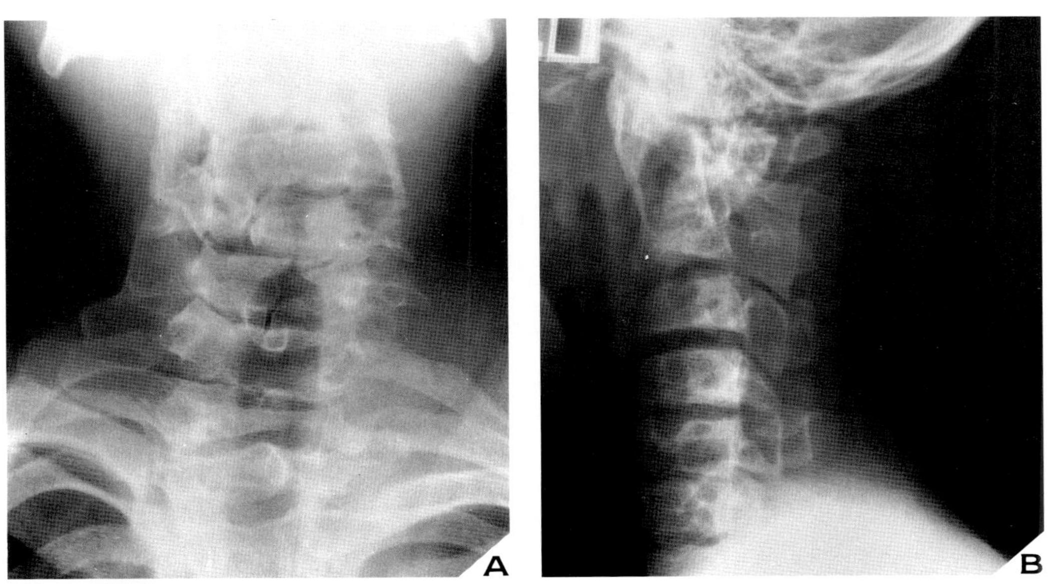

Fig. 5.7 Noonan's syndrome. (A) Frontal and (B) lateral projections of cervical spine in a patient with Noonan's syndrome show segmentation abnormalities of the cervical vertebrae (Klippel–Feil anomaly). Skeletal malformations are not uncommon in this autosomal dominant disorder. The patient had a small ostium secundum atrial septal defect. Other cardiac abnormalities commonly associated with Noonan's syndrome are pulmonic stenosis and abnormalities of the left ventricle.

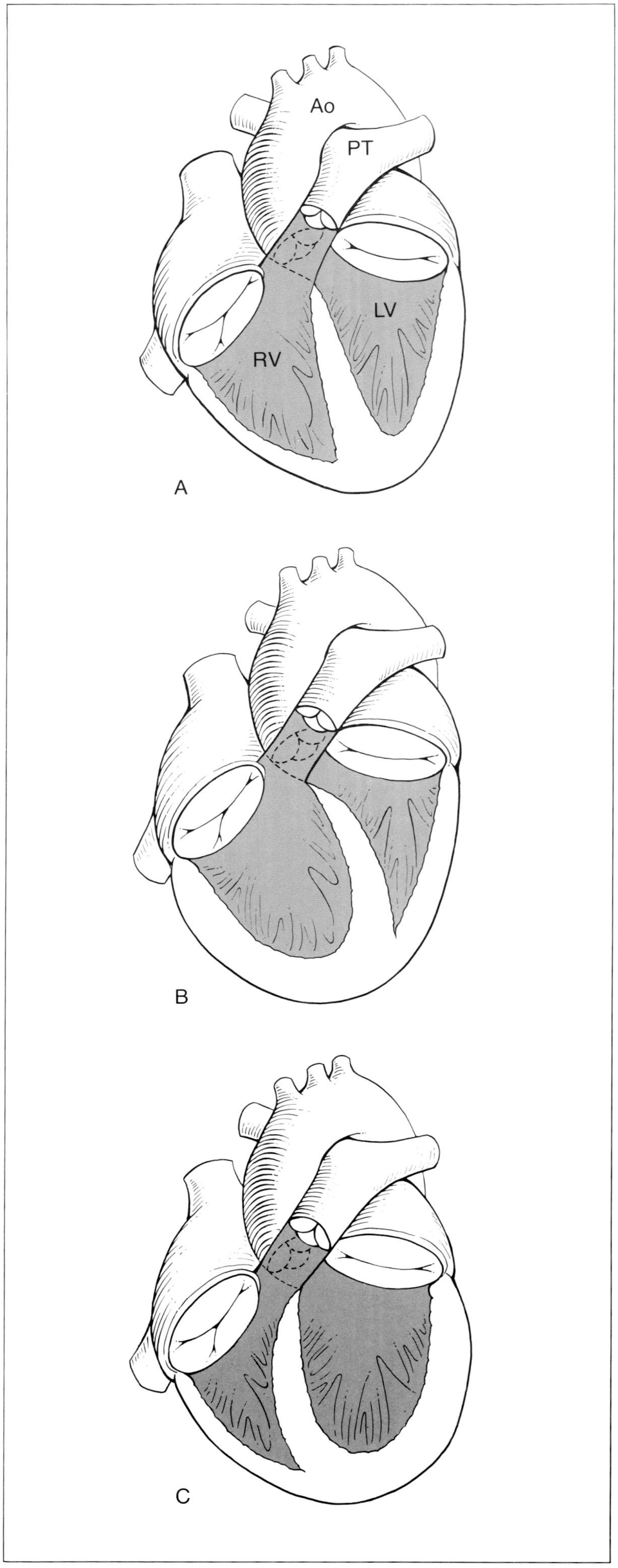

Fig 5.8 Effect of left and right ventricular hypertrophy on the ventricular septum. (A) At birth, development of both ventricles is usually balanced; the ventricular septum is not deviated towards either ventricle. (B) Right ventricular hypertrophy. The ventricular septum is displaced to the left. (C) Left ventricular hypertrophy. The ventricular septum is displaced to the right. Note in B and C that the ventricular septum is concave towards the more powerful ventricle.

formations often represent a combination of developmental errors.

Blood flow, which begins early in cardiogenesis, modifies the anatomic defect, stimulating the growth of some cardiovascular segments and delaying or inhibiting the development of others. Hemodynamic abnormalities associated with certain cardiac malformations may alter somatic growth and development. In extreme instances the cardiac defect may be incompatible with intrauterine or postnatal life.

The initial stage of myocardial development is cell multiplication. As the number of myocardial cells increases, there is concomitant development of a capillary network. The developing myocardium adapts to the hemodynamic alterations caused by a cardiovascular malformation by structural modifications that maximize the functional capacity of the deformed heart.

The fetal myocardium can also adapt to abnormal conditions by undergoing hypertrophy (enlargement of myocytes) and/or dilatation. Myocardial hypertrophy and dilatation of the cardiac chambers may induce compensatory mechanisms, which in turn can give rise to secondary complications and structural changes. For example, right ventricular dilatation leading to tricuspid insufficiency may be associated with marked dilatation of the right atrium. In children with concentric hypertrophy of the right ventricle (eg, secondary to pulmonic valvular stenosis), the interventricular septum may have a nearly straight configuration. Conversely, severe left ventricular hypertrophy may cause the interventricular septum to bulge into the right ventricle, sometimes compromising right ventricular function (Fig. 5.8).

Severe left ventricular hypertrophy secondary to pressure or volume overload can cause impaired myocardial perfusion; the resulting decrease in transmural perfusion pressure may interfere with oxygenation of the subendocardial myocardium. Marked dilatation of the left ventricle secondary to volume overload increases the risk of myocardial injury. Chronic volume overload sets up a vicious cycle of myocardial ischemia followed by further left ventricular dilatation with an increase in pressure and end diastolic volume. Left ventricular failure exacerbates the myocardial ischemia, resulting in further dilatation of the left ventricle (Fig. 5.9).

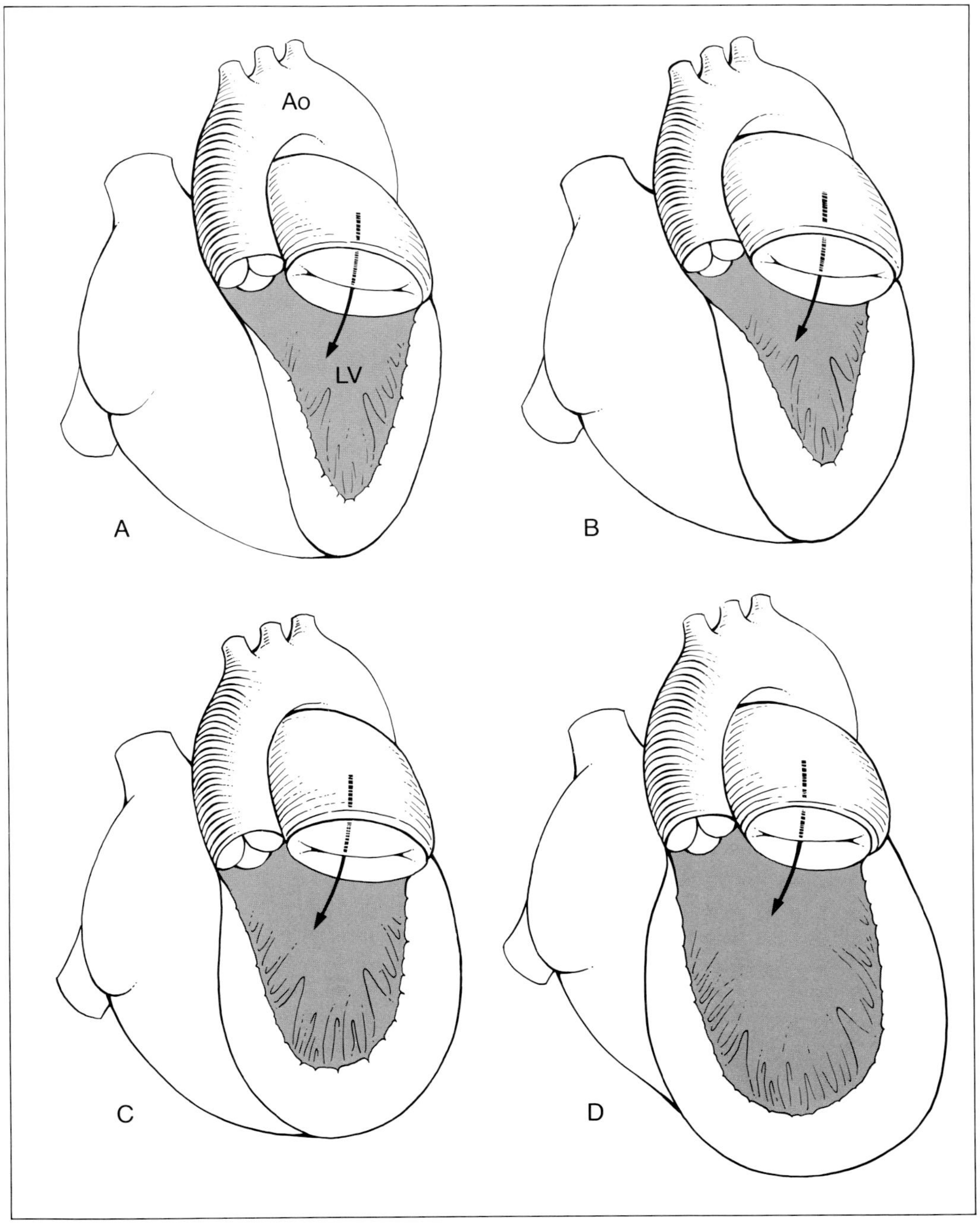

Fig. 5.9 Effect of volume overload on the left ventricle. (A) Normal; (B) hypertrophy only; (C) hypertrophy plus dilatation; (D) massive dilatation.

POSTNATAL ADAPTATIONS

The fetal circulatory pattern differs in a number of important ways from the postnatal circulatory pattern (Fig. 5.10). In the fetus, blood flows from the placenta to the right atrium. Most of the right atrial volume passes across the tricuspid valve into the right ventricle. Owing to the high pulmonary vascular resistance, most of the right ventricular output is shunted across the ductus arteriosus, bypassing the lungs. A portion of the right atrial volume flows across the foramen ovale into the left atrium. Left atrial blood passes across the mitral valve into the left ventricle. The left ventricular output enters the aorta and is distributed to the systemic circulation.

The physiologic status of the cardiopulmonary system undergoes a dramatic change at the moment of birth (Fig. 5.11). As the lungs expand, pulmonary vascular resistance decreases and the pulmonary circulation assumes its normal postnatal pattern, and the foramen ovale ceases to function as a pathway between the right and left atria. During the first few days of life the ductus arteriosus, which played a crucial role in intrauterine life, decreases in size and eventually becomes occluded. In some infants, pulmonary vascular resistance fails to decrease after birth, resulting in right to left shunting across the ductus arteriosus and/or foramen ovale. This physiologic aberration, known as *persistent fetal circulation* or *pulmonary hypertension of the newborn,* may occur as an isolated phenomenon or as a complication of another neonatal disorder (eg, meconium aspiration or congenital diaphragmatic hernia).

The left ventricular myocardium hypertrophies in response to the marked increase in systemic resistance. Because pulmo-

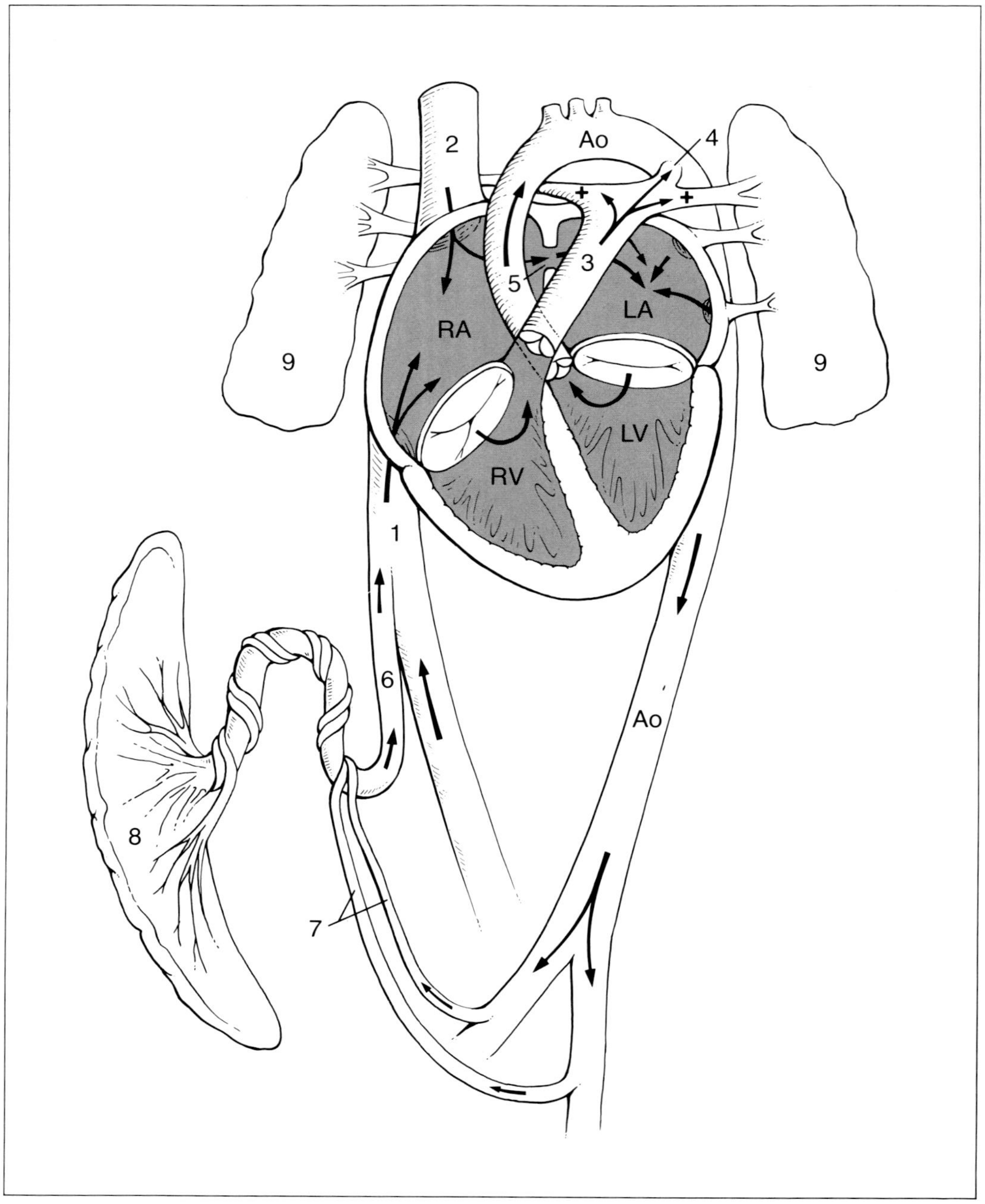

Fig. 5.10 Normal fetal circulation at the end of gestation.

1 inferior vena cava
2 superior vena cava
3 pulmonary artery
4 patent ductus arteriosus
5 patent foramen ovale
6 umbilical vein
7 umbilical artery
8 placenta
9 lungs

nary resistance is only one tenth that of systemic resistance, the right ventricular myocardium hypertrophies more slowly and to a much lesser degree than the left. In an infant with a large left to right shunt, pulmonary resistance begins to rise immediately after birth, progressively increasing until it reaches systemic or suprasystemic levels. (These hemodynamic changes reflect hypertrophy of the acinar and preacinar arteries in response to increased pulmonary arterial pressure and increased pulmonary blood flow.) Increased pulmonary resistance causes the right ventricle to hypertrophy and may eventually lead to right ventricular failure and decreased perfusion of the pulmonary vascular bed.

These and other postnatal adjustments account for variations in the clinical manifestations of congenital heart disease and in their time of onset. Some defects result in severe hemodynamic aberrations that are incompatible with extrauterine life; the affected infants die soon after birth unless appropriate support is provided. (Some defects are incompatible with life despite treatment.) In general, infants who survive the neonatal period have less severe defects than those who die. Postnatal hemodynamic adaptations that permit adequate tissue perfusion may allow some infants with potentially lethal defects to survive. Certain malformations result in only minimal alteration of cardiopulmonary physiology; in such patients growth and development may be normal or only slightly impaired. Many cardiac defects are well tolerated early in life; in such cases the first clinical manifestations may not appear until late in childhood or during adolescence.

CLINICAL MANIFESTATIONS OF CONGENITAL HEART DISEASE

CARDIAC FAILURE

Either ventricle may fail as a result of volume overload, pressure overload, or impairment of the myocardium itself. Congestive heart failure (CHF) occurs when the systemic pumping ventricle (usually the left) is unable to provide enough blood to satisfy peripheral demands. When the pulmonary pumping ventricle (usually the right) fails, the heart cannot pump an adequate volume of blood through the pulmonary circulation. Patients with right ventricular failure typically present with cyanosis secondary to peripheral desaturation.

Right or left ventricular failure can lead, respectively, to pulmonary or systemic venous hypertension. Pulmonary or systemic venous hypertension can also be caused by lesions that obstruct pulmonary or systemic venous drainage; in such pa-

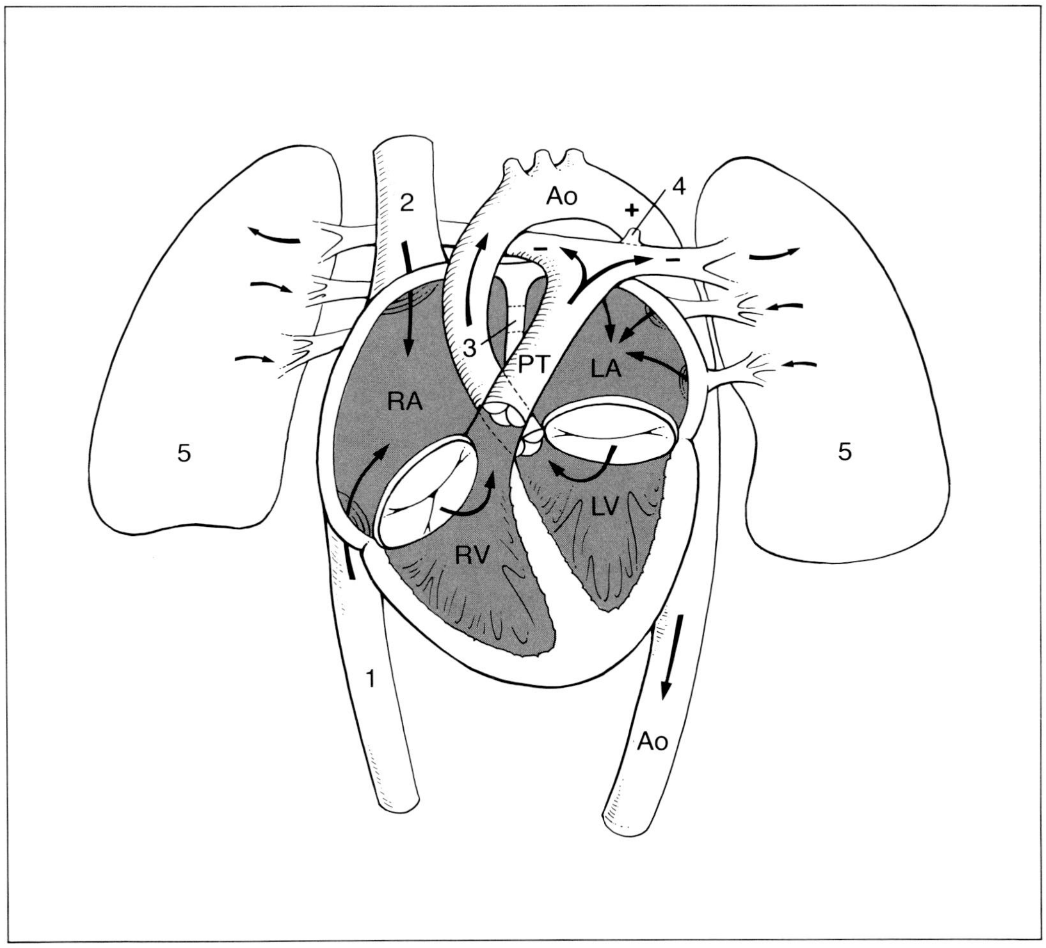

Fig. 5.11 Normal transitional circulation at birth.

1 inferior vena cava
2 superior vena cava
3 patent foramen ovale
4 ductus arteriosus
5 expanded lungs

tients the pumping function of the ventricles is not impaired. The many causes of pulmonary venous hypertension in the neonatal period and early infancy are listed in Fig. 5.12.

PERIPHERAL DESATURATION

Cyanosis, a generalized bluish coloration of the trunk and extremities, indicates the presence of peripheral desaturation. Because cyanosis is usually not appreciated when the hemoglobin saturation is greater than 85 percent, mild desaturation may go undetected on physical examination. Digital clubbing is common in children and adults with severe, longstanding peripheral desaturation, but is seldom seen in infants. Severe longstanding desaturation leads to polycythemia, which may be complicated by thrombosis of systemic and small pulmonary arteries, as well as hypertrophic pulmonary osteoarthropathy.

Many children with tetralogy of Fallot prefer to assume a squatting position, an adaptation that appears to lessen the desaturation associated with this malformation. These patients may also experience episodes during which the cyanosis becomes more severe *(cyanotic crises* or *spells),* often resulting in impaired perfusion of the brain and kidneys. The mechanism of cyanotic crises is uncertain; transient closure of the narrowed subpulmonic segment is the most attractive hypothesis for this phenomenon.

Cyanosis associated with congenital heart disease is nearly always caused by a right to left shunt. Such shunts may be intracardiac, at the atrial level, at the ventricular level, or extracardiac. [Most extracardiac shunts occur at the level of the great arteries (eg, pulmonary arteriovenous fistula)]. The severity of the cyanosis reflects the magnitude of the right to left shunt and the amount of oxygenated blood in the peripheral circulation. This combination of factors accounts for the relatively mild cyanosis typically observed in patients with transposition of the great arteries and other malformations associated with a right to left shunt and pulmonary plethora (Fig. 5.13). Because pulmonary blood flow is increased, there is a relatively large amount of oxygenated blood in the peripheral circulation; therefore, these patients are usually not severely desaturated.

In patients with congenital defects, failure of the pumping function of the systemic ventricle (usually the left) may aggravate the previously existing cyanosis by increasing the right to left shunt. Patients with such lesions, which include truncus arteriosus with hypoplasia of the aortic arch and total anomalous pulmonary venous connection (infradiaphragmatic type) typically present with both CHF and cyanosis.

METABOLIC ABERRATIONS

Metabolic aberrations are common in patients with severe congenital cardiac defects. For example, perfusion of the kidneys is often impaired in neonates with hypoplastic left ventricle, severe stenosis of the left ventricular outflow tract, or interruption of the aortic arch. Infants with such lesions typically present in heart failure owing to the combined effects of the right ventricular volume overload imposed by closure of the ductus arteriosus and inadequacy or absence of the left ventricular pumping function. A low-output syndrome, manifested by systemic hypotension and decreased peripheral pulses, may also be present in such cases, quickly followed by renal failure (anuria) and metabolic acidosis.

CLINICAL PRESENTATION AT VARIOUS AGES

The clinical manifestations of congenital heart disease vary with the age of the patient and the nature of the malformation.

NEWBORNS AND YOUNG INFANTS

The usual manifestations of congenital heart disease in the newborn period are congestive heart failure, cyanosis, or a combination of the two. Cyanosis can be associated with cardiomegaly or a normal-sized heart, depending on the nature of the underlying lesion (Fig. 5.14). Neonates and young infants with

FIG. 5.12 CAUSES OF PULMONARY VENOUS HYPERTENSION IN NEONATES AND YOUNG INFANTS

First Week	Second and Third Weeks	Fourth to Sixth Weeks
Overhydration	Coarctation of the aorta	Coarcation of the aorta
Tachyarrythmia	Interrupted aortic arch	Critical aortic stenosis
Bradyarrhythmia	Critical aortic stenosis	Endocardial fibroelastosis
Hypoplastic left ventricle	Endocardial fibroelastosis	Anomalous origin of the left coronary artery
Critical aortic stenosis	Hypertrophic cardiomyopathy	Hypertrophic cardiomyopathy
Obstructive total pulmonary venous connection	Cor triatriatum	Cor triatriatum
Stenotic or atretic pulmonary veins	Congenital mitral valvular atresia or stenosis	Congenital mitral valvular stenosis or atresia
Peripheral arteriovenous fistula [eg, liver, brain (vein of Galen aneurysm)]	Peripheral arteriovenous fistula	
Myocarditis (intrauterine)		

Fig. 5.12 Causes of pulmonary venous hypertension in neonates and young infants.

CHF typically present with respiratory distress, easy fatigability during feeding, and/or growth retardation. The usual findings on physical examination are tachycardia, tachypnea, cardiomegaly, and hepatomegaly. Infants with large VSDs and atrioventricular septal defects typically present with CHF during the second week, when pulmonary vascular resistance decreases. Neonates with hypoplastic left ventricle or interruption of the aortic arch commonly present with signs and symptoms of cardiogenic shock, including diminished pulses, low blood pressure, anuria, and metabolic acidosis.

OLDER INFANTS (2 TO 12 MONTHS)

Patients with congenital heart disease who are asymptomatic during the neonatal period may present later in infancy with cyanosis, CHF, failure to thrive, or a combination of these symptoms. The disorders encountered in the older infant are the same as those seen in the neonate (those with the most severe malformations have already succumbed). VSD, atrioventricular septal defect (atrioventricular canal), and PDA are the acyanotic disorders most frequently encountered at this age. Cyanotic disorders associated with pulmonary plethora (eg, transposition of the great arteries, truncus arteriosus, total anomalous pulmonary venous connection), as well as those associated with pulmonary oligemia (eg, tetralogy of Fallot, tricuspid atresia), commonly present at this age. Anomalous origin of the left coronary artery from the pulmonary trunk, which may cause massive ischemia of the left ventricle with resulting left ventricular failure, and isolated coarctation of the aorta may also appear at this age.

CHILDREN AND ADOLESCENTS

Children and adolescents with congenital heart disease typically present with cyanosis, CHF, and/or growth failure. The severity of the clinical picture varies according to the structural abnormality and the pathophysiology. Some congenital malformations may manifest for the first time at this age. For example, isolated coarctation of the aorta may go undetected until the patient begins to experience symptoms of sytemic hypertension (eg, headache). A patient with anomalous origin of the left cornary artery from the pulmonary trunk may be asymptomatic until signs of cardiac failure secondary to myocardial ischemia appear. The onset of cyanosis, clubbing, and/or hemoptysis in an older child or adolescent may be the first evidence of a pulmonary arteriovenous fistula. A heart murmur, arrhythmia, or elevated blood pressure detected on a pre-school or pre-camp physical examination may lead to the diagnosis of congenital heart disease in an asymptomatic child or teenager.

ADULTS

Occasionally, patients with congenital heart disease may remain asymptomatic until adult life. Such patients typically present with systemic hypertension, arrhythmias, or heart failure secondary to longstanding volume overload. Malformations that are asymptomatic until adult life tend to be less severe than those that are symptomatic earlier.

The clinical picture may change over time in a patient with a previously diagnosed congenital defect. For example, an individual with a large VSD or other large left to right shunt may

FIG. 5.13 CARDIAC MALFORMATIONS ASSOCIATED WITH CYANOSIS AND PULMONARY PLETHORA

- Transposition of the great arteries
- Truncus arteriosus
- Total anomalous pulmonary venous connection
- Univentricular atrioventricular connection
- Double outlet right ventricle
- Double outlet left ventricle

Fig. 5.13 Cardiac malformations associated with cyanosis and pulmonary plethora.

FIG. 5.14 CARDIAC MALFORMATIONS ASSOCIATED WITH CYANOSIS IN NEONATE AND INFANT

Cyanosis with Cardiomegaly	Cyanosis with Normal-sized Heart
Critical pulmonary valvular stenosis	Tetralogy of Fallot with pulmonary atresia
Pulmonary atresia with intact ventricular septum	Tetralogy of Fallot with pulmonary stenosis
Ebstein's anomaly	Tricuspid atresia
Tricuspid atresia	Total anomalous venous return to portal system or inferior vena cava

Fig. 5.14 Cardiac malformations associated with congestive heart failure and cyanosis.

develop pulmonary arterial hypertension secondary to progressive obliteration of the pulmonary arterial tree. Such patients typically present with cyanosis. In extreme instances, the pulmonary resistance is so high that there is reversal of the left to right shunt, leading to marked cyanosis, clubbing, and polycythemia (Eisenmenger syndrome). Complications, including paradoxical peripheral embolization via a right to left shunt, endocarditis, or arrhythmias, are not uncommon in adults with congenital heart disease. Occasionally such complications may lead to the discovery of an unsuspected congenital defect.

The clinical and radiologic findings in adults with congenital heart disease are discussed further in Chapter 17.

DIAGNOSIS OF CONGENITAL HEART DISEASE

The existence and the general nature of a congenital cardiac malformation are usually suggested by the history and the findings at physical examination. Judicious use of the diagnostic modalities described in earlier chapters will define the pathologic anatomy and functional derangements and serve as a guide to appropriate therapy. The chapters that follow will consider the diagnosis of congenital malformations of the heart and great vessels by invasive and noninvasive techniques.

CHAPTER 6

Cardiac Anatomy Relevant to Congenital Heart Disease

NORMAL ANATOMY

The normal heart consists of three segments connected in sequence: the atria, the ventricles, and the great arteries (Fig. 6.1). Normally, there are two morphologically distinct atria; each is connected to a ventricle, which in turn is connected to a great artery (pulmonary trunk or aorta).

THE ATRIA

The morphological "rightness" or "leftness" of the atrial chambers is determined by their internal architecture and by the configuration of the atrial appendages. Normally the atria are dissimilar (*asymmetrical* or *lateralized*); the morphologic right atrium lies to the right of the morphologic left atrium, an arrangement known as *atrial situs solitus*. In some individuals the morphologic right atrium lies to the left of the morphologic left atrium (*atrial situs inversus*). In other individuals the atria are morphologically similar (isomeric), in which event the isomeric atria may both resemble either a right atrium (*right atrial isomerism*) or a left atrium (*left atrial isomerism*). Thus, there are four possible arrangements of the atria: normal atrial situs (atrial situs solitus), mirror image atrial situs (atrial situs inversus), right atrial isomerism, and left atrial isomerism (Fig. 6.2).

THE VENTRICLES

The left and right ventricles are morphologically distinct (Fig. 6.3). Each ventricle consists of three segments: inlet, trabecular, and outlet. Certain malformations are characterized by the

CHAPTER LABELING KEY	
RA right atrium	RV right ventricle
LA left atrium	LV left ventricle

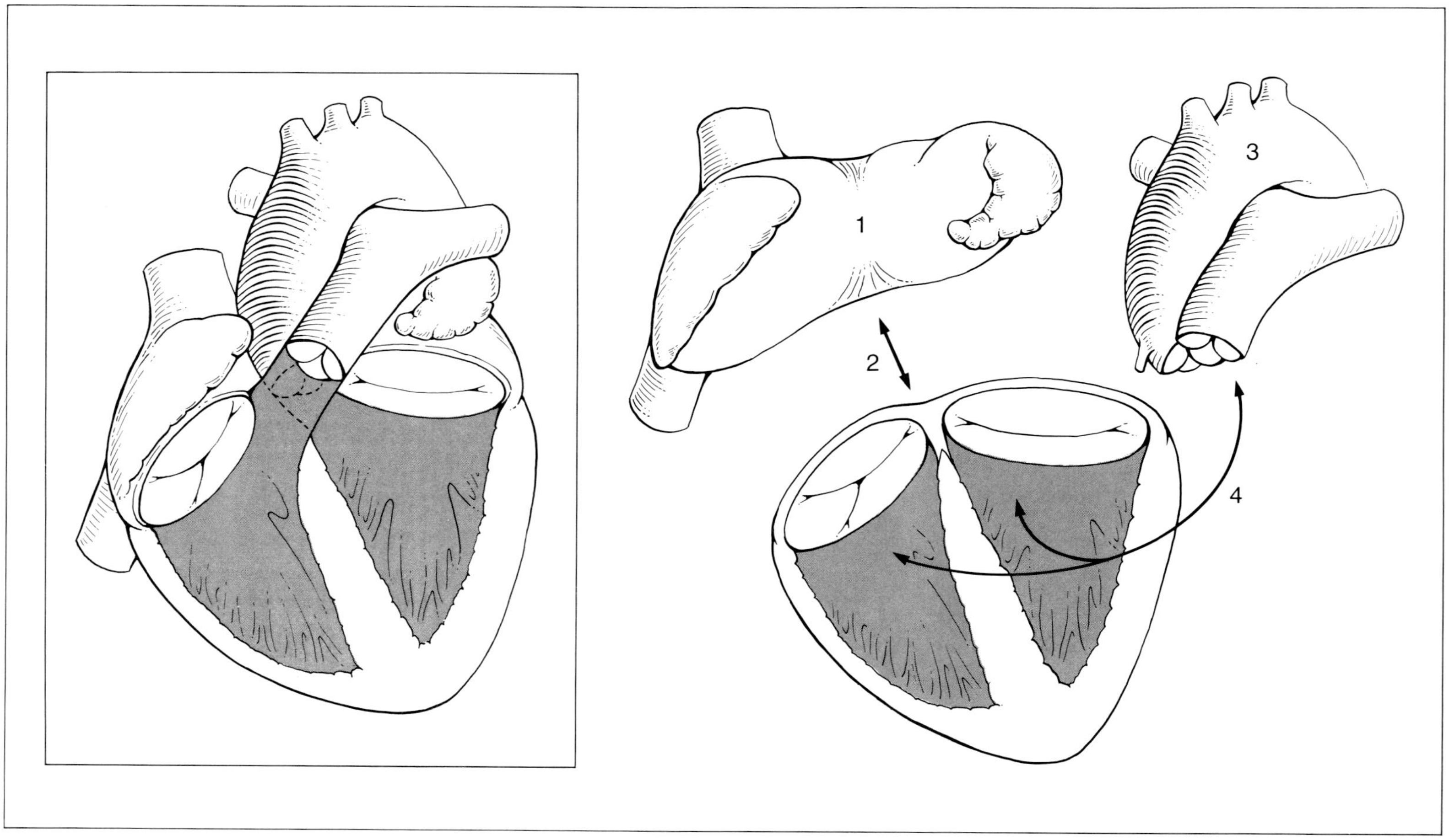

Fig. 6.1 The three cardiac segments.

1 atrial segment	3 arterial segment
2 atrioventricular junction	4 ventriculoarterial junction

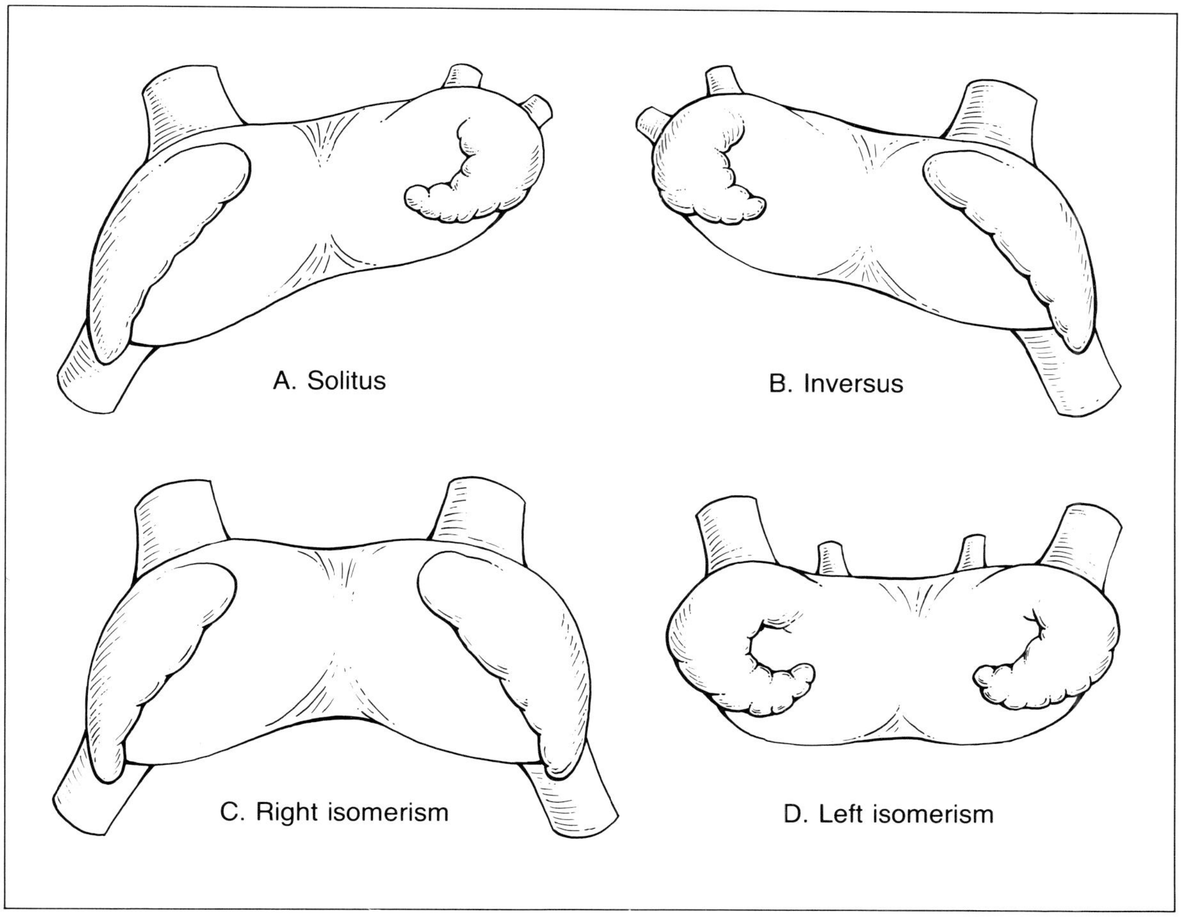

Fig. 6.2 Atrial morphology. (A) Solitus; (B) inversus; (C) right isomerism; (D) left isomerism. The morphologic right atrial appendage is short and blunt, whereas the morphologic left atrial appendage is long and fingerlike.

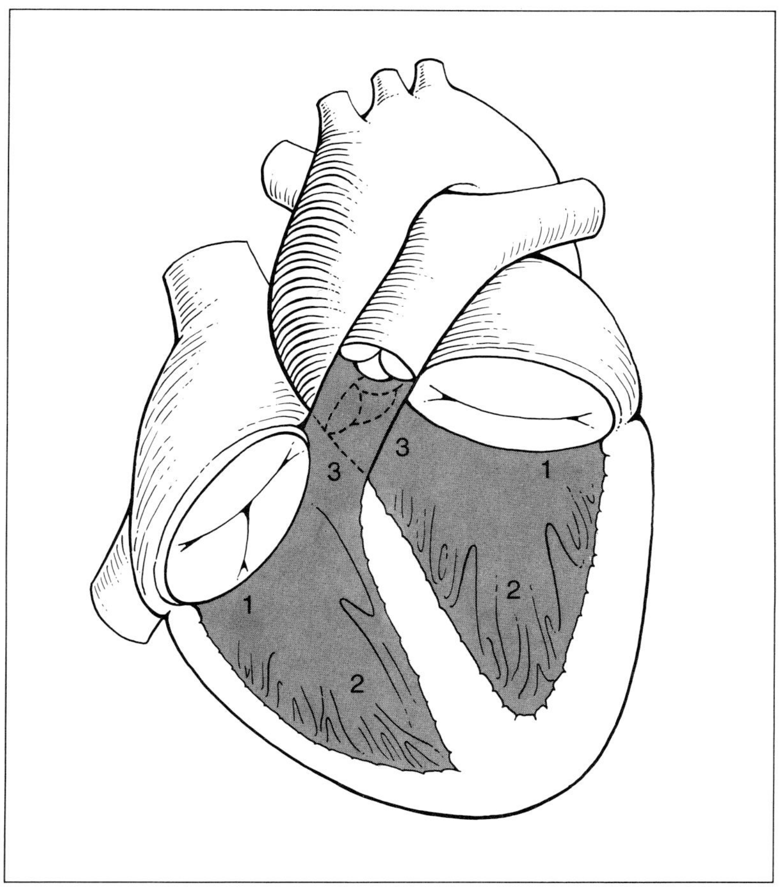

Fig. 6.3 The ventricles and their components.

1 inlet   2 trabecular   3 outlet

absence of one or more of these segments (Fig. 6.4). The two ventricles are separated by a septum consisting of membranous and muscular portions.

Abnormal folding of the primitive ventricular loop can result in abnormal spatial orientation of the ventricles. In normal development, the primitive ventricle buckles to the right (D-loop) so that the right ventricle comes to lie to the right of and anterior to the left ventricle. If the primitive ventricle buckles to the left

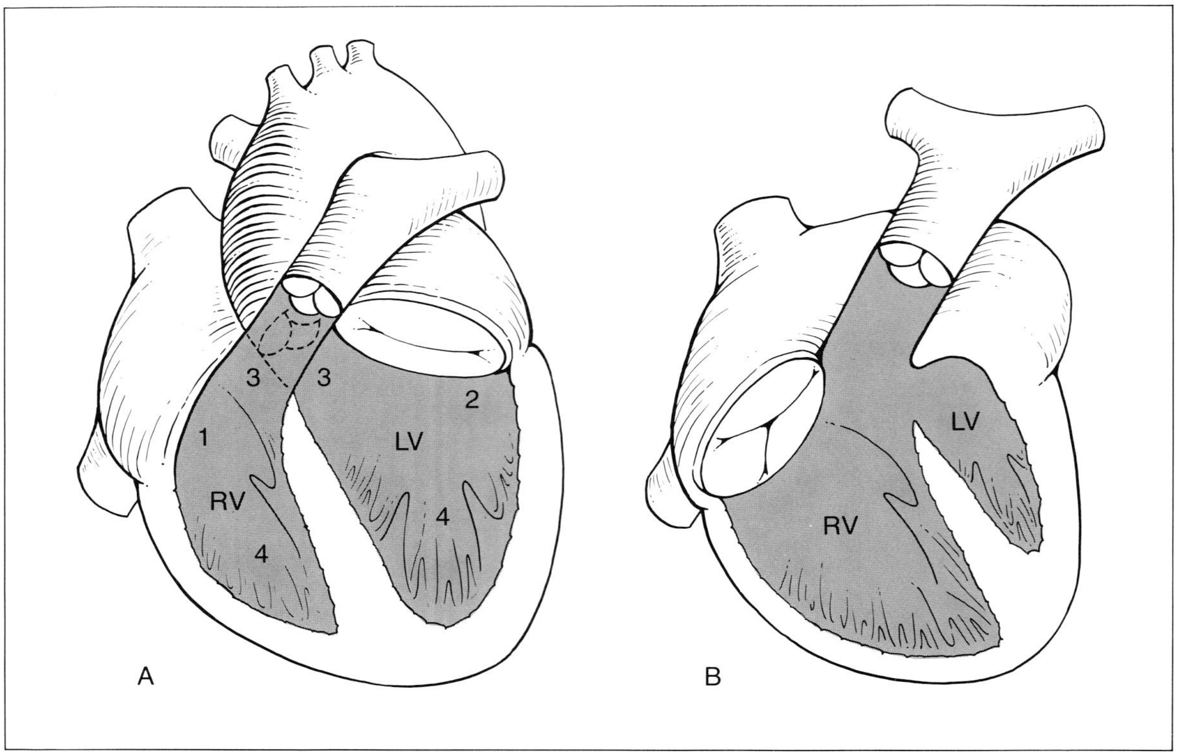

Fig. 6.4 Incomplete ventricles. (A) Incomplete right ventricle with absent inlet segment. (B) Incomplete left ventricle with absent inlet and outlet segments.

1	absent inlet	3	outlet
2	inlet	4	trabecular

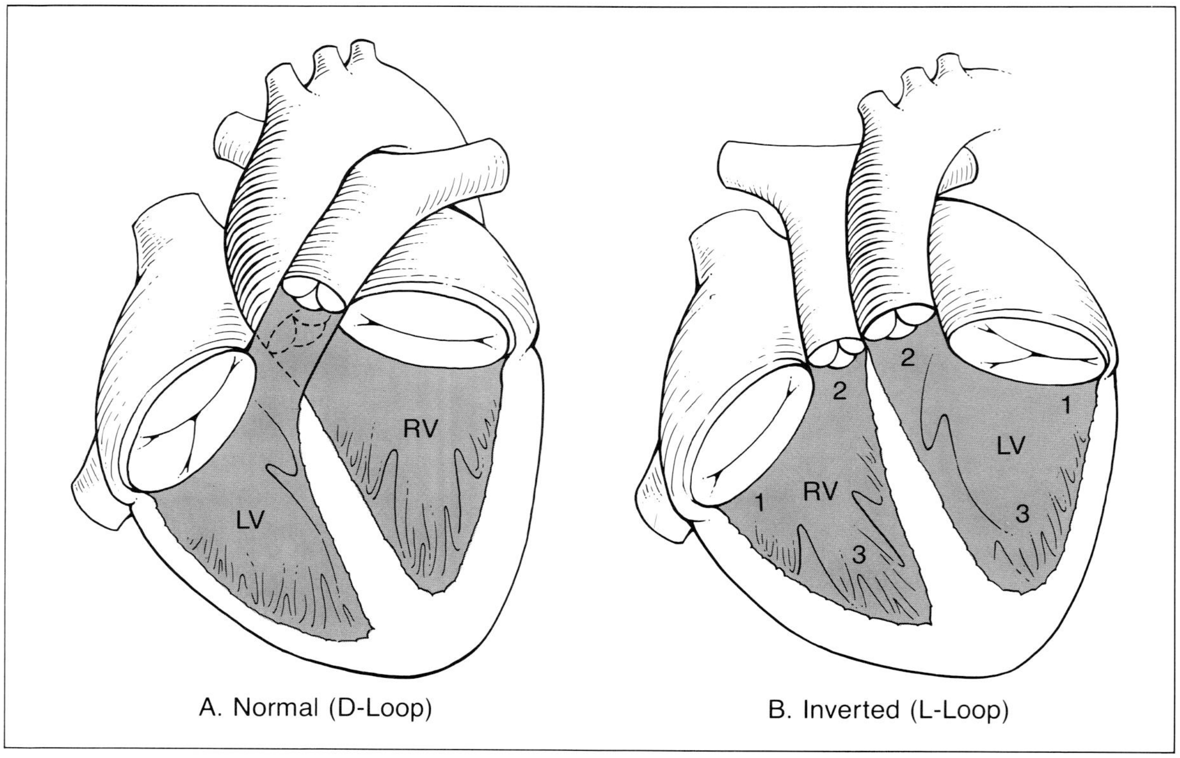

Fig. 6.5 Spatial relations of the ventricles. (A) Normal (D-loop). (B) Inverted (L-loop).

1	inlet	3	trabecular
2	outlet		

(L-loop), the morphologic right ventricle will come to lie to the left of the morphologic left ventricle, a condition known as *ventricular inversion* (Fig. 6.5).

THE ATRIOVENTRICULAR CONNECTIONS

In a normal heart, the atrioventricular connections are *concordant*, ie, the right-sided right atrium is connected with the right-sided right ventricle (via the tricuspid valve) and the left-sided left atrium is connected with the left-sided left ventricle (via the mitral valve). In certain cardiac malformations, the atrioventricular connections are *discordant*, ie, each atrium is connected to an inappropriate ventricle. A third possible type of atrioventricular connection is *univentricular connection*, an anomaly in which both atria are connected to a single ventricular chamber. Finally, either the left or the right atrioventricular connection may be absent (tricuspid or mitral atresia) (Fig. 6.6).

In hearts with atrial isomerism the atrioventricular connections cannot be characterized as "concordant" or "discordant." In such cases the atrioventricular connections are described as "ambiguous." There are two varieties of ambiguous atrioventricular connection, depending on the ventricular relationships: normally related or with inverted ventricles.

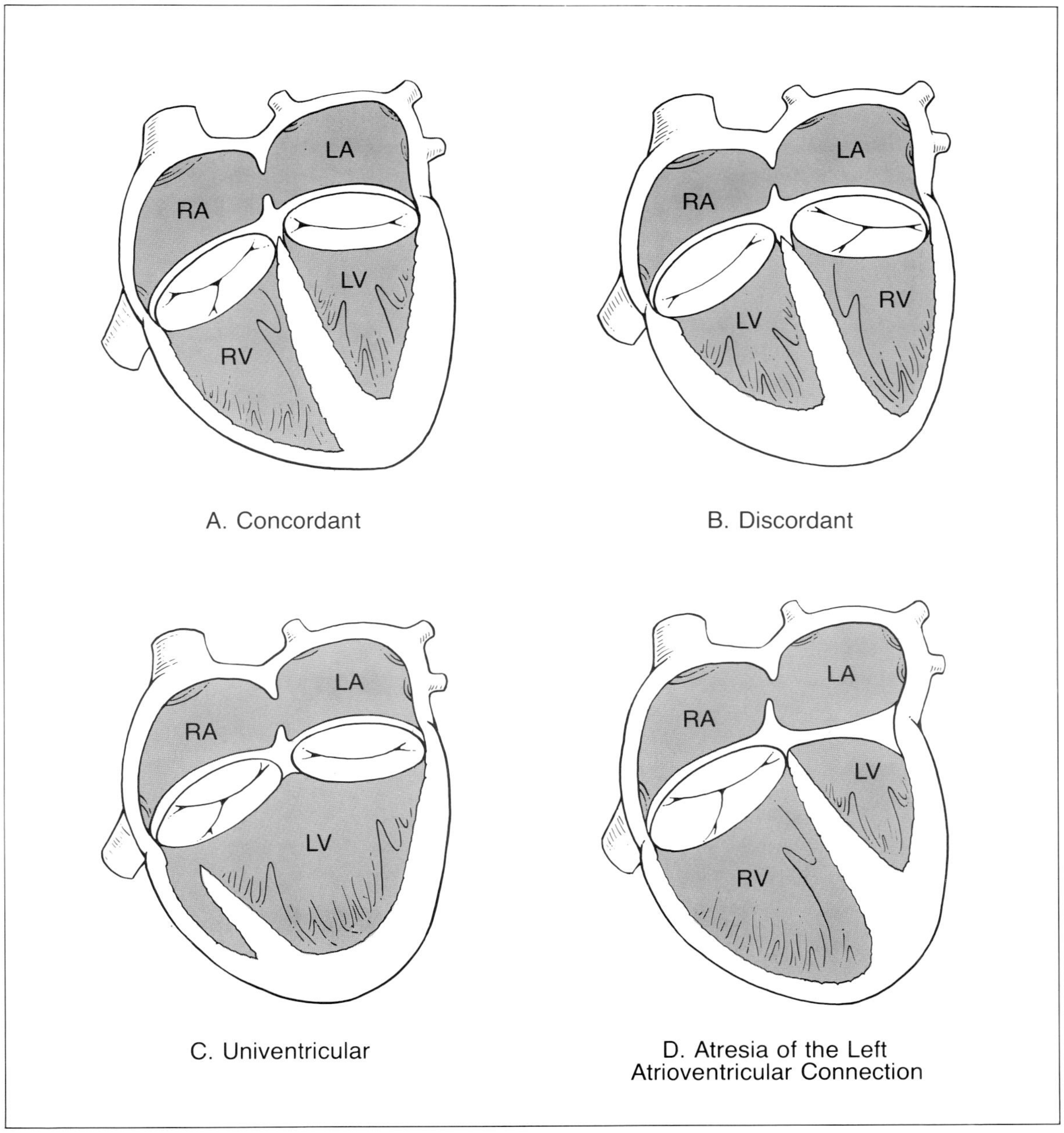

Fig. 6.6 The four possible atrioventricular connections. (A) Concordant; (B) discordant; (C) univentricular; (D) atresia of the left atrioventricular connection.

THE VENTRICULOARTERIAL CONNECTIONS

In a normal heart, the ventriculoarterial connections are concordant: the right ventricle is connected with the pulmonary artery and the left ventricle is connected to the aorta as shown in Fig. 6.7. The right and left ventriculoarterial connections each have distinct morphologic features. A portion of the left ventricular outlet segment is fibrous, and the annuli of the mitral and aortic valves are continuous. In contrast, the outlet segment of the right ventricle is wholly muscular; the pulmonary valve is seated in muscle and is entirely separate from the tricuspid valve. However, several abnormal types of ventriculoarterial connection may be seen. These include discordant ventriculoarterial connection (transposition), double outlet left ventricle, double outlet right ventricle, and single outlet left or right ventricle with atresia of a great artery (Figs. 6.7 and 6.8). Truncus arteriosus is also included in this category.

THE GREAT ARTERIES

The ascending aorta normally lies posterior and to the right of the pulmonary trunk. The proximal portion of the aortic arch lies anterior and to the right of the trachea, while its distal portion lies posterior and to the left of the trachea. The pulmonary trunk lies to the left of and anterior to the ascending aorta; on frontal chest films it forms a portion of the left mediastinal border, just caudal to the projection of the aortic arch.

THE VENOATRIAL CONNECTIONS

The normal venoatrial connections consist of the superior and inferior caval veins (venae cavae), which enter the right atrium, and four pulmonary veins (two left and two right), which enter the left. This anatomic arrangement creates two separate circulatory systems (pulmonary and systemic) which work in series. Abnormal venoatrial connections are not uncommon; some (or all) of the systemic or pulmonary veins may be affected.

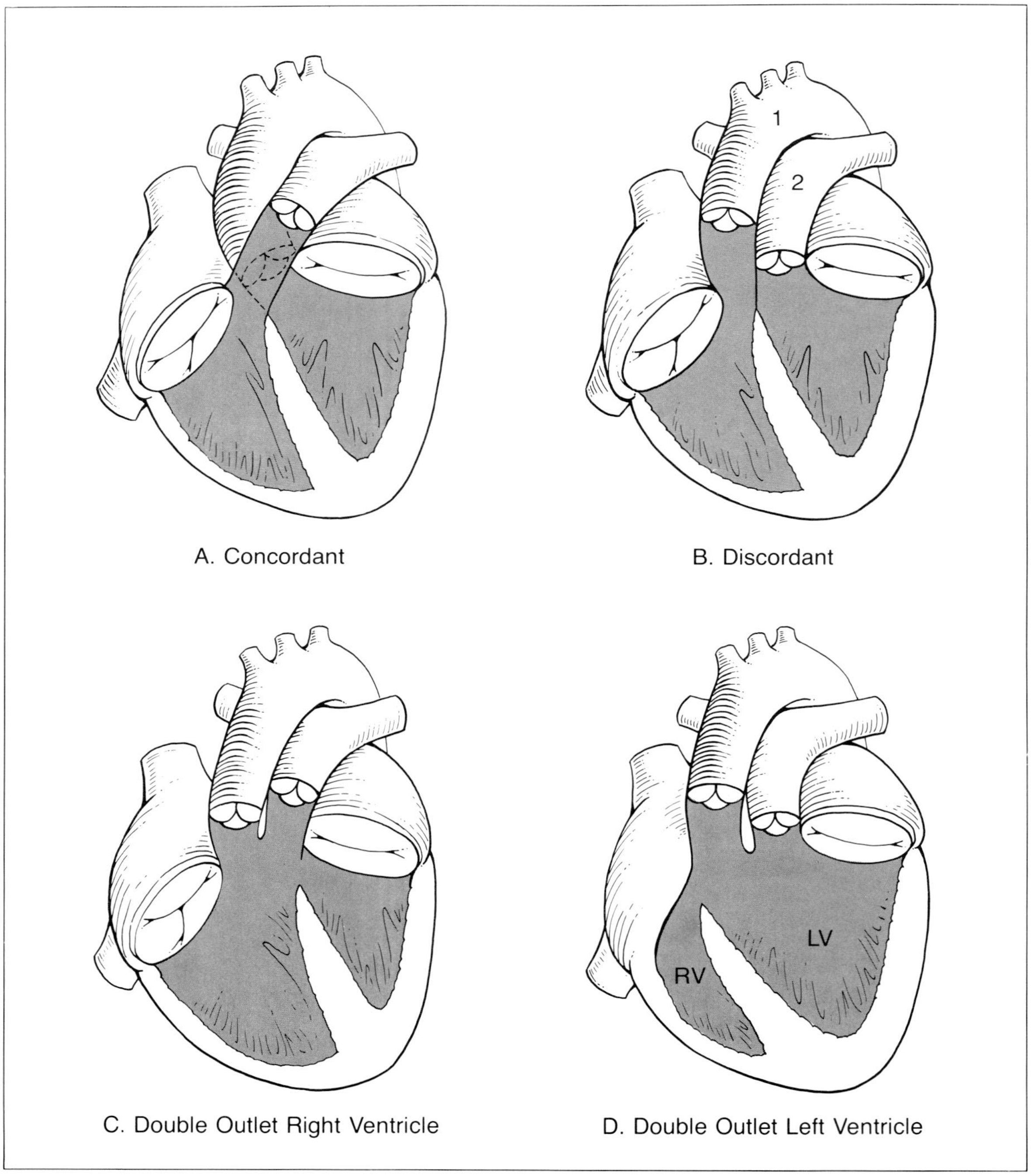

Fig. 6.7 Four varieties of ventriculoarterial connection. (A) Concordant; (B) discordant; (C) double outlet right ventricle; (D) double outlet left ventricle.

1 aorta 2 pulmonary trunk

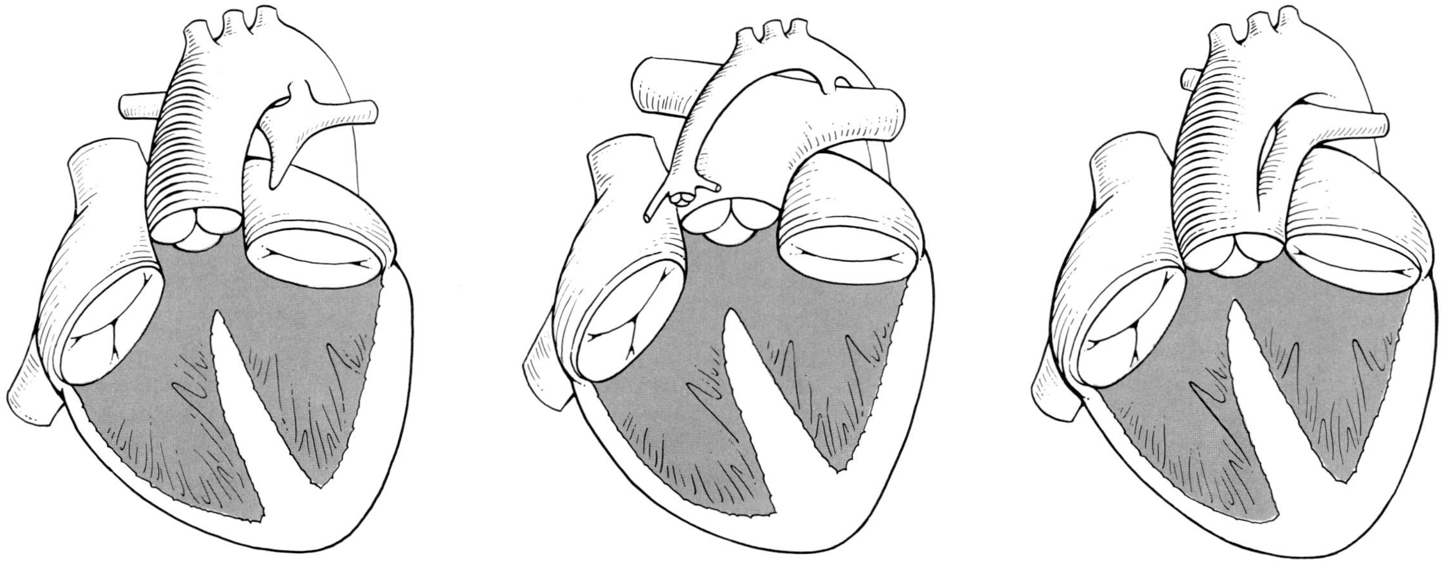

Fig. 6.8 Single outlet ventricle. A single arterial outlet constitutes the fifth variety of ventriculoarterial connection. (A) Pulmonary atresia; (B) aortic atresia; (C) truncus arteriosus.

CHAPTER 7

Plain Film Evaluation

Armed with a clear understanding of normal cardiac anatomy and physiology, as well as knowledge of the aberrations associated with various pathologic states, one can often derive important information from plain films in a patient with suspected congenital heart disease. By judiciously employing one or more additional imaging modalities [eg, two-dimensional echocardiography, angiocardiography, cine computed tomography, or magnetic resonance imaging (MRI)], one can generally define the nature of the defect with considerable precision.

NORMAL CARDIAC ANATOMY

THE FRONTAL PROJECTION

Normally, most of the cardiac volume occupies the left hemithorax and the cardiac axis is directed to the left (Figs. 7.1A and 7.2A). In some individuals the heart lies predominantly in the right hemithorax and the cardiac axis is directed to the right (Fig. 7.3). Because atrial situs can be normal or abnormal in such cases, the presence of "dextrocardia" or "dextroposition" cannot be taken as an indicator of atrial situs. (As these terms have been employed in a variety of contexts, with resultant confusion, we will characterize abnormal heart position according to the direction of the *cardiac axis* and type of *atrial situs* in subsequent chapters.)

CARDIAC AXIS

The cardiac axis is usually directed to the left in individuals with normal atrial situs (atrial situs solitus), whereas it is usually directed to the right in those with atrial situs inversus.

CARDIOVASCULAR SILHOUETTE

On the right, the border of the cardiovascular silhouette is formed superiorly by the superior vena cava, which is sometimes superimposed on the ascending aorta, and inferiorly by the right atrium (Fig. 7.2A). On the left, the aortic arch forms the upper border of the cardiovascular silhouette. (Occasionally, the left subclavian artery contributes to the cardiovascular

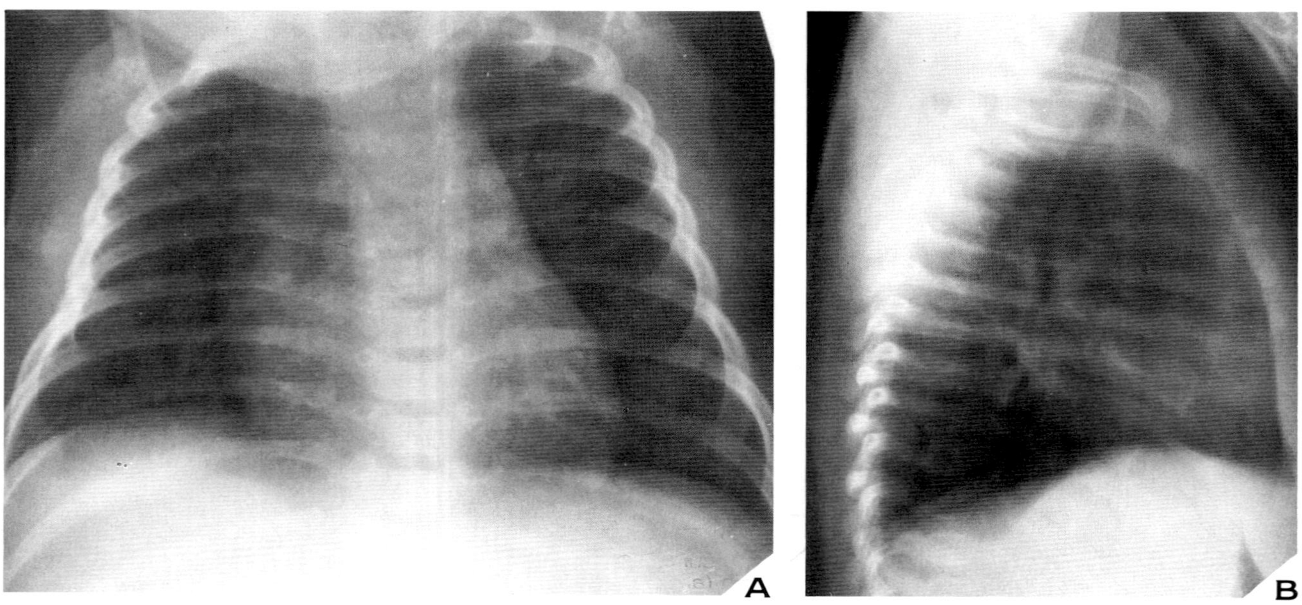

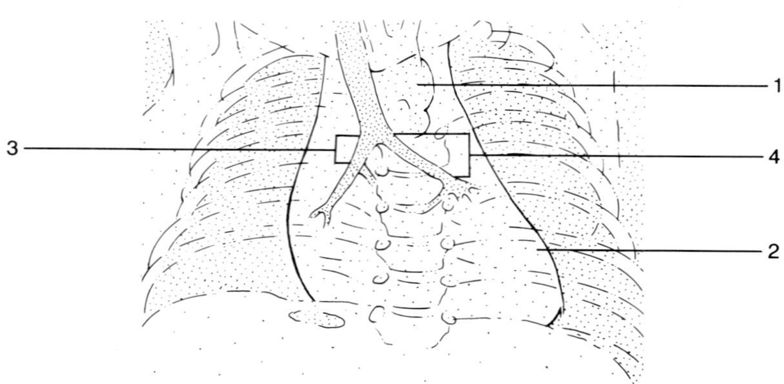

1 aortic arch;
2 left ventricle;
3 right main bronchus;
4 left main bronchus; L/R bronchia length ratio = 2 : 1

Fig. 7.1 Normal chest. (a) Supine chest film of a normal 3-year-old child shows normal mediastinal relationships. The aortic arch and descending thoracic aorta are both on the left. The right mainstem bronchus is shorter than the left, indicating normal thoracic and atrial situs (atrial situs solitus). The pulmonary vessels are normally distributed throughout the lung fields. The cardiac silhouette is normal in size and shape. The left cardiac contour is formed by the left ventricle. The liver is on the right and the stomach bubble on the left (abdominal situs solitus). (b) On the lateral view, the majority of the cardiac mass is located in the anterior and inferior thorax, placing the anterior aspect of the heart in contact with the inferior third of the anterior chest wall. The left pulmonary artery is located superior and posterior to the left mainstem bronchus.

silhouette, appearing as a discrete structure just cephalad to the arch.) The pulmonary trunk forms a discrete prominence just below the aortic arch. The left ventricle forms the remainder of the left heart border, extending from below the pulmonary trunk to the level of the diaphragm. In some normal individuals the left atrial appendage forms part of the left heart border, appearing as a localized convexity between the pulmonary trunk and the left ventricle.

The aortic arch is easily identified in older infants and children; however, it is inconspicuous or invisible in young infants. Close scrutiny of the tracheal air column may be helpful at this age: when the aortic arch is on the left, there is a corresponding

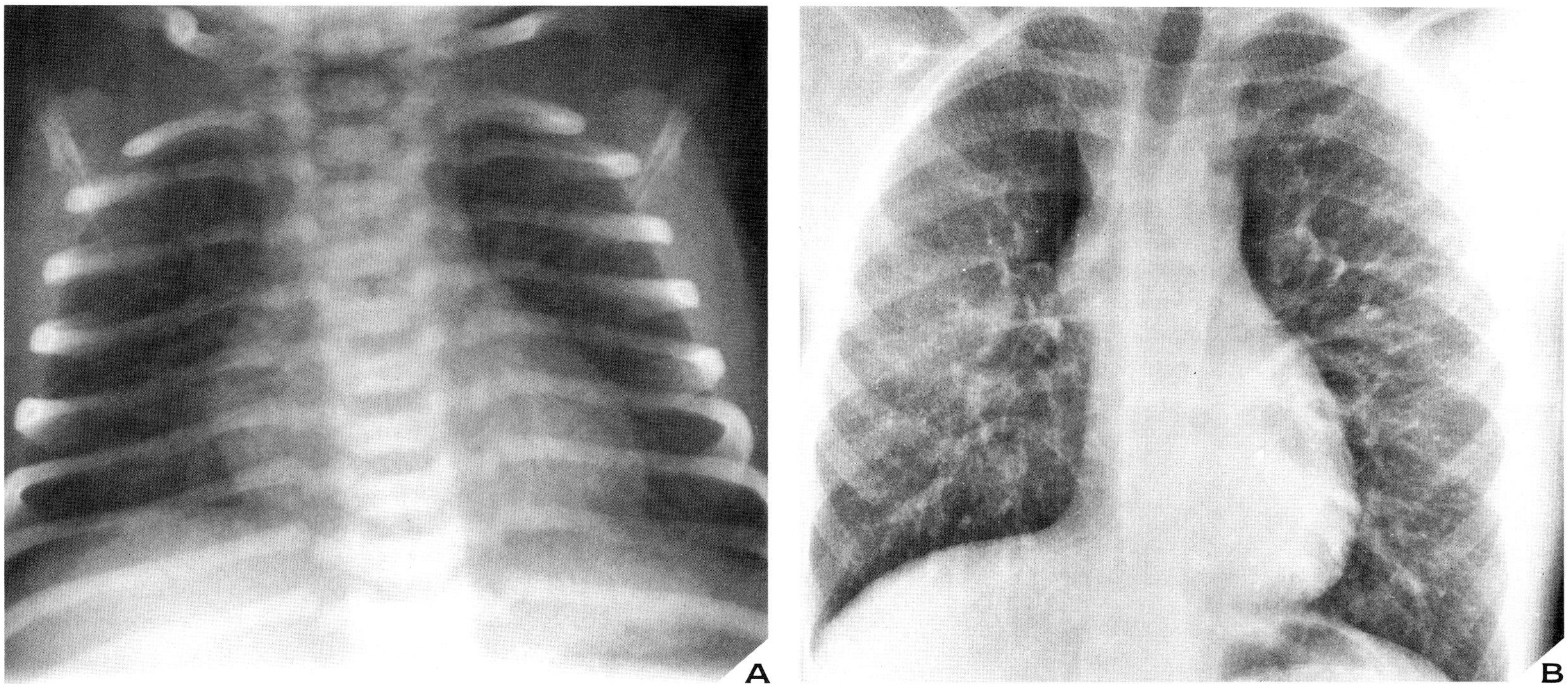

Fig. 7.2 Low versus high kVp. (A) Erect posteroanterior chest film in a normal 3-month-old infant using low kVp technique. Although the cardiac and mediastinal contours and pulmonary vascularity are well demonstrated, details of the mediastinal structures cannot be appreciated. The tracheobronchial tree is not well seen. (B) A supine chest with high kVp technique in a 1-year-old child clearly demonstrates the tracheobronchial tree, left aortic arch, and descending thoracic aorta. The pulmonary vascular pattern is much better seen with the high kVp technique.

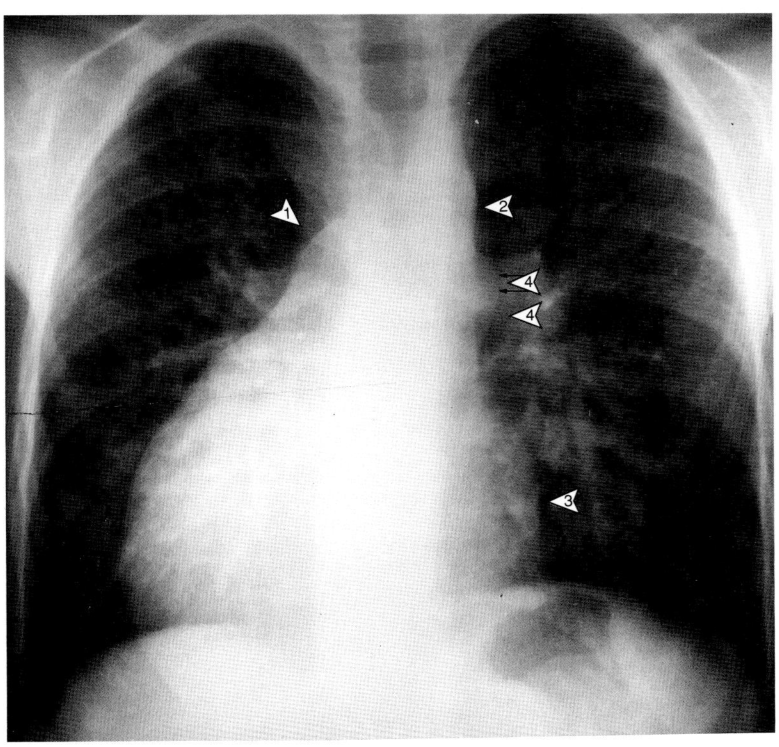

Fig. 7.3 Abnormal cardiac axis with thoracic isomerism. On this posteroanterior chest film, the cardiac axis is directed to the right. Most of the cardiac mass lies in the right hemithorax. The tracheobronchial tree is symmetrical (thoracic isomerism). Both main bronchi are of the left type, indicating left atrial isomerism. The azygos vein (*arrow* 1) is distended. There is a left aortic arch (*arrow* 2). The right ventricle is indicated by *arrow* 3. (The ascending aorta is indicated by *arrows* 4).

impression on the left side of the tracheal air column (in infants with a right aortic arch it is usually on the right) (Fig. 7.4B). The proximal portion of the descending thoracic aorta, which can usually be identified even in newborns, is almost always on the left in infants with a left aortic arch, whereas it is nearly always on the right in infants with a right arch.

The normal thymus can overlie portions of the mediastinal and cardiac border, especially in infants and young children, in which event it may be mistaken for a dilated ascending aorta or an enlarged main pulmonary artery (see below).

TRACHEOBRONCHIAL TREE

In normal subjects, the respiratory and cardiovascular systems have a characteristic pattern of asymmetry that can be appreciated on plain films (Figs. 7.1 and 7.2A). Normally, the left mainstem bronchus is longer than the right, with a left:right ratio of at least 1.4:1. Characteristic abnormalities of the tracheobronchial tree associated with abnormal atrial situs (see Chapter 8) can often be appreciated on routine chest films and are easily identified on high-kilovoltage radiographs or tomograms (Fig. 7.2B).

THYMUS

In infants and young children, the normal thymus can produce marked mediastinal widening, simulating a mediastinal mass or cardiomegaly; in some instances it may appear as a juxtacardiac mass (Fig. 7.4A). Because the thymus shrinks rapidly in response to stress, simply repeating the film a few days later will often exclude mediastinal or cardiac pathology (Fig. 7.4B).

THE LATERAL PROJECTION

The heart normally occupies the angle between the anterior chest wall and the diaphragm (Fig. 7.1B). It occupies the anterior third of the chest and "silhouettes" the anterior portion of the left hemidiaphragm, on which it rests. Other cardiovascular structures that can be routinely identified on the lateral projection include the anterior aspect of the proximal pulmonary trunk, the central pulmonary arteries, a portion of the ascending aorta, and the convex (anterosuperior) border of the aortic arch. The right pulmonary artery lies anterior to the right main bronchus and anterior to the plane of the trachea. The left pulmonary artery lies superior and posterior to the left main bronchus. In infants and young children the right ventricular outflow tract, proximal pulmonary trunk, and ascending aorta may be obscured by the thymus.

The posterior heart border is formed by the left ventricle, which extends inferiorly to join the diaphragm. Normally, the left atrium does not contribute to the posterior heart border on the lateral projection. However, the posterosuperior aspect of the left atrium abuts the left main bronchus, and posterior displacement of this structure usually indicates left atrial enlargement.

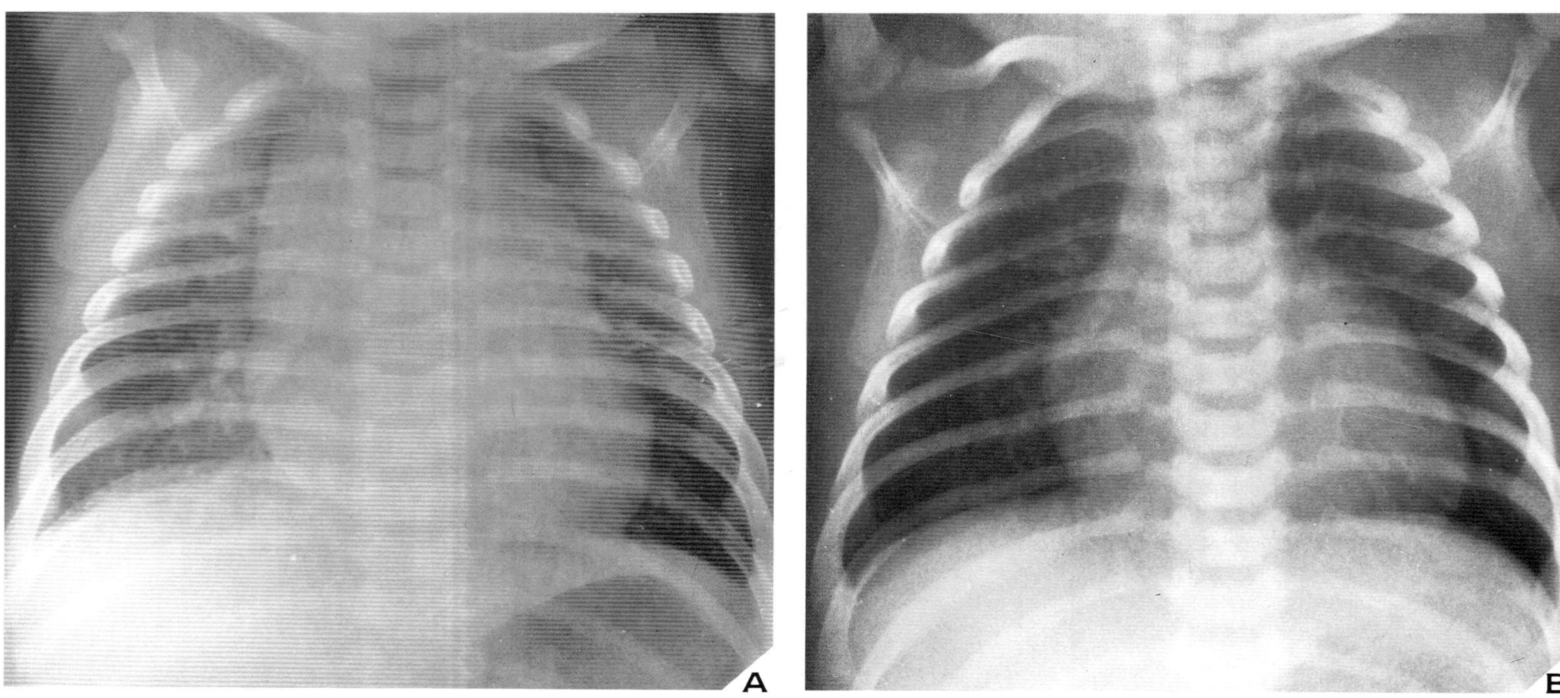

Fig. 7.4 Thymus mimicking mediastinal mass. (A) In this 1-month-old with transposition of the great arteries, the frontal film shows cardiac enlargement and increased pulmonary circulation. There is an apparent mass along the right cardiomediastinal border. (B) Several days later the apparent mass is much smaller. There is persistent cardiomegaly and pulmonary overcirculation. The "mass" represented normal thymus, which has undergone spontaneous involution owing to stress in this seriously ill infant.

NORMAL AND ABNORMAL PULMONARY VASCULARITY

NEONATE

The lungs of a normal neonate typically appear oligemic on chest films, owing to the physiologic elevation of pulmonary vascular resistance which is normally present during the first weeks of life. The elevated resistance limits the amount of blood that can flow into the lungs across a ventricular septal defect or patent ductus arteriosus; therefore, the presence of a left to right shunt may not be appreciated at this age. In general, increased pulmonary vascularity resulting from a left to right shunt cannot be appreciated radiographically until the pulmonary vascular resistance drops to more "adult" levels.

Elevated pulmonary venous pressure leads to accumulation of fluid in the interstitium, which can usually be detected on chest films. However, vascular redistribution to the upper lung fields ("cephalization"), a useful radiologic sign of pulmonary venous hypertension in older patients, is seldom evident on the supine films that are usually obtained in neonates.

INFANTS AND OLDER CHILDREN

Characteristic alterations of the normal pulmonary vascular pattern occur in many types of congenital or acquired heart disease. In general, these patterns are more easily appreciated after the neonatal period.

Abnormalities of the pulmonary vasculature associated with congenital heart disease include plethora, oligemia, pulmonary venous hypertension, asymmetrical or uneven distribution of pulmonary vessels, and a disordered pulmonary vascular pattern.

Pulmonary plethora reflects pulmonary overcirculation. Chest films show an increase in the size and number of pulmonary vessels. Pulmonary plethora in a cyanotic patient indicates the presence of an admixture lesion (eg, truncus arteriosus) (Fig. 7.5).

Pulmonary oligema reflects pulmonary undercirculation. Plain films show a decrease in the size and number of identifiable pulmonary vessels (Fig. 7.6).

The radiographic manifestations of *pulmonary venous hypertension* vary with the age of the patient. Infants exhibit in-

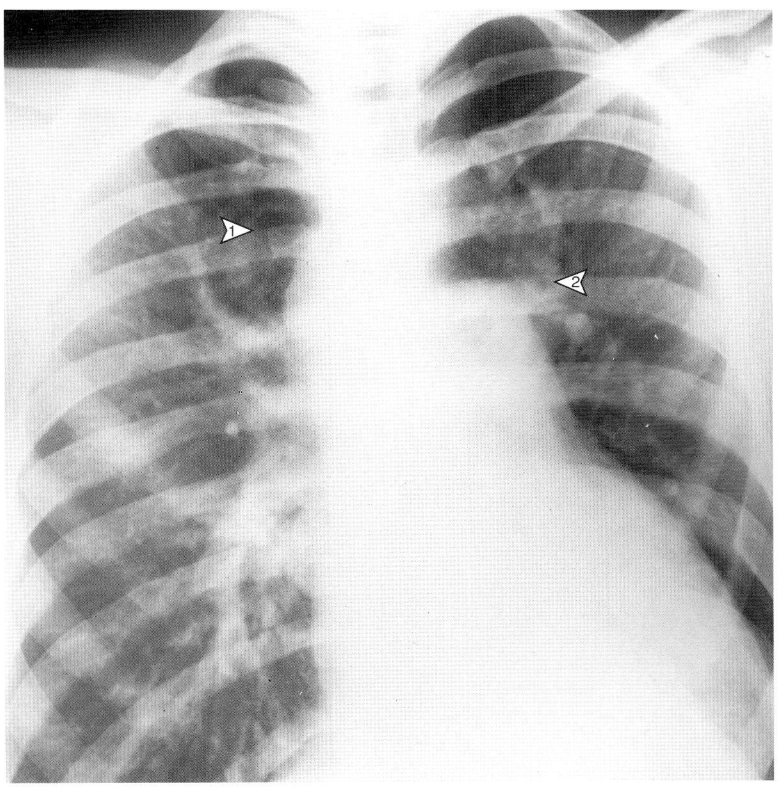

Fig. 7.5 Pulmonary plethora (truncus arteriosus). Anteroposterior supine chest film in a cyanotic 10-year-old patient. Although the pulmonary vessels are uniformly distributed, they are dilated and more numerous than normal. The presence of a right aortic arch (*arrow* 1), taken in conjunction with the cephalic displacement of the left pulmonary artery (*arrow* 2), strongly suggests the diagnosis of truncus arteriosus in a cyanotic patient.

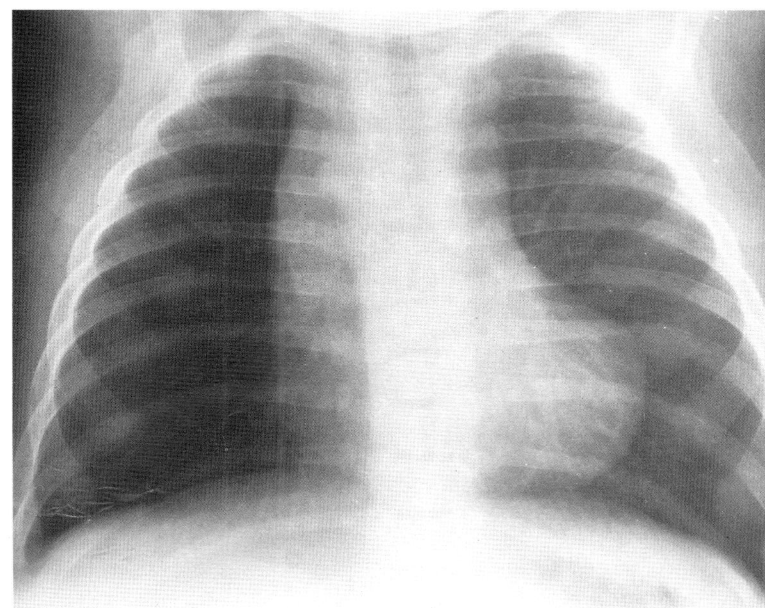

Fig. 7.6 Severe pulmonary oligemia. Supine chest film in a 2-day-old infant with severe cyanosis shows small, indistinct pulmonary vascular markings throughout both lungs.

terstitial or alveolar pulmonary edema; the former causes the pulmonary vessels to appear indistinct, whereas the latter produces central or generalized airspace opacification (Fig. 7.7). In older children, the radiographic signs of pulmonary venous hypertension are similar to those seen in adults, ie, septal (Kerley A, B, and C) lines and redistribution of blood flow to the upper zones ("cephalization").

Certain cardiac malformations are associated with an *asymmetric or uneven distribution* of pulmonary vessels. For example, asymmetric or uneven pulmonary perfusion (due to hypoplasia or aplasia of portions of the pulmonary arterial tree) is commonly seen in patients with tetralogy of Fallot (Fig. 7.8).

A *disordered pulmonary vascular pattern* is characteristic of certain cardiac malformations. In patients with pulmonary atresia and ventricular septal defect (VSD), for example, the lungs are perfused by collateral vessels which arise from the descending thoracic aorta and enter the lungs at various levels. Owing to their peculiar horizontal course, these aortopulmonary collaterals can often be identified on chest films (Fig. 7.9). Some patients with pulmonary atresia and VSD also exhibit pulmonary plethora.

ABNORMAL MEDIASTINAL CONFIGURATION

Malformations or disorders resulting in an abnormal mediastinal configuration include pulmonary atresia, left superior vena cava, azygos distension, and right aortic arch. A concavity of the left mediastinal contour caudad to the level of the aortic arch usually indicates hypoplasia or atresia of the main pulmonary trunk (Figs. 7.8 and 7.10). A straight, vertically oriented

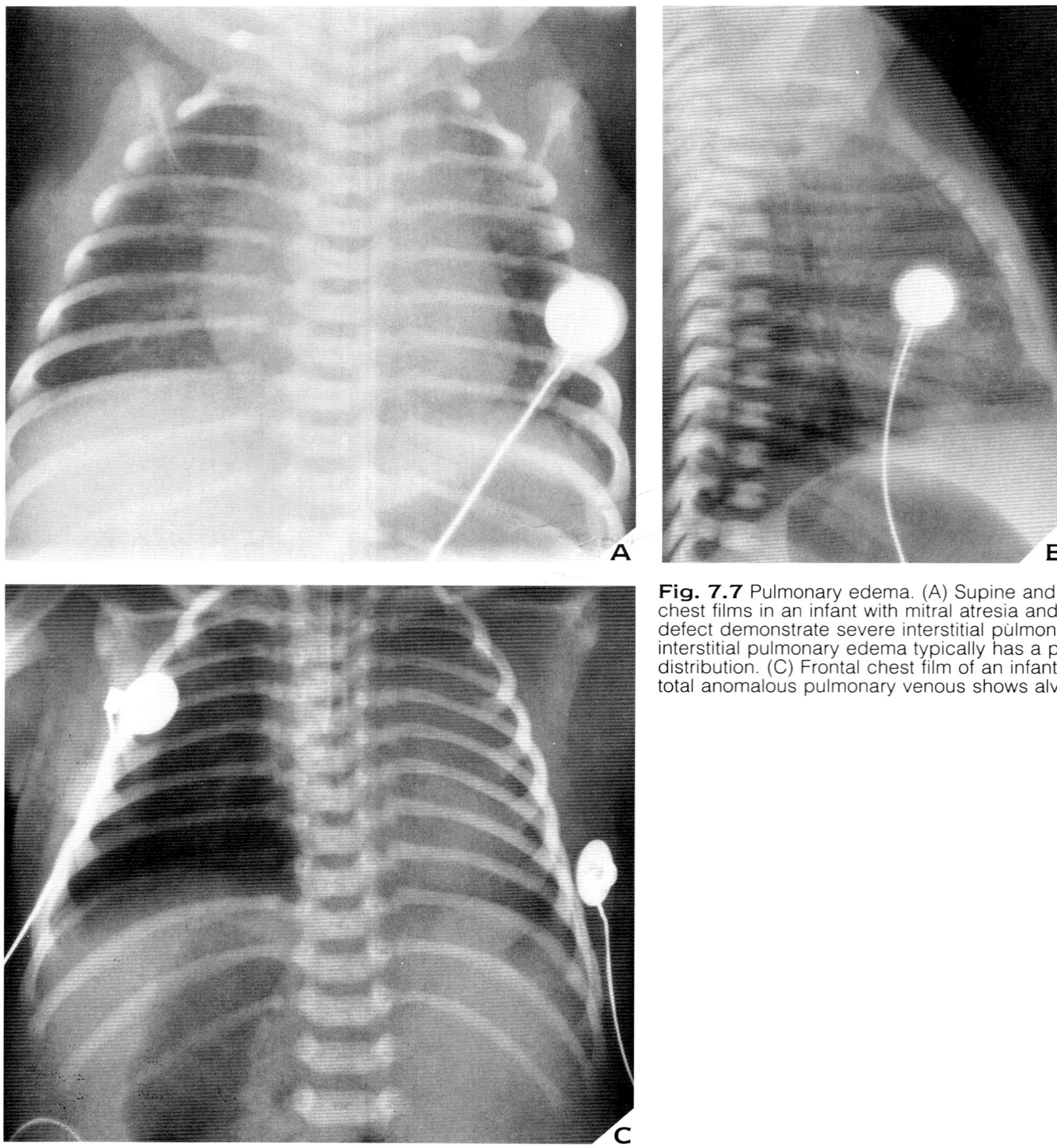

A B C

Fig. 7.7 Pulmonary edema. (A) Supine and (B) recumbent lateral chest films in an infant with mitral atresia and restricted atrial septal defect demonstrate severe interstitial pulmonary edema. In infants, interstitial pulmonary edema typically has a perihilar and retrosternal distribution. (C) Frontal chest film of an infant with infradiaphragmatic total anomalous pulmonary venous shows alveolar pulmonary edema.

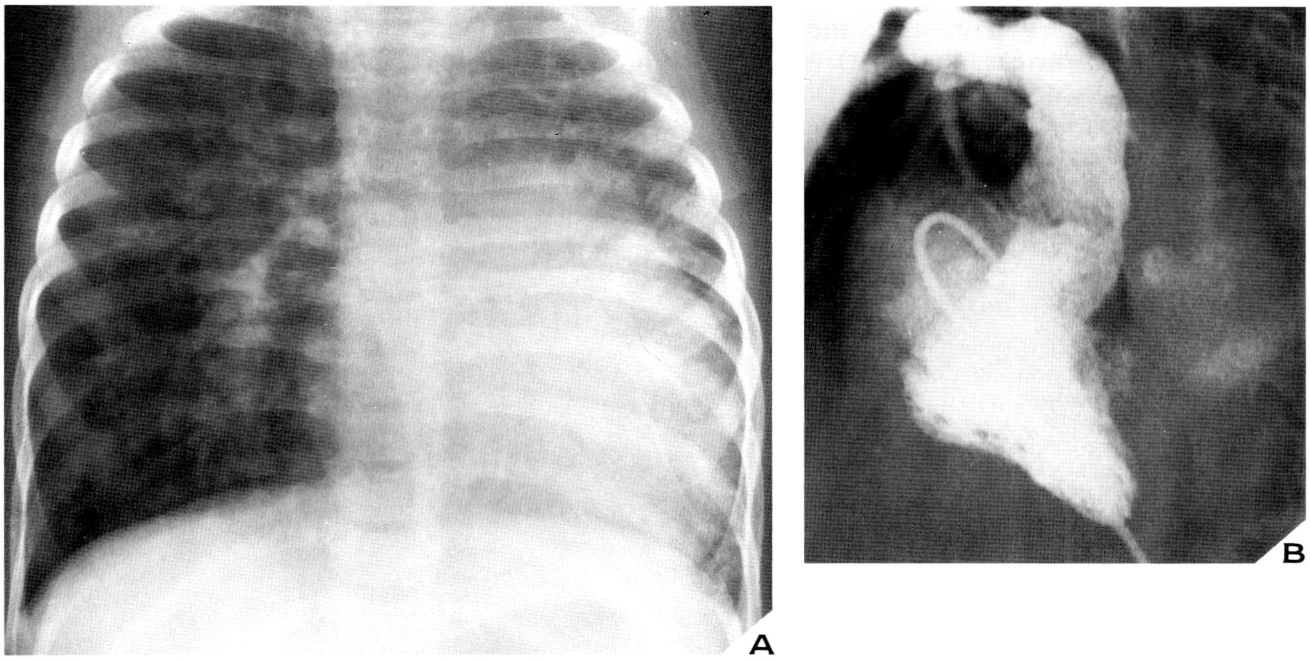

Fig. 7.8 Asymmetrical pulmonary perfusion. (A) Upright frontal chest film shows asymmetrical pulmonary perfusion: the left lung is oligemic and the right plethoric. The mediastinum is displaced to the left. The configuration of the left heart border indicates right ventricular enlargement. (B) Right ventriculogram (left anterior oblique projection) demonstrates absence of the left pulmonary artery, accounting for the pulmonary oligemia on the left.

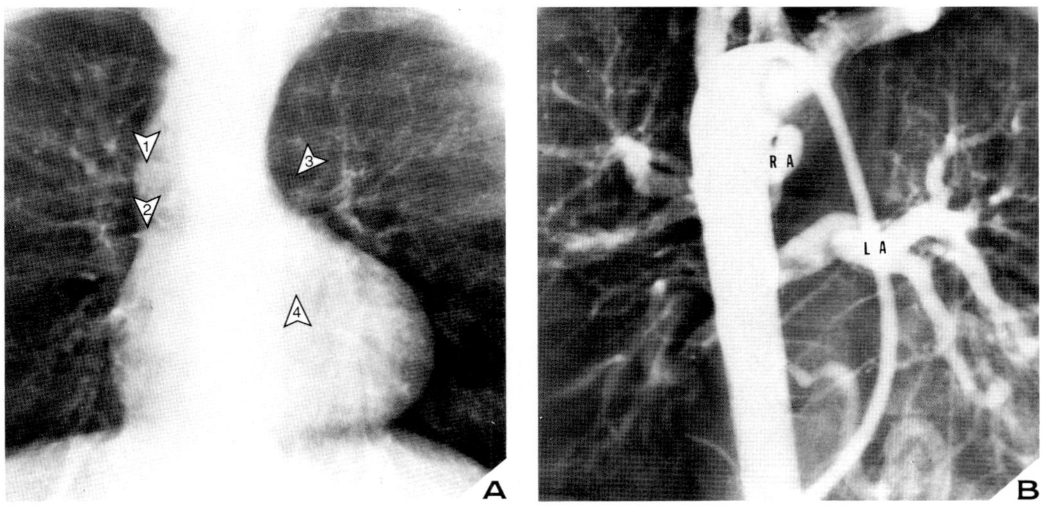

Fig. 7.9 Pulmonary atresia with aortopulmonary collaterals. (A) Upright posteroanterior chest film in a patient with pulmonary atresia, ventricular septal defect, right aortic arch, and right descending thoracic aorta. The pulmonary trunk is absent. The arteries supplying the right lung (*arrows* 1 and 2) arise at different levels. The blood supply to the left lung is provided by two separate arteries (*arrows* 3 and 4). The branches to the right upper zone are normally distributed. (B) Thoracic aortogram demonstrates aortopulmonary collaterals corresponding to the abnormally positioned pulmonary vessels seen on the chest film. (RA = right aorto-pulmonary collaterals; LA = left aorto-pulmonary collaterals)

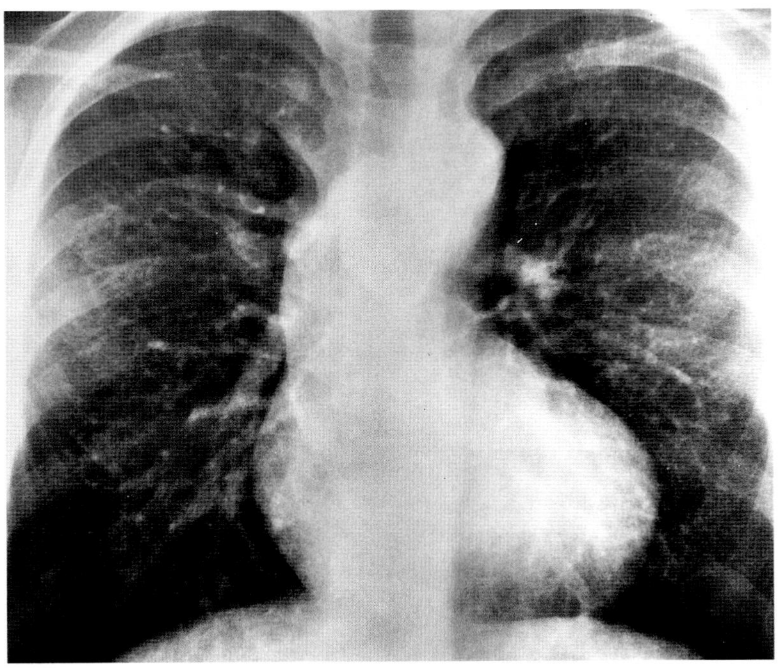

Fig. 7.10 Pulmonary atresia with hypoplastic main pulmonary artery. Supine chest film in a cyanotic patient demonstrates pulmonary oligemia. Note the concavity in the region normally occupied by the main pulmonary artery. The uplifted apex is formed by the hypertrophied right ventricle in this patient with pulmonary atresia and ventricular septal defect. The aortic arch is on the left.

contact between the anterior margin of the heart and the anterior chest wall (Fig. 7.14B). In patients with left ventricular enlargement, plain films show prominence of the left cardiac border and inferior displacement of the apex (Fig. 7.15). Radiographic findings of left atrial enlargement include a double density within the right side of the cardiac silhouette, widening of the carinal angle, posterior displacement of the left main bronchus, and an anterior impression on the barium-filled esophagus (Fig. 7.16).

ABNORMALITIES OF THE BONY THORAX

Some cardiac malformations are commonly associated with abnormalities of the ribs, sternum, and/or thoracic spine; conversely, certain skeletal abnormalities are associated with specific cardiac malformations. Abnormalities of the bony thorax and cardiovascular system occur together in several genetic syndromes and chromosomal disorders (Fig. 7.17). For exam-

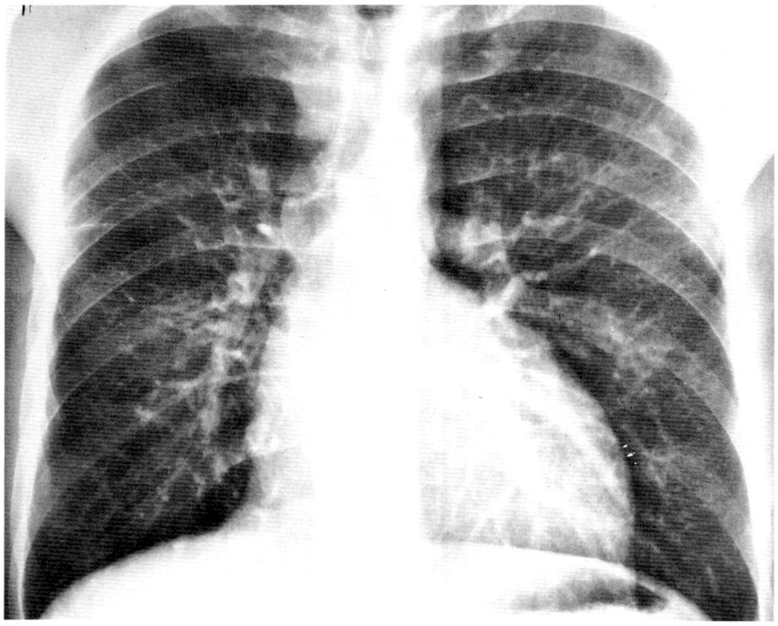

Fig. 7.15 Left ventricular enlargement. Posteroanterior film shows the characteristic appearance of left ventricular enlargement in a patient with tricuspid atresia. The apex is displaced downward.

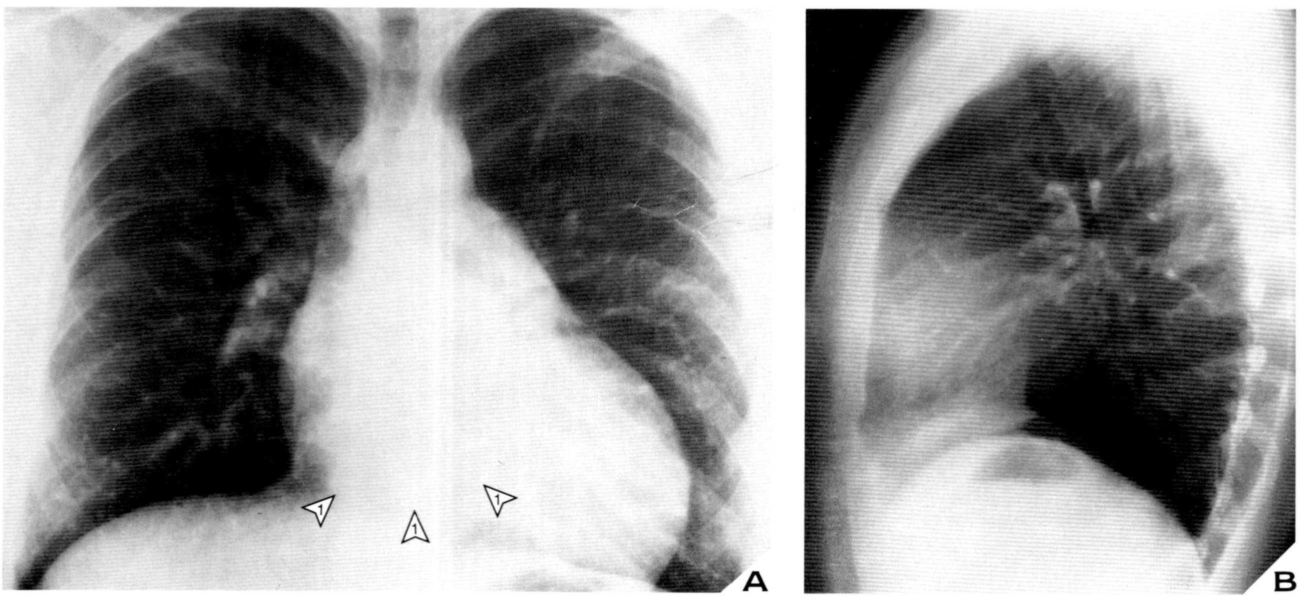

Fig. 7.16 Left atrial and right ventricular enlargement. (A) Frontal chest film of a patient with a ventricular septal defect show an enlarged left atrium [manifested by a double density within the right heart border (*arrows* in A)], a prominent pulmonary trunk, right ventricular enlargement (note upturned apex), and pulmonary plethora. (B) The lateral projection reveals increased contact between the heart and the anterior chest wall caused by the enlarged right ventricle.

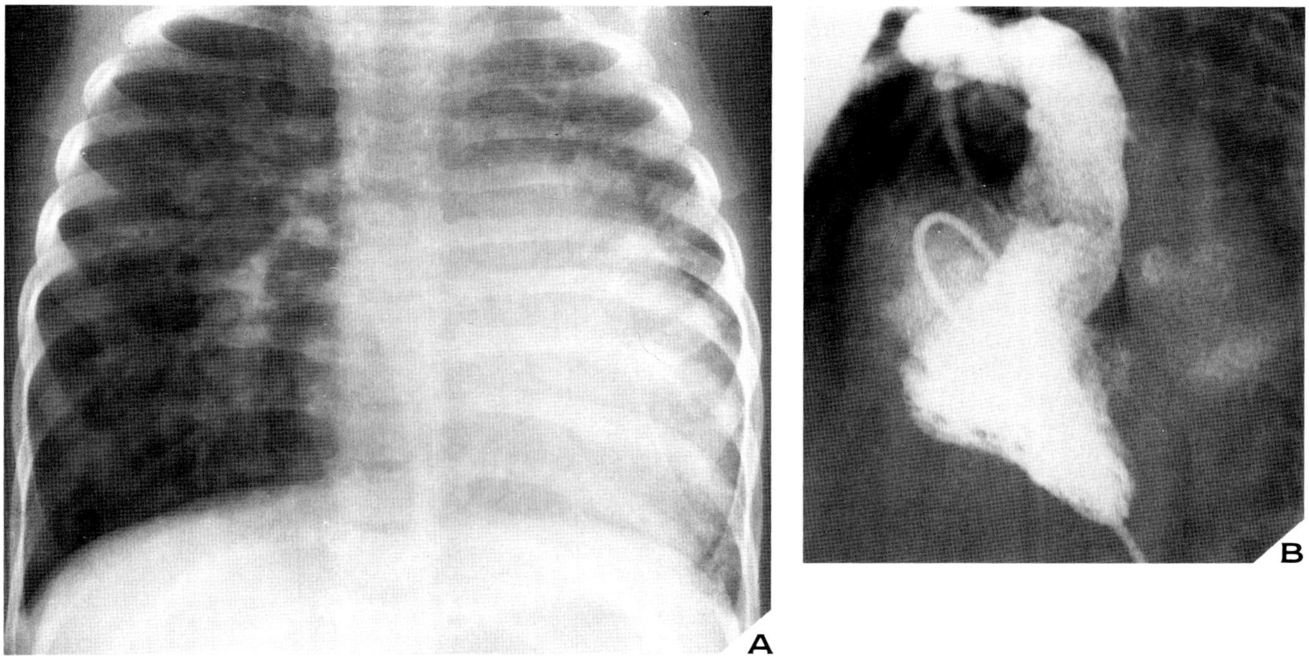

Fig. 7.8 Asymmetrical pulmonary perfusion. (A) Upright frontal chest film shows asymmetrical pulmonary perfusion: the left lung is oligemic and the right plethoric. The mediastinum is displaced to the left. The configuration of the left heart border indicates right ventricular enlargement. (B) Right ventriculogram (left anterior oblique projection) demonstrates absence of the left pulmonary artery, accounting for the pulmonary oligemia on the left.

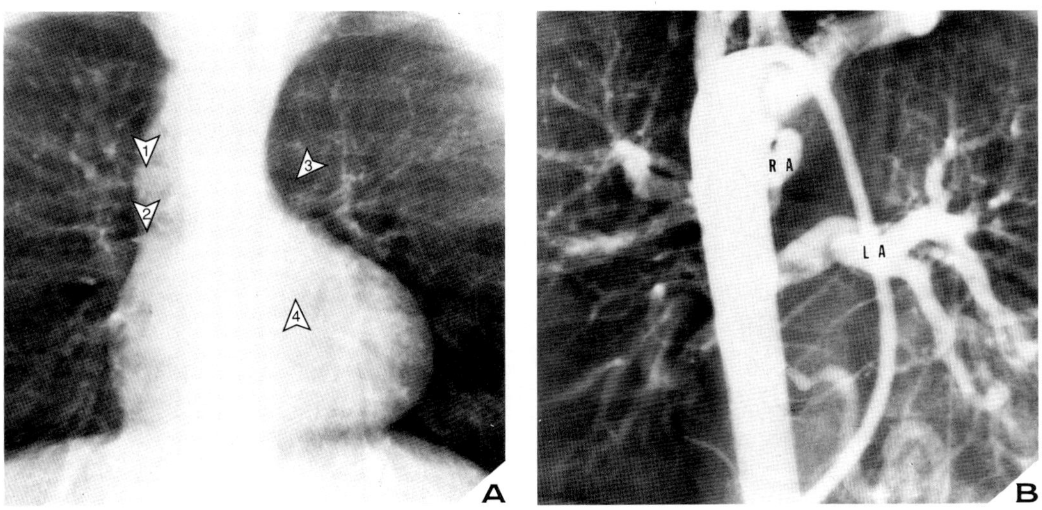

Fig. 7.9 Pulmonary atresia with aortopulmonary collaterals. (A) Upright posteroanterior chest film in a patient with pulmonary atresia, ventricular septal defect, right aortic arch, and right descending thoracic aorta. The pulmonary trunk is absent. The arteries supplying the right lung (*arrows* 1 and 2) arise at different levels. The blood supply to the left lung is provided by two separate arteries (*arrows* 3 and 4). The branches to the right upper zone are normally distributed. (B) Thoracic aortogram demonstrates aortopulmonary collaterals corresponding to the abnormally positioned pulmonary vessels seen on the chest film. (RA = right aorto-pulmonary collaterals; LA = left aorto-pulmonary collaterals)

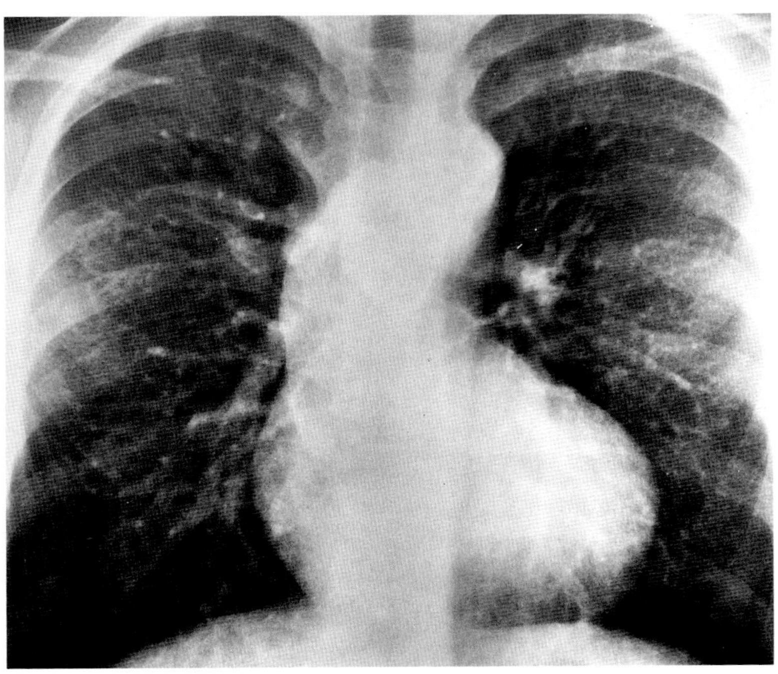

Fig. 7.10 Pulmonary atresia with hypoplastic main pulmonary artery. Supine chest film in a cyanotic patient demonstrates pulmonary oligemia. Note the concavity in the region normally occupied by the main pulmonary artery. The uplifted apex is formed by the hypertrophied right ventricle in this patient with pulmonary atresia and ventricular septal defect. The aortic arch is on the left.

left upper mediastinal border that lies lateral to the aortic arch suggests the presence of a left superior vena cava (Fig. 7.11). A dilated azygos vein appears as a soft tissue opacity within the right tracheobronchial angle; it may be quite large (Fig. 7.12; see also Fig. 7.3). (In a child, the presence of a dilated azygos vein usually indicates interruption of the suprarenal portion of the inferior vena cava, an anomaly in which blood from the lower half of the body returns to the heart via the azygos and hemiazygos systems.) A localized indentation of the right side of the trachea, just above the carina, usually indicates the presence of a right aortic arch (see Fig. 7.10). This anomaly is generally associated with an aberrant (anomalous) left subclavian artery, which produces an oblique indentation on the posterior aspect of the esophagus (Fig. 7.13; see also Chapter 15).

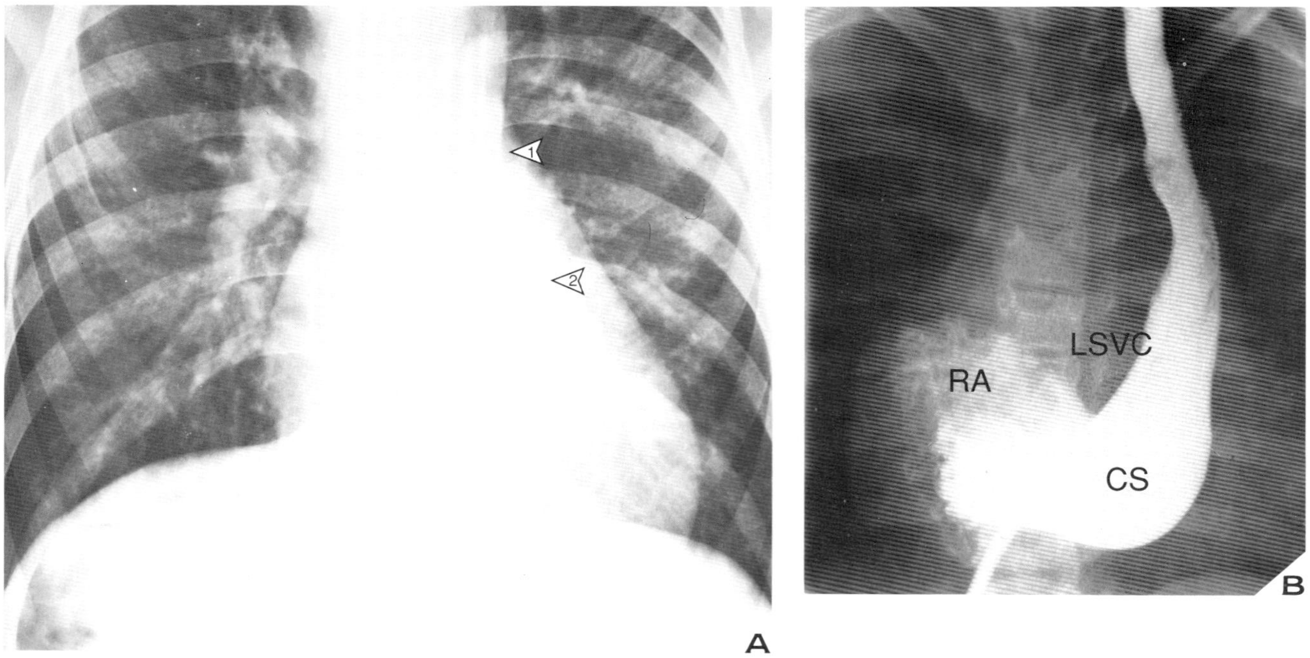

Fig. 7.11 Left superior vena cava. (A) Upright posteroanterior chest film in a 15-year-old patient with a large left superior vena cava (*arrow* 1) that enters the coronary sinus. There is pulmonary plethora secondary to an associated atrial septal defect. The pulmonary trunk is indicated by *arrow* 2. (B) Angiogram in a different patient demonstrates a left superior vena cava (LSVC) emptying into the coronary sinus (CS) and thence into the right atrium (RA).

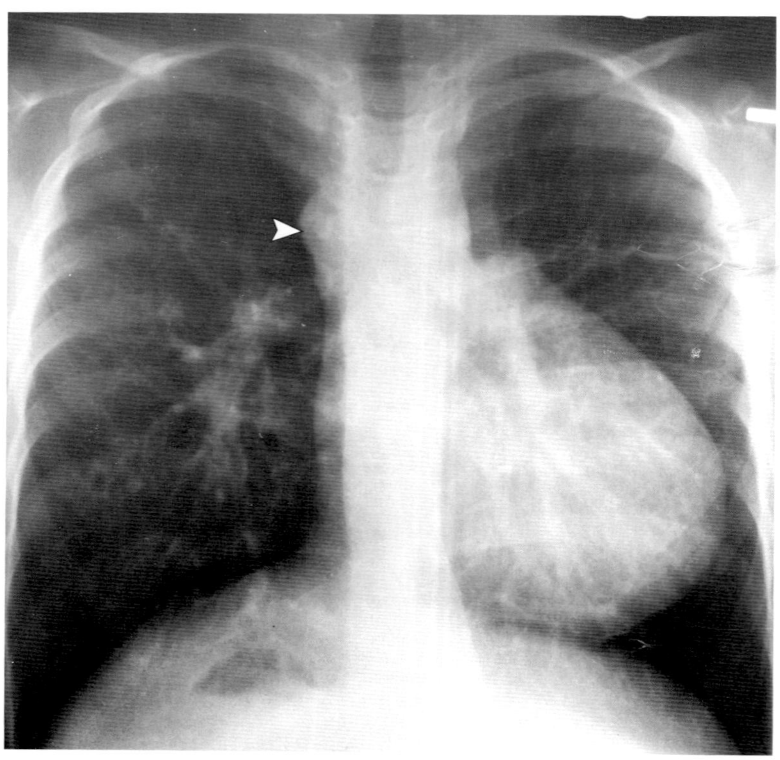

Fig. 7.12 Dilated azygos vein. Posteroanterior chest film demonstrates cardiac enlargement and plethora. Note the large soft tissue mass (*arrow*) which bulges the mediastinal contour at the level of the right tracheobronchial angle. The "mass" represents a dilated azygos vein which is receiving all of the venous return from the right lung in this patient with left atrial isomerism and interruption of the inferior vena cava. A gastric air bubble is on the right.

ABNORMAL CARDIOVASCULAR SILHOUETTE

Enlargement of one or more chambers produces characteristic alterations of the cardiac silhouette. In general, only gross cardiac enlargement can be appreciated on plain films. Mild to moderate cardiac enlargement is more readily detected by 2-D echocardiography (see Chapter 2).

Right atrial enlargement results in prominence of the right cardiac border (Fig. 7.14A). With right ventricular enlargement, the cardiac apex is upturned on the frontal view (Figs. 7.8 to 7.10, 7.12, and 7.14A), and the lateral view reveals increased

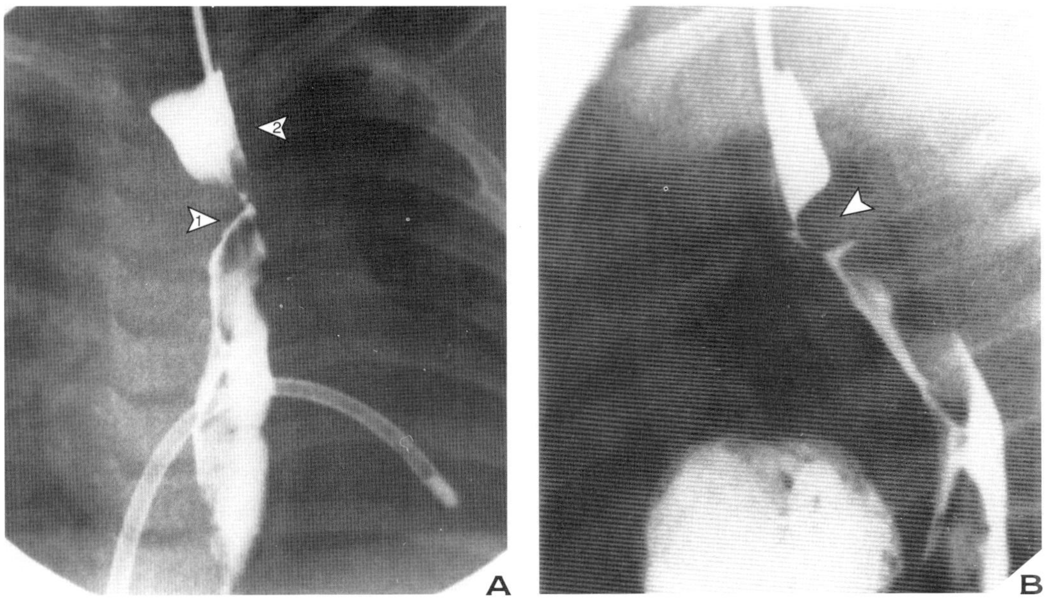

Fig. 7.13 Right aortic arch and aberrant left subclavian artery. (A) Frontal and (B) lateral views of cardiac series show a right aortic arch (*arrow* 1 in A). The aberrant subclavian artery produces a prominent impression on the posterior aspect of the esophagus (*arrow* in B) and a more subtle impression on the left side of the esophagus (*arrow* 2 in A) at the level of the aortic arch.

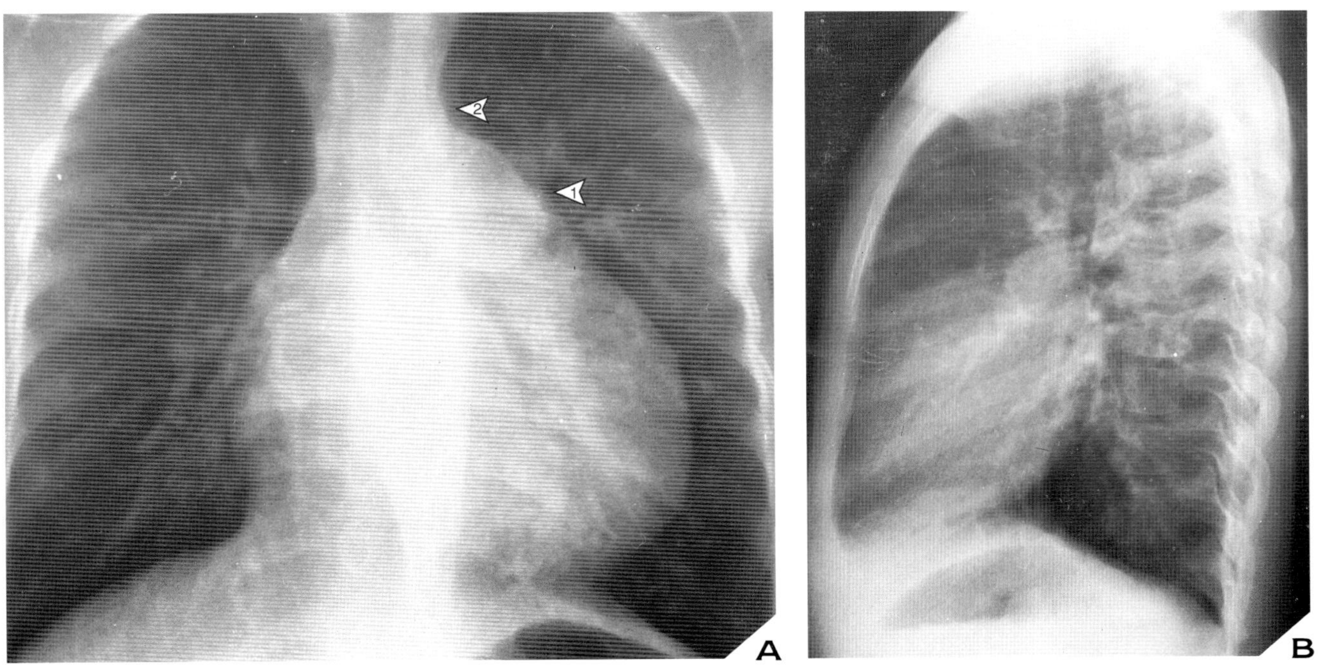

Fig. 7.14 Right atrial and right ventricular enlargement. (A) Anteroposterior chest film in a child with an atrial septal defect shows prominence of the right cardiac border, indicating right atrial enlargement. The upturned apex is evidence of right ventricular enlargement. The bulge of the left upper heart border (*arrow* 1) represents a dilated pulmonary trunk. The aortic arch is on the left *arrow* 2. (B) Lateral projection. Note the increased contact between the heart and the anterior chest wall owing to right ventricular enlargement.

contact between the anterior margin of the heart and the anterior chest wall (Fig. 7.14B). In patients with left ventricular enlargement, plain films show prominence of the left cardiac border and inferior displacement of the apex (Fig. 7.15). Radiographic findings of left atrial enlargement include a double density within the right side of the cardiac silhouette, widening of the carinal angle, posterior displacement of the left main bronchus, and an anterior impression on the barium-filled esophagus (Fig. 7.16).

ABNORMALITIES OF THE BONY THORAX

Some cardiac malformations are commonly associated with abnormalities of the ribs, sternum, and/or thoracic spine; conversely, certain skeletal abnormalities are associated with specific cardiac malformations. Abnormalities of the bony thorax and cardiovascular system occur together in several genetic syndromes and chromosomal disorders (Fig. 7.17). For exam-

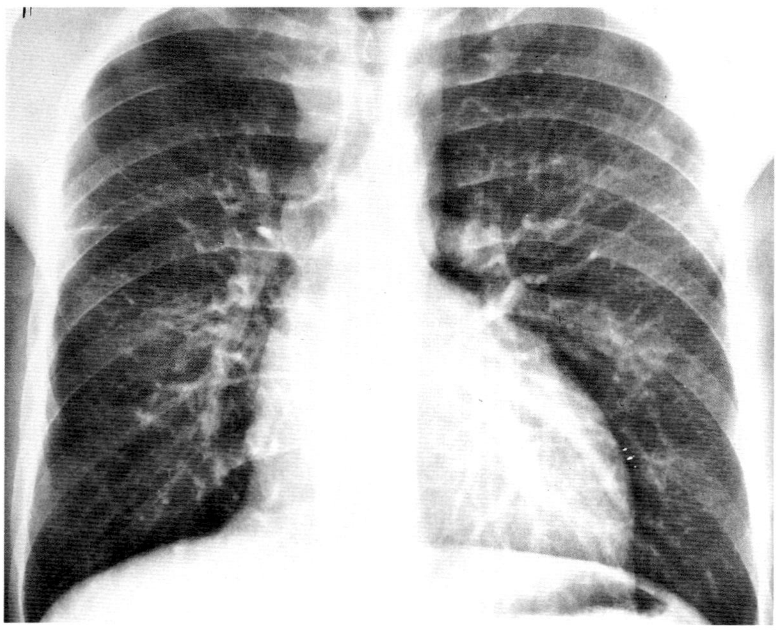

Fig. 7.15 Left ventricular enlargement. Posteroanterior film shows the characteristic appearance of left ventricular enlargement in a patient with tricuspid atresia. The apex is displaced downward.

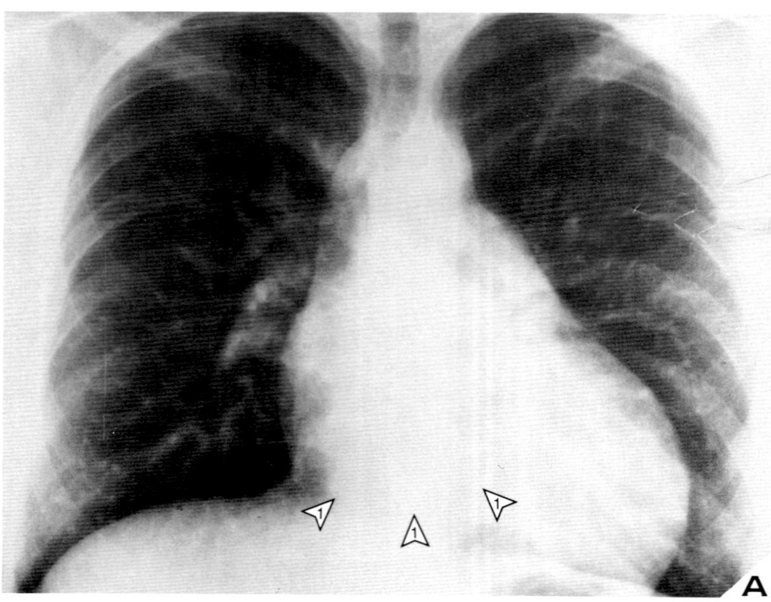

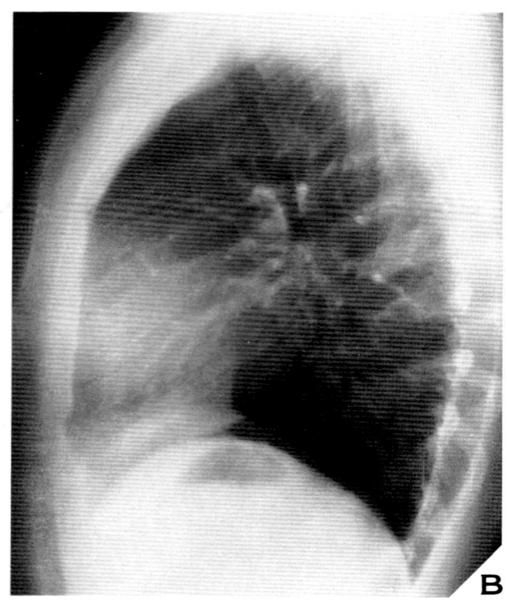

Fig. 7.16 Left atrial and right ventricular enlargement. (A) Frontal chest film of a patient with a ventricular septal defect show an enlarged left atrium [manifested by a double density within the right heart border (*arrows* in A)], a prominent pulmonary trunk, right ventricular enlargement (note upturned apex), and pulmonary plethora. (B) The lateral projection reveals increased contact between the heart and the anterior chest wall caused by the enlarged right ventricle.

FIG. 8.17 THORACIC ABNORMALITIES ASSOCIATED WITH CARDIAC DISORDERS

Abnormality (Syndrome/Disease)	Cardiac Disorder
Abnormal configuration	
Bell-shaped in infant [Down syndrome (trisomy 21)]	ASD, secundum ASD, atrioventricular canal, tetralogy of Fallot
Bell-shaped in older child or adult (muscular dystrophy)	Cardiomyopathy
Sternum	
Double or triple manubrial center (trisomy 21)	VSD, secundum ASD, atrioventricular canal, tetralogy of Fallot
Premature fusion of sternal centers	Cyanotic CHD (various defects)
Prominent lower sternum	VSD
Spine	
Scoliosis (Marfan syndrome)	Dilated aortic root, myxomatous degeneration of aortic and mitral valves
Scoliosis (paralytic secondary to muscular dystrophy)	Cardiomyopathy
Scoliosis (idiopathic)	Various cyanotic and acyanotic defects
Abnormal segmentation (Rubenstein–Taybi syndrome; Goldenhar syndrome; Turner syndrome; Noonan–Ulrich syndrome)	Various defects
Calcified intervertebral discs (alkaptanuria)	Early degeneration of valves with calcification (stenosis and insufficiency)
Vertebral deformities resembling Scheurmann's disease [Turner syndrome (XO karyotype); Noonan–Ulrich syndrome]	*Turner syndrome:* aortic coarctation *Noonan–Ulrich syndrome:* pulmonic stenosis, secundum ASD
Ribs	
Notching, hyperostosis or inferior rib margins	Coarctation of the aorta
Short ribs [Ellis–van Crevald syndrome (chondroectodermal dysplasia)]	VSD, ASD, atrioventricular canal, single atrium
Absent or dysmorphic ribs [Goldenhar syndrome (oculoauriculovertebral dysplasia)]	Various defects
Gracile ribs (trisomy 18)	VSD
Scapula	
Abnormal rotation (Holt–Oram syndrome)	Secundum ASD, conduction defect (prolonged P-R interval)
Clavicles	
"Handlebar" clavicles (trisomy 18)	VSD
Generalized bone disease	
Osteoporosis, fractures (osteogenesis imperfecta)	Aortic insufficiency (secondary to premature degeneration of leaflets)
Bizarre modeling disturbances, paddle ribs, deformed vertebrae [mucopolysaccharidosis I (Hurler) and II (Hunter)]	Valve lesions (especially mitral), cardiomyopathy
Coarse trabecular pattern, thin cortices (congenital anemias: thalassemia, sickle cell anemia)	High-output states
Decreased cortical bone formation, retarded bone area	Cyanotic CHD

Abbreviations: CHD = congenital heart disease; VSD = ventricular septal defect; ASD = atrial septal defect.

Fig. 7.17 Thoracic abnormalities associated with cardiac disorders.

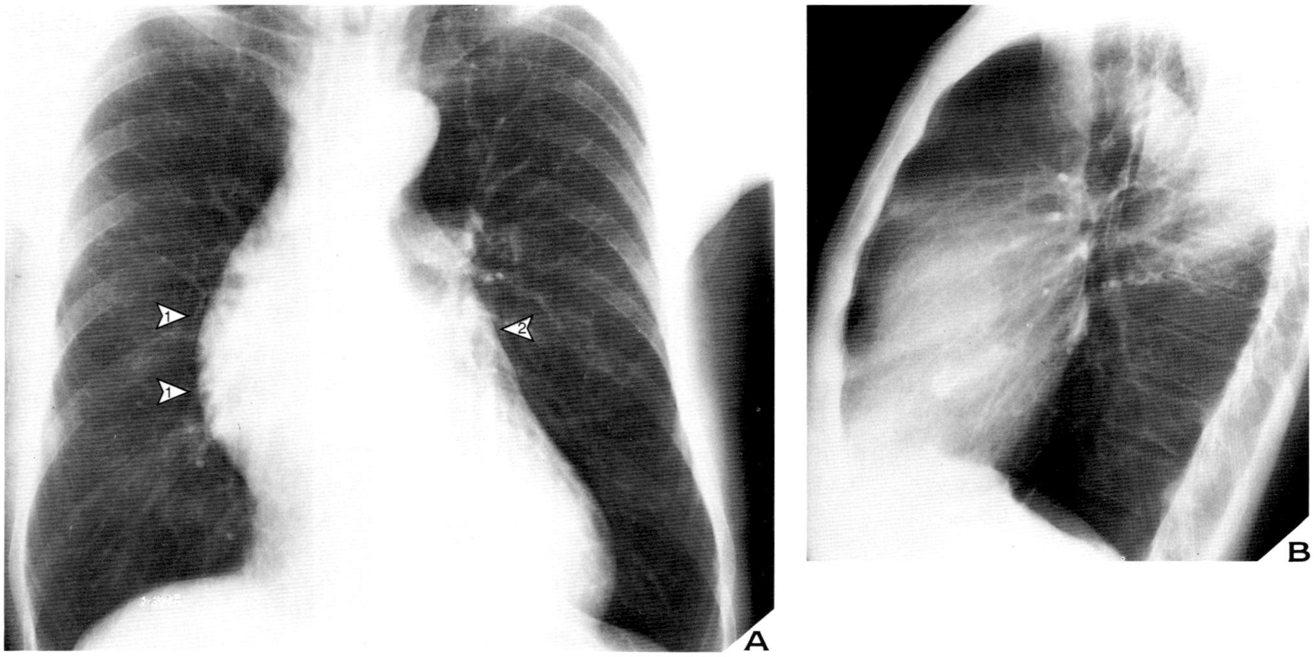

Fig. 7.18 Thoracic abnormalities secondary to Marfan syndrome. (A) Frontal and (B) lateral chest radiographs show a markedly elongated thorax and dextroscoliosis, characteristic features of Marfan syndrome. Note prominent contours produced by the dilated ascending aorta (*arrows* 1) and displaced pulmonary trunk (*arrow* 2) secondary to an aneurysm of the aortic root, a frequent complication of this genetic connective tissue disorder.

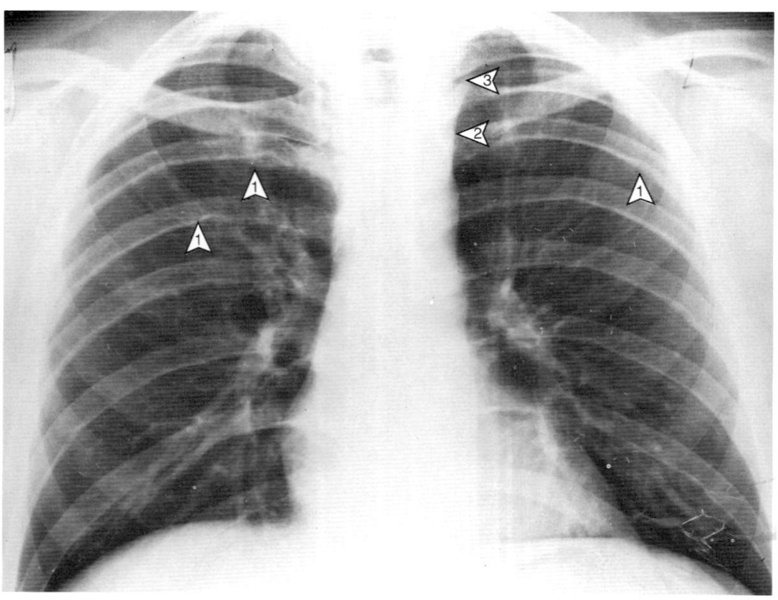

Fig. 7.19 Bilateral rib notching. Frontal projection of the chest in a patient with coarctation of the aorta demonstrates bilateral rib notching (*arrows* 1) caused by dilated, tortuous intercostal arteries. The diminutive aortic arch (*arrow* 2) and dilated left subclavian artery (*arrow* 3) are other classical features of coarctation of the aorta.

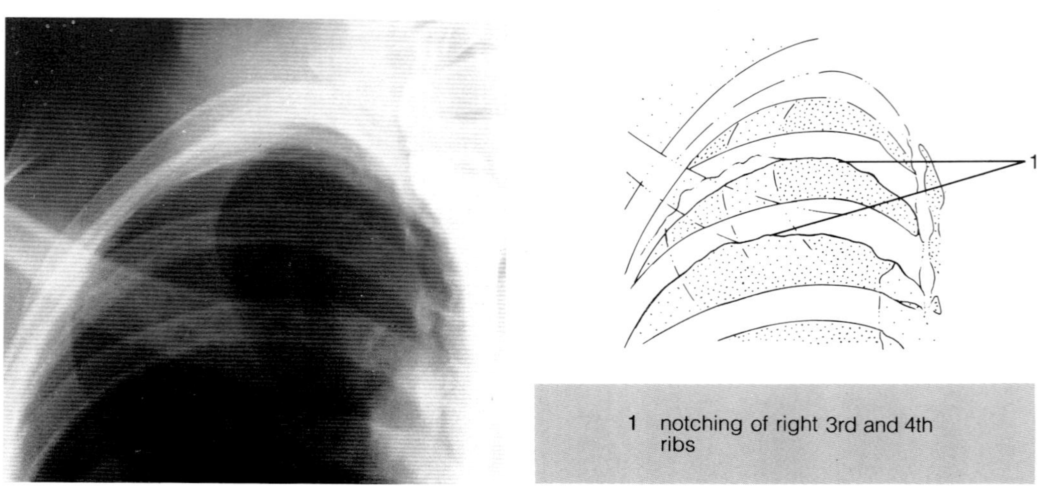

Fig. 7.20 Unilateral rib notching after palliative shunt. Chest film of a 20-year-old patient with tetralogy of Fallot who had previously undergone a left Blalock–Taussig anastomosis shows notching of the inferior borders of the right third and fourth ribs.

ple, hypersegmentation of the sternum, 11 ribs, and scoliosis are commonly seen in patients with trisomy 21 (Down syndrome), which is associated with VSD, atrioventricular septal defect (atrioventricular canal), tetralogy of Fallot, and secundum ASD (the first three of these account for more than 90 percent of the symptomatic congenital heart disease encountered in infants with this chromosomal defect). Thoracic abnormalities are also an important marker for certain types of acquired heart disease. Kyphoscoliosis and anterior chest wall deformities, for example, are common in patients with Marfan syndrome (Fig. 7.18).

RIBS

Rib notching is a common finding in patients with coarctation of the aorta (Fig. 7.19; see also Chapter 12). Caused by dilated and tortuous intercostal arteries, rib notching is manifested radiographically by erosions of the inferior aspect of the fourth and more caudal ribs. (Although rib notching secondary to aortic coarctation is almost always bilateral, it may be unilateral in the rare patient whose coarcted segment is proximal to the origin of either the left of the right subclavian artery.) Unilateral rib notching on the side of the thoracotomy is quite common in patients with cyanotic congenital heart disease who have had a palliative Blalock–Taussig shunt (pulmonary artery to subclavian artery anastomosis) performed early in life (Fig. 7.20).

STERNUM

Sternal abnormalities may be a clue to the presence of congenital heart disease. Early fusion of the sternal segments (manubrial–sternal joint or mesosternum) occurs more often in patients with cyanotic congenital malformations than in the general population, whereas delayed fusion is associated with various cardiac defects (Fig. 7.21). Hypersegmentation of the sternum (multiple ossification centers with delayed fusion) is not uncommon in children with trisomy 21.

SPINE

Scoliosis occurs in 6 percent of patients with cyanotic disorders and in 0.8 percent of those with acyanotic defects. It is much more frequent in females with cyanotic conditions than in males with acyanotic disorders. The spinal curvature usually involves the thoracolumbar segment, although in some instances only the thoracic segment is affected (Fig. 7.22). An underlying structural malformation (eg, butterfly vertebra, hemivertebrae) is present in a small percentage of cases.

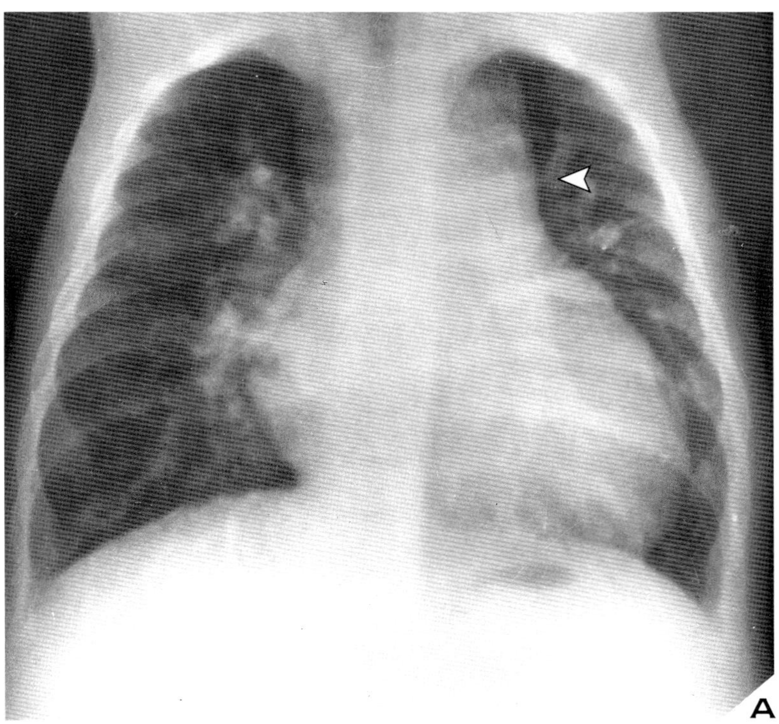

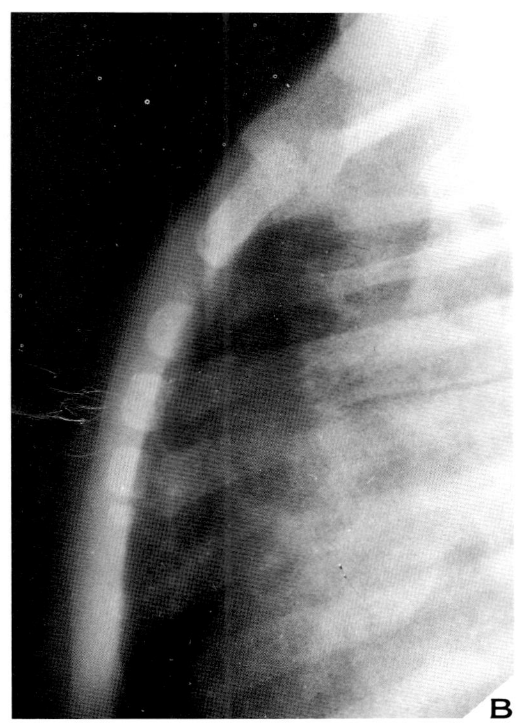

Fig. 7.21 Sternal malformation associated with atrioventricular septal defect. Frontal (A) and lateral (B) projections show hypersegmentation of the sternum in a child with an atrioventricular septal defect ("atrioventricular canal"). The enlarged right ventricle (note elevated cardiac apex), pulmonary plethora, and enlarged pulmonary trunk indicate the presence of a left-to-right shunt. A persistent left superior vena cava (*arrow*) is common in patients with atrioventricular septal defects.

CHAPTER 8

Abnormalities of the Atrial Segment

NORMAL ATRIAL MORPHOLOGY

The atrial chambers are normally asymmetrical, each having its own unique morphologic features. The atria can be characterized as *left-type* or *right-type* on the basis of their distinctive internal architecture and the configuration of the atrial appendage.

ATRIAL ISOMERISM

Atrial isomerism refers to a condition in which the atria, normally anatomically distinct, are morphologically similar, each having the anatomic characteristics of a normal right atrium or a normal left atrium. Atrial isomerism is commonly associated with major cardiovascular and extracardiac malformations.

MORPHOLOGY

RIGHT ATRIAL ISOMERISM

In right atrial isomerism, both atria resemble a normal right atrium (Fig. 8.1). The atrial appendages are triangular in shape and have a broad connection to the body of the atrium. Internally, each atrium has a crista terminalis, and the trabecular structure of the atrial wall is characteristic of the normal right atrium. Only rarely is the atrial septum intact; in most instances there is a large atrial septal defect (ASD) which includes the inferior and middle portion of the septum. (At first glance, right atrial isomerism with a giant ASD can be mistaken for a single atrium; however, the presence of two atrial appendages indicates the correct diagnosis.)

The most common associated cardiac anomaly is total anomalous pulmonary venous connection (TAPVC). This is not surprising, because the pulmonary veins normally connect with the morphologic left atrium, which is absent in these hearts. TAPVC associated with right atrial isomerism is usually of the supracardiac type, in which the pulmonary veins drain into the right superior vena cava (SVC), left SVC, or innominate vein. Less often, the pulmonary veins drain into the azygos system or inferior vena cava (IVC). In some instances, the pulmonary veins drain into a common channel which is connected to the posterior aspect of the chamber through a narrow aperture, an arrangement that can be considered a variety of cor triatriatum (see Chapter 12). Finally, the pulmonary veins may drain directly into each atrium in which case those pulmonary veins that drain into the right atrium are anomalous.

Abnormalities of the systemic veins are very common in patients with right atrial isomerism. Bilateral superior venae cavae are present in about 70 percent (occasionally the right SVC is hypoplastic). Not infrequently, the coronary sinus is absent, in which case the left SVC drains directly into the left-sided atrial chamber. The abdominal segment of the IVC often lies to the left of the aorta.

Right atrial isomerism is commonly, but not always, associated with absence or (rarely) hypoplasia of the spleen and abdominal heterotaxia. [The latter term refers to malposition and malfixation of the stomach and incomplete rotation of the intestine, with variable abdominal symmetry and displacement and dysmorphism of asymmetric structures.] Extracardiac abnormalities associated with right isomerism include imperforate anus, diaphragmatic hernia, symmetrical liver (right and left lobes of almost equal size), midline gallbladder, agenesis of the gallbladder, kidney abnormalities (renal dysplasia, cystic kidneys, fused kidneys), adrenal abnormalities (fused or horseshoe adrenals, unilateral absence of the adrenal gland), and bicornuate uterus.

It should be emphasized that there is a poor correlation between the morphology of the spleen and the morphology of the atria, whereas there is a strong correlation between the appearance of the tracheobronchial tree (to be discussed later) and atrial morphology. For this reason, we prefer to use the term *right atrial isomerism* when describing the cardiovascular malformations that are commonly found in patients with asplenia and heterotaxy but which may also occur in patients with a normal spleen and normal abdominal situs.

LEFT ATRIAL ISOMERISM

In left atrial isomerism, both atria have the morphologic features of a left atrium. Each atrial appendage is a long channel with a narrow connection to the body of the atrium (Fig. 8.2). Both atria have a relatively smooth, poorly trabeculated endo-

CHAPTER LABELING KEY			
RA	right atrium	RV	right ventricle
LA	left atrium	LV	left ventricle

cardial surface with absence of the crista terminalis, which are characteristic features of the normal left atrium.

The most important cardiovascular malformation associated with left atrial isomerism is anomalous connection of the systemic veins. The suprarenal segment of IVC is commonly absent, the hepatic veins connecting to one or both atria. Not infrequently, the abdominal segment of the IVC lies to the left of the aorta. Bilateral superior venae cavae and absence or hypoplasia of the right SVC are also common. The coronary sinus is absent in about two thirds of cases. Unlike right atrial isomerism, the pulmonary veins connect to the left atrium (usually to the left-sided atrium); however, variations in the site of the connection are common.

Left atrial isomerism is commonly (but not invariably) associated with polysplenia and abdominal heterotaxia. Extracardiac abnormalities associated with the left isomerism/polysplenia/heterotaxia complex (''polysplenia syndrome'') include a right-sided stomach, hepatic symmetry, intestinal malrotation, absent gallbladder, extrahepatic biliary atresia, preduodenal portal vein, esophageal atresia, renal abnormalities, and vertebral abnormalities.

As noted above, there is a poor correlation between the morphology of the spleen and the morphology of the atria. For this reason, we prefer to use the term *left atrial isomerism* to describe the cardiovascular malformations commonly found in patients with multiple splenules, but which may also occur in patients with a normal spleen.

CARDIAC MALFORMATIONS ASSOCIATED WITH ATRIAL ISOMERISM

In general, atrial isomerism indicates the presence of a severe malformation of the pulmonary or systemic venous connection; right atrial isomerism is typically associated with TAPVC, whereas left atrial isomerism is typically associated with anomalous systemic venous connection. Both right and left isomerism are frequently associated with other cardiac malformations. Most patients with right isomerism have a univentricular heart with a common atrioventricular valve. Absence of one atrioventricular valve is common in right isomerism but rare in left isomerism. The ventriculoarterial connection is frequently abnormal in patients with atrial isomerism. The most common abnormality is double-outlet ventricle, which occurs in about half the cases. Transposition of the great arteries occurs in 20 percent and pulmonary atresia in 9 percent. Transposition is more commonly seen with left isomerism, and pulmonic atresia with right isomerism.

CLINICAL FEATURES

The clinical manifestations of atrial isomerism are related to the associated cardiac defects, which are discussed elsewhere. Patients with the ''asplenia syndrome'' frequently have Howell–Jolly bodies and Heinz bodies in the peripheral blood. As with patients who have undergone splenectomy, patients with congenital asplenia have a high incidence of sepsis (about 25 per-

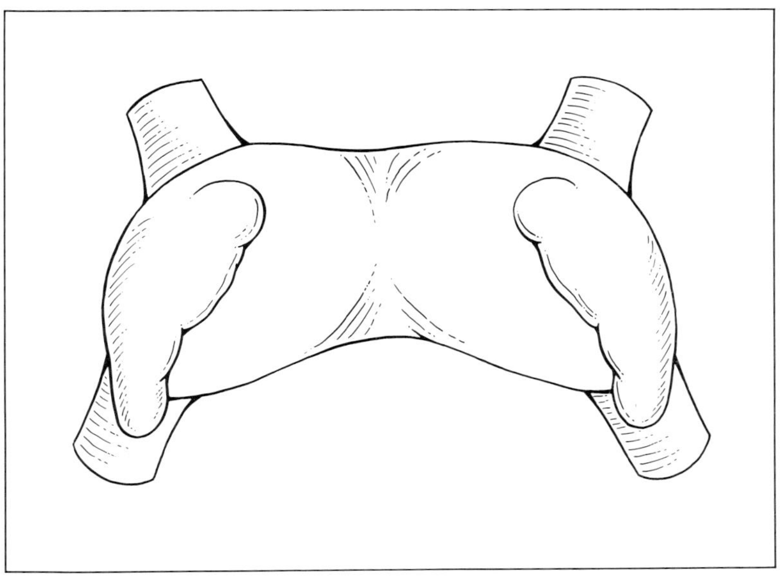

Fig. 8.1 Right atrial isomerism: appearance of atrial appendages. The right- and left-sided atrial appendages have the configuration of the normal right atrial appendage, ie, a triangular shape and a wide connection to the body of the atrium.

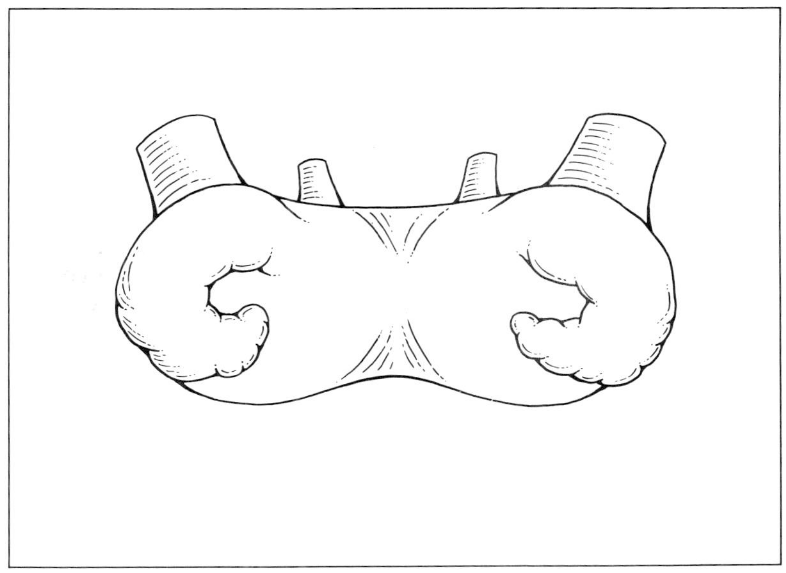

Fig. 8.2 Left atrial isomerism: appearance of atrial appendages. The right- and left-sided atrial appendages have the configuration of a normal left atrial appendage; both are large, somewhat elongated channels with a relatively narrow connection to the body of the atrium.

cent). An occasional patient with right or left isomerism may present with vomiting or acute abdominal signs secondary to obstructing duodenal bands or midgut volvulus.

IMAGING AND INVASIVE DIAGNOSIS

PLAIN FILMS

If the trachea and main bronchi can be identified on the chest film, one can predict the morphology and relationships of the atria (see Chapter 7). High-kilovoltage films show large airways more clearly than conventional plain films, and may be helpful when the latter are inconclusive. The large airways, as well as their relationship to the main pulmonary arteries, are clearly seen on MRI.

The main bronchi are normally of unequal length, the lung on the side of the longer bronchus representing the morphologic left lung. In *atrial situs solitus* (the normal relationship) the lungs are asymmetrical; the left main bronchus is considerably longer than its mate, with a left to right ratio of 1.4 to 1 or greater (Fig. 8.3). In *atrial situs inversus,* the lungs and mainstem bronchi are also asymmetrical; however, the morphologic left lung is on the right and the morphologic right lung is on the left. The right-sided (morphologic left) main bronchus is considerably longer than the left-sided (morphologic right) main bronchus, ie, the ratio of the right main bronchus to the left main bronchus is 1.4 to 1 or greater (Fig. 8.4).

Symmetry of the main bronchi (ie, left bronchus to right bronchus ratio less than 1.4 to 1) strongly suggests the presence of atrial isomerism. In *right thoracic isomerism,* both main bronchi are of the "right" type and both lungs are morphologic right lungs (three lobes, eparterial bronchus) (Fig. 8.5). On the frontal chest film the left and right pulmonary arteries lie infe-

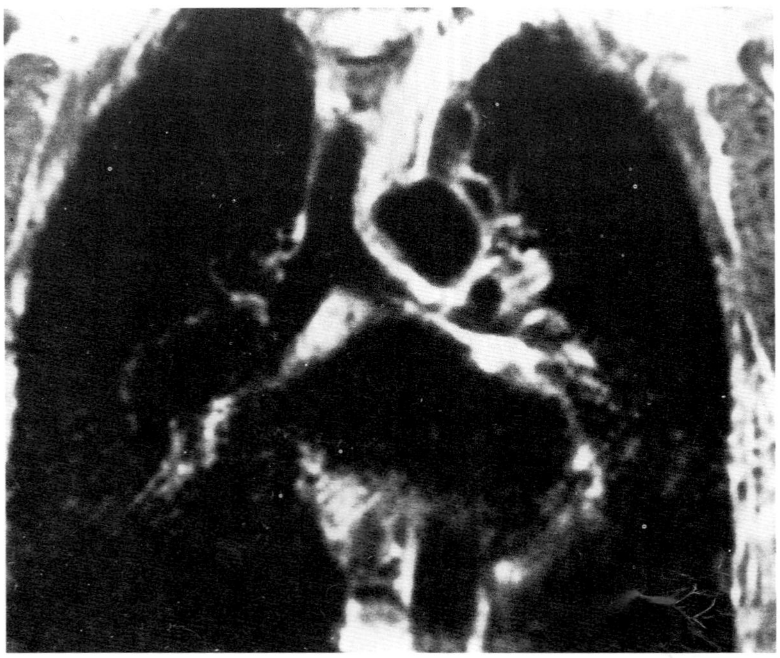

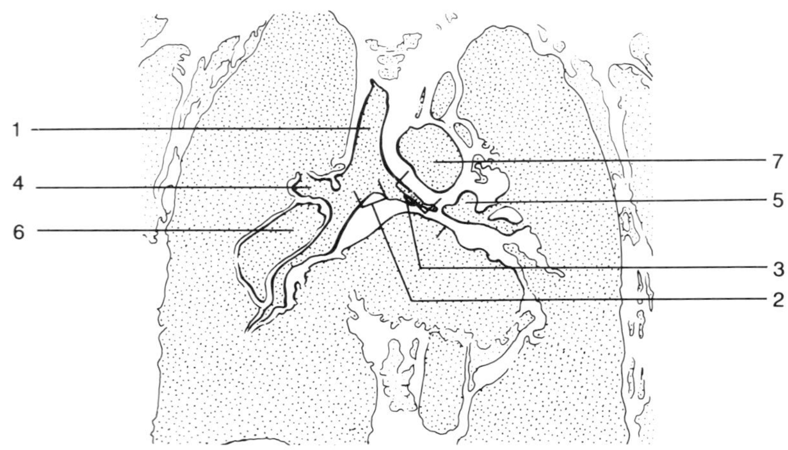

1 trachea
2 right main bronchus
3 left main bronchus
4 right upper lobe bronchus
5 left upper lobe bronchus
6 right pulmonary artery
7 left pulmonary artery

Fig. 8.3 Normal anatomy of tracheobronchial tree. Coronal spin-echo MR image. The right main bronchus is shorter than the left (left bronchus: right bronchus ratio is about 1.4:1). The upper border of the right pulmonary artery lies below the upper border of right upper lobe bronchus ("eparterial bronchus"). The left pulmonary artery lies above the left main bronchus (hyparterial bronchus). Although the right bronchus is often called the "eparterial bronchus," it does not sit atop the right pulmonary artery; rather, the artery is anterior to and at a slightly lower level than the bronchus.

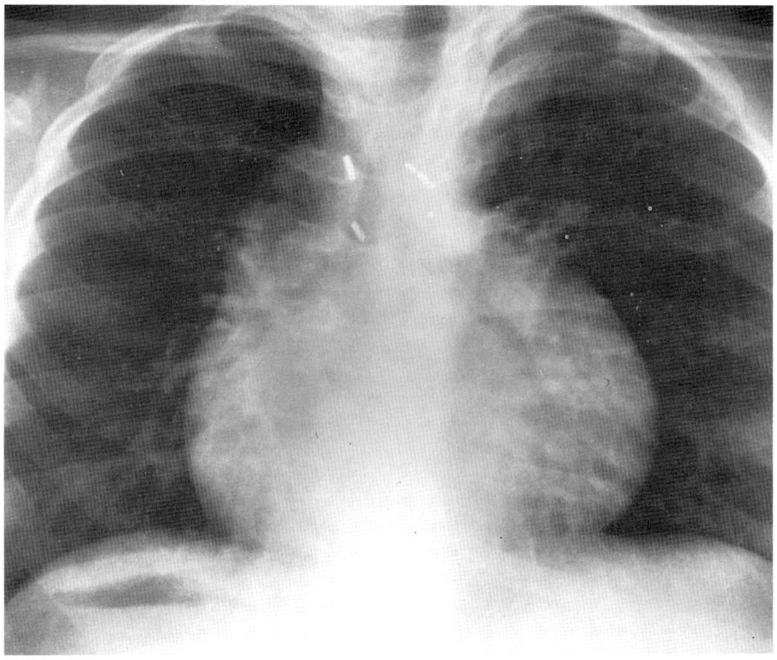

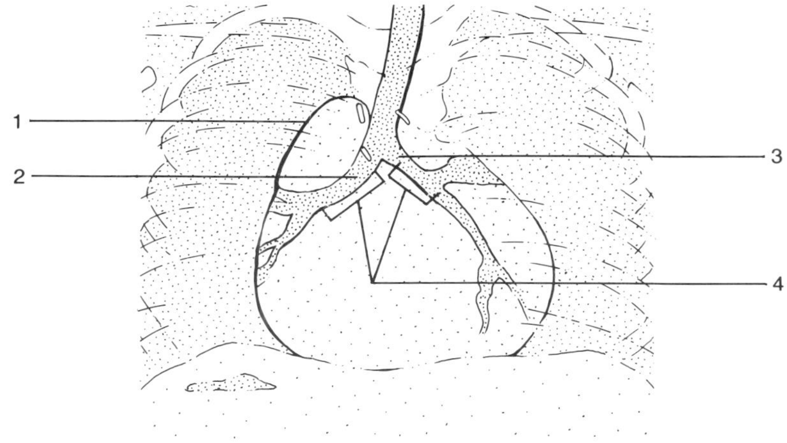

1 right aortic arch
2 right-sided morphologic left bronchus
3 left-sided morphologic right bronchus
4 ratio of left and right main bronchi

Fig. 8.4 Atrial situs inversus. Posteroanterior film of a patient with thoracic and atrial situs inversus. The right main bronchus is longer than the left. The cardiac axis is oriented to the left. The liver is on the left and the gastric air bubble is on the right, indicating the presence of abdominal situs inversus. The metallic clips are from previous surgery to close a patent ductus arteriosus.

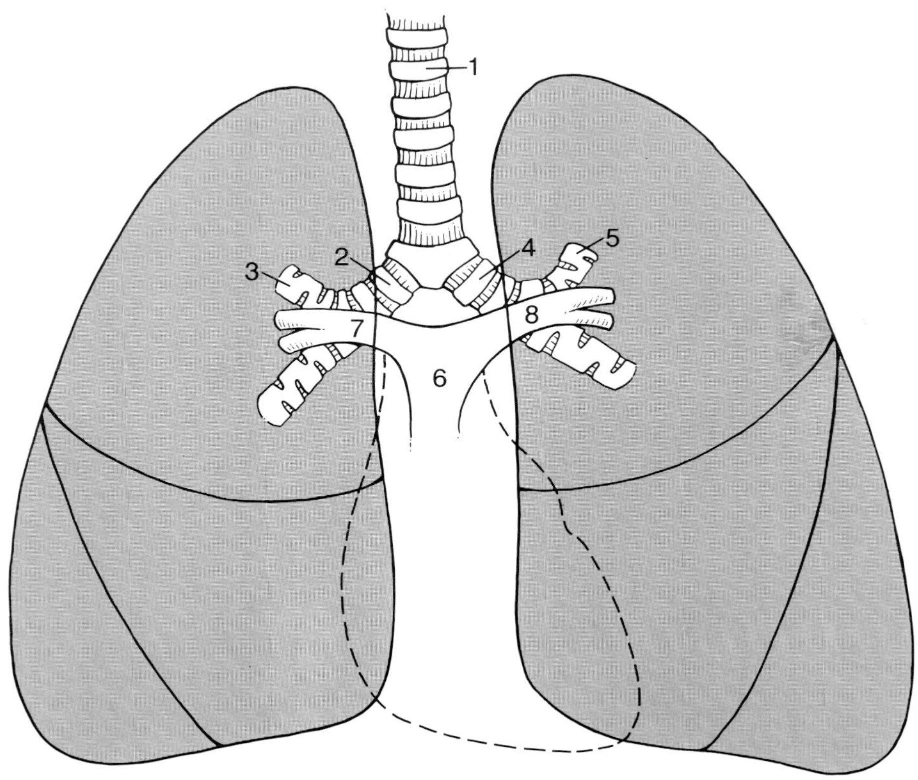

Fig. 8.5 Right thoracic isomerism. In this anomaly, which is almost always associated with right atrial isomerism, both lungs have the appearance of a right lung. The right and left main bronchi are of equal length; both upper lobe bronchi take off at a relatively acute angle; the pulmonary arteries are anterior and slightly inferior to the main bronchus; and each lung has three lobes (two interlobar fissures).

1 trachea
2 right main bronchus
3 right upper lobe bronchus
4 left main bronchus
5 left upper lobe bronchus
6 pulmonary trunk
7 right pulmonary artery
8 left pulmonary artery

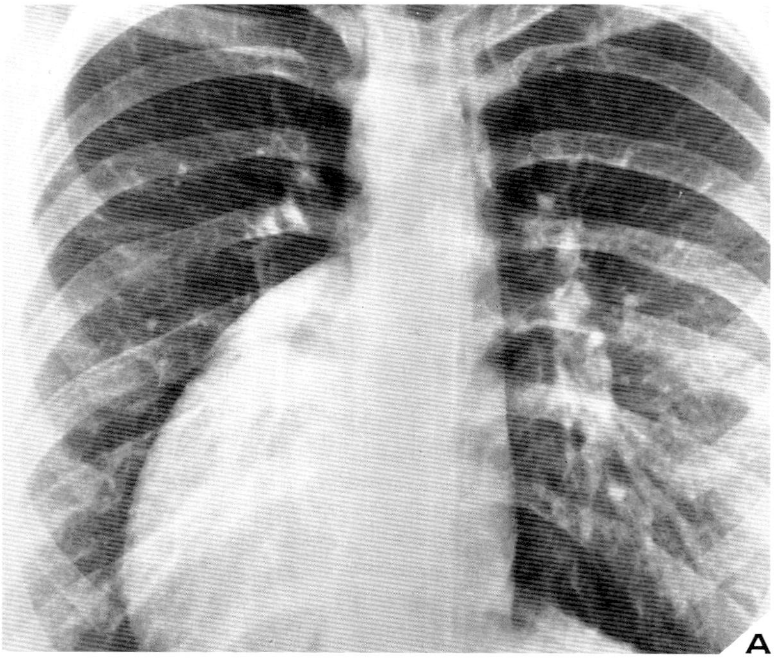

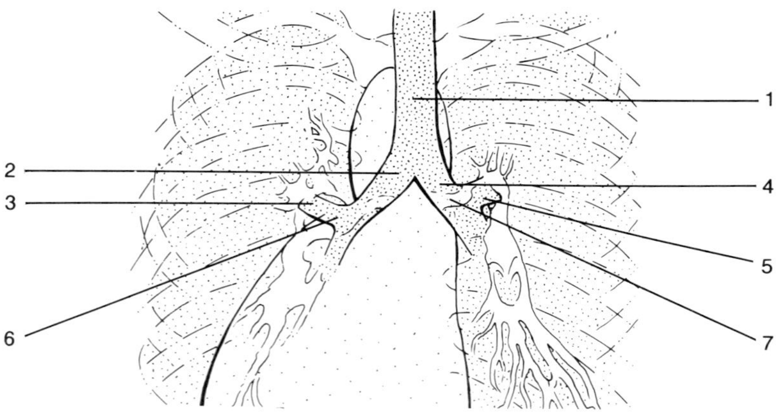

1	trachea
2	right main bronchus
3	right upper lobe bronchus
4	left main bronchus
5	left upper lobe bronchus
6	right pulmonary artery
7	left pulmonary artery

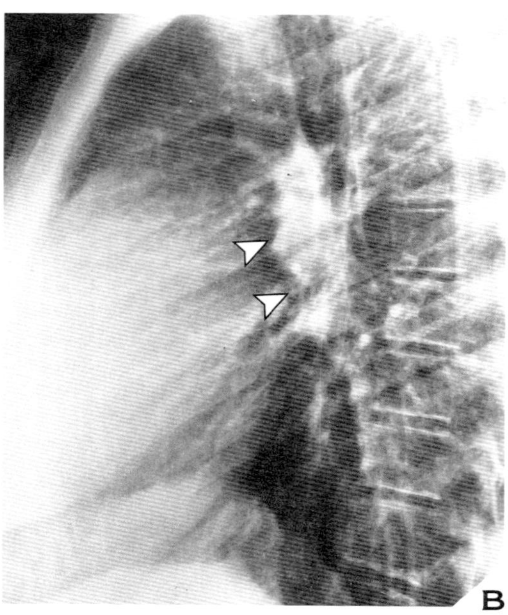

Fig. 8.6 Right thoracic isomerism. (A, B) Chest films are shown of a patient with right atrial isomerism. The posteroanterior film (A) shows symmetry of the main bronchi (left bronchus to right bronchus ratio is 1:1). Both upper lobe bronchi take off at a relatively acute angle, which is characteristic of a right upper lobe bronchus. The left and right pulmonary arteries are projected beneath the upper border of the corresponding main bronchus. The cardiac axis is to the right and there is a right aortic arch. On the lateral projection (B) both pulmonary arteries (*arrows*) lie anterior to the plane of the tracheobronchial tree. The right and left upper lobe bronchi are superimposed owing to the presence of bronchial isomerism.

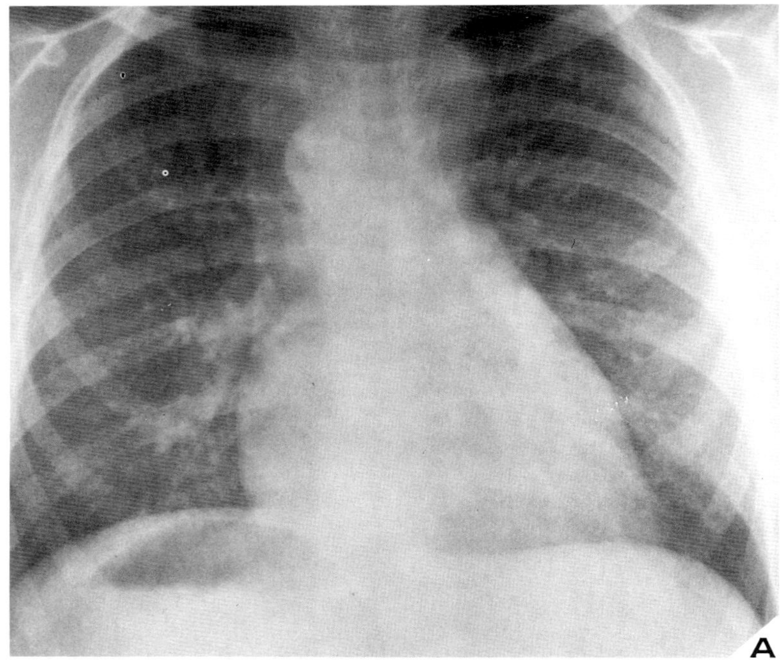

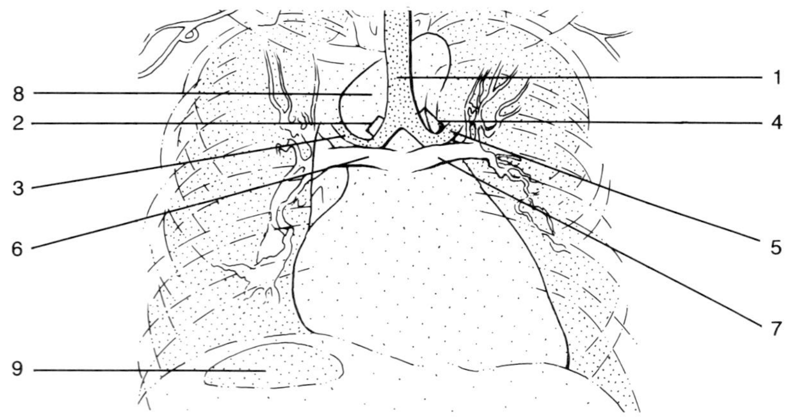

1	trachea
2	right main bronchus
3	right upper lobe bronchus
4	left main bronchus
5	left upper lobe bronchus
6	right pulmonary artery
7	left pulmonary artery
8	right aortic arch
9	gastric air bubble (on right)

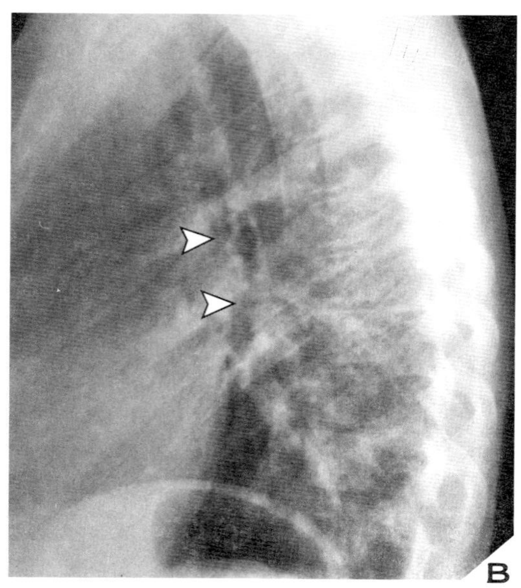

Fig. 8.7 Right thoracic isomerism. (A, B) Chest films are of a 7-year-old child with right atrial isomerism. The postero–anterior film (A) shows symmetrical short (right-type) main bronchi. The upper margins of the pulmonary arteries are inferior to the upper margin of the ipsilateral main bronchus. The gastric air bubble is on the right (abdominal situs inversus), indicating incongruent visceroatrial situs. There is a right aortic arch. The cardiac axis is to the left. On the lateral projection (B) the images of the pulmonary arteries (*arrows*) are superimposed and lie anterior to the tracheobronchial tree.

rior to the ipsilateral main bronchus (Figs. 8.6A and 8.7A). On the lateral chest film, the superimposed images of the pulmonary arteries are seen as a prominent density anterior to the tracheobronchial tree (Figs. 8.6B and 8.7B). (Normally, the right pulmonary artery is in front of the tracheobronchial tree and the left pulmonary artery is behind it.)

In *left thoracic isomerism,* both main bronchi are of the "left" type and both lungs are morphologic left lungs (two lobes, hyparterial bronchus) (Fig. 8.8). On the frontal chest film, both pulmonary arteries are superior to the ipsilateral

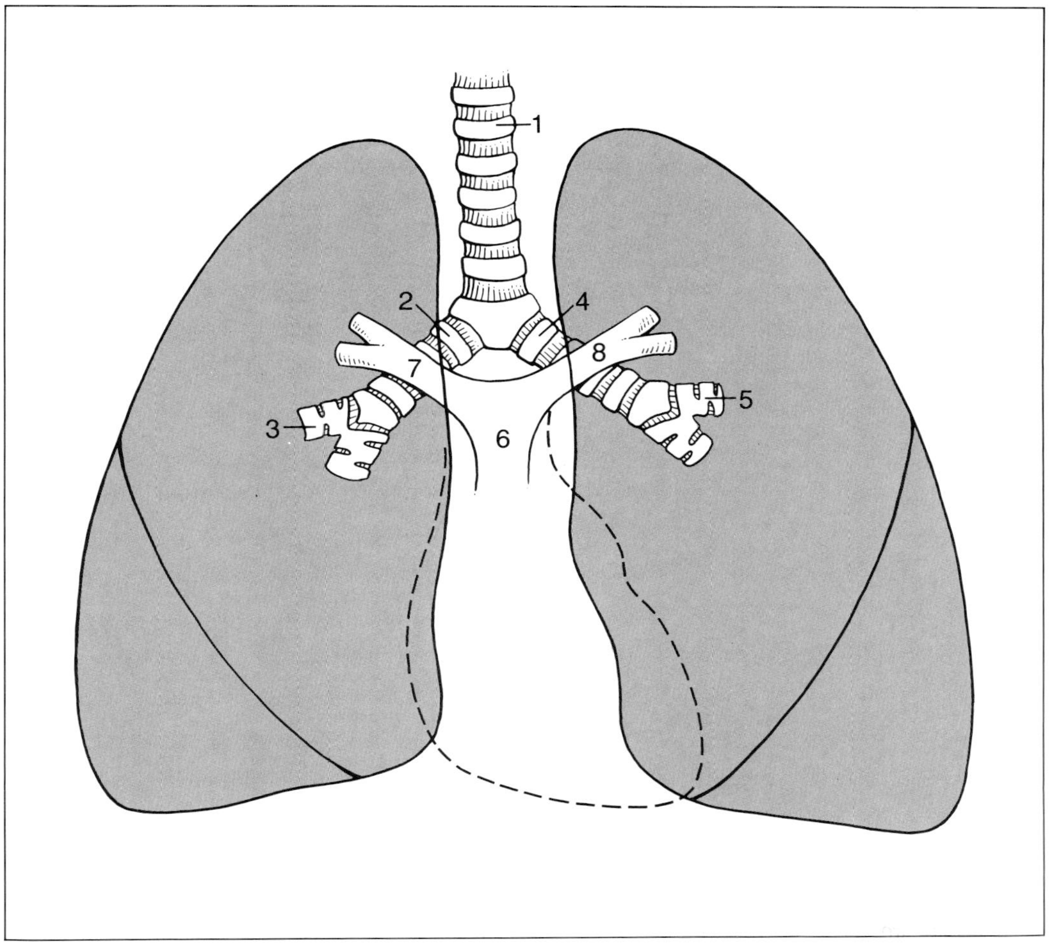

Fig. 8.8 Left thoracic isomerism. In this anomaly, which is almost always associated with left atrial isomerism, both lungs have the appearance of a left lung. The right and left main bronchi are of equal length; the upper lobe artery takes off at a relatively obtuse angle; the pulmonary arteries are anterior and superior to the upper lobe bronchi; and each lung has two lobes (one interlobar fissure).

1 trachea
2 right main bronchus
3 right upper lobe bronchus
4 left main bronchus
5 left upper lobe bronchus
6 pulmonary trunk
7 right pulmonary artery
8 left pulmonary artery

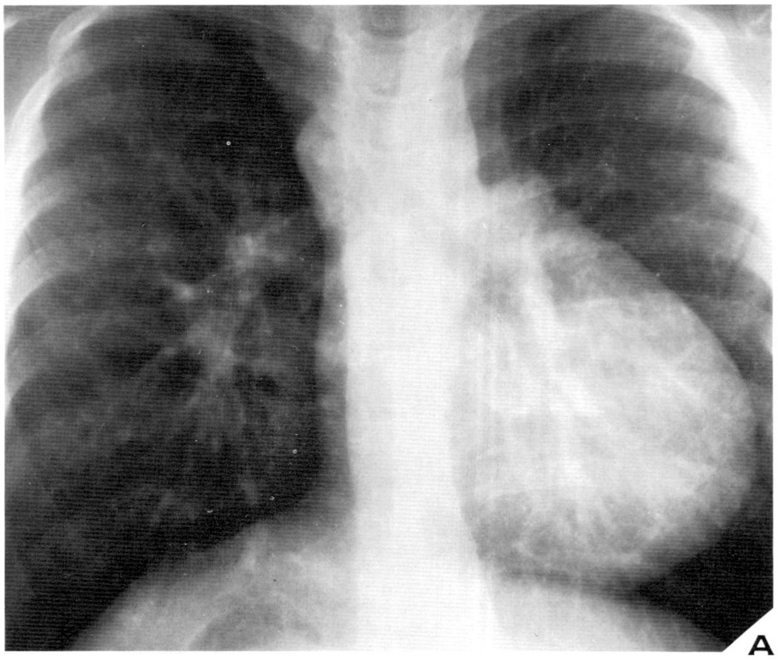

A

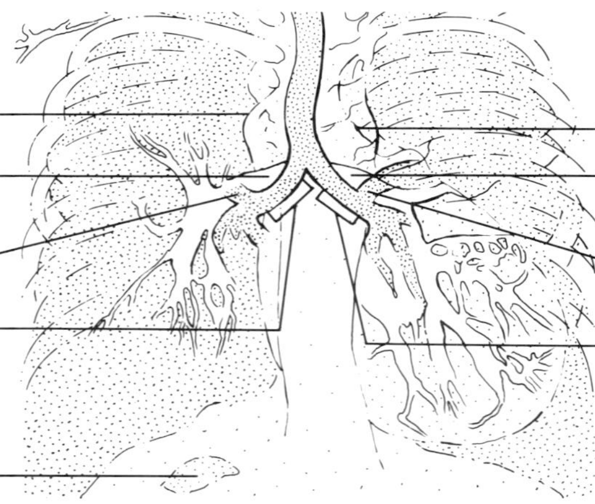

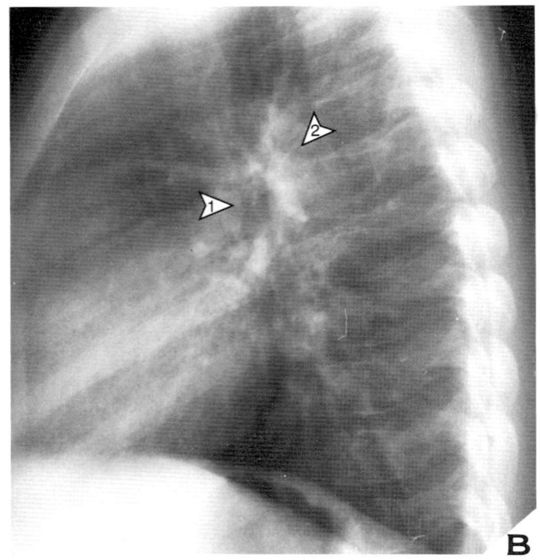

B

Fig. 8.9 Left thoracic and left atrial isomerism. (A) Upright posteroanterior chest film demonstrates left-type thoracic isomerism with two hyparterial (left-type) mainstem bronchi of equal length. The transverse liver and right-sided, somewhat centrally positioned gastric bubble (incongruent visceroatrial situs) suggest that abdominal heterotaxy is also present. Note marked distenstion of azygos vein resulting from azygos continuation of the inferior vena cava. The aortic arch is on the left. (B) Lateral view of another patient with left isomerism. The left and right pulmonary arteries are superimposed (*arrows 1*) and lie superior and posterior to the ipsilateral mainstem bronchus. The aortic arch is indicated by *arrow 2*.

1	right pulmonary artery	6	left upper lobe bronchus
2	"left-type" right main bronchus	7	azygos vein
3	right upper lobe bronchus	8	left aortic arch
4	"right-type" left main bronchus	9	gastric air bubble
5	left pulmonary artery		

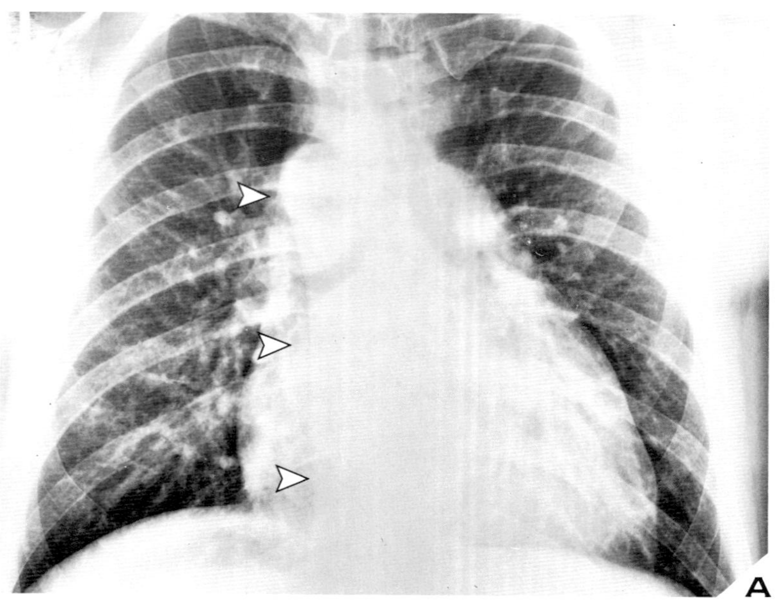

A

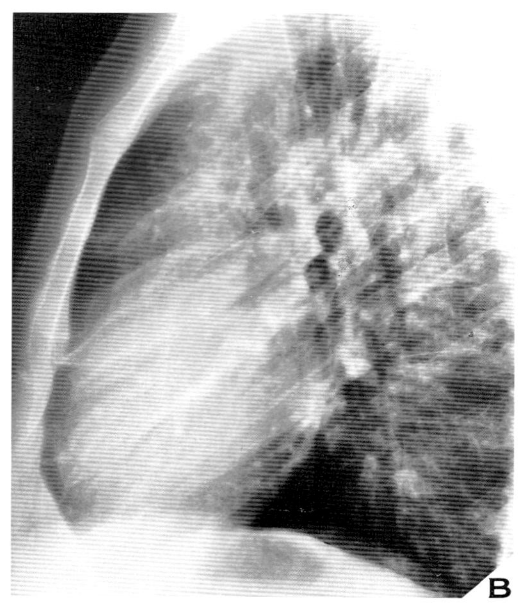

B

Fig. 8.10 Left thoracic and left atrial isomerism. (A) Posteroanterior chest film show a left cardiac axis and a left aortic arch. The left and right main bronchi are nearly equal in length (ratio 1.3:1). The right and left pulmonary arteries lie above the ipsilateral main bronchus, corresponding to the relations of the normal left hilum. The azygos vein (*arrows*), which is markedly dilated, can be followed down into the abdomen. The stomach is slightly to the right of the midline and the liver is transverse. (B) Lateral view. The right and left pulmonary arteries are posterior to the tracheobronchial tree. (Note absence of major pulmonary arterial branches anterior to the tracheobronchial tree.) The plain film findings are consistent with left atrial isomerism, which is usually associated with polysplenia; however, other studies revealed that this patient had a single, normally formed spleen.

main bronchus (Figs. 8.9–8.11; see also Figs. 7.2B and 7.3). On the lateral film, the pulmonary arteries are posterior to the tracheobronchial tree (Figs. 8.9B and 8.10B)

Patients with right atrial isomerism typically have radiographic features of TAPVC of the supracardiac or infracardiac type (see below). Many patients have pulmonary plethora secondary to a left to right shunt at the atrial or ventricular level. Pulmonary vascularity is decreased in those patients with pulmonic stenosis or atresia. About one third of patients with right atrial isomerism have a right cardiac axis.

Patients with left atrial isomerism typically have marked enlargement of the azygos and/or hemiazygos vein, which carry the systemic venous return from the lower part of the body in this anomaly (Figs. 8.9A and 8.10A). About one third have a right cardiac axis. There is usually evidence of a left to right shunt. (Owing to the rarity of pulmonic valvular obstruction, pulmonary oligemia is very uncommon in patients with left isomerism.)

Infants with major cardiac defects typically have abnormalities of the cardiac silhouette characteristic of the associated condition.

ECHOCARDIOGRAPHY

Echocardiography clearly depicts the configuration of the atrial appendages, and is the method of choice for detecting and characterizing atrial isomerism. TAPVC (associated with right isomerism) and anomalous systemic venous connection (associated with right or left atrial isomerism) can be identified with either the transthoracic or transesophageal approach.

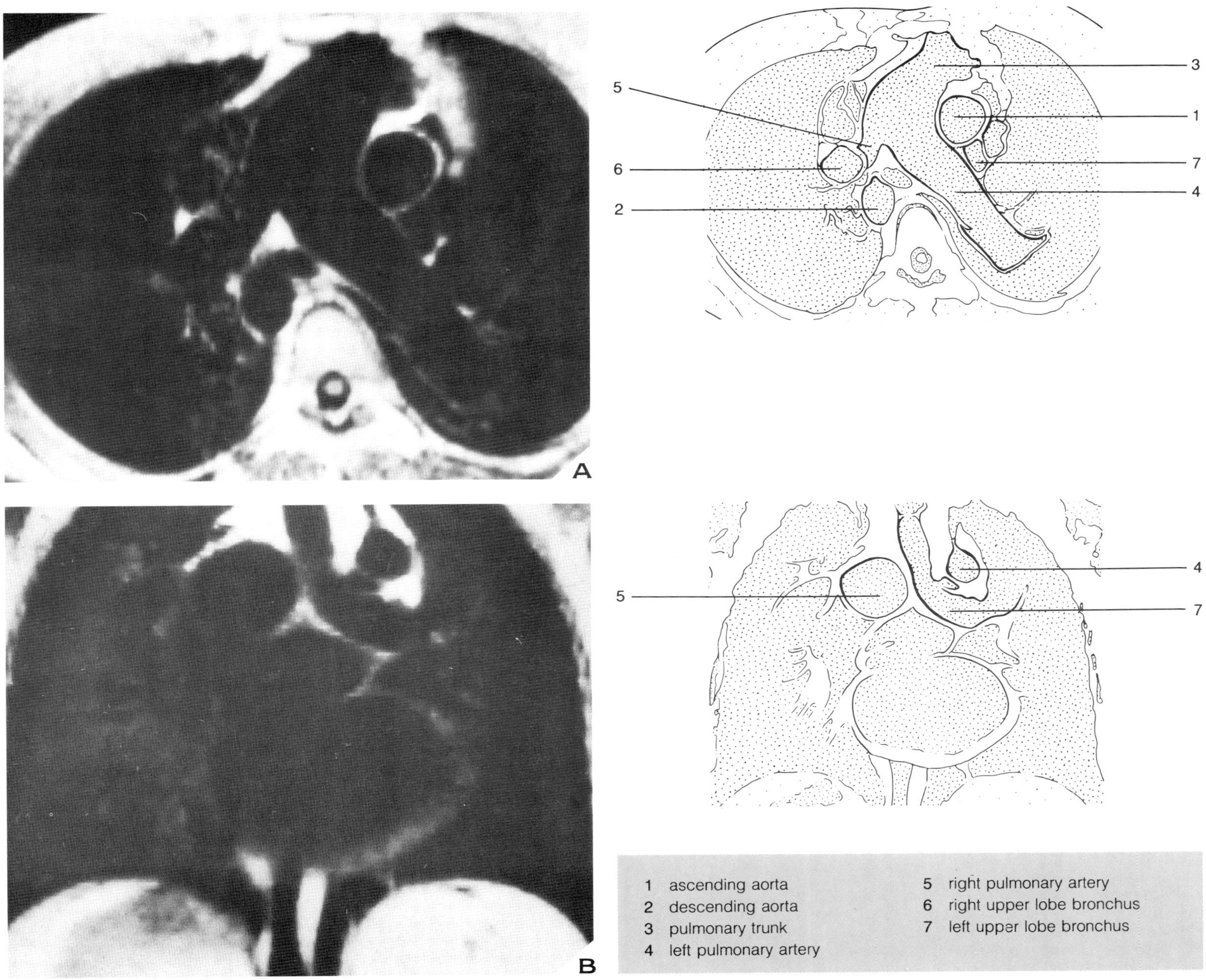

Fig. 8.11 Left thoracic isomerism. (A) Transverse (axial) and (B) coronal spin–echo MR images show an enlarged pulmonary trunk. The right and left pulmonary arteries lie posterior to the corresponding bronchi, ie, both bronchi are of the "left" type. Left thoracic isomerism is almost always associated with left atrial isomerism.

CT AND MRI

Cross-sectional imaging techniques are useful in diagnosing thoracic and atrial isomerism. The enlarged azygos vein associated with anomalous systemic venous drainage is readily demonstrated by contrast enhanced CT or MRI in patients with left isomerism (Figs. 8.11–8.13; see also Fig. 8.25). Anomalies of the systemic veins, eg, persistent left superior vena cava, are clearly shown by either technique (Fig. 8.21). MRI also clearly shows the anomalous pulmonary venous connections in patients with right atrial isomerism. The atrial appendages can be characterized as left-type or right-type on axial spin–echo images. (Multiple sections may be necessary owing to the variable orientation of the atrial appendages.) As noted earlier, MRI clearly depicts the tracheobronchial tree and main pulmonary arteries (see Figs. 8.3 and 8.11), and thus can provide indirect evidence of atrial isomerism.

CARDIAC CATHETERIZATION AND ANGIOCARDIOGRAPHY

In general, catheterization and angiocardiography are performed to evaluate the associated cardiac malformations rather than to confirm the diagnosis of atrial isomerism. However, in some instances, angiocardiographic demonstration of the atrial appendages may be necessary (Fig. 8.14). In patients with left isomerism, inferior vena cavography will demonstrate absence of the suprarenal segment of the IVC with azygos continuation (see Fig. 8.24). (The presence of this anomaly, which can be predicted if the plain film shows enlargement of the azygos vein, precludes cardiac catheterization via the femoral venous route.) Persistence of the left superior vena cava, which is associated with both right and left isomerism, can be demonstrated by injecting contrast material into the left subclavian vein. The angiographic demonstration of TAPVC in patients with right isomerism requires special techniques (see below).

ABDOMINAL IMAGING IN THE DIAGNOSIS OF ATRIAL ISOMERISM

Identification of the infrahepatic IVC and its location with respect to the aorta and the midline can be made noninvasively by means of sonography and MRI. Both modalities will demonstrate interruption of the infrahepatic IVC with right or left azygos continuation or confirm the presence of the intrahepatic segment of the IVC. The IVC and aorta commonly lie on the same side of the spine in both right and left isomerism. In some patients with left isomerism the IVC lies to the left of the abdominal aorta and can be seen to cross over anterior to the aorta in piggyback fashion in order to enter the common atrium. Various vascular abnormalities associated with right isomerism, including anomalous hepatic venous connection and subdiaphragmatic TAPVC, can be demonstrated by sonography or MRI.

ANOMALIES OF THE VENOATRIAL CONNECTION

ANOMALOUS PULMONARY VENOUS CONNECTION

In this group of malformations, the pulmonary veins are connected to the right atrium or its tributaries. The anomalous pulmonary venous connection may be total, affecting all of the pulmonary veins, or partial, in which case only one or several pulmonary veins are affected. Total anomalous pulmonary venous connection (TAPVC) is classified according to whether the anomalous connection is supracardiac, cardiac, or infracardiac. The diagnosis of TAPVC is suggested by typical plain film findings and confirmed by angiocardiography or MRI.

SUPRACARDIAC TAPVC

In this anomaly, the pulmonary veins join to form a common venous sinus which drains into the left vertical vein. The latter drains into the innominate vein and thence into the right superior vena cava; it may also drain directly into the caval veins.

Hemodynamic Features

Cardiac catheterization demonstrates increased saturation in the superior vena cava and right atrium and decreased systemic saturation (below 75 percent). In the absence of pulmonary venous obstruction, right ventricular and pulmonary artery pressure is mildly or moderately elevated; when pulmonary venous

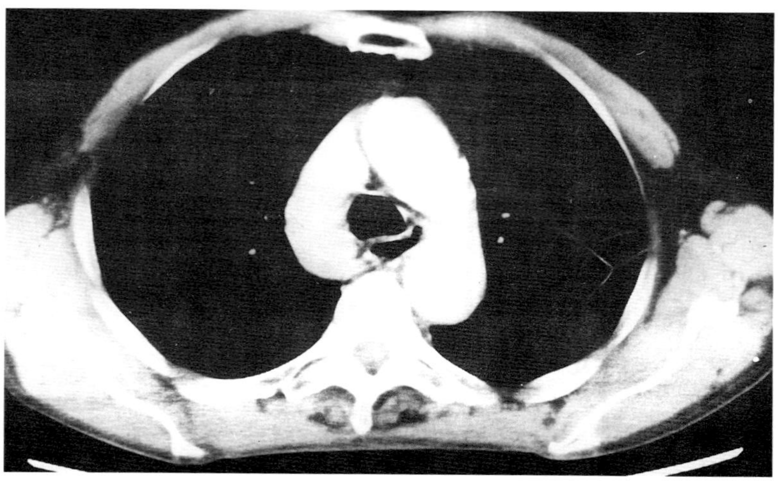

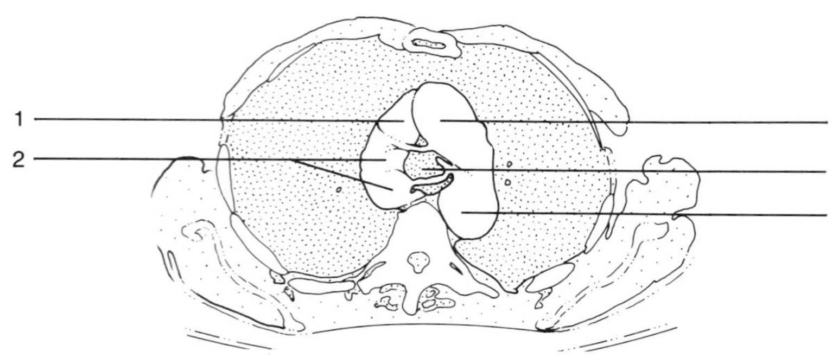

1 right superior vena cava
2 right azygos vein
3 ascending aorta
4 descending thoracic aorta
5 trachea

Fig. 8.12 Left atrial isomerism; interruption of the IVC with right azygos continuation (CT findings). Contrast-enhanced scan of the upper mediastinum demonstrates a left aortic arch. The azygos vein lies anterior and to the right of the spine and courses anteriorly to reach the SVC.

drainage is obstructed (eg, at the entrance of the veins into a common pulmonary venous channel or at the point where the left vertical vein passes between the left main bronchus and the left pulmonary artery), both the right ventricular and pulmonary artery pressure are markedly elevated.

Clinical Features

Most patients with suparacardiac TAPVC present with tachypnea during the first few weeks or months of life. The most common manifestation is unexplained tachypnea. In the absence of marked pulmonary venous obstruction or a wide-open PDA, cyanosis is usually absent or mild. The physical examination is usually unremarkable. Auscultation may reveal a precordial systolic murmur and a gallop rhythm. The second heart sound is usually single or narrowly split.

The main differential diagnosis at this age is lung disease, which can also present with unexplained tachypnea. Premature infants with idiopathic respiratory distress syndrome (hyaline membrane disease) typically exhibit intercostal and substernal retractions; cyanosis is usually not very impressive unless there is marked pulmonary venous obstruction or marked right to left shunting through a patent ductus arteriosus. Transient tachypnea of the newborn (type 2 respiratory distress syndrome) is usually of very short duration, the symptoms subsiding within a few days. Differentiation from acute pulmonary infection is usually possible on clinical and radiologic grounds.

Children with supracardiac TAPVC have signs and symptoms of a large atrial septal defect. They typically present with right ventricular precordial hyperactivity, which is usually accompanied by a soft systolic ejection murmur along the left sternal border. A systolic murmur indicating tricuspid insufficiency is occasionally heard.

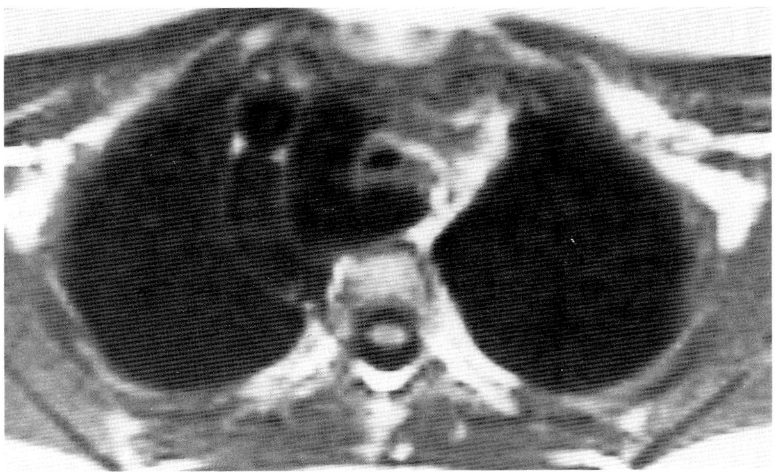

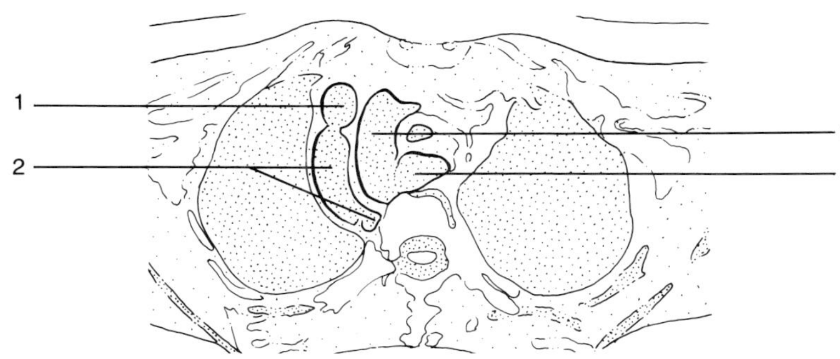

1 right superior vena cava
2 azygos vein
3 right aortic arch
4 anomalous origin of the left subclavian artery

Fig. 8.13 Left atrial isomerism; interruption of IVC with right azygos continuation (MRI findings). Axial spin–echo image shows the right azygos vein coursing anteriorly to join the SVC. Also note the right aortic arch with anomalous origin of the left subclavian artery.

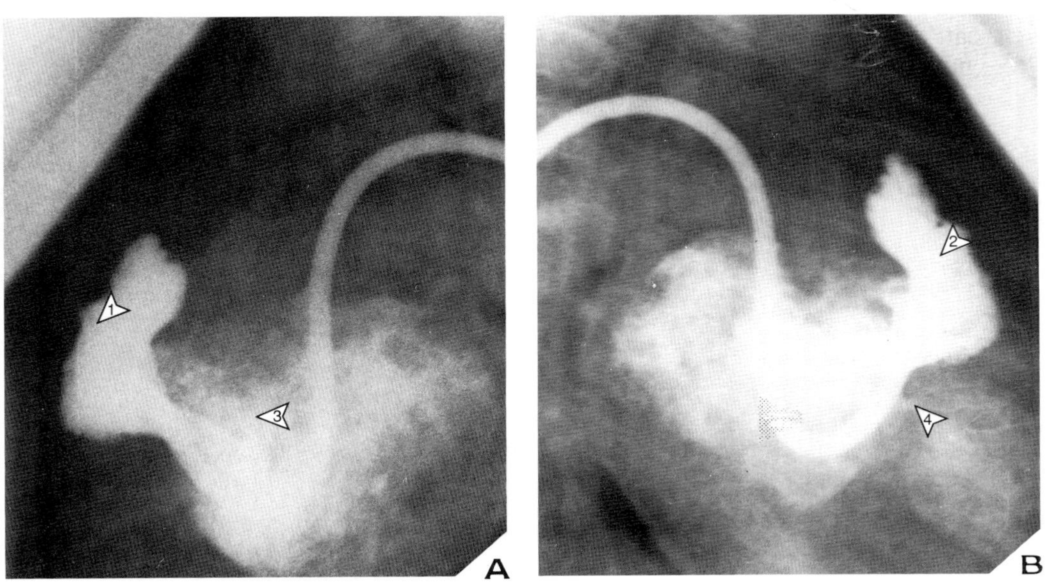

Fig. 8.14 Left atrial isomerism (angiocardiographic findings). Selective injections of the right (A) and left (B) atrial chambers show similar morphology of the atrial appendage (*arrows* 1 and 3) on each side. Its enlongated configuration and its narrow junction with the body of the atrium (*arrows* 2 and 4) are characteristic of a left atrial appendage.

Imaging and Invasive Diagnosis

On the frontal chest film, the dilated venous structures (vertical vein, innominate vein, and right SVC) appear as a round opacity which has been likened to the "head" of a squat snowman whose "body" is formed by the cardiac mass. On the lateral view, the dilated supracardiac venous structures appear as an opacity anterior to the plane of the trachea (Fig. 8.15). In patients with TAPVC to the right superior vena cava, the latter structure is markedly enlarged. The pulmonary vasculature is usually plethoric. The anomalous venous structures are clearly depicted by angiography, cine CT, or MRI.

TAPVC AT THE CARDIAC LEVEL

In this anomaly all four pulmonary veins usually drain into a common venous sinus which lies posterior to the heart (Fig. 8.16). The common sinus may empty into the coronary sinus or

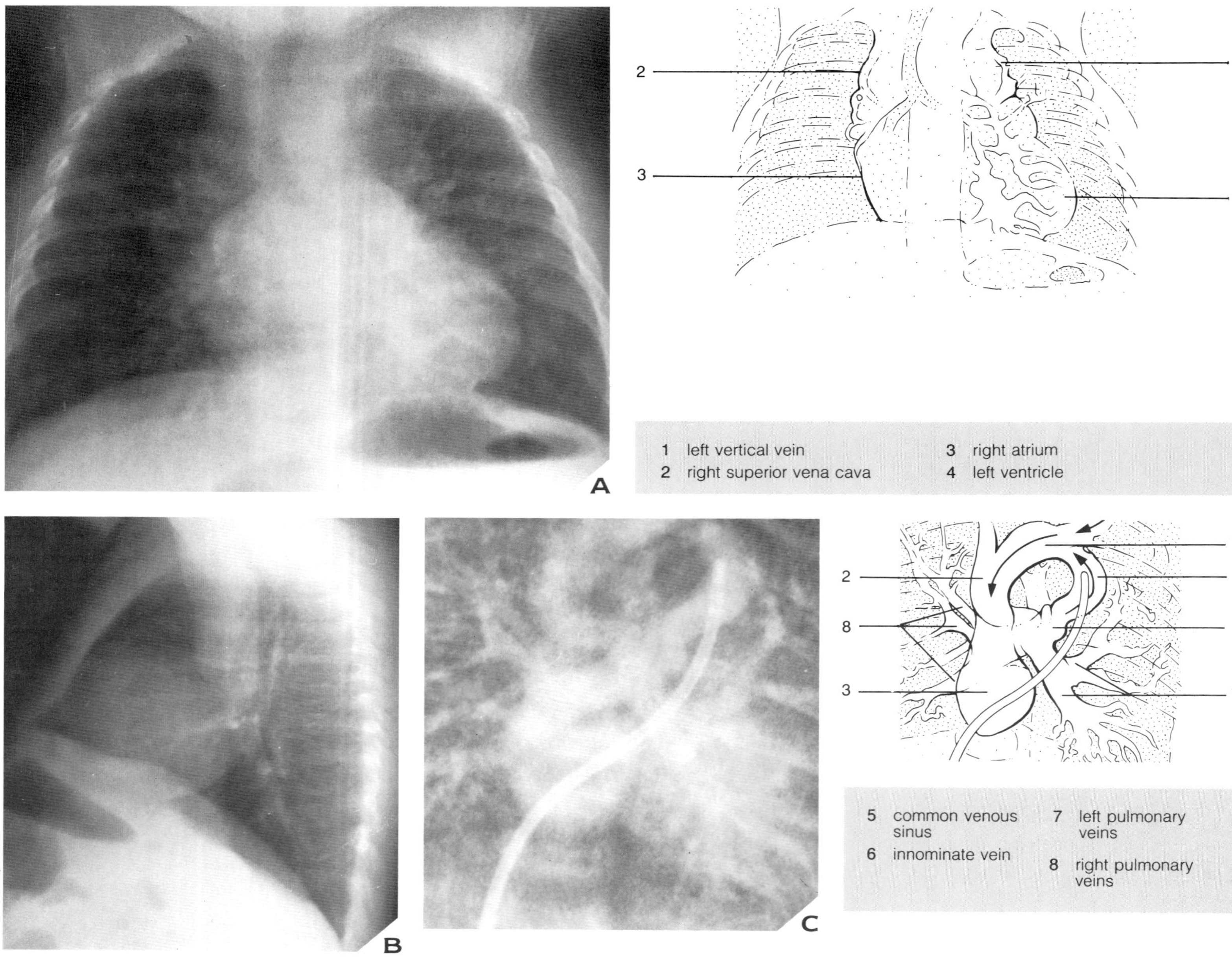

Fig. 8.15 Supracardiac anomalous pulmonary venous connection ("snowman heart"). (A) Supine chest film of a cyanotic 3-month-old infant with TAPVC to the left vertical vein shows marked enlargement of the left vertical vein and the right SVC. The widened upper mediastinum (caused by the enlarged veins) and the cardiac mass resemble the head and body of a snowman. (B) Lateral projection reveals a large soft tissue opacity anterior to the trachea. (C) Levophase of a pulmonary arteriogram in another patient shows the pulmonary veins draining into a common venous sinus, which in turn drains into the left vertical vein, innominate vein, right SVC, and eventually into the right atrium.

directly into the right atrium. In a small percentage of cases the pulmonary veins enter the right atrium directly and independently.

Hemodynamic Features

As in the case of TAPVC at the supracardiac level, right atrial saturation is increased. An increase in saturation in the caval veins may also be sometimes observed owing to reflux from the right atrium. Systemic saturation is also diminished, but cyanosis may not be apparent in compensated cases with a large VSD. Right ventricular and pulmonary artery pressure is usually mildly to moderately elevated. Pulmonary hypertension may develop when the pulmonary veins are obstructed at their entrance into the right atrium.

Imaging and Invasive Diagnosis

Chest films show an enlarged heart and pulmonary plethora (Fig. 8.16A). Although these findings are compatible with any large left to right shunt at the atrial level, the presence of cyanosis suggests IAPVC at the cardiac level. The diagnosis is confirmed by pulmonary arteriography (Fig. 8.16B).

INFRADIAPHRAGMATIC FORM OF TAPVC

In this malformation, all four pulmonary veins drain into an anomalous vein that crosses the diaphragm through the esophageal hiatus to enter the portal vein or, less often, the IVC.

Hemodynamic and Clinical Features

Compression of the anomalous vein at the level of the esophageal hiatus and the increased resistance of the portal circulation result in obstruction of the pulmonary venous return, which in turn leads to severe pulmonary venous hypertension. Patients with infradiaphragmatic TAPVC typically present soon after birth with profound cyanosis.

Cardiac catheterization reveals increased saturation in the inferior vena cava. Because of streaming of systemic venous blood in the right atrium, inferior vena caval blood tends to pass through the foramen ovale and across the mitral valve, whereas superior vena caval blood tends to flow across the tricuspid valve; consequently, systemic venous saturation is typically greater than pulmonary arterial saturation. The relationship between arterial saturation, pulmonary blood flow, and pulmonary vascular resistance has prognostic significance in patients with all types of TAPVC who survive the neonatal period. Because the pulmonary–systemic blood flow ratio (QP/QS) is determined primarily by the magnitude of the pulmonary blood flow, and because pulmonary vascular resistance is inversely related to pulmonary blood flow, the arterial oxygen saturation serves as a rough guide to the patient's operability. In a child or adult whose arterial oxygen saturation is less than 80 percent, QP/QS is likely to be less than 1.4 and the pulmonary vascular resistance is likely to be greater than 10 U/square meter of body surface. Such a patient can be considered inoperable.

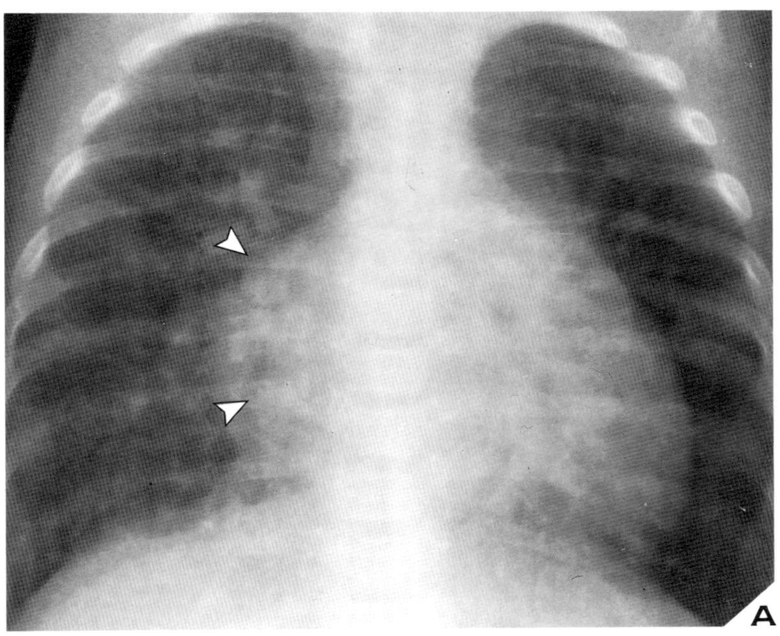

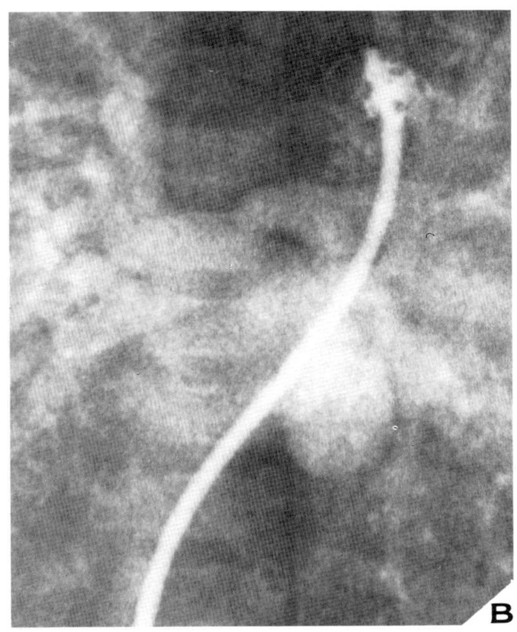

Fig. 8.16 Total anomalous venous connection (TAPVC) at the cardiac level. (A) Supine film demonstrates pulmonary plethora and cardiomegaly with right atrial (*arrows*) and right ventricular enlargement in a cyanotic child. These findings indicate the presence of a large left to right shunt at atrial level; in a cyanotic patient, they strongly suggest the diagnosis of TAPVC at the cardiac level. (B) Levophase of pulmonary arteriogram shows the pulmonary veins of both lungs draining into a common venous sinus, located posterior to the heart. The common venous sinus empties into the coronary sinus, and thence into the right atrium.

Imaging and Invasive Diagnosis

Chest films ordinarily show a normal-sized heart and pulmonary edema; a generalized reticular pattern is occasionally seen (Figs. 8.17A and 8.17B). Angiography (Fig. 8.17C) or MRI confirms the diagnosis.

PARTIAL ANOMALOUS PULMONARY VENOUS CONNECTION (PAPVC)

Although this anomaly can involve any of the four pulmonary veins, it usually occurs on the right, in which case one or both right pulmonary veins may be affected. The anomalous connection may be infracardiac (to the inferior vena cava) (Fig. 8.18A), at the level of the heart (to the right atrium) (Fig. 8.18B), or supracardiac (to the superior vena cava, innominate vein, or azygos vein) (Fig. 8.18C). Anomalous connection of the right pulmonary veins to the inferior vena cava (the so-called *scimitar syndrome*) is typically associated with a hypogenetic right lung (Fig. 8.18A). Although anomalous pulmonary venous connection of the scimitar type may occur as an isolated anomaly, it is usually associated with a secundum ASD.

Clinical Features

Patients with partial anomalous venous connection and ASD present with a wide variety of symptoms, depending on the magnitude of the shunt. Patients with shunts (QP/QS) of less than 1.5 to 1 are usually asymptomatic; on the other hand, those with shunts greater than 1.8 to 1 are usually symptomatic. Shortness of breath with exercise and recurrent respiratory infections, typically beginning in early adulthood, are the usual presenting complaints. Older adults may present with chronic congestive heart failure with fluid retention, hepatomegaly, and marked cardiomegaly. Patients with large ASDs of the sinus venosus type may present with cyanosis owing to partial connection of the SVC to the left atrium. Brain abscess or a peripheral embolus is a potential complication and may be the presenting complaint.

Invasive Diagnosis

Cardiac catheterization demonstrates increased saturation in the right atrium; in patients with a left to right shunt across an ASD, left ventricular saturation is normal. In patients with ele-

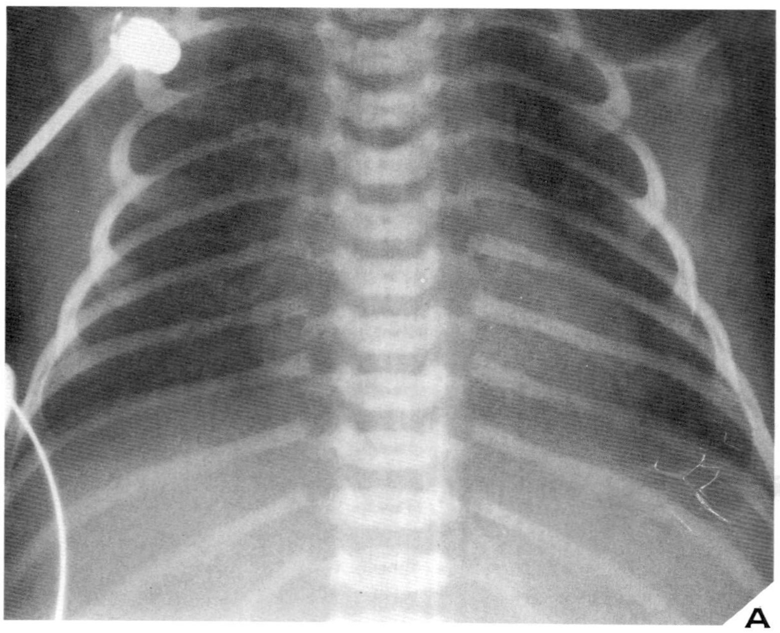

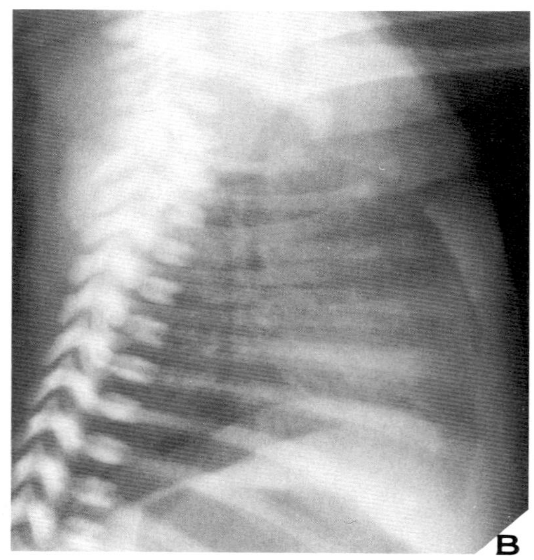

Fig. 8.17 TAPVC (infradiaphragmatic type). (A) Antero–posterior supine chest film of a cyanotic 1-day-old infant demonstrates interstitial edema, indicating obstructed pulmonary venous return. The heart is of normal size. Owing to the interstitial edema, the posterior cardiac border is not well seen on the lateral projection (B). (C) Levophase of pulmonary angiogram shows the entire pulmonary venous return entering a common venous sinus which communicates (via an anomalous vein) with the portal vein.

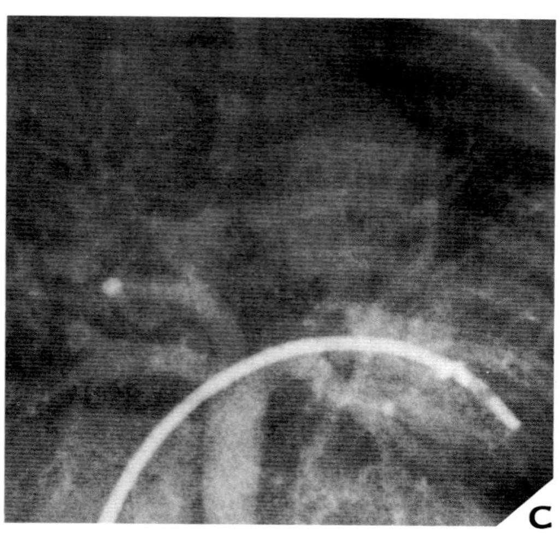

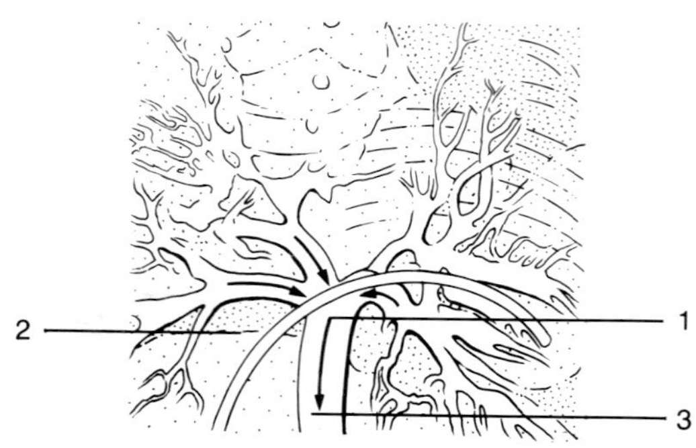

1 common venous sinus
2 diaphragm
3 anomalous vein draining into portal vein

vated pulmonary vascular resistance (6–12 U/m^2 of body surface), it is important to determine whether there is a further increase in resistance with exercise. QP/QS of 1.5 at rest and 0.85 with exercise indicates that pulmonary vascular resistance is unchanged or increased during exercise and that systemic vascular resistance is decreased. Such patients will not benefit from operative repair. It is particularly important to measure QP/QS in patients with isolated partial anomalous venous connection involving only a portion of one lung. In such cases, surgical repair of the anomalous vein is not indicated if QP/QS is less than 1.8. (QP/QS may be less than 1.8 when only the right pulmonary vein enters the superior vena cava and the atrial septum is intact; in this arrangement, the measured QP/QS may not accurately reflect the magnitude of the shunt because superior vena caval and right atrial pressure are lower than left atrial pressure, resulting in a venous gradient that is greater than usual.)

ANOMALOUS SYSTEMIC VENOUS CONNECTION

PERSISTENT LEFT SUPERIOR VENA CAVA

The most common type of anomalous systemic venous connection is persistent left SVC. In this anomaly, the left jugular and left subclavian veins join to form the left SVC. The latter structure descends through the mediastinum, anterior to the left pulmonary artery, and connects with the coronary sinus, which is enlarged (see Fig. 7.11). Thus, the venous drainage from the left side of the upper body passes through the persistent left SVC into the coronary sinus and right atrium.

Bilateral superior caval veins are present in the great majority of patients with persistent left SVC. The caval veins are usually connected by a bridging vein (if there is none, all of the venous drainage from the left upper part of the body returns to the

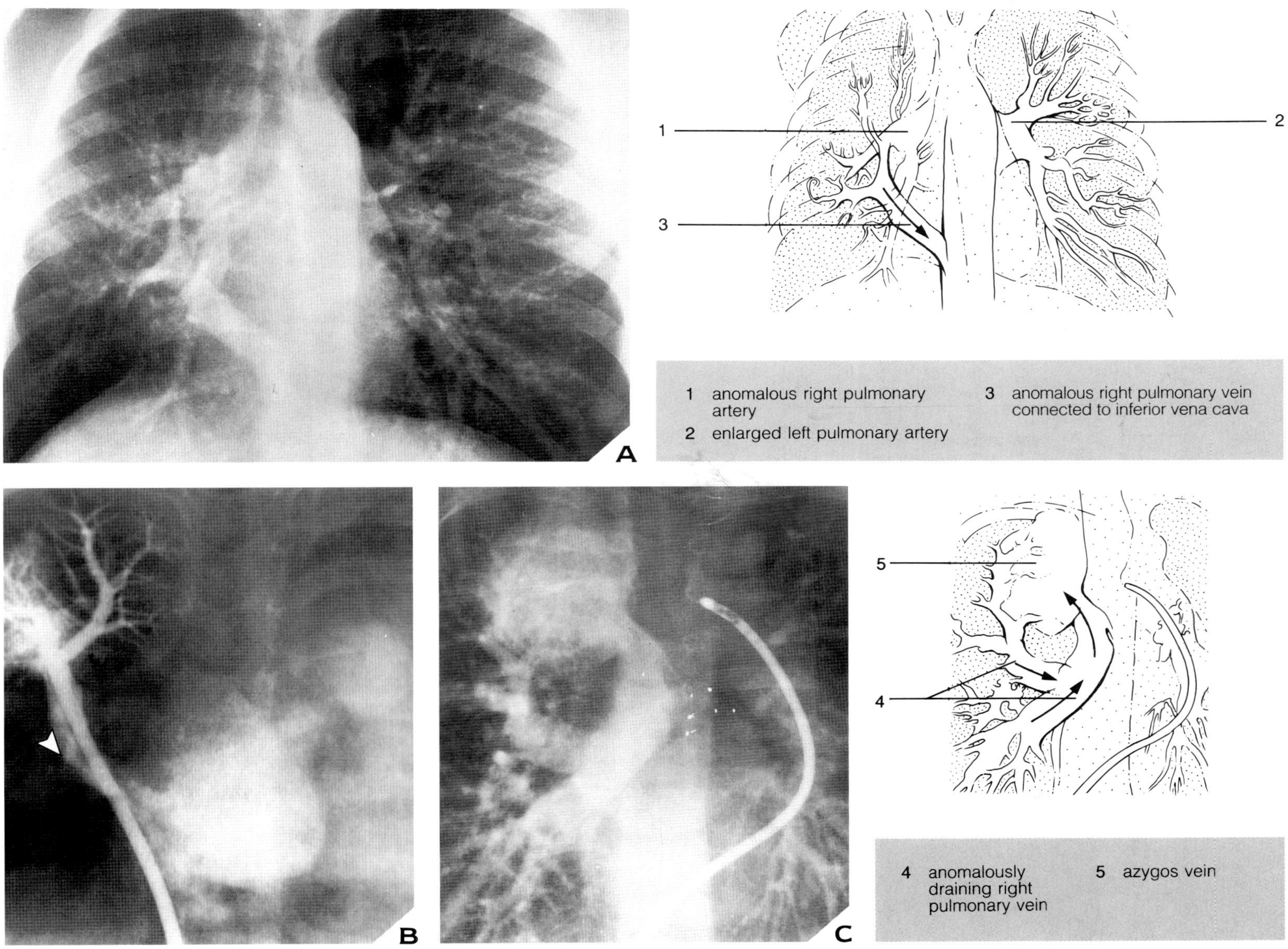

Fig. 8.18 Partial anomalous pulmonary connection; findings in three patients with different patterns of partial anomalous pulmonary connection. (A) In the first patient, a postero–anterior chest film shows the right pulmonary veins converging to form a single anomalous vein which runs inferiorly and medially to join the IVC. The heart is shifted to the right owing to the presence of right pulmonary hypoplasia in this patient with the scimitar syndrome. (B) A retrograde pulmonary venogram in another patient shows the right upper pulmonary veins entering directly into the right atrium (*arrow* indicates direction of blood flow). (C) Levophase of a right pulmonary arteriogram in a third patient shows all the right pulmonary veins joining to form a channel that drains into the azygos vein.

heart via the left SVC). Occasionally the right SVC is hypoplastic or atretic. When it is atretic, all of the venous drainage from the upper part of the body is via the left SVC; a bridging or innominate vein must be present in such cases (Fig. 8.19).

Persistent left SVC may be associated with cardiac malformations such as ASD (*unroofed coronary sinus syndrome;* see below) or atrioventricular septal defect *(endocardial cushion defect)* (see Fig. 9.13).

Hemodynamic and Clinical Features

Except for peripheral desaturation (cyanosis), isolated anomalous systemic venous connection is usually asymptomatic. Patients with isolated total connection of the left SVC to the left atrium may present in adulthood with a brain abscess or peripheral thromboembolism. Those with an associated ASD have a bidirectional shunt with hemodynamic features similar to those of an isolated ASD. Isolated persistent left SVC connected to

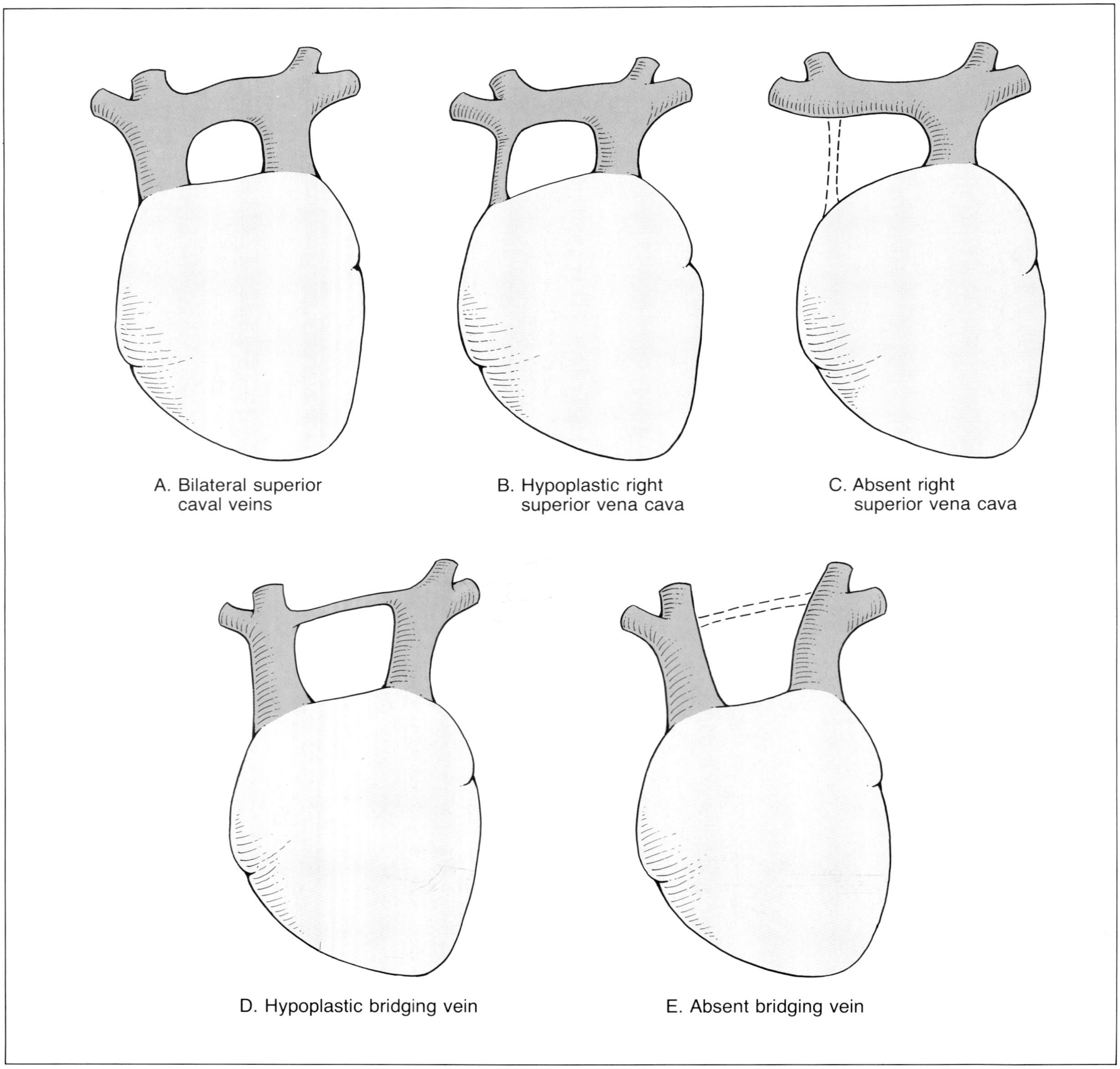

Fig. 8.19 Anomalies of the superior caval veins. (A) Bilateral superior venae cavae, (B) hypoplastic right SVC, (C) Absent right SVC, (D) hypoplastic bridging vein, and (E) absent bridging vein are illustrated.

the coronary sinus is clinically silent unless there is an associated defect in the roof of the coronary sinus, in which case the symptoms reflect the resulting left to right shunt. (If the shunt is large enough, it may produce right atrial and right ventricular overload in the same way as an ASD of comparable size.)

No hemodynamic aberrations are associated with isolated persistent left SVC connected to the coronary sinus. Therefore, cardiac catheterization and angiocardiography are not indicated in patients with this anomaly.

Imaging and Invasive Diagnosis

Chest films may show left atrial isomerism. The left SVC can usually be identified as a discrete structure on the frontal projection, particularly when it is dilated. The lateral border of the left SVC forms a sharp interface with the lung from the atrioventricular groove (inferiorly) to the level of the clavicle (superiorly), usually projecting laterally to the aortic arch and pulmonary artery (Fig. 8.20). (In 20 to 30 percent of cases the left SVC is displaced medially and cannot be identified on the frontal projection.) On the lateral projection, the left SVC can often be identified as a soft tissue density anterior to the trachea.

Left SVC and the accompanying anomalies are readily confirmed by angiography (Fig. 8.21) or MRI (Fig. 8.22).

ANOMALIES OF THE CORONARY SINUS

Anomalies of the coronary sinus include atresia, stenosis of its distal portion, and defective formation of its roof. The latter results in a left to right shunt in patients with a persistent left SVC. When the roof of the coronary sinus is absent, the left SVC drains directly into the left atrium, so that the entrance of the coronary sinus functions as an ASD. In patients with this anomaly, often called the *unroofed coronary sinus syndrome,* plain

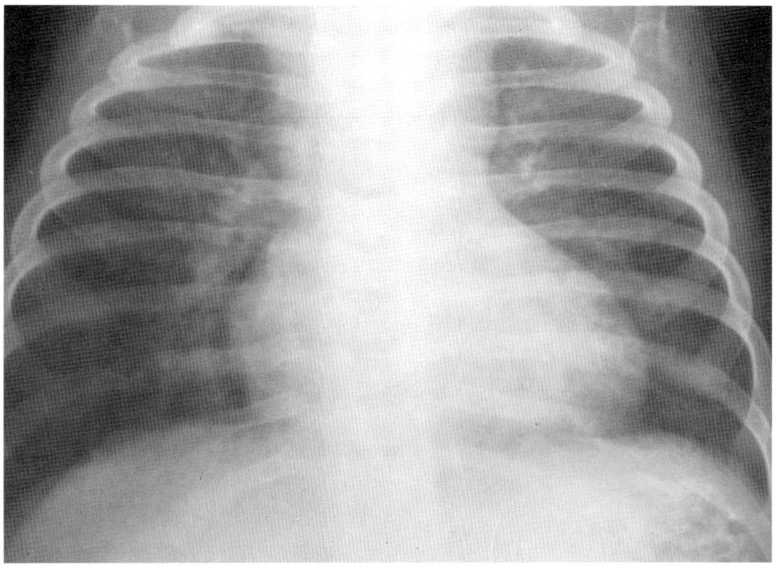

Fig. 8.20 Left superior vena cava. Frontal chest film of a patient with tetralogy of Fallot (note right ventricular enlargement and inapparent pulmonary trunk) shows a persistent left SVC, which appears as a density with a straight border extending upward from the atrioventricular groove.

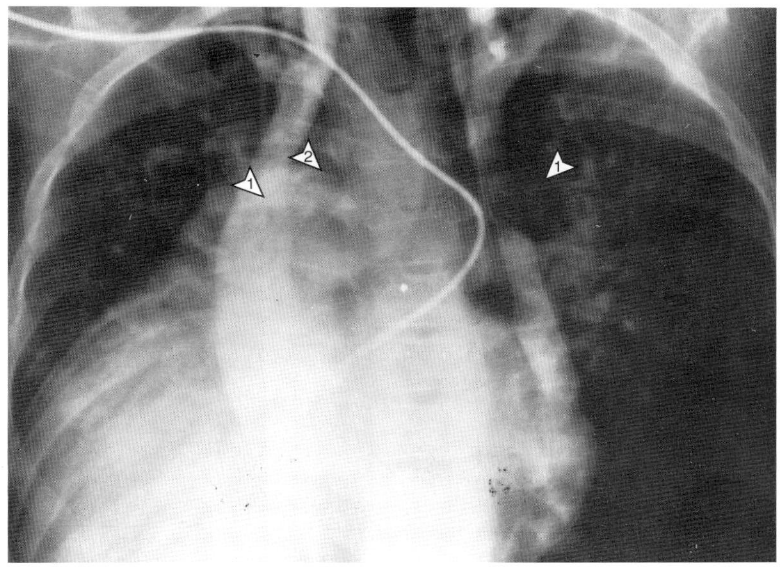

Fig. 8.21 Bilateral superior venae cavae without a bridging vein. Plain films (not illustrated) showed left isomerism with the cardiac axis directed to the right. Venous phase of aortogram demonstrates bilateral superior venae cavae (*arrows* 1) without a bridging innominate vein (ie, absence of the left innominate vein). The azygos vein is indicated by *arrow* 2.

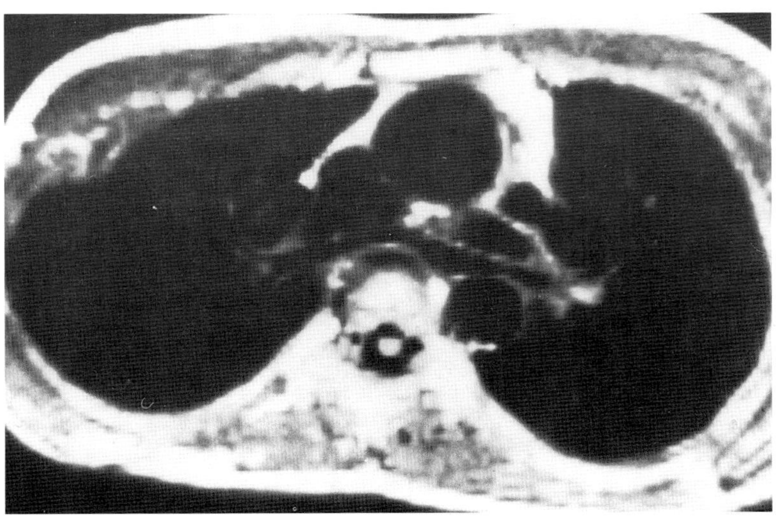

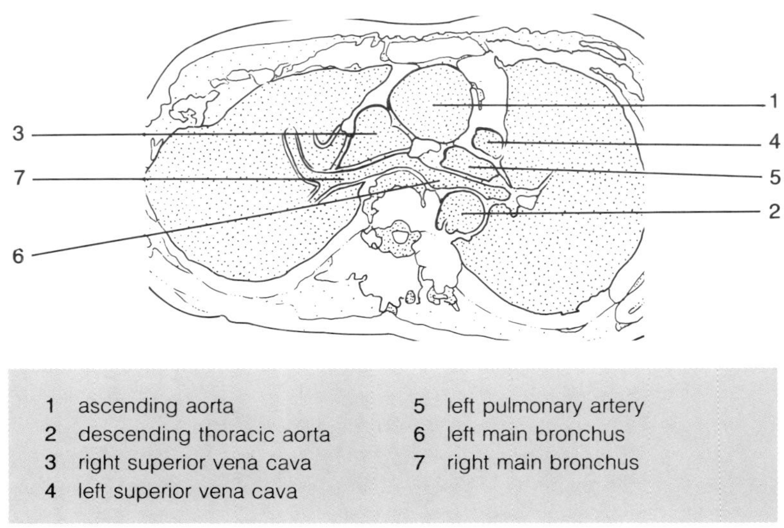

Fig. 8.22 Bilateral superior venae cavae (persistent left SVC); MRI findings. Transverse (axial) spin–echo image through the upper mediastinum demonstrates the left and right superior venae cavae, which appear as echo-free channels anterior to the pulmonary arteries and main bronchi.

films show evidence of a left to right shunt at the atrial level. The unroofed coronary sinus and associated left to right shunt can be demonstrated angiographically by injecting contrast material into the left SVC or left atrium (Fig. 8.23). Echocardiography and color Doppler imaging can also demonstrate the pertinent anatomy and pathophysiology.

ANOMALIES OF THE INFERIOR VENA CAVA

The most common anomaly of the IVC is absence of its infrahepatic segment with azygos continuation. In this anomaly, which may occur as an isolated malformation or in association with left isomerism, the venous return from the lower part of the body drains into the SVC (which may be on the left or right).

Partial or total connection of the IVC with the left atrium is a rare anomaly. Both forms are usually accompanied by a large ASD. In the partial form, the ASD, which involves the posterior portion of the limbus of the fossa ovalis, is located in the inferior portion of the atrial septum.

Hemodynamic and Clinical Features

Isolated interruption of the IVC with azygos continuation is usually an asymptomatic condition, detected as an incidental finding on plain films or at autopsy. When it is associated with major cardiac malformations, as is often the case in patients with left isomerism, the clinical picture is that of the associated defects.

Patients with total anomalous connection of the IVC to the left atrium typically present with cyanosis secondary to arterial desaturation. Although there are no hemodynamic changes, paradoxical peripheral embolization of thrombi originating in the veins of the lower extremities is a potential complication.

Imaging and Invasive Diagnosis

Frontal and lateral chest films in patients with azygos continuation of the IVC typically show a prominent azygos vein at the point where it enters the right or left SVC. On the frontal projection, the dilated azygos vein, which may be on the right or the left, can sometimes be identified as a shadow overlying or just

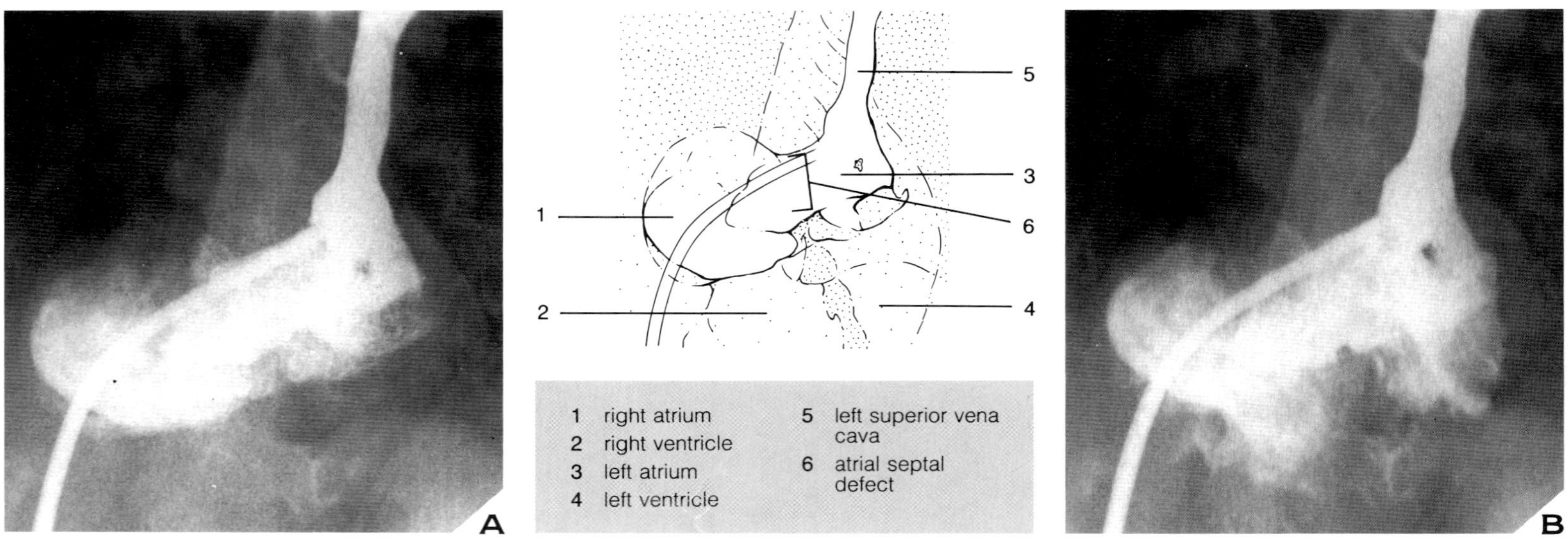

Fig. 8.23 Unroofed coronary sinus syndrome; selective cineangiography of the left SVC (left anterior oblique projection). Early (A) and late (B) phases of show the left SVC connecting with the left atrium and a large "coronary sinus-type" ASD connecting the left and right atria.

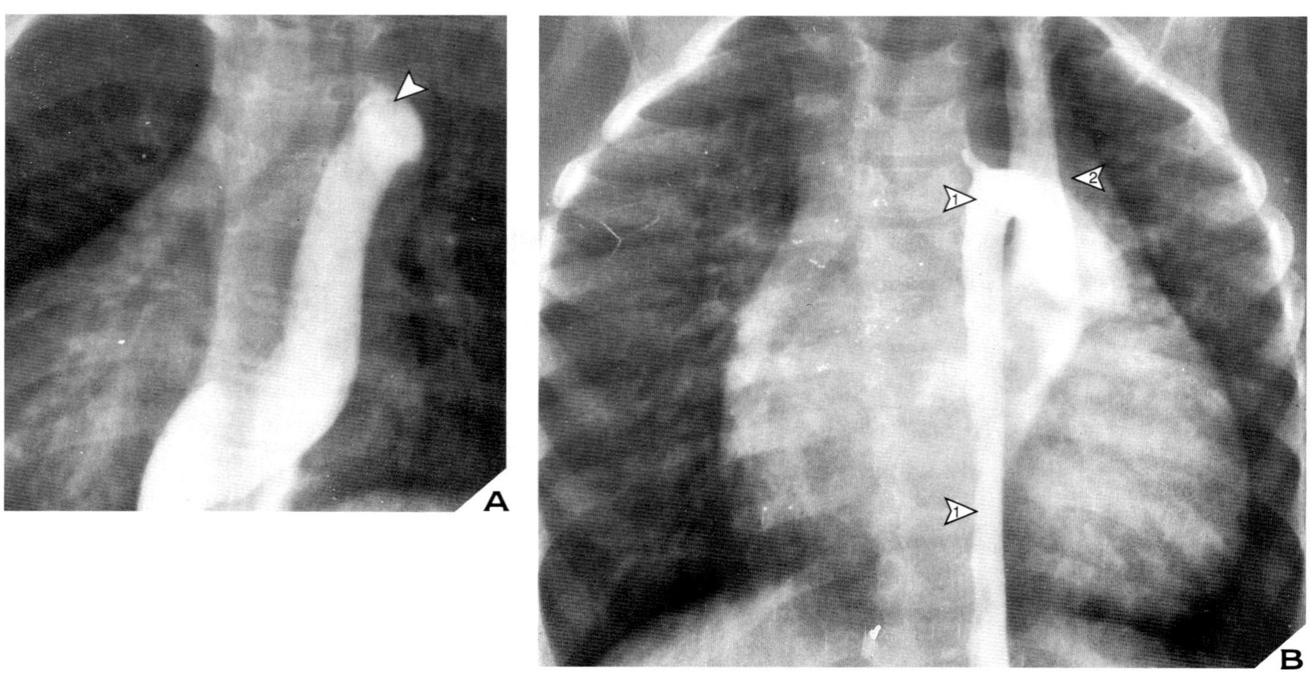

Fig. 8.24 Absence of the inferior vena cava with azygos continuation. (A) Inferior venacavogram in a patient with a right cardiac axis and situs inversus. The azygos vein (which functions as the continuation of the infrahepatic segment of the IVC) ascends along the left mediastinal border and empties into a persistent left SVC (*arrow*). (B) In another patient, selective opacification of the azygos vein (*arrows* 1) shows its connection with the left SVC (*arrow* 2).

lateral to the thoracic spine; it is not visible on the lateral projection. Although the portion of the cardiac silhouette normally formed by the suprahepatic segment of IVC is absent (see Fig. 7.3), a similar density may be formed by the hepatic veins entering the corresponding atria.

The abnormal vascular structures are clearly demonstrated by angiography (Fig. 8.24) or MRI (Fig. 8.25).

ANOMALOUS HEPATIC VENOUS CONNECTION

The hepatic veins normally enter the IVC directly, via a common channel or via two separate and independent connections. In total anomalous hepatic venous connection (AHVC), all of the hepatic veins connect directly with the atria, either separately or through a common channel. The anomalous hepatic venous connection may be to the left- or to the right-sided atrium, or occasionally to both; it may be partial or complete. The great majority of cases of AHVC are associated with more complex cardiac malformations, such as left atrial isomerism; in such cases the suprarenal segment of the IVC is usually absent. Total AHVC is found in most patients with left atrial isomerism, whereas partial AHVC is more common in patients with right atrial isomerism.

Hemodynamic and Clinical Features

Isolated AHVC is usually asymptomatic unless the connection is to the atrium that receives the pulmonary venous return, in which case peripheral desaturation is present. Owing to the low flow through the hepatic veins, clinical cyanosis is uncommon and hemodynamic effects on the heart are rarely evident.

Imaging and Invasive Diagnosis

In both forms of AHVC, selective injection of contrast material into the affected atrium demonstrates reflux into the hepatic vein (Fig. 8.26). The anomalous connection can also be shown by echocardiography or MRI (Fig. 8.27).

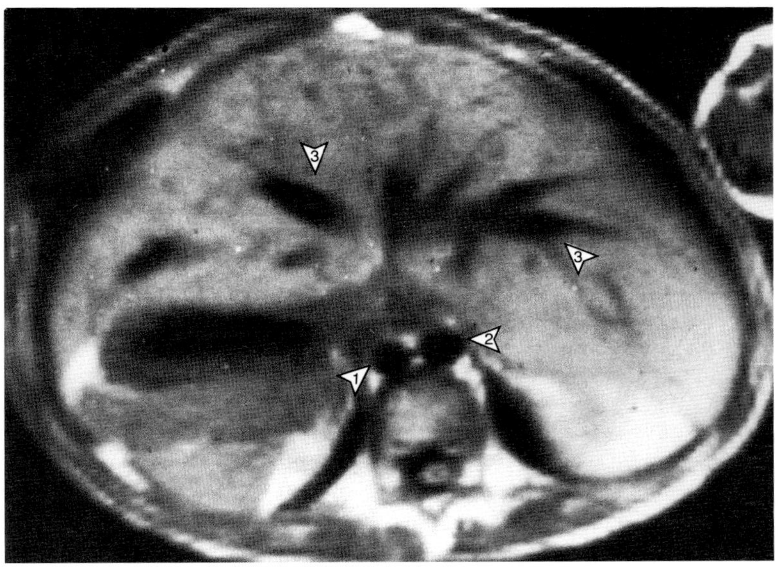

Fig. 8.25 Absence of the inferior vena cava with azygos continuation (MRI findings). On this transverse (axial) spin–echo image of the upper abdomen, the azygos vein (*arrow* 1) lies to the right of the abdominal aorta (*arrow* 2) and the IVC is absent. On other cuts the hepatic veins (*arrow* 3) were seen to drain directly into the right atrium.

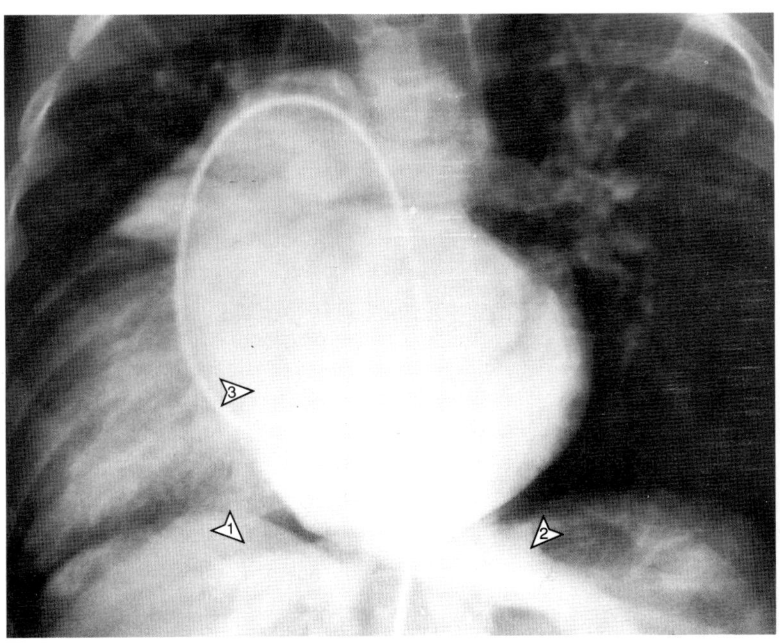

Fig. 8.26 Totally anomalous hepatic venous connection. Atrial injection is shown in a patient with a common atrium, abdominal heterotaxia, and interruption of the IVC with azygos continuation. The left (*arrow 1*) and right (*arrow 2*) hepatic veins enter the common atrial chamber (*arrow 3*) directly via two separate channels.

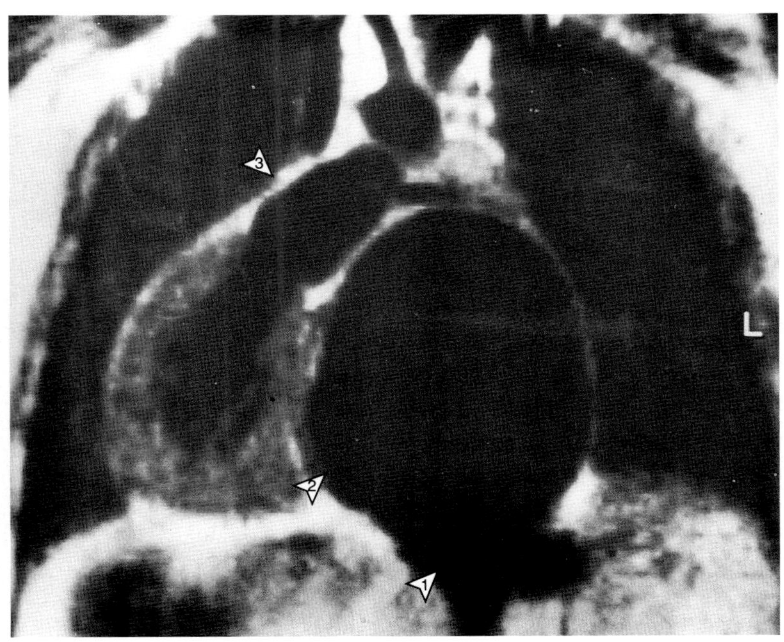

Fig. 8.27 Anomalous systemic venous connection (MRI findings). Coronal spin–echo image shows a left-sided liver. The hepatic veins (*arrow* 1) empty into a large left-sided left atrium (*arrow* 2). The right ventricle lies to the right of the left atrium and supports the ascending aorta (*arrow* 3).

ATRIAL SEPTAL DEFECT

Atrial septal defect (ASD) is one of the most frequently encountered cardiac malformations. There are three types of ASD: the *sinus venosus type,* located in the vicinity of the entrance of the superior vena cava; the *fossa ovalis (ostium secundum) type,* located in the midportion of the atrial septum and unrelated to the atriventricular valves; and the *ostium primum type,* located in the most caudal portion of the atrial septum and related to the atrioventricular valves (Fig. 8.28). Certain other malformations (eg, unroofed coronary sinus, partial anomalous pulmonary venous connection, coronary artery–right atrial fistula) can function hemodynamically as an ASD.

Hemodynamic Features

The hemodynamic changes associated with ASD depend on the size of the defect. Small ASDs with small left to right shunts are well tolerated and produce few adverse hemodynamic consequences; left atrial pressure is higher than right atrial pressure, and saturation in the right heart chambers and pulmonary trunk is low. Patients with small left to right shunts (QP/QS less than 1.5) are usually asymptomatic. When the ASD is large, atrial pressures are equal and there is a predominant left to right shunt at atrial level; right ventricular volume overload is common, resulting in right atrial and right ventricular enlargement. The right ventricular end diastolic pressure typically remains normal for many years, reflecting the pressure in the atrial chambers. With marked right ventricular dilatation, the ventricular septum is displaced posteriorly, compressing the left ventricular lumen and impeding diastolic filling.

The magnitude of the left to right shunt is largely determined by the relative compliance of the ventricles. A very compliant, distensible right ventricle will allow a very large left to right shunt (large QP/QS), whereas a less compliant right ventricle will accommodate a shunt of more modest size. Left ventricular compliance tends to decrease with age, which tends to increase the QP/QS; similarly, disorders that decrease left ventricular compliance (eg, systemic hypertension), as well as mitral insufficiency and mitral stenosis, will increase the magnitude of the left to right shunt. Progressive elevation of pulmonary vascular resistance associated with a longstanding large left to right shunt may eventually lead to reversal of the shunt (Eisenmenger syndrome) (see Chapter 5).

Congestive heart failure is not uncommon in adult patients

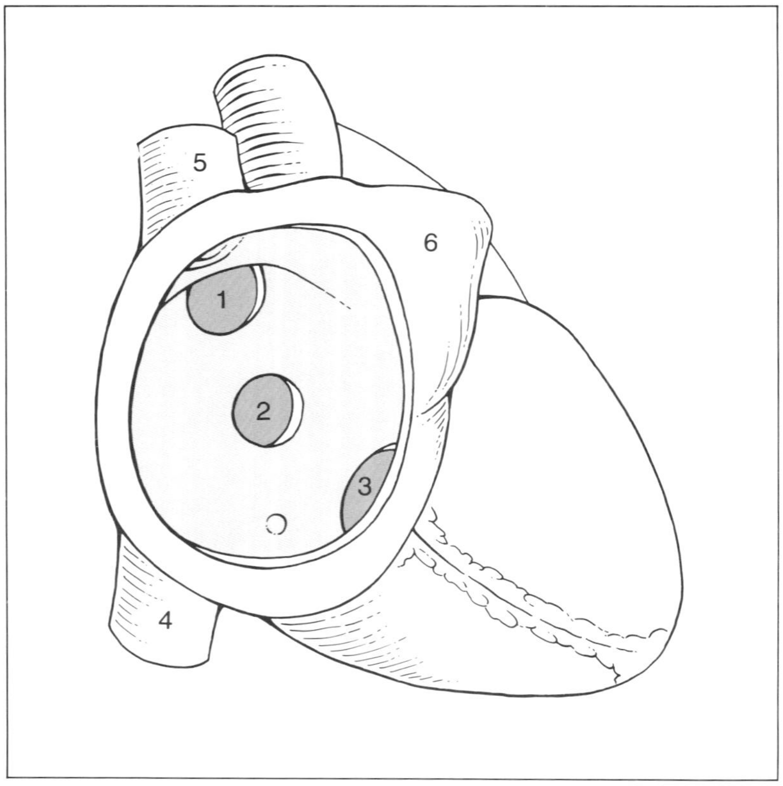

Fig. 8.28 Atrial septal defect. The three most common types of ASD (as seen from the right atrium) are illustrated.

1 sinus venosus defect
2 fossa ovalis (ostium secundum) defect
3 ostium primum defect
4 inferior vena cava
5 superior vena cava
6 right atrial appendage

with large ASDs. The main contributory factors are compression of the left ventricle by the enlarged right ventricle, which interferes with diastolic filling of the former, and tricuspid insufficiency secondary to right ventricular failure.

Clinical Features

The clinical manifestations depend on the size of the defect. Patients with small ASDs may remain asymptomatic throughout their lives; even those with large defects may remain asymptomatic for many years. Infants and children with large ASDs typically present with shortness of breath and recurrent respiratory infections. Older adults with large ASDs typically present with manifestions of congestive heart failure (eg, fluid retention, hepatomegaly, severe cardiac dilatation).

Imaging and Invasive Diagnosis

Plain Films. Chest radiographs show evidence of pulmonary plethora and of right atrial and right ventricular enlargement; in an acyanotic patient, this combination of findings favors the diagnosis of ASD (see Fig. 7.14). Unlike other types of left to right shunt (eg, ventricular septal defect or patent ductus arteriosus), the left atrium is usually of normal size. The various types of ASD usually cannot be differentiated on plain films. A wide right hilum, seen in some patients with partial anomalous pulmonary venous connection of the right upper pulmonary vein, favors the diagnosis of ASD of the sinus venosus type.

Echocardiography. The pathologic anatomy is best seen in the four-chamber view, which demonstrates the entire atrial septum in its anatomic orientation. The fossa ovalis type of ASD appears as an echo-free region in the midportion of the septum. Ostium primum ASD (absence of the atrioventricular septum) appears as a defect in the inferior portion of the septum which is bordered by the atrioventricular valve (Fig. 8.29). Sinus venosus (subcaval) ASD appears as an echo-free area in the upper part of the septum, close to the point where the superior vena cava enters the right atrium. In each type of ASD, color Doppler imaging will confirm the orientation and the magnitude of the shunt.

MRI. The various types of ASD are clearly seen on spin–echo images obtained in the transverse (axial) plane. The fossa ovalis type of ASD appears as a discontinuity in the midportion of the atrial septum (Fig. 8.30). Owing to absence of the atrioventricular septum, the septal leaflets of the right and left atrioventricular valves lie at the same level in patients with ostium primum

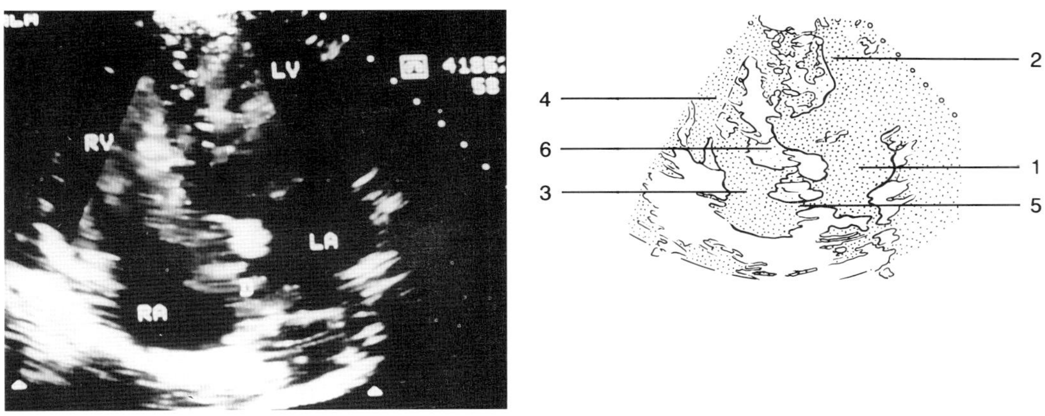

Fig. 8.29 Atrial septal defect (fossa ovalis type) (echocardiographic findings). Four-chamber view (Doppler image) shows a defect in the midportion of the atrial septum. The turbulent flow in the right atrium indicates the presence of a left to right shunt.

1 left atrium
2 left ventricle
3 right atrium
4 right ventricle
5 atrial septal defect
6 turbulence in right atrium caused by left to right shunt

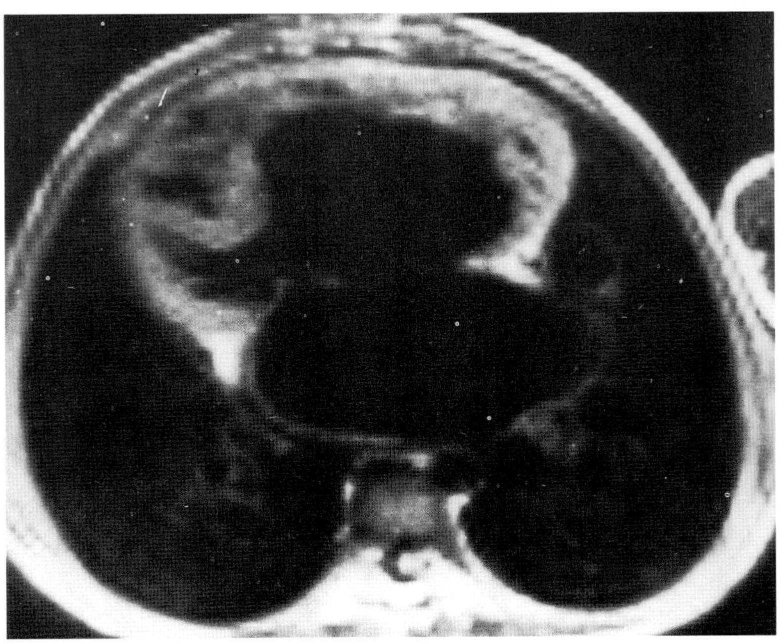

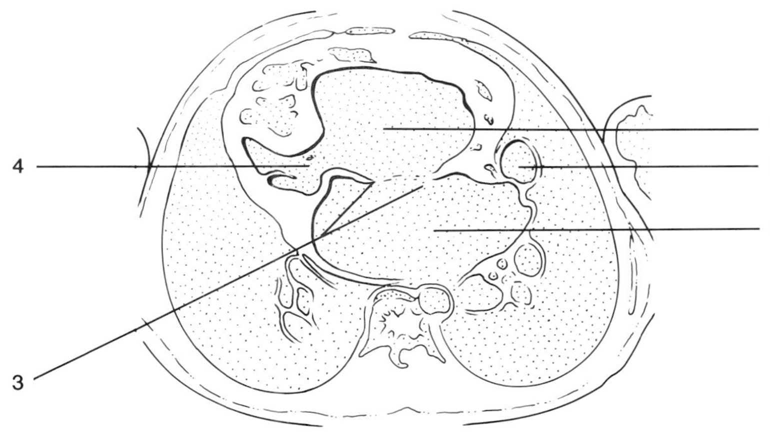

1 anterior ("right") atrium
2 posterior ("left") atrium
3 atrial septal defect (ostium primum type)
4 appendage of anterior ("right") atrium
5 appendage of posterior ("left") atrium

Fig. 8.30 Atrial septal defect (ostium primum type) (MRI findings); transverse (axial) spin–echo image. The atrium receiving the systemic venous return ("right atrium") is anterior. Its appendage resembles that of a normal left atrium. The atrium receiving the pulmonary venous return ("left atrium") is posterior. The atrial septum is parallel to the transverse axis. The ASD is within the inferior part of the septum, and therefore is of the ostium primum type.

defects. (This abnormal relationship is also clearly demonstrated on coronal and coronal oblique images.) The characteristic location of sinus venosus ASDs, immediately beneath the orifice of the superior vena cava, is clearly shown on MR images. Although cine MRI can theoretically improve diagnostic accuracy, it is seldom performed because echocardiography with color Doppler provides comparable information.

Angiocardiography. All three types of ASD are clearly depicted in the four-chamber view (Fig. 8.31).

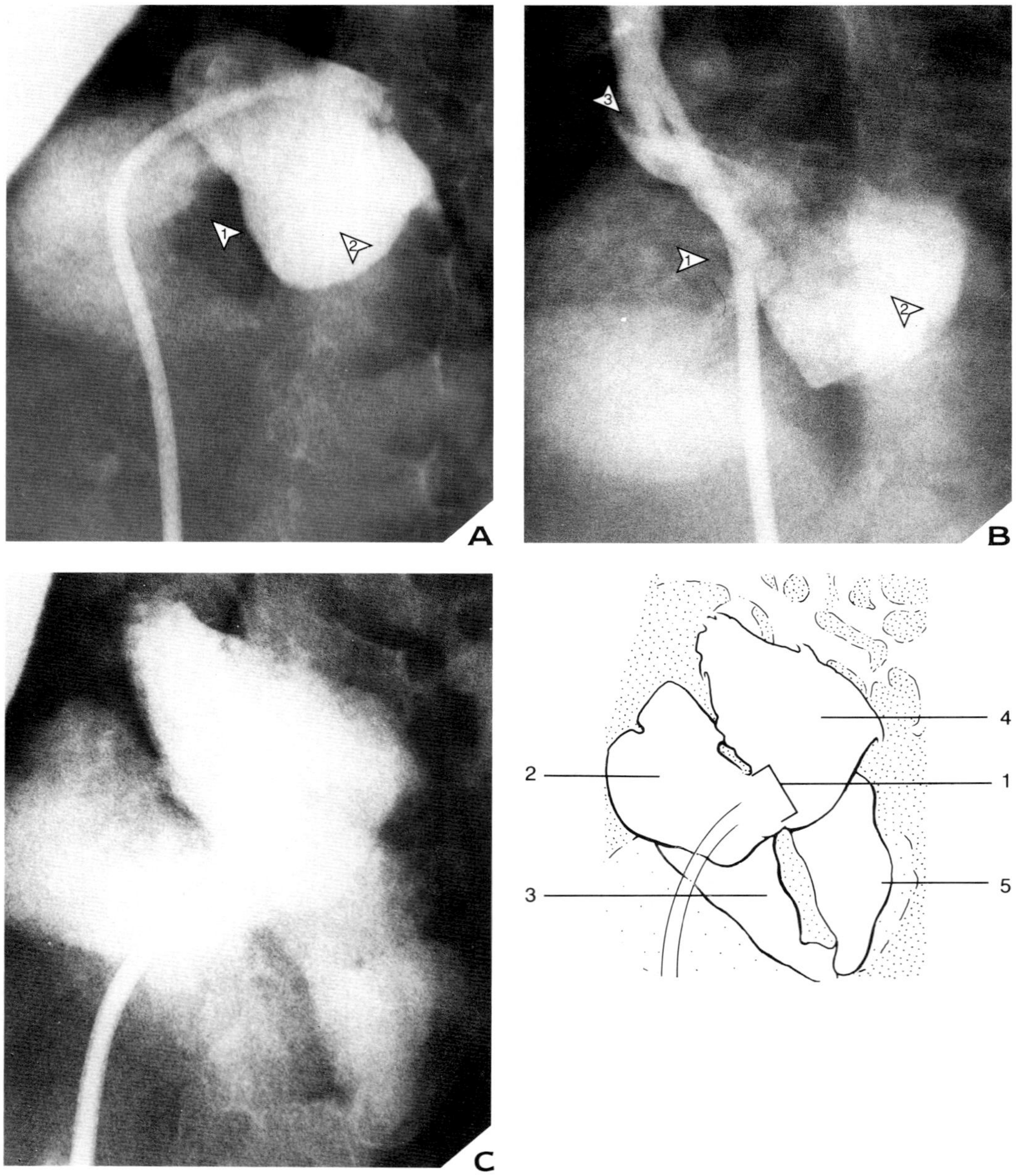

Fig. 8.31 Atrial septal defect; angiographic demonstration of the three most common types of ASD. Each study was obtained in the four-chamber projection with the catheter tip in the left atrium. (A) Sinus venosus type (*arrow* 1) is located in the upper portion of the atrial septum (*arrow* 2 indicates left atrium). (B) Fossa ovalis type (*arrow* 1) is located in the middle portion of the septum, ie, the area of the fossa ovalis (*arrow* 2 = left atrium; *arrow* 3 = right upper pulmonary vein). (C) Ostium primum type is located in the most inferior portion of the interatrial septum and is related to the atrioventricular valves.

1 atrial septal defect
2 right atrium
3 right ventricle
4 left atrium
5 left ventricle

CHAPTER 9

Ventricular and Atrioventricular Septal Defects

VENTRICULAR SEPTAL DEFECT

MORPHOLOGY

The term *ventricular septal defect* (VSD) denotes a group of congenital malformations characterized by a hole in the ventricular septum. VSDs are classified, according to their location, as perimembranous, muscular, or juxtaarterial (Figs. 9.1 and 9.2).

Perimembranous VSDs are located close to the central fibrous body. Therefore, they are related to the membranous septum, tricuspid valve, mitral valve, and aortic valve (all of which border the defect). This type of VSD, which nearly always extends into the trabecular, inlet, or outlet portion of the muscular septum, is more accurately described as "perimembranous" than "membranous."

Muscular VSDs are confined to the muscular portion of the septum. They may be located in the inlet, trabecular, or outlet regions of the muscular septum. A large defect may involve two or all three regions.

Juxtaarterial VSDs are related to the aortic pulmonic valves. The roof of the defect is formed by the arterial valve; the rest of the defect is bordered by the outlet portion of the muscular septum.

HEMODYNAMIC AND CLINICAL FEATURES

Patients with normal pulmonary vascular resistance have a pure left to right shunt with biventricular volume overload. With increasing pulmonary resistance, the shunt becomes bidi-

CHAPTER LABELING KEY

RA	right atrium	LV	left ventricle
LA	left atrium	Ao	aorta
RV	right ventricle		

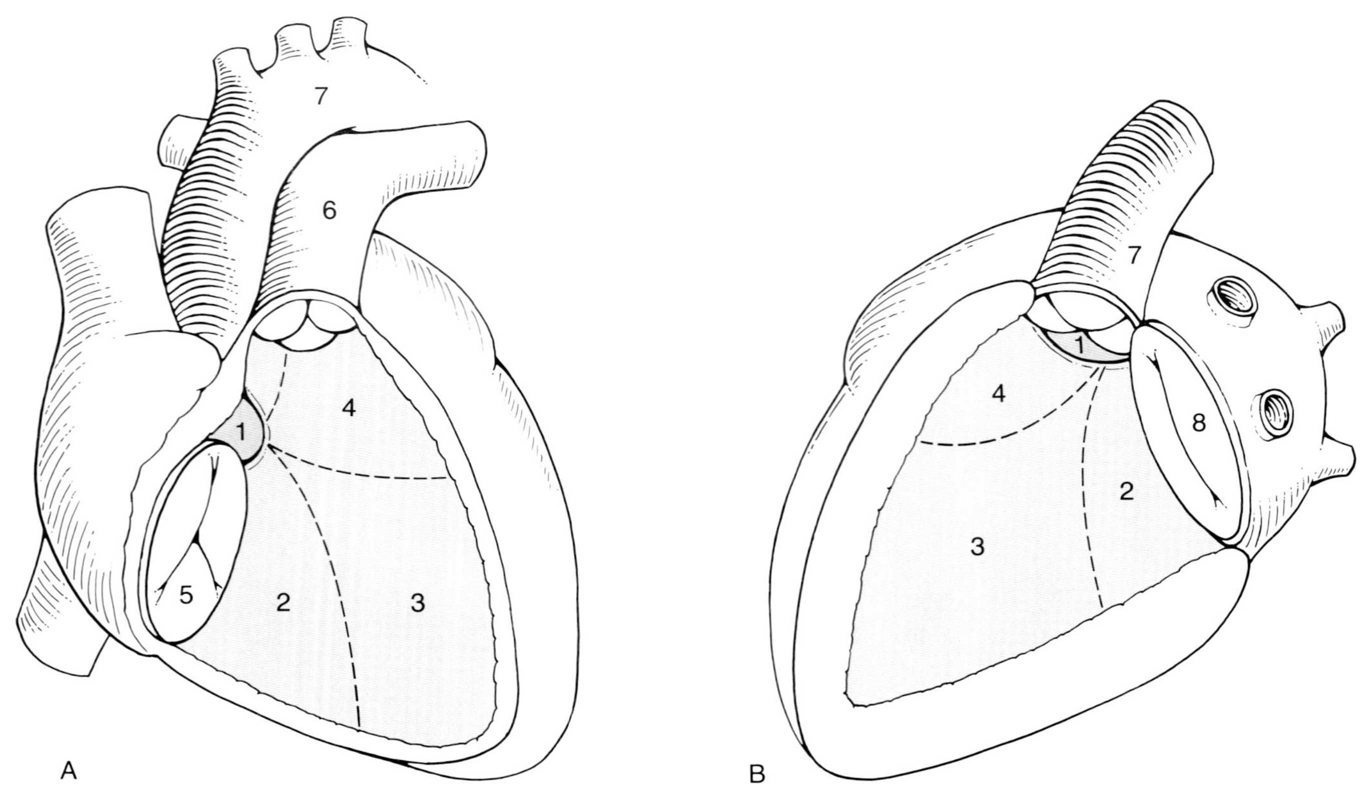

Fig. 9.1 Components of the ventricular septum. (A) Septal aspect of the right ventricle. (b) Septal aspect of the left ventricle.

1	membranous septum	5	tricuspid valve
2	muscular inlet septum	6	pulmonary trunk
3	muscular trabecular septum	7	aorta
4	muscular outlet septum	8	mitral valve

rectional and right ventricular work increases; plain films and cardiac catheterization reveal evidence of pulmonary arterial hypertension. With a further increase in pulmonary resistance, there is a net right to left shunt with severe right ventricular volume overload. The increased pulmonary blood flow at systemic or suprasystemic pressure leads to muscular hypertrophy of the acinar and pre-acinar arteries. When pulmonary vascular resistance is high enough, there may be reversal of the shunt with cyanosis (Eisenmenger syndrome).

Infants with large VSDs typically present with signs and symptoms of congestive heart failure (eg, tachypnea, hepatomegaly) and growth failure. Physical examination reveals a precordial systolic murmur and a hyperactive heart. A mitral diastolic murmur, reflecting increased flow through the mitral valve, is often heard. The ECG usually shows biventricular hypertrophy.

In older patients with a large VSD the clinical picture is usually nonspecific. Physical examination reveals biventricular enlargement and a systolic murmur, best heard in the left third or fourth interspace. In patients with a moderate increase in pulmonary resistance, resulting in a bidirectional shunt, the systolic murmur is soft or absent. The ECG reveals moderate to severe right ventricular hypertrophy. Patients with a marked increase in pulmonary resistance are cyanotic, with ECG evidence of marked right ventricular hypertrophy.

Patients with a small VSD are usually asymptomatic; a pansystolic murmur may be the only abnormality on physical examination. The ECG may reveal right ventricular hypertrophy.

IMAGING AND INVASIVE DIAGNOSIS

PLAIN FILMS

The plain film findings depend on the magnitude (volume) of the shunt and the presence or absence of pulmonary arterial hypertension (PAH).

Small Shunt Without PAH

The chest film is usually normal in patients with a small left to right shunt (2:1 or less) and normal right ventricular pressure. In general, shunts of this magnitude are not associated with right ventricular enlargement or pulmonary plethora; hence, they cannot be appreciated on plain films.

Large Shunt Without PAH

In patients with a large left to right shunt (3:1 or greater) in whom pulmonary artery pressure is only moderately elevated, chest films show right ventricular and left atrial enlargement and a normal left ventricle. The central pulmonary arteries, as well as their lobar, segmental, and subsegmental branches, are enlarged. Subsegmental branches, which normally cannot be

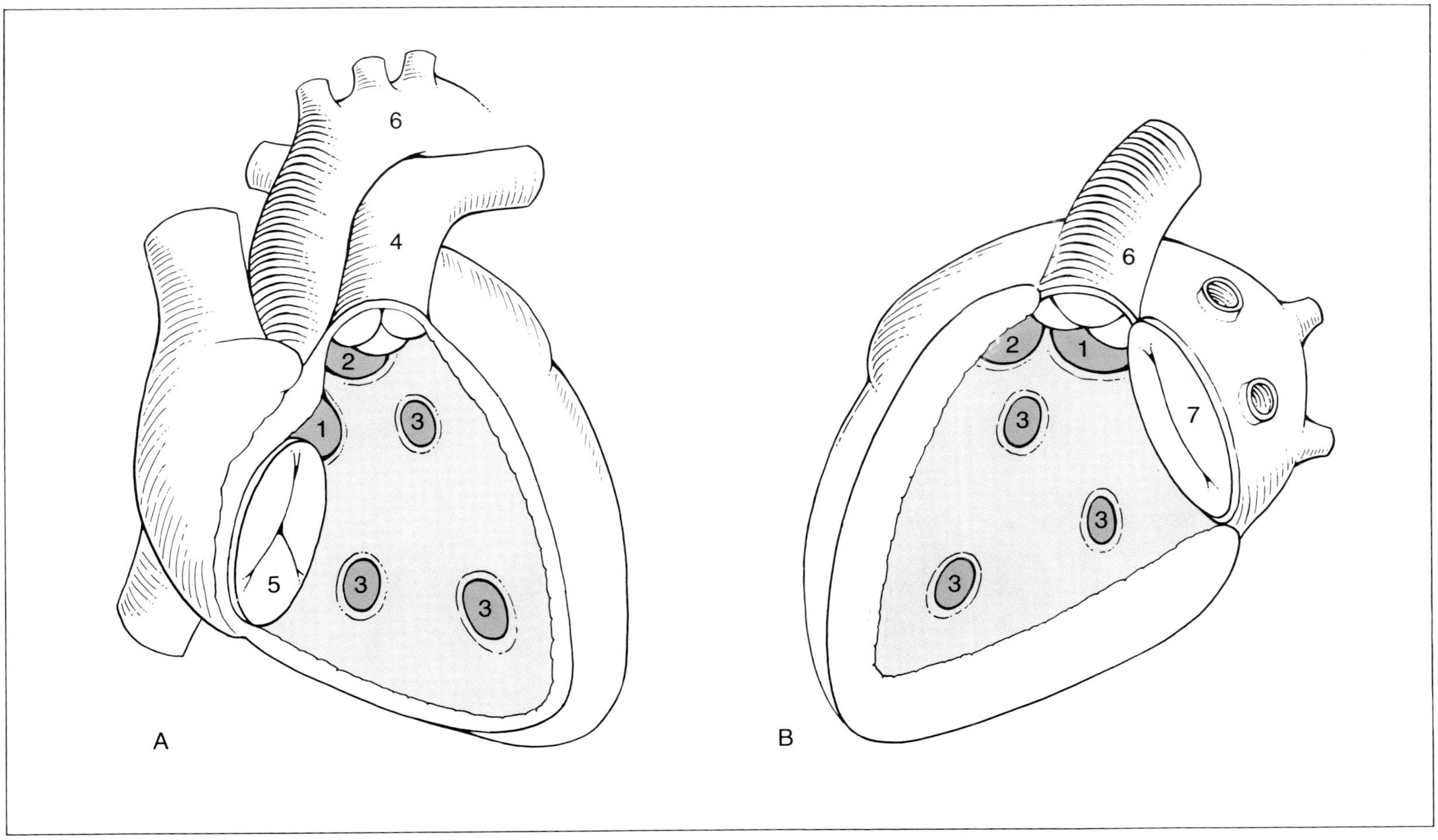

Fig. 9.2 Types of VSD. (A) Right ventricular aspect. (B) Left ventricular aspect.

1 perimembranous VSD
2 juxtaarterial VSD
3 muscular VSD
4 pulmonary artery
5 tricuspid valve
6 aorta
7 mitral valve

identified in the outer third of the lung fields, can be followed out to the periphery (Fig. 9.3). (When seen end on, the tortuous segmental and subsegmental branches can mimic lung nodules.) Medium-sized pulmonary veins, normally invisible or inconspicuous on chest films, can be quite prominent, especially in the upper zones. Left lower lobe atelectasis is not uncommon.

Large Shunt with PAH (Eisenmenger Syndrome)

When right ventricular pressure equals or exceeds left ventricular pressure, chest films show right ventricular enlargement, dilatation of the pulmonary trunk and central pulmonary branches, and a decrease in the size and number of small peripheral arteries (Fig. 9.4).

ECHOCARDIOGRAPHY

Perimembranous VSDs are most readily identified on long axial and short axial projections as an echo-free area related to the aortic, mitral, and tricuspid valves. A muscular VSD appears as an echo-free defect in the muscular septum, although small defects may not be appreciated. Juxtaarterial VSDs are best seen on short axis views. In this projection the VSD appears as an echo-free area at the junction between the aortic and pulmonic valves, which is clearly separate from the mitral and tricuspid valves (Fig. 9.5). The magnitude and direction of the shunt can be assessed on color-flow Doppler images (Fig. 9.6; see Appendix).

MAGNETIC RESONANCE IMAGING

VSDs in various anatomic locations can be demonstrated and localized by gated spin–echo and cine MRI (Figs. 9.7 and 9.8). The latter also provides important functional information regarding blood flow and right and left ventricular function. In some instances, the signal loss resulting from the turbulent blood flow may indicate the presence of a VSD that cannot be visualized on spin–echo images. By determining the difference between the left and right ventricular stroke volumes as demonstrated on cine MRI, it is possible to arrive at a quantification of the net shunt size.

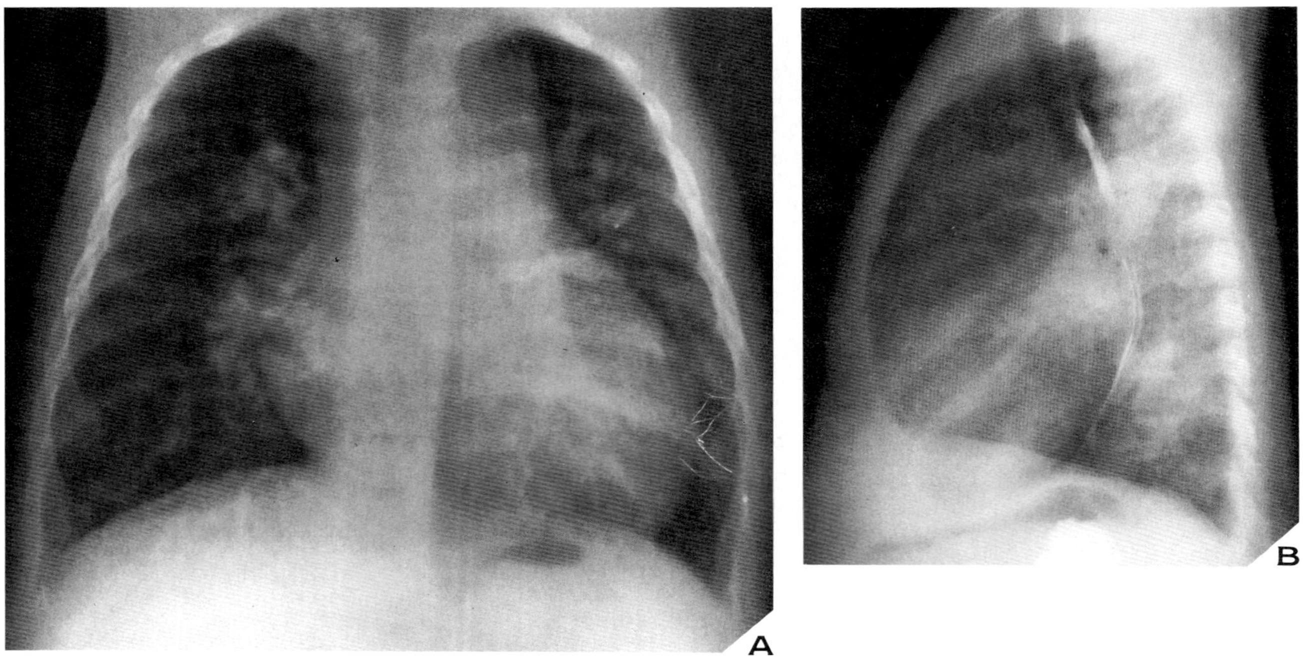

Fig. 9.3 Large VSD without a significant increase in pulmonary resistance. (A) Frontal and (B) lateral chest films show right ventricular and left atrial enlargement and plethoric pulmonary vasculature.

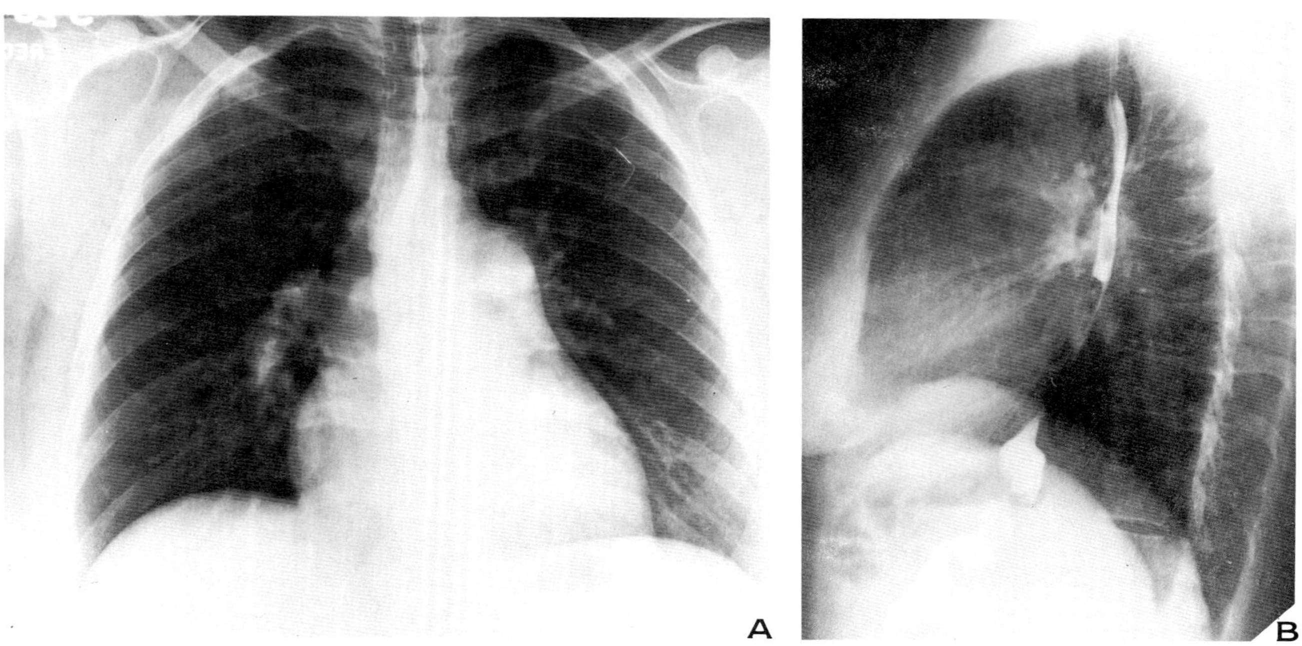

Fig. 9.4 Large VSD with a significant increase in pulmonary resistance (Eisenmenger syndrome). (A) Frontal and (B) lateral chest films show right ventricular enlargment, dilatation of the pulmonary trunk, and enlargement of the left and right pulmonary branches. The peripheral pulmonary branches are smaller than normal.

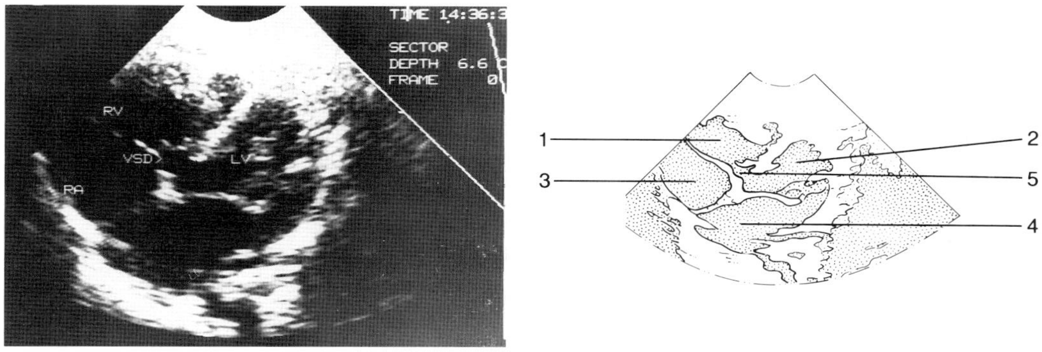

Fig. 9.5 Perimembranous VSD. Communication between the right and left ventricles is clearly seen in the four-chamber view of this 2-D echocardiogram.

1 right ventricle
2 left ventricle
3 right atrium
4 left atrium
5 ventricular septal defect

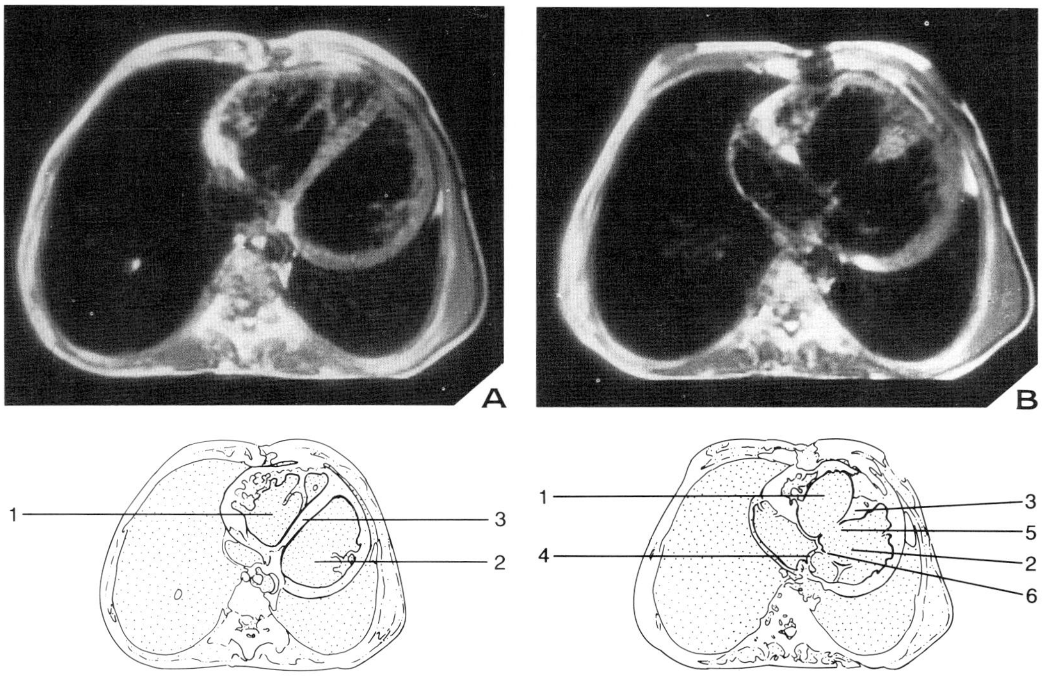

Fig. 9.7 Perimembranous VSD. ECG-gated spin–echo images; transverse sections. (A) A section through the posteroinferior part of the ventricular septum shows that the septum is intact at this level. (B) A more cephalic section shows a VSD at the level of the central fibrous body. Note that the VSD is in continuity with the septal leaflet of the tricuspid valve.

1 right ventricle
2 left ventricle
3 ventricular septum
4 atrial septum
5 perimembranous VSD
6 septal leaflet of tricuspid valve

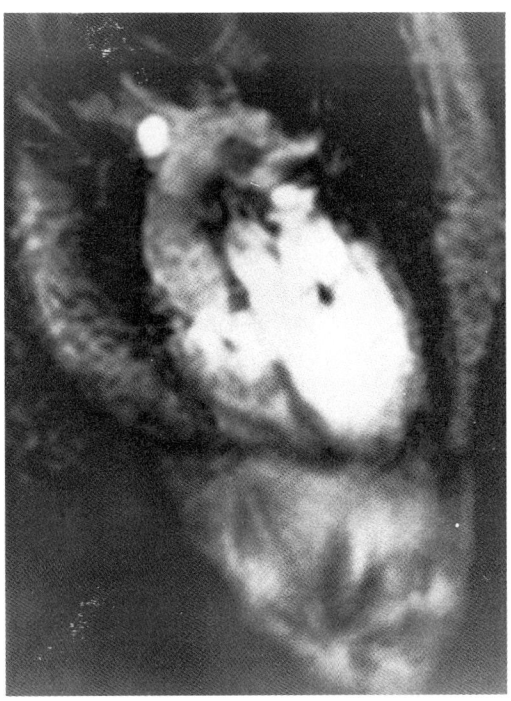

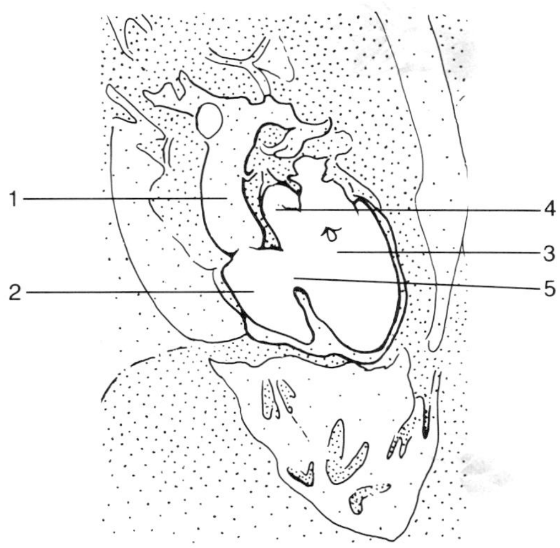

Fig. 9.8 Muscular VSD associated with transposition of the great arteries. Cine MRI (flowing blood appears white). The ventricular septum is seen in profile on this oblique craniocaudal section. The VSD is entirely surrounded by the muscular portion of the ventricular septum (low signal). The aorta arises from the morphologic right ventricle and the pulmonary trunk from the morphologic left ventricle in this patient with transposition of the great arteries.

1 ascending aorta
2 right ventricle
3 left ventricle
4 pulmonary trunk
5 ventricular septal defect

CARDIAC CATHETERIZATION

A thorough quantitative assessment of the hemodynamic status is necessary to plan surgical treatment in patients with large VSDs. The catheterization data should include right ventricular systolic and diastolic pressures; main pulmonary artery pressure; pulmonary wedge pressure; systemic arterial pressure; oxygen consumption, oxygen content, and saturation in the right atrium, main pulmonary artery, aorta, and peripheral arterial blood; and left atrial pressure and oxygen content. With these data one can calculate the systemic (Qs) and pulmonary

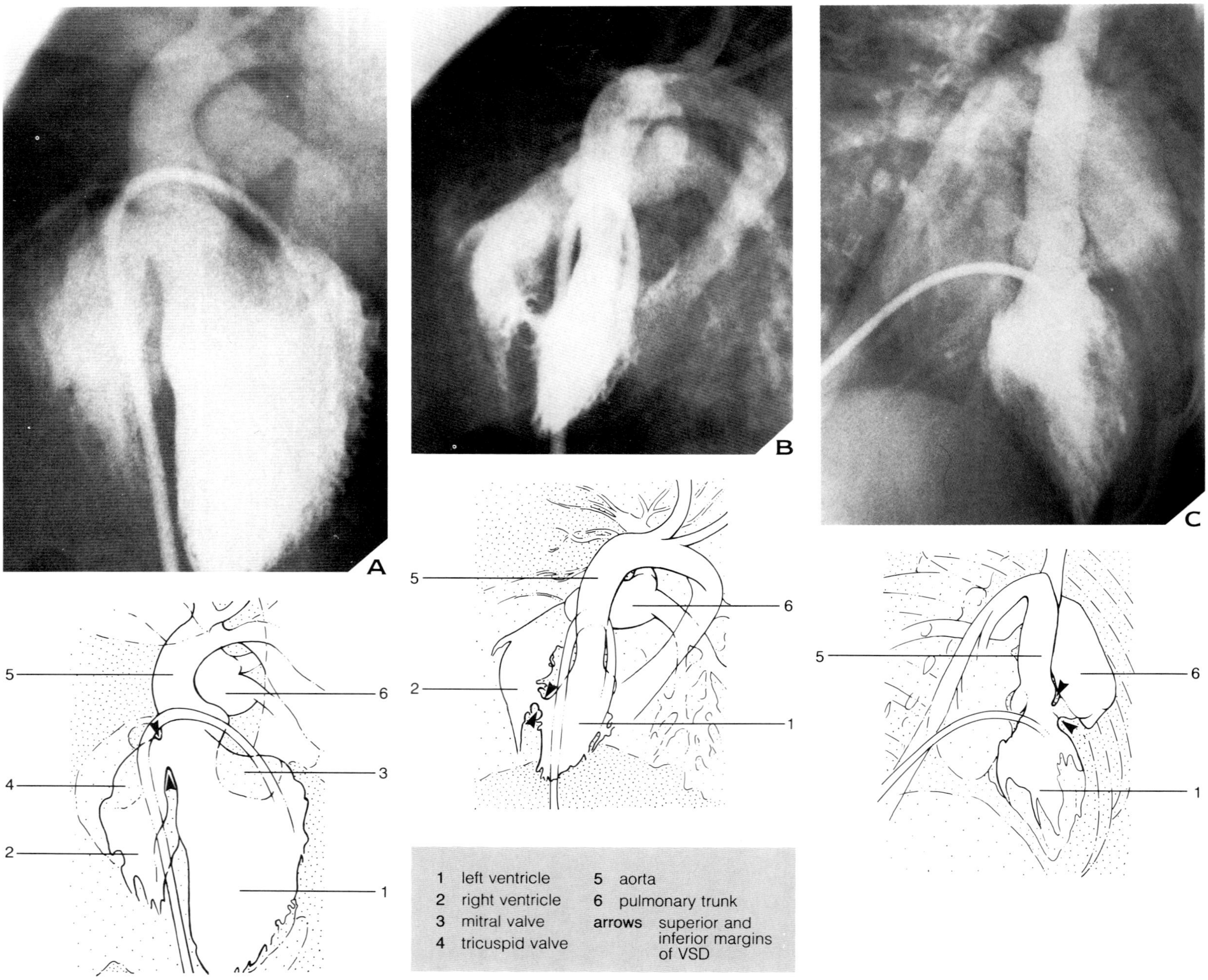

Fig. 9.9 Angiographic appearance of various types of VSD. (A) Perimembranous VSD (long axis projection). Contrast material delineates the margins of the VSD, which is located beneath the aortic valve and is related to the tricuspid valve. (B) Muscular VSD (long axis projection). The septal defect is in the midportion of the trabecular part of the muscular septum. (C) Juxtaarterial VSD (elongated right anterior oblique projection). The septal defect is immediately beneath the aortic and pulmonic valves.

(Qp) flow and the pulmonary/systemic blood flow ratio (Qp/Qs), as well as the pulmonary vascular resistance (expressed as absolute units × body surface area). The calculated pulmonary vascular resistance is the most reliable parameter for predicting operability.

ANGIOCARDIOGRAPHY

Perimembranous and muscular VSDs are best seen on left ventriculography in the long axial projection. As noted above, perimembranous VSDs are related to the aortic, mitral, and tricuspid valves; they may extend for a variable distance into the adjacent muscular portions of the ventricular septum (Fig. 9.9A). Muscular VSDs are located within the inlet, trabecular, and/or outlet portions of the muscular septum; they are not related to the valvular structures (Fig. 9.9B). Juxtaarterial VSDs are located just beneath the right coronary cusp of the aortic valve and below the right and left cusps of the pulmonic valve. They are best seen on left ventriculograms obtained in the right anterior oblique projection (Fig. 9.9C).

ATRIOVENTRICULAR SEPTAL DEFECT (AVSD) ("ENDOCARDIAL CUSHION DEFECT")

MORPHOLOGY

This group of congenital malformations involves structures that are derived from the endocardial cushions, ie, the atrioventricular septum and portions of the mitral and tricuspid valves (Fig. 9.10). The septal leaflet of the mitral valve has two components: an anterior portion (derived from the anterior endocardial cushion) and a posterior portion (derived from the posteroinferior endocardial cushion). The mural leaflet of the mitral valve is derived from the lateral endocardial cushion. The tricuspid valve has three components: a septal leaflet (derived from the posteroinferior endocardial cushion), an inferior cusp (derived from the lateral endocardial cushion), and an anterior leaflet (derived from the conus).

Failure of fusion of the endocardial cushions results in an abnormal communication between the left and right sides of the heart. The abnormal communication may be restricted to the atrial level *(ostium primum ASD)* or the ventricular level; most commonly, however, there is communication at both the atrial and ventricular levels. Because the atrioventricular septum is absent, the left ventricle and right atrium always communicate with each other *(atrioventricular septal defect)*. In the most severe anomaly, all four cardiac chambers communicate *(complete atrioventricular canal)*. The morphology and attachments of the atrioventricular valves are abnormal as well.

The malformation of the atrioventricular valves may be complete or partial. In the *complete form* there is a common atrio-

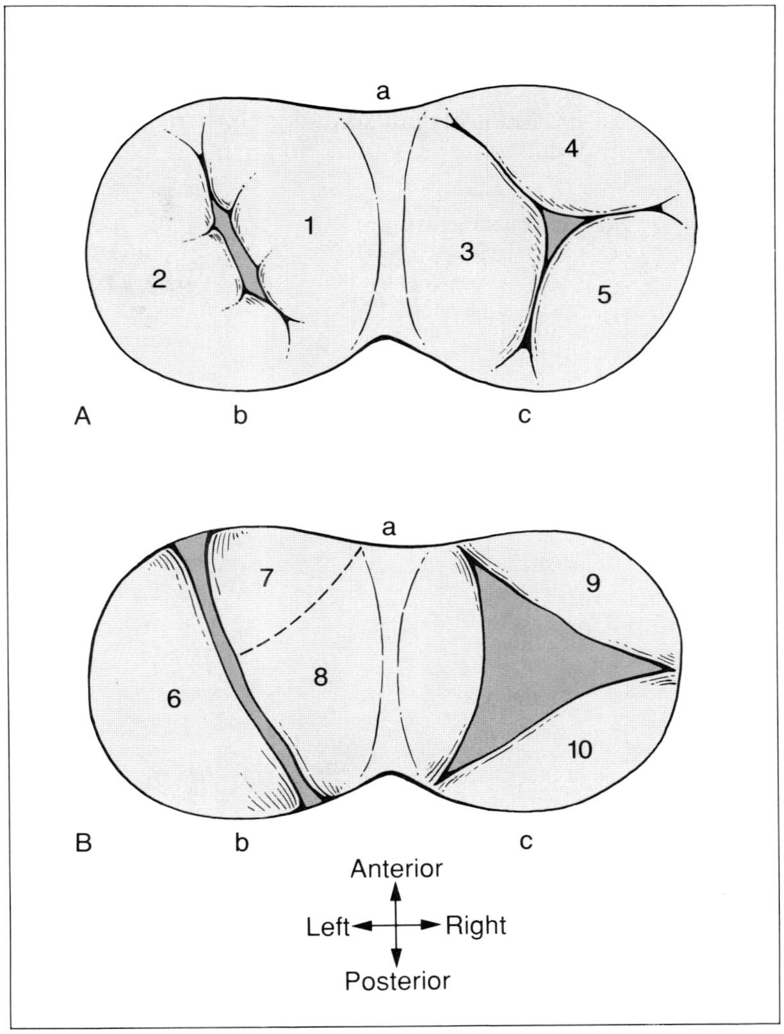

1 septal mitral leaflet
2 mural (posterior) leaflet
3 septal tricuspid leaflet
4 anterior tricuspid leaflet
5 inferior tricuspid leaflet
6 left lateral endocardial cushion
7 anterosuperior endocardial cushion
8 posteroinferior endocardial cushion
9 conal component
10 lateral endocardial cushion
a ventricular septum
b mitral valve
c tricuspid valve

Fig. 9.10 Morphogenesis of the atrioventricular valves: contribution of the endocardial cushions. (A) Normal mitral and tricuspid valves (viewed from above). (B) Portions of the endocardial cushions contributing to the formation of the normal mitral and tricuspid valves.

ventricular valve (Figs. 9.11 and 9.11B). It is convenient, from an anatomic and practical standpoint, to consider the common atrioventricular valve as a structure with a single annulus which is related to both ventricles, an arrangement that results in a common orifice. The common atrioventricular valve—which is neither a mitral nor a tricuspid valve—has either four or five leaflets.

In the *partial form* there are two separate atrioventricular valves (Fig. 9.11C). The common atrioventricular orifice is divided by the attachments of the anterior and posterior bridging leaflets, which insert at the top of the ventricular septum. The valve that connects the left atrium with the left ventricle *(left atrioventricular valve)* usually has three leaflets: the *superior leaflet,* which is attached to the ventricular septum and is related to the aortic valve; the *inferior leaflet,* which is also attached to the septum but is related to the crux cordis; and the *lateral leaflet,* which represents the normal mural leaflet of the mitral valve. The commissure separating the superior and inferior leaflets faces the ventricular septum and has a cleft appearance owing to the absence of a papillary muscle attachment. The valve that connects the right atrium with the right ventricle *(right atrioventricular valve)* usually has four components, one of which is atretic. The anterior leaflet is in continuity with the superior leaflet of the left atrioventricular valve, creating a structure known as the *anterior bridging leaflet.* The posterior leaflet of the right atrioventricular valve and the posterior or inferior leaflet of the left atrioventricular valve are also fused, creating a structure known as the *posterior bridging leaflet.*

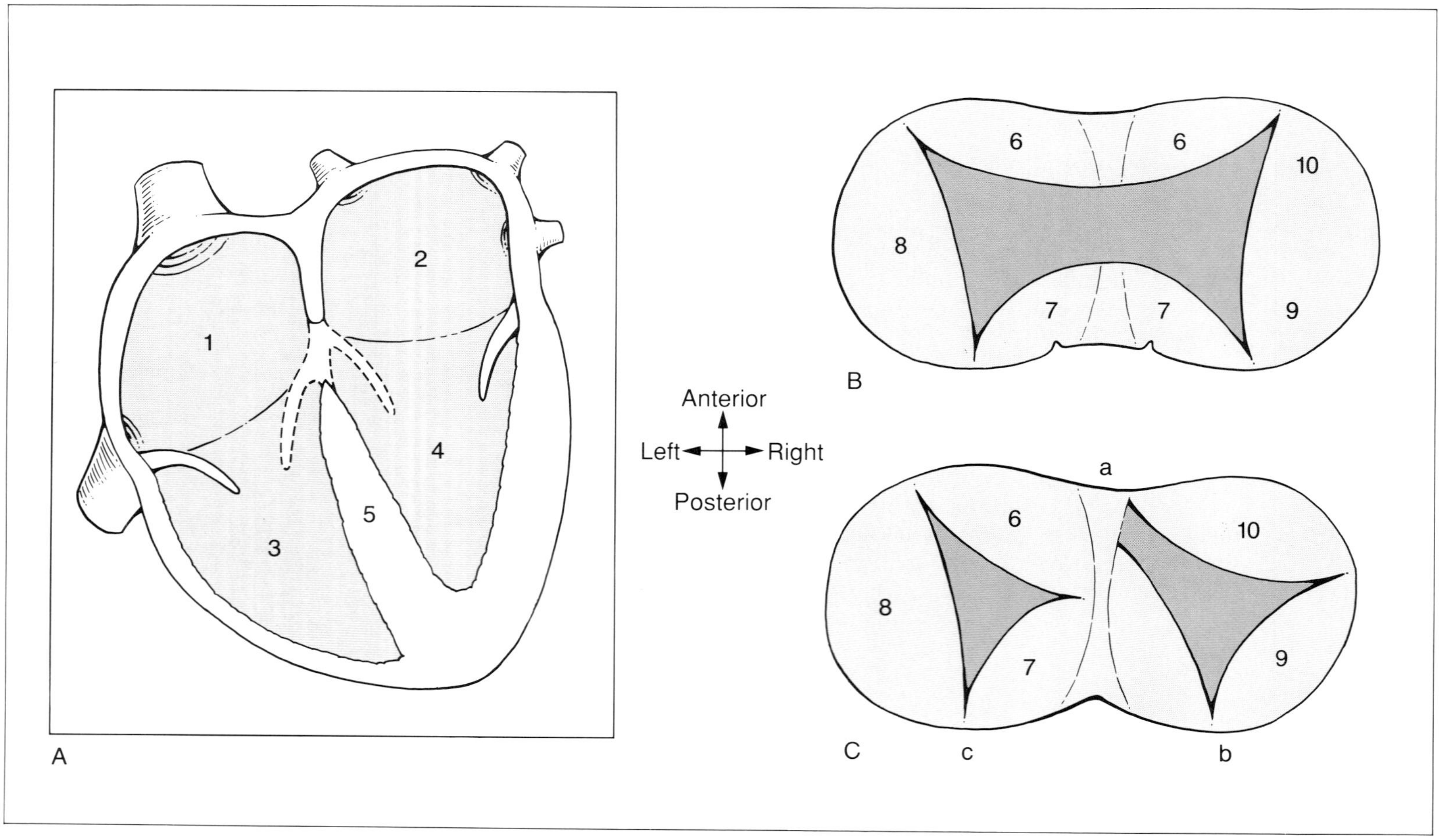

1 right atrium (RA)
2 left atrium (LA)
3 right ventricle (RV)
4 left ventricle (LV)
5 ventricular septum (VS)
6 superior bridging leaflet (anterior endocardial cushion)
7 inferior bridging leaflet (posterior endocardial cushion)
8 left lateral leaflet (left lateral endocardial cushion)
9 right lateral leaflet (right lateral endocardial cushion)
10 right anterior leaflet (conal component)
a ventricular septum
b right atrioventricular valve
c left atrioventricular valve

Fig. 9.11 Atrioventricular septal defect (AVSD). (A) *Complete AVSD (complete A-V canal).* Interrupted line indicates the portions of the septum that are missing (the atrioventricular septum and portions of the atrial septum and ventricular septum). (B) *Common atrioventricular valve (complete form of AVSD).* There are usually four leaflets: one anterior, one posterior, and two lateral. Occasionally the anterior leaflet (superior bridging leaflet) is divided into two parts at the level of the septum; valves of this type have five leaflets. (C) *Divided atrioventricular valve (incomplete or partial form of AVSD).* There are two separate atrioventricular valves, one related to each ventricular chamber.

HEMODYNAMIC AND CLINICAL FEATURES

The hemodynamic consequences of this anomaly reflect the patency of the various potential shunts. Insufficiency of the left or right atrioventricular valves may be an additional factor in some instances. About 50 percent of patients with the complete form of AVSD have trisomy 21 (Down syndrome).

Infants and children with AVSD typically present with congestive heart failure and growth failure, which are manifestations of the large left to right shunt that is usually present. The magnitude of the shunt is determined by the size of the interatrial and interventricular communications. Except for a small percentage of patients in whom the atrioventricular leaflets are attached to the remnant of the atrial septum, an interatrial communication is always present. Patients with complete form (atrioventricular canal) almost always have a large interventricular communication; however, this is not the case in patients with partial defects. The size of the defect is of great prognostic significance. Patients with a large one develop increased pulmonary resistance early in life, eventually culminating in an Eisenmenger syndrome, whereas those with no interventricular communication, or a very small VSD, have a relatively benign course similar to that of a secundum ASD.

Insufficiency of the left atrioventricular valve may contribute to the early onset of congestive heart failure. A large left to right shunt at the atrial level will usually mask mild to moderate insufficiency of the left atrioventricular valve.

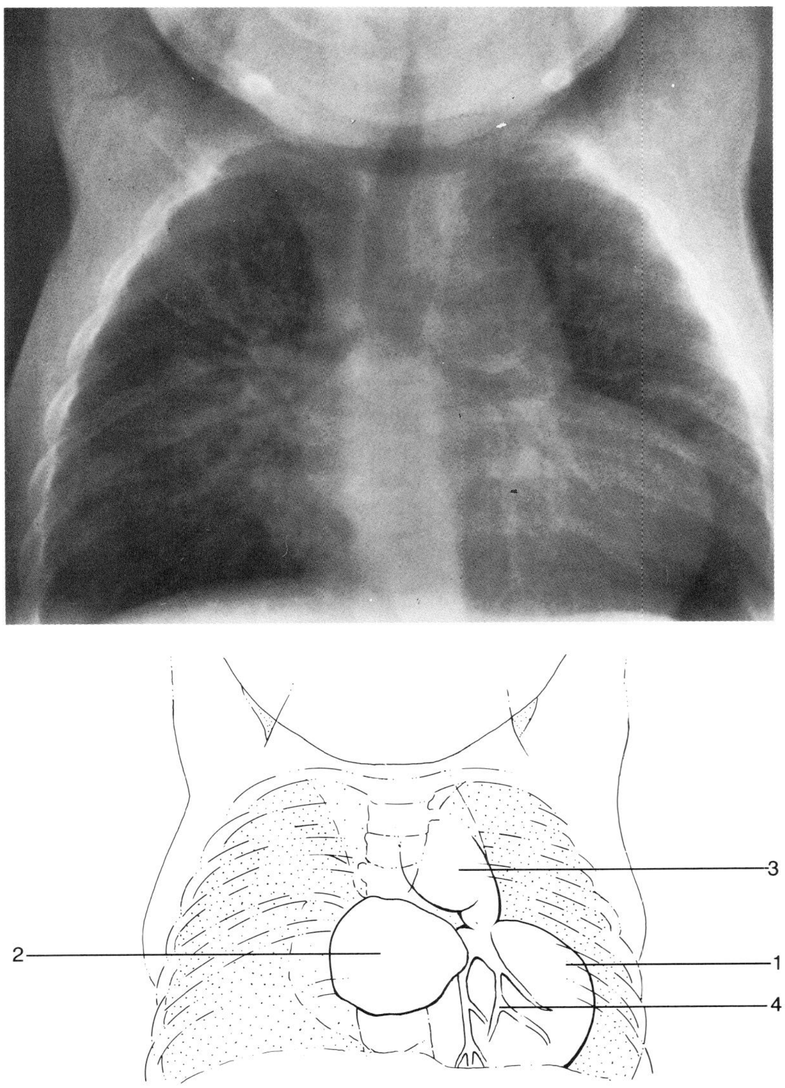

1 upturned apex indicating right ventricular enlargement
2 normal-sized left atrium
3 left superior vena cava
4 enlarged pulmonary vessels

Fig. 9.12 Complete AVSD in a neonate. Anteroposterior chest film in a one-week-old infant shows cardiomegaly with right ventricular prominence and a persistent left superior vena cava. The lungs are plethoric.

IMAGING AND INVASIVE DIAGNOSIS

PLAIN FILMS

Symptomatic infants commonly have radiographic evidence of congestive heart failure. Although some infants with complete AVSD have marked right atrial enlargement, in most instances the cardiac configuration is nonspecific. Additional findings that favor the diagnosis of AVSD include a left superior vena cava and thoracic abnormalities commonly seen in trisomy 21 (eg, hypersegmentation of the sternum, 11 ribs) (Fig. 9.12).

The plain film findings in most older children and teenagers resemble those of a secundum ASD: moderate cardiomegaly, with right atrial and right ventricular enlargement, and pulmonary plethora, the pulmonary vessels reaching far into the periphery (Fig. 9.13). Marked right atrial enlargement caused by incompetence of the common atrioventricular valve favors the diagnosis of AVSD.

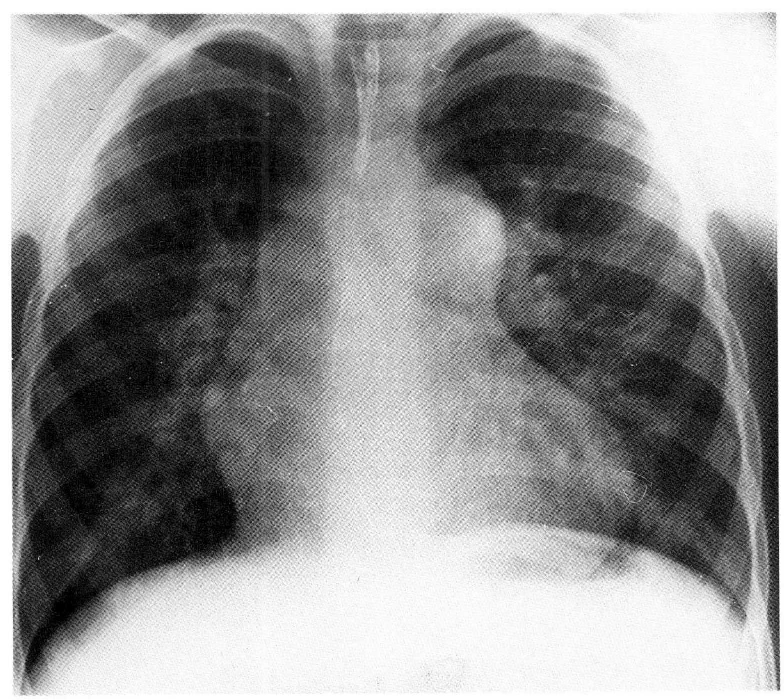

Fig. 9.13 Complete AVSD. Frontal film of a 5-year-old patient shows mild cardiomegaly with prominence of the right ventricle and pulmonary trunk and right atrial enlargement. The lungs are plethoric. The aortic arch is hypoplastic.

ECHOCARDIOGRAPHY

The morphologic features of this anomaly are clearly shown by two-dimensional echocardiography. The AVSD and the anomalous atrioventricular valve are clearly depicted in four-chamber views obtained with various degrees of angulation (Fig. 9.14). The anterior bridging leaflet is seen to pass through the AVSD, connecting the anterior papillary muscle of the left ventricle with the medial (anterior) papillary muscle of the right ventricle. Continuity of the posterior bridging leaflet, which extends (via the AVSD) from the posterior papillary muscle of the right ventricle to the posterior papillary muscle of the left ventricle, is seen on four-chamber views obtained with less angulation. (The attachment of the posterior bridging leaflet to the top of the ventricular septum is also well seen on these images.) Long axis views demonstrate other characteristic features of this malformation, including malposition of the papillary muscles, narrowing of the left ventricular outflow tract, and malposition of the aortic valve. Interatrial and interventricular shunting and insufficiency of the atrioventricular valves can be detected and quantified with color Doppler imaging.

MAGNETIC RESONANCE IMAGING

Spin–echo images accurately depict the morphologic features of this complex malformation. The absence of the atrioventricular septum and the relations of the common atrioventricular valve are best seen on transverse (axial) images. The interatrial and interventricular communications are clearly shown by cine MRI.

CARDIAC CATHETERIZATION

Cardiac catheterization provides important data needed to plan surgical treatment, eg, the magnitude and direction of the shunt, the pulmonary and systemic pressures, pulmonary resistance, and flow. Patients with complete AVSD typically have a large interventricular communication with equalization

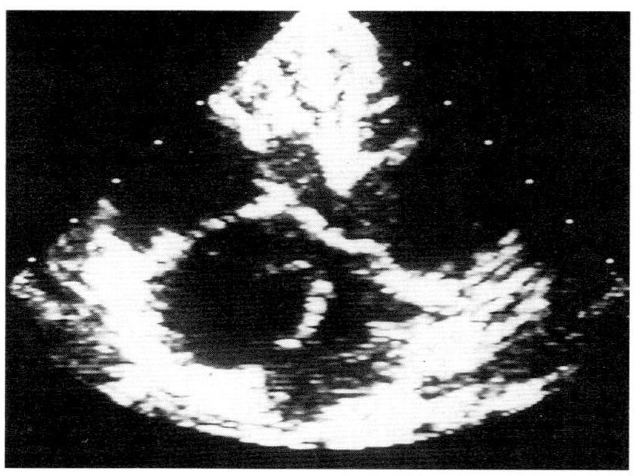

Fig. 9.14 Complete AVSD. Four-chamber projection of echocardiogram shows absence of the atrioventricular septum, resulting in an ostium primum ASD and deficiency of the inlet portion of the muscular ventricular septum (muscular VSD). The superior bridging leaflet passes from one ventricle to the other.

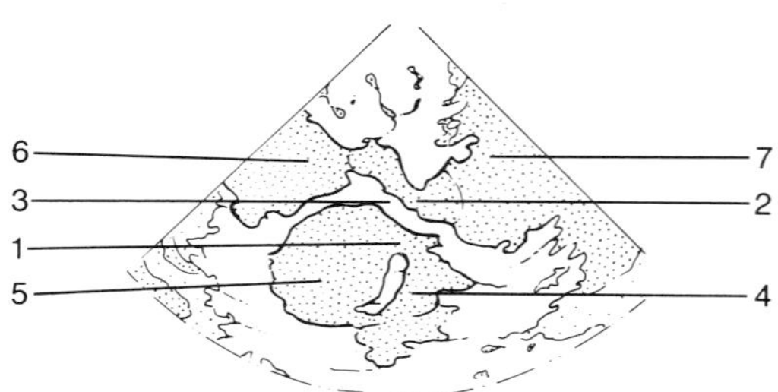

1 ostium primum ASD (absence of atrial portion of atrioventricular septum
2 deficient inlet portion of muscular ventricular septum
3 superior bridging leaflet (attached to both ventricles)
4 left atrium
5 right atrium
6 right ventricle
7 left ventricle

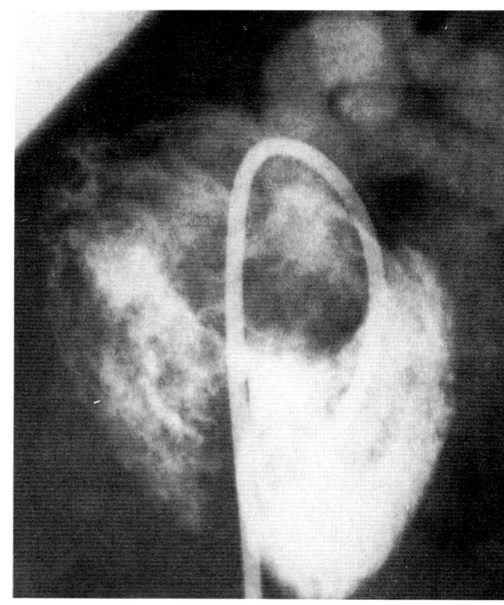

Fig. 9.15 Complete atrioventricular canal. Left ventriculogram (four-chamber projection) shows a large round filling defect, which represents the common atrioventricular valve, straddling the left and right ventricles.

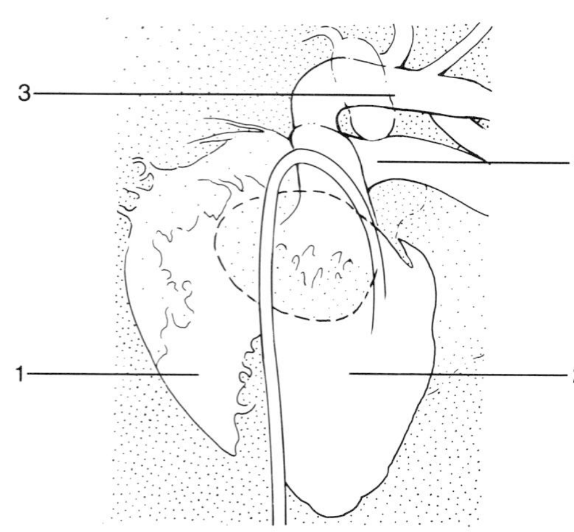

1 right ventricle
2 left ventricle
3 aorta
4 pulmonary trunk

of right and left ventricular pressures. The high right ventricular and pulmonary arterial pressure stimulates an increase in pulmonary vascular resistance. In general, patients with trisomy 21 tend to develop increased pulmonary resistance more rapidly than patients with normal karyotypes.

In most patients with partial AVSD, right ventricular pressure is normal or only slightly elevated; this is because the leaflets of the common atrioventricular valve are attached to the top of the ventricular septum, an arrangement that prevents interventricular shunting. Therefore, patients with partial defects are unlikely to develop early increased pulmonary resistance.

ANGIOCARDIOGRAPHY

Left and right ventriculograms obtained in the four-chamber and elongated right anterior oblique projections demonstrate the pertinent anatomy. The left ventricle is of normal size, but the outlet segment is markedly deformed owing to the absence of the atrioventricular septum and the abnormal position of the corresponding atrioventricular valve. Because the aorta is usually deviated anteriorly, the left ventricular outflow tract usually appears elongated. Because of the large left to right shunt the aorta is usually smaller than normal. In most cases the right and left pulmonary arteries are enlarged and the lungs are plethoric.

The atrioventricular valves are best seen in the four-chamber projection. Patients with a complete AVSD have a common atrioventricular valve, which appears as a negative round shadow during diastole (Fig. 9.15), whereas those with partial defects have a separate atrioventricular valve for each ventricle (Fig. 9.16). Ventricular and atrial septal defects are best seen in the four-chamber projection (Fig. 9.17), whereas those in the atrioventricular septum are best demonstrated in the four-

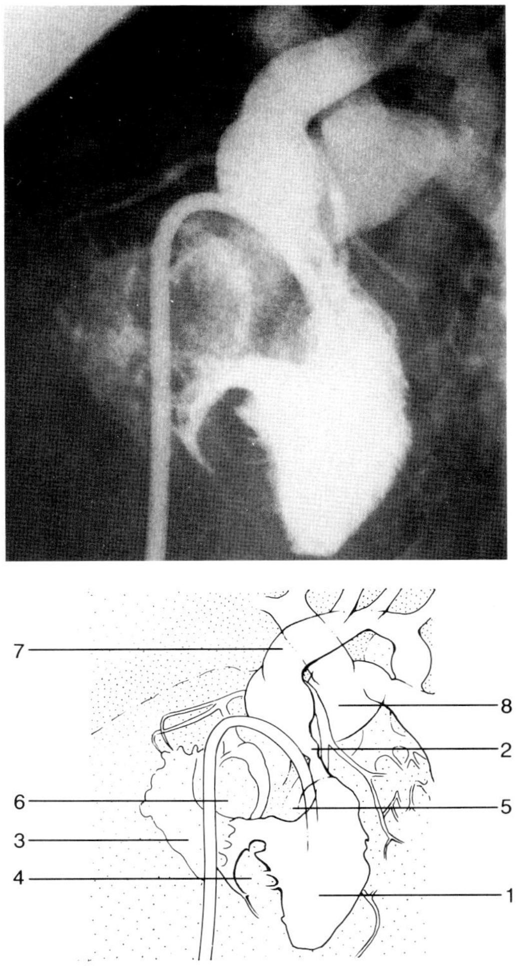

Fig. 9.16 Partial AVSD. Four-chamber projection of left ventriculogram shows deformity of the left ventricular outflow tract resulting from absence of the atrioventricular septum. There are two atrioventricular valves, one related to each ventricle. The junction of the atrioventricular valves is represented by a fibrous structure atop the ventricular septum.

1 left ventricle
2 deformed left ventricular outflow tract
3 right ventricle
4 ventricular septum
5 left atrioventricular valve
6 right atrioventricular valve
7 aorta
8 pulmonary trunk

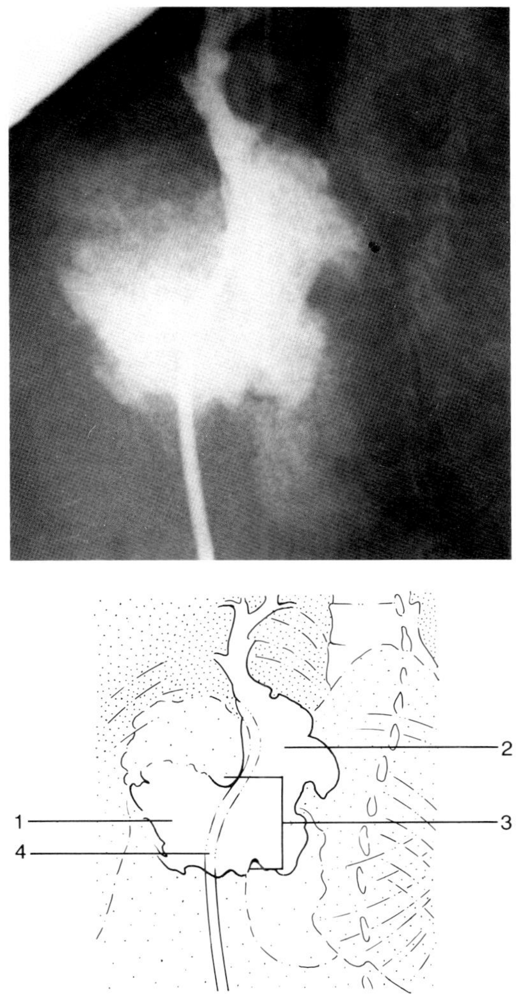

Fig. 9.17 Atrioventricular septal defect: primum ASD. Four-chamber view of left atrial angiogram shows a defect in the inferior part of the atrial septum. The catheter traverses the atrial septal defect.

1 right atrium
2 left atrium
3 atrial septal defect
4 catheter

chamber and elongated right anterior oblique projections (Figs. 9.16 to 9.18).

Many patients have some degree of atrioventricular valve insufficiency owing to the deficiency of leaflet tissue or the abnormal attachment of the leaflets to the top of the ventricular system. Regurgitant flow through the atrioventricular valve is best seen on left and right ventriculograms obtained in the lateral or elongated right anterior oblique projection (Fig. 9.19).

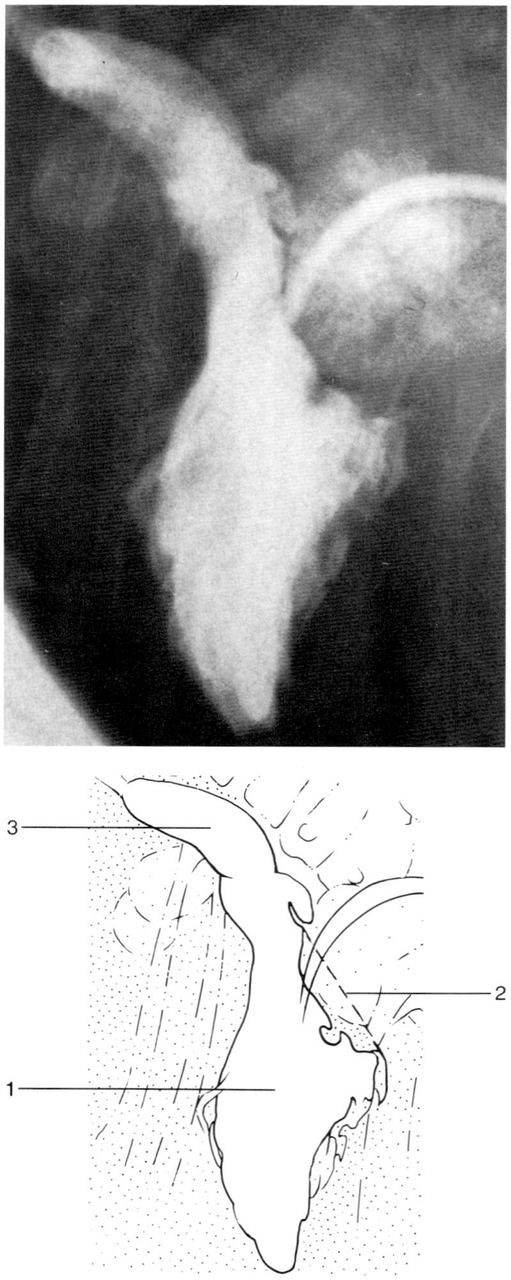

1 left ventricle	3 aorta
2 border normally formed by atrioventricular septum	

Fig. 9.18 Complete AVSD. Elongated right anterior oblique projection of left ventriculogram shows deformity of the inlet and outlet portions of the left ventricle resulting from absence of the atrioventricular septum and the adjacent portions of the atrial and ventricular septa. The border normally formed by the atrioventricular septum is absent.

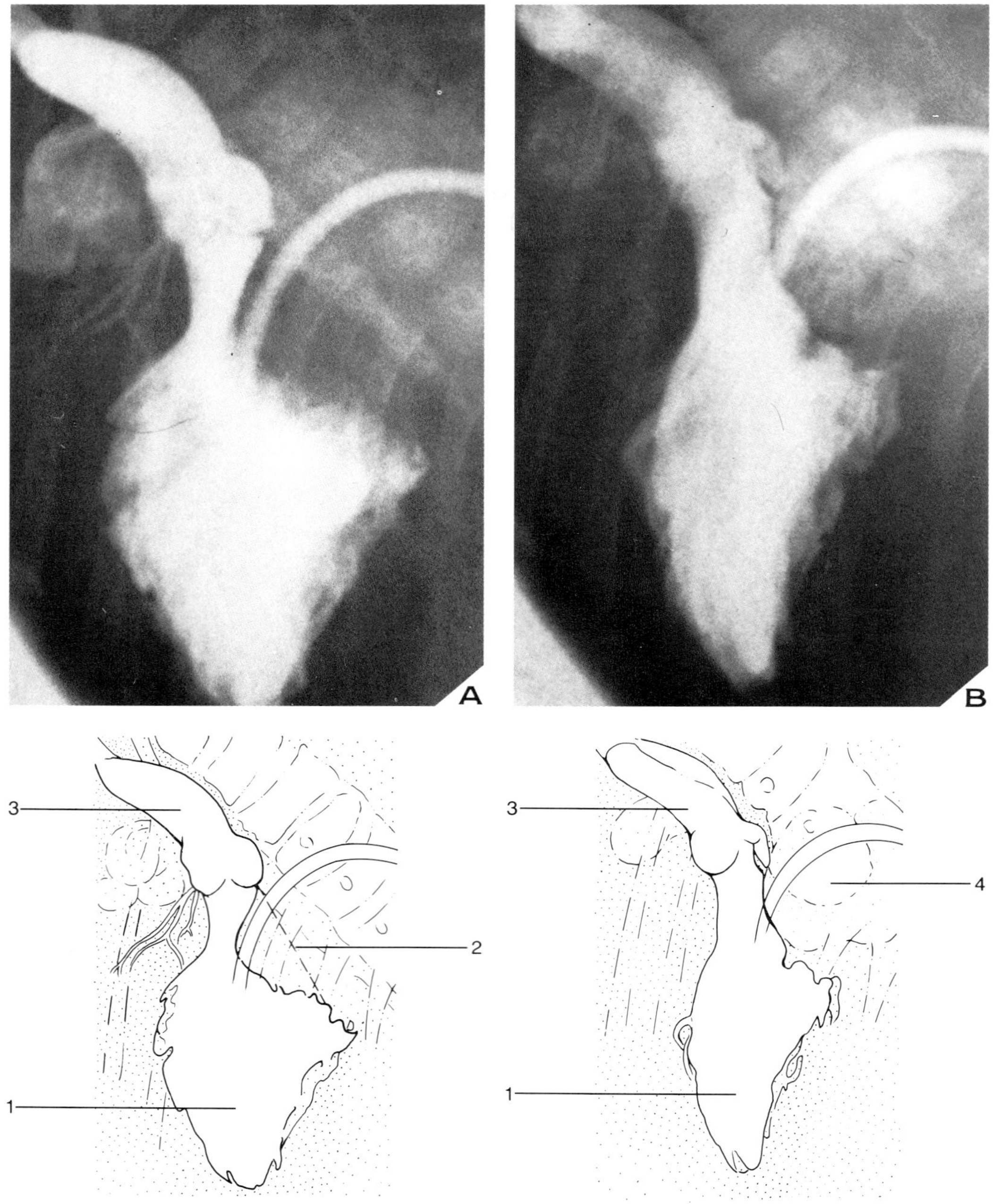

Fig. 9.19 Elongated right anterior oblique projection of left ventriculogram in diastole (A) and systole (B). Absence of the contour normally formed by the atrioventricular septum produces a "goose-neck" deformity. Note opacification of the left atrium in B, indicating that the left atrioventricular ("mitral") valve is incompetent.

1 left ventricle	3 aorta
2 normal position of atrioventricular septum	4 left atrium

CHAPTER 10

Abnormal Atrioventricular Connection

Anomalies of the ventricles may be related to their components, number, and/or relationships. The ventricles have three portions: inlet, trabecular, and outlet. One or occasionally two portions of either ventricle may be absent.

VENTRICULAR INVERSION

Ventricular inversion denotes an abnormal relationship of the ventricular chambers with respect to the septum. In a normal heart, the ventricle that is anterior and on the right is the morphologic right ventricle and the ventricle that is posterior and on the left is the morphologic left ventricle. When examining an anatomic specimen, one can use the "hand rule" to verify that the ventricles are normally related to each other. In a normal heart, one can place one's right hand (but not the left) in the opened right ventricle so that the thumb lies within the atrioventricular (tricuspid) valve, the palm covers the septum, and the fingers occupy the outlet (Fig. 10.1A). The left hand, but not the right, can be applied to the opened left ventricle so that with the thumb in the atrioventricular (mitral) valve, the palm overlies the septum, and the fingers are in the outlet (Fig. 10.1B). If the ventricles are inverted, only the left hand will "fit" the morphologic right ventricle (which is on the left), and only

CHAPTER LABELING KEY			
RA	right atrium	RV	right ventricle
LA	left atrium	LV	left ventricle

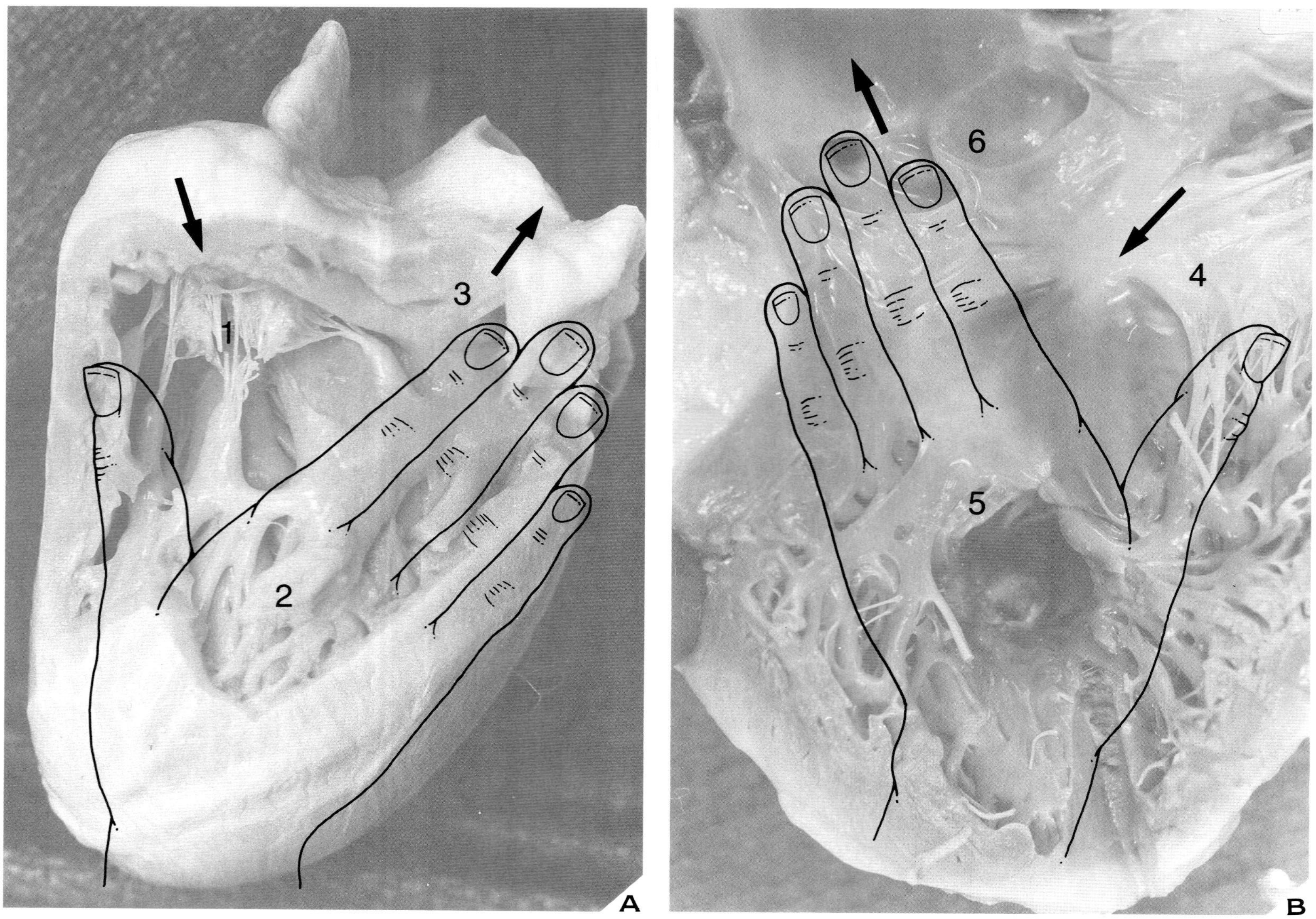

1	tricuspid valve	4	mitral valve
2	septal aspect of right ventricle	5	septal aspect of left ventricle
3	pulmonic valve	6	aortic valve

Fig. 10.1 Morphology of normally positioned ventricles ("the hand rule"). (A) Normally positioned right ventricle. When the right hand is applied to the opened right ventricle, the thumb occupies the inlet portion, the palm overlies the septum, and the fingers occupy the outlet. (B) Normally positioned left ventricle. When the left hand is applied to the opened left ventricle, the thumb occupies the inlet portion, the palm overlies the septum, and the fingers occupy the outlet.

the right hand will "fit" the morphologic left ventricle (which is on the right). This abnormal relationship of the ventricles is independent of the atrioventricular and ventriculoarterial connections.

Ventricular inversion is an integral feature of congenitally corrected transposition (Fig. 10.2; see below). However, it may also occur as an isolated malformation or in association with double-outlet right ventricle, double-outlet left ventricle, or pulmonary atresia.

DISCORDANT ATRIOVENTRICULAR CONNECTION

Discordant atrioventricular connection denotes a malformation in which the atria are connected to the inappropriate ventricles, the right atrium connecting with the morphologic left ventricle through a mitral valve and the left atrium connecting with the morphologic right ventricle through a tricuspid valve. In most hearts with discordant atrioventricular connection, the ventricles are inverted (see Fig. 10.2). In a person with atrial situs solitus (ie, normal atrial situs), the connection between the right atrium and the morphologic left ventricle lies to the right of that between the left atrium and the morphologic right ventricle. The atrioventricular connections are spatially oriented in parallel fashion (ie, as in a normal heart). The morphologic left ventricle lies anterior, inferior, and to the right of the morphologic right ventricle. Both the inlet and outlet portions of the morphologic left ventricle are on the right and the trabecular portion of the chamber is inferior. The morphologic right ventricle lies posterior, superior, and to the left of the morphologic left ventricle. In most cases of ventricular inversion, the inlet of the morphologic right ventricle is enlarged and the tricuspid valve is dysplastic.

The ventriculoarterial connections largely determine the clinical presentation of patients with ventricular inversion. The great majority of patients with discordant atrioventricular connection also have transposition of the great vessels (TGA). In this arrangement, commonly known as *congenitally corrected transposition,* the morphologic right ventricle connects with the aorta and the morphologic left ventricle with the pulmonary

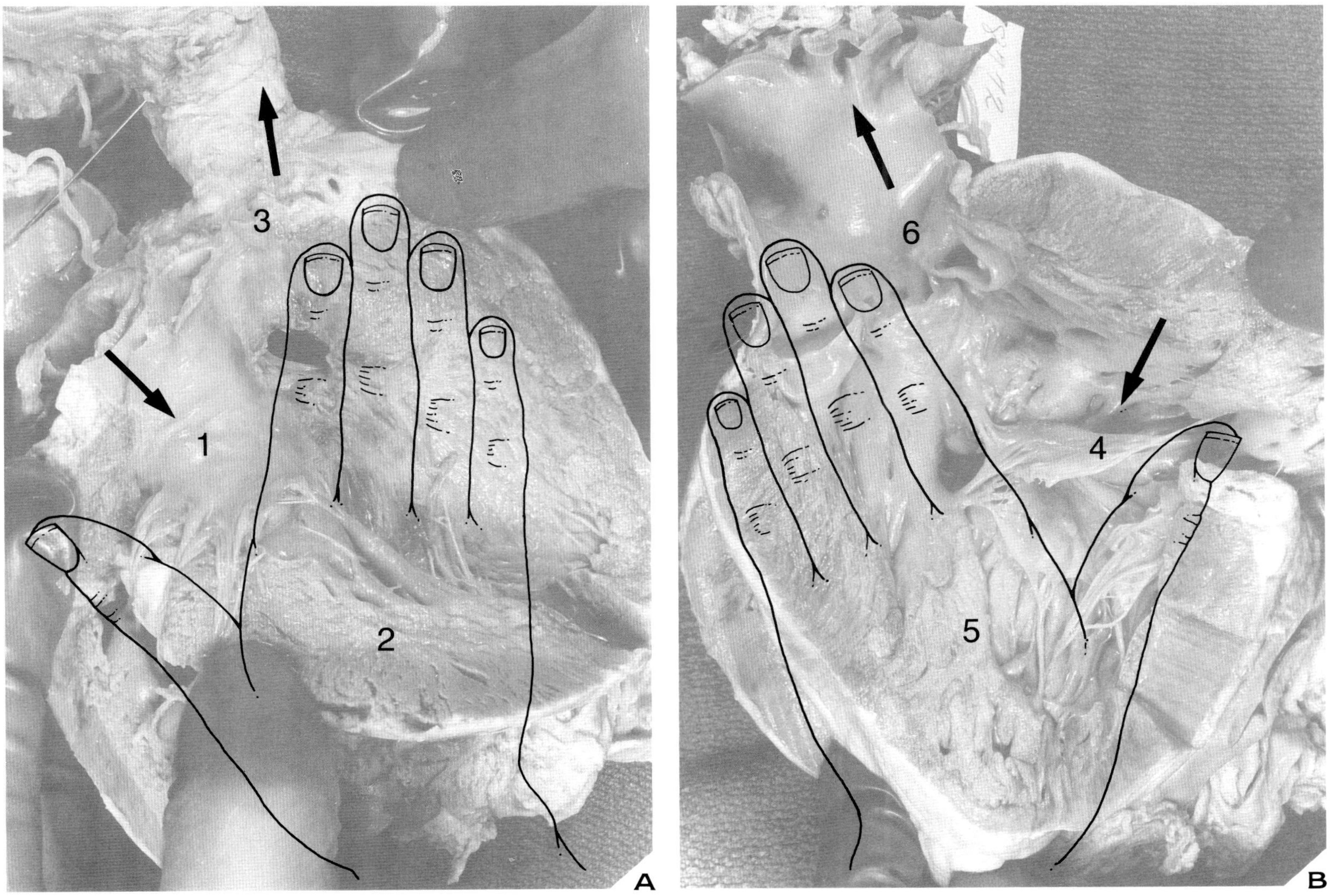

Fig. 10.2 Morphology of inverted ventricles ("the hand rule"). Autopsy specimen from a patient with congenitally corrected transposition. (A) Right-sided morphologic left ventricle. The right hand "fits," ie, the thumb is in the inlet (mitral valve), the palm overlies the septum, and the fingers are in the outlet (pulmonic valve). (B) Left-sided morphologic right ventricle. The left hand "fits."

1 mitral valve
2 septal aspect of left ventricle
3. pulmonary trunk
4 tricuspid valve
5 septal aspect of right ventricle
6 aortic valve

artery (Fig. 10.3). Therefore, desaturated systemic venous blood is pumped by the morphologic left ventricle into the pulmonary artery and oxygenated pulmonary venous blood is pumped by the morphologic right ventricle into the aorta. The net physiologic result is the same as that of a normal heart.

Less common types of abnormal ventriculoarterial connection include double-outlet right ventricle and ventricular inversion with concordant ventriculoarterial connection. In some instances, one of the great arteries (usually the pulmonary artery) is atretic. This type of malformation can also be classified as pulmonary atresia with discordant AV connection (Fig. 10.3).

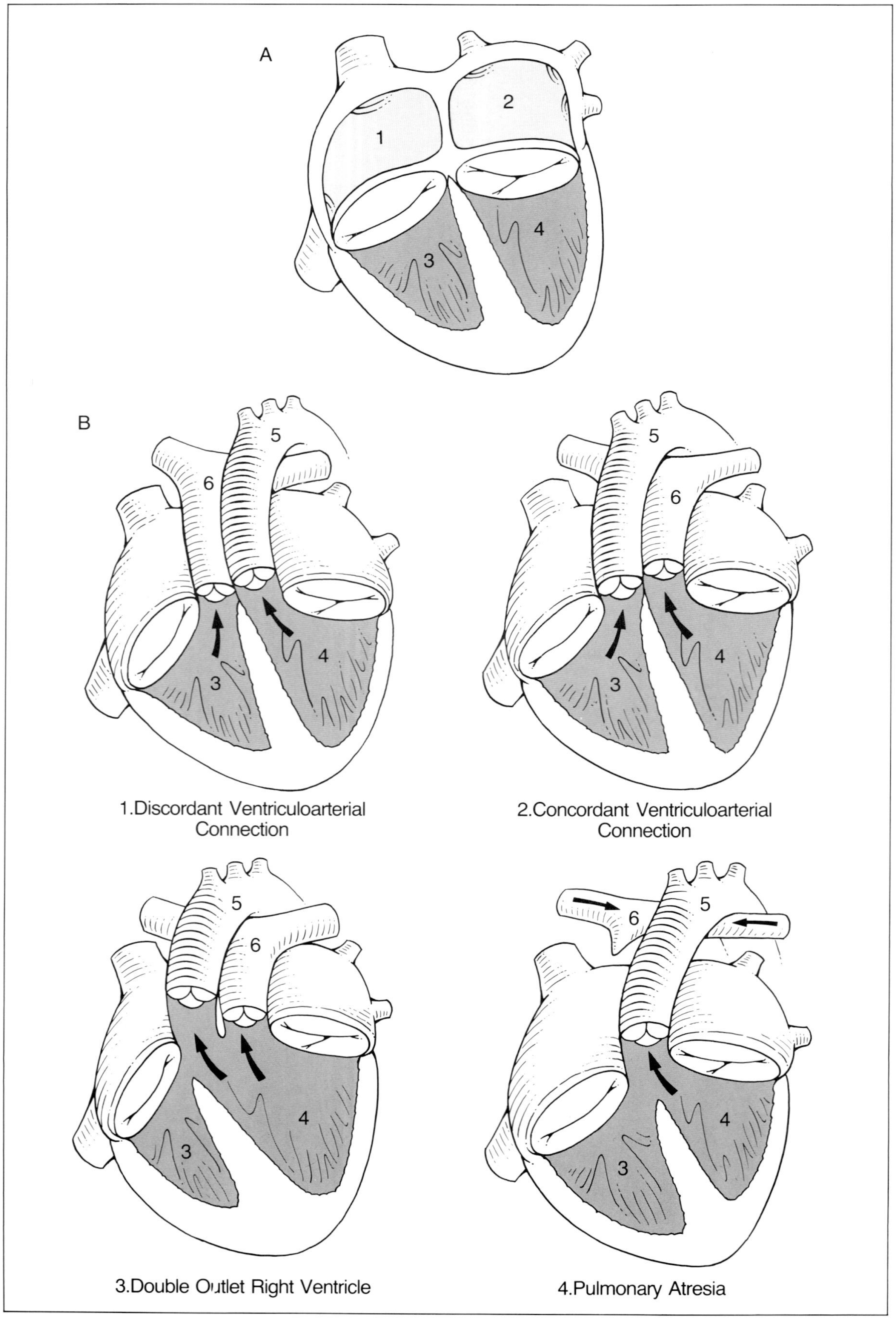

Fig. 10.3 Discordant atrioventricular connection. (A) Discordant atrioventricular connection. (B) Possible ventriculoarterial connections associated with discordant atrioventricular connection. 1, Discordant; 2, concordant, 3, double-outlet right ventricle; 4, atresia of the pulmonary artery with the aorta originating from both ventricles.

1	right atrium
2	left atrium
3	left ventricle
4	right ventricle
5	aorta
6	pulmonary trunk

CONGENITALLY CORRECTED TRANSPOSITION

IMAGING AND INVASIVE DIAGNOSIS

Plain Films

Provided there are no additional cardiac malformations, patients with congenitally corrected transposition and atrial situs solitus have a normal-sized heart. The frontal chest film typically shows prominence of the left lower cardiac contour, with a convexity in the vicinity of the atrioventricular groove (occasionally the apex is indented). In about one third of cases the cardiac apex is displaced medially (mesocardia) or to the right (dextrocardia).

In 60 to 70 percent of patients with congenitally corrected TGA, the ascending aorta forms the left upper mediastinal border; in the remainder, it is displaced towards the midline and cannot be identified on plain films. The main pulmonary artery is usually displaced to the right. Because it is obscured by other mediastinal structures, it cannot be identified as a discrete structure along the left mediastinal border. The right and left pulmonary arteries lie at the same level (Fig. 10.4).

The probability of congenitally corrected TGA is very high in a patient with atrial situs solitus (ratio of main bronchi $\geq 1.4:1$) and a right cardiac axis, in whom the ascending aorta forms the left upper mediastinal border. It should be noted, however, that this pattern can also be seen in patients with other malformations, including the so-called "criss-cross heart," anatomically corrected malposition, and certain types of double-outlet right ventricle.

Angiocardiography

The morphologic left ventricle is anterior and to the right of the morphologic right ventricle and supports the pulmonary trunk, which lies to the right of the aorta (Fig. 10.5). The right and left

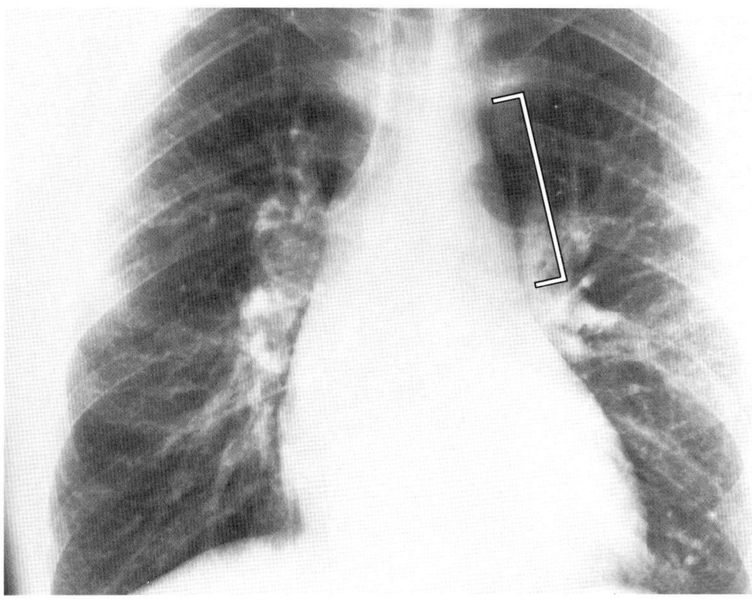

Fig. 10.4 Congenitally corrected transposition and VSD. Frontal chest film shows cardiomegaly with convexity of the left lower heart border. The left upper mediastinal border, which is formed by the ascending aorta, is straight and merges with the aortic arch superiorly (*brace*). The left and right pulmonary arteries are enlarged and lie at the same level, reflecting the medial displacement of the pulmonary trunk.

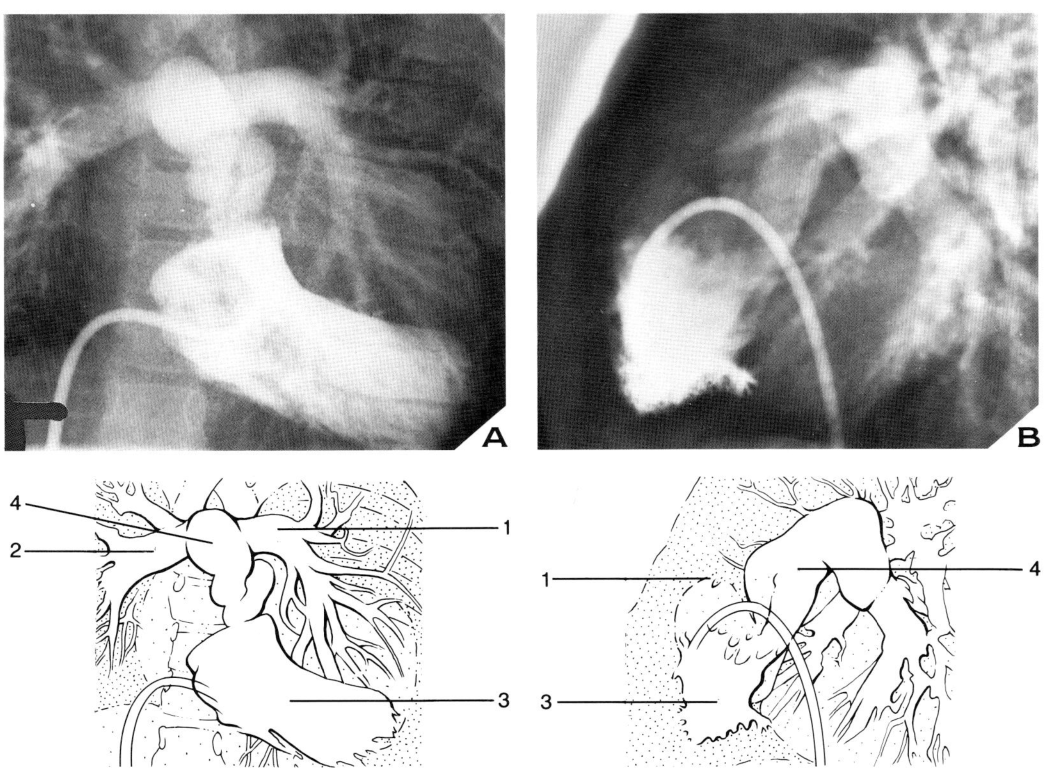

Fig. 10.5 Congenitally corrected transposition. Frontal (A) and lateral (B) projections of left ventriculogram. The catheter has been advanced from the inferior vena cava into the right atrium, across the triscuspid valve, and into the left ventricle, which is located anterior, inferior, and to the right of its normal position and has an anterior recess. The pulmonary trunk is medially and posteriorly located, and the right and left pulmonary arteries are at the same level.

1 left pulmonary artery
2 right pulmonary artery
3 left ventricle
4 pulmonary trunk

pulmonary arteries lie at the same level (in a normal subject the left is higher than the right). The morphologic right ventricle connects with the left atrium and supports the aorta, which lies to the left of the pulmonary artery; its ascending segment forms the left upper mediastinal border. The aortic arch and descending thoracic aorta are usually on the left (Fig. 10.6).

Anatomic details, as well as associated anomalies (eg, tricuspid insufficiency, VSD, or stenosis of the left ventricular outflow tract) are best appreciated on axial projections obtained after selective injection of each ventricle (Fig. 10.7).

UNIVENTRICULAR ATRIOVENTRICULAR CONNECTION

In this malformation both atria connect with only one ventricular chamber. The nature of the atrioventricular connection ranges from two well-separated atrioventricular valves, through a common atrioventricular valve (which represents the fused left and right atrioventricular valves), to a single isolated atrioventricular valve (with atresia of its mate). There are also anatomic variations in ventricular morphology. The ventricle that receives the total atrial output is called the *main ventricular chamber.* There is usually an *accessory ventricular chamber,* consisting of an incomplete ventricle lacking one or two components. (Rarely, there is only a single ventricular chamber.) The main and accessory ventricular chambers can be either normally related or inverted.

The classification of this group of malformations is based on the morphology of the main ventricular chamber: (1) univentricular atrioventricular connection to a morphologic right ventricle; (2) univentricular atrioventricular connection to a morphologic left ventricle; or (3) univentricular atrioventricular connection to an indeterminate ventricle (Fig. 10.8). The ventriculoarterial connection may be discordant (the most common arrangement) or concordant, or there may be atresia of either of the great arteries.

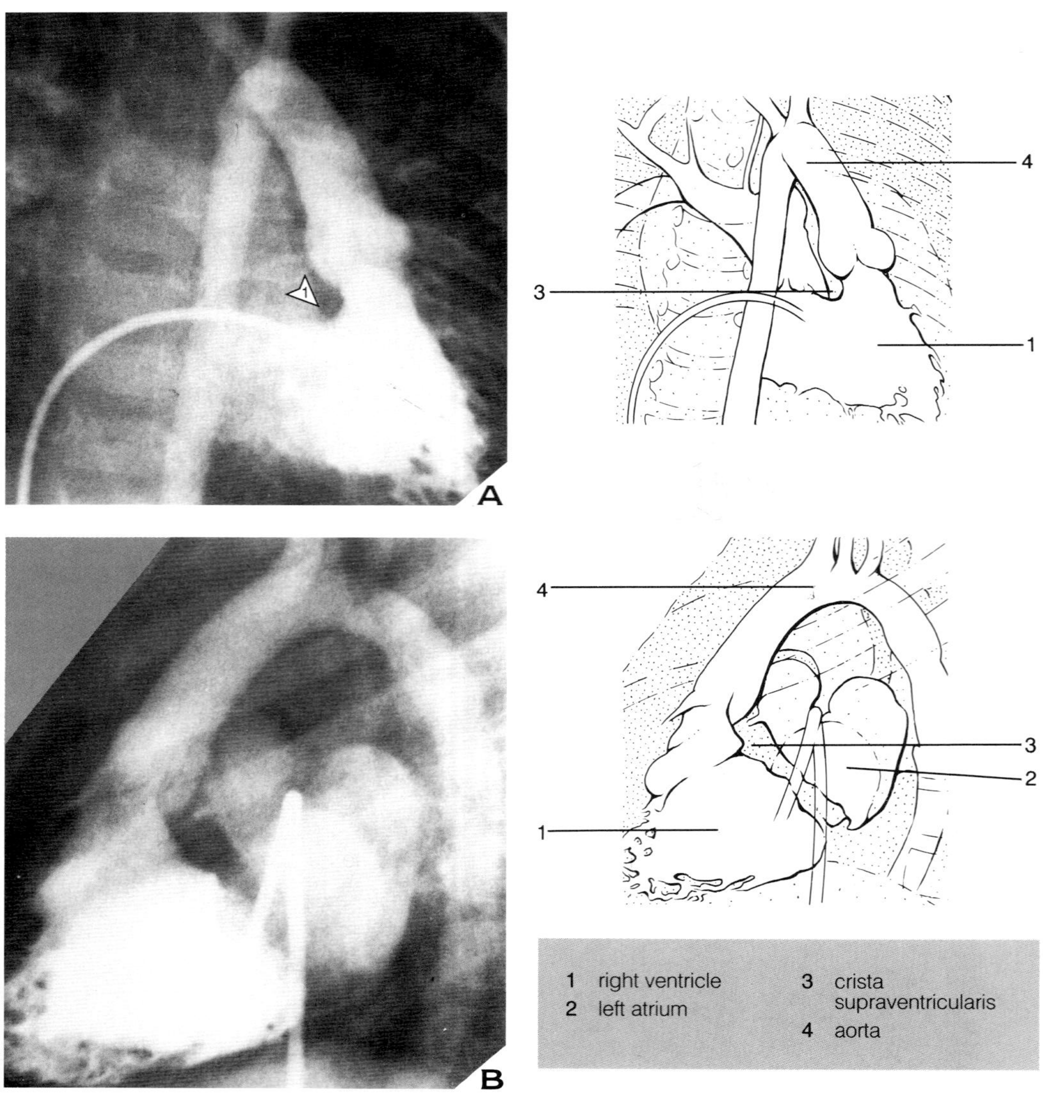

Fig. 10.6 Congenitally corrected transposition. The catheter has been advanced from the inferior vena cava into the right atrium, and across the triscuspid valve into the right ventricle. Frontal (A) and lateral (B) projections show the right ventricle to the left of the left ventricle and connected to the left atrium. The right ventricle is connected to the aorta via a muscular infundibulum with a large crista supraventricularis (*arrow* 1 in A). The ascending aorta lies anteriorly and to the left, forming the left upper mediastinal border.

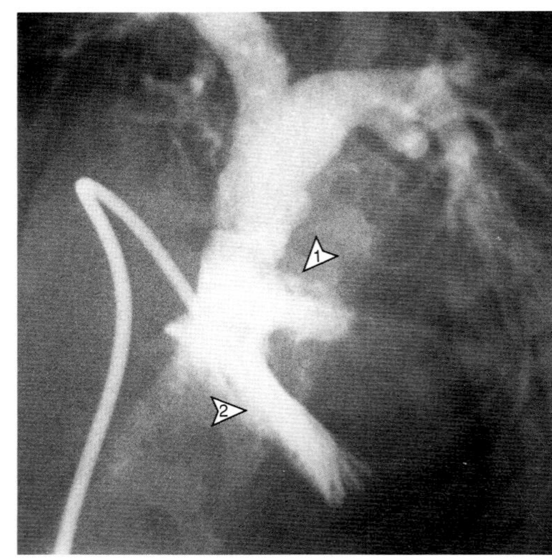

Fig. 10.7 Congenitally corrected transposition and VSD. Left ventriculogram (long axis view) shows a jet of opacified blood crossing the VSD (*arrow* 1), which is located just beneath the pulmonic valve. Note the medially positioned pulmonary trunk. The left and right pulmonary arteries lie at the same level. (*Arrow* 2 = left ventricle.)

In the great majority of cases the main ventricular chamber is a morphologic left ventricle and the ventriculoarterial connection is discordant. In this arrangement the morphologic right ventricle supports the aorta and the morphologic left ventricle supports the pulmonary trunk. When the main ventricular chamber is a morphologic right ventricle, the ventriculoarterial connection is nearly always a double-outlet right ventricle. Although univentricular atrioventricular connection with pulmonary atresia has been described, it is rare.

ANATOMIC FEATURES

The most frequently encountered anatomic pattern in patients with univentricular atrioventricular connection consists of: atrial situs solitus; a dominant morphologic left ventricle; a rudimentary left-sided morphologic right ventricle; two independent, well-separated atrioventricular valves; a discordant ventriculoarterial connection; and a muscular VSD connecting the dominant morphologic left ventricle with the small (or rudimentary) morphologic right ventricle.

Other anatomic patterns are present in approximately 30 to 35 percent of patients with univentricular atrioventricular connection. The radiographic findings vary, and the plain film findings seldom allow a specific diagnosis.

IMAGING AND INVASIVE DIAGNOSIS

Plain Films

Plain films typically show atrial situs solitus (ratio of main bronchi $\geq$1.4:1). The cardiac axis is oriented to the left and the aortic arch is usually left-sided. The small, incomplete ventricular mass is represented by a prominence along the left heart border, near the atrioventricular groove. The ascending aorta forms the left upper mediastinal border; the main pulmonary artery does not form any part of the mediastinal contour. The right and left pulmonary arteries lie at the same level (Fig. 10.9).

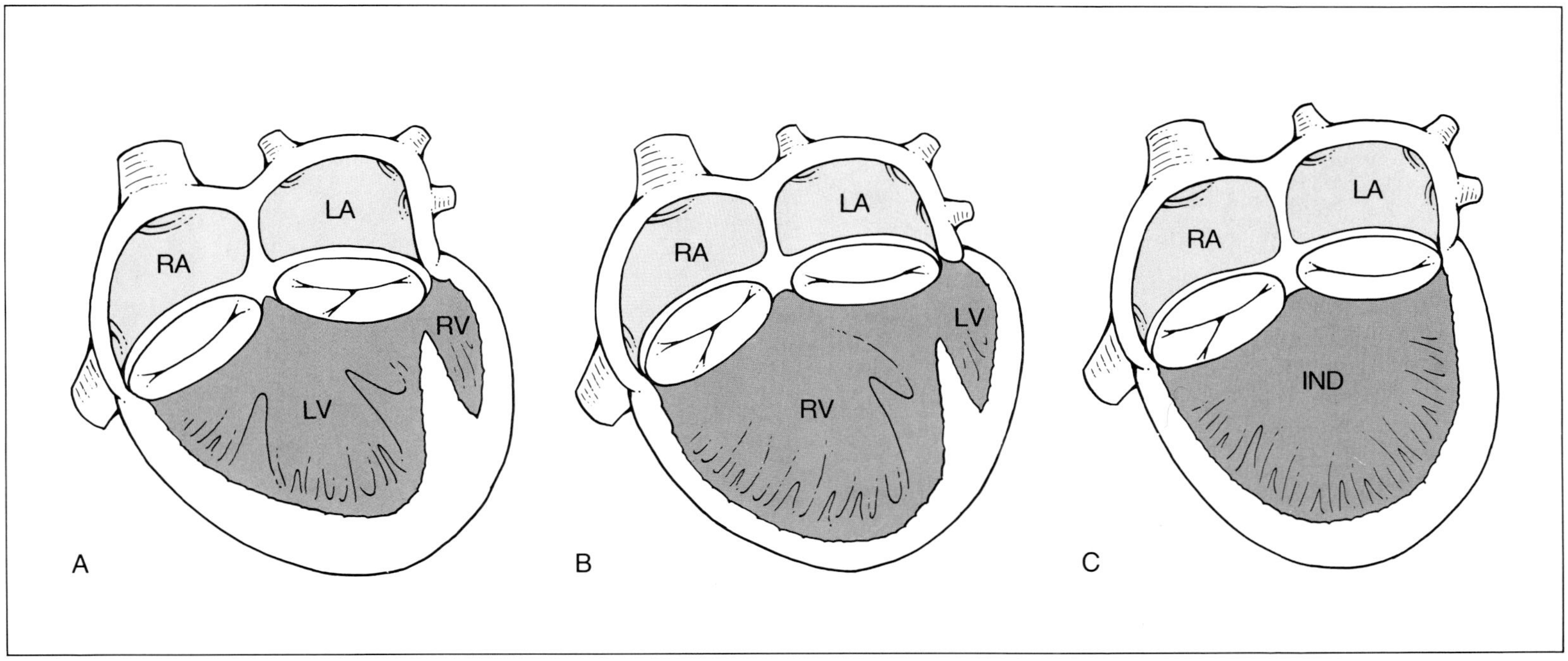

Fig. 10.8 Univentricular atrioventricular connection through two atrioventricular valves. (A) Both atria connected to the left ventricle. (B) Both atria connected to the right ventricle. (C) Both atria connected to a ventricle of indeterminate type.

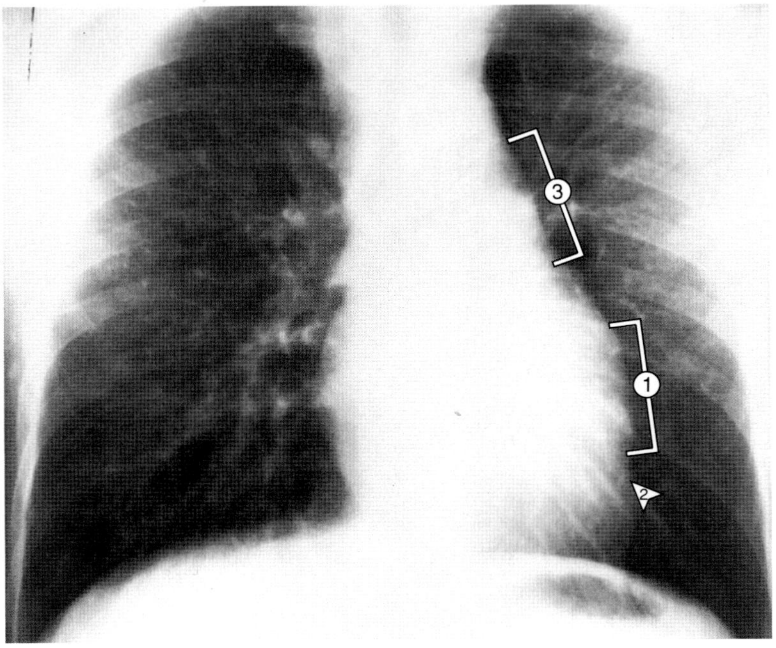

Fig. 10.9 Univentricular atrioventricular connection to a left ventricle. Frontal film shows atrial situs solitus, a left cardiac axis, and a left aortic arch. The lower portion of the left heart border is deformed (*brace* 1) with an identation inferiorly (*arrow* 2). The ascending aorta (*brace* 3) forms the left upper heart border. The left and right pulmonary arteries are at the same level at the hilum, indicating that the pulmonary trunk is displaced medially.

Angiocardiography

In the most common arrangement there are two discrete atrioventricular valves, and the main ventricular chamber is a morphologic left ventricle with smooth borders and fine trabeculation thoughout most of the ventricular mass. The small morphologic right ventricle, which lies along the left border of the morphologic left ventricle, appears angiographically as a small cavity formed by the trabecular and outlet portions of the chamber. The aorta lies anterior and to the left of the pulmonary trunk and forms the left upper mediastinal border. The pulmonary trunk, which lies posterior and to the right of the aorta, is projected over the spine. The right and left pulmonary arteries lie at the same level (Fig. 10.10). The precise nature of the atrioventricular connection, the size and position of the VSD, and any associated intracardiac malformations are best demonstrated by long axis projections obtained with the catheter in the right or left ventricle (Fig. 10.10).

Although the plain film findings are atypical in patients with univentricular atrioventricular connection to a morphologic right ventricle, this diagnosis is easily made angiographically, because both great arteries can be seen to arise from a chamber with a discrete infundibulum (Fig. 10.11).

ATRIOVENTRICULAR VALVE ATRESIA

As noted above, either the left or the right atrioventricular valve may be absent (atretic) in some patients with univentricular atrioventricular connection. However, because tricuspid atresia and mitral atresia have characteristic clinical and radiologic features, it is appropriate to consider these malformations separately. Hypoplastic left ventricle, a distinctive malformation complex associated with an atretic or hypoplastic mitral valve, will also be discussed.

TRICUSPID ATRESIA

Tricuspid atresia is the unifying feature of a group of cardiac malformations in which the right ventricle does not connect with the atria. The most common arrangement is *atrial situs solitus with right-sided tricuspid atresia.* In this anomaly there is no connection between the right atrium and the right ventricle. Less common variations include *atrial situs solitus with left-sided tricuspid atresia,* in which there is no connection between the left atrium and the inverted subjacent right ventricle, and *atrial isomerism with left- or right-sided tricuspid atresia.* In the latter variation, right-sided tricuspid atresia is present in hearts with normally related ventricles (Fig. 10.12), and left-sided tricuspid atresia is present in hearts with inverted ventricles.

ANATOMIC FEATURES

In the great majority of hearts lacking a right atrioventricular connection, the atrioventricular arrangement is concordant. The right ventricle, which lies to the right of or anterior to the left ventricle, is a small chamber formed exclusively by the trabecular and outlet segments (ie, it lacks an inlet segment). In such hearts the patent atrioventricular valve is related to the left ventricle, which is large and normally developed (ie, all three segments are present) and connects with the left atrium via a normal mitral valve. The atrial septum is usually incomplete, the left and right atria communicating via a large ASD of the fossa ovalis type. A VSD is generally present as well.

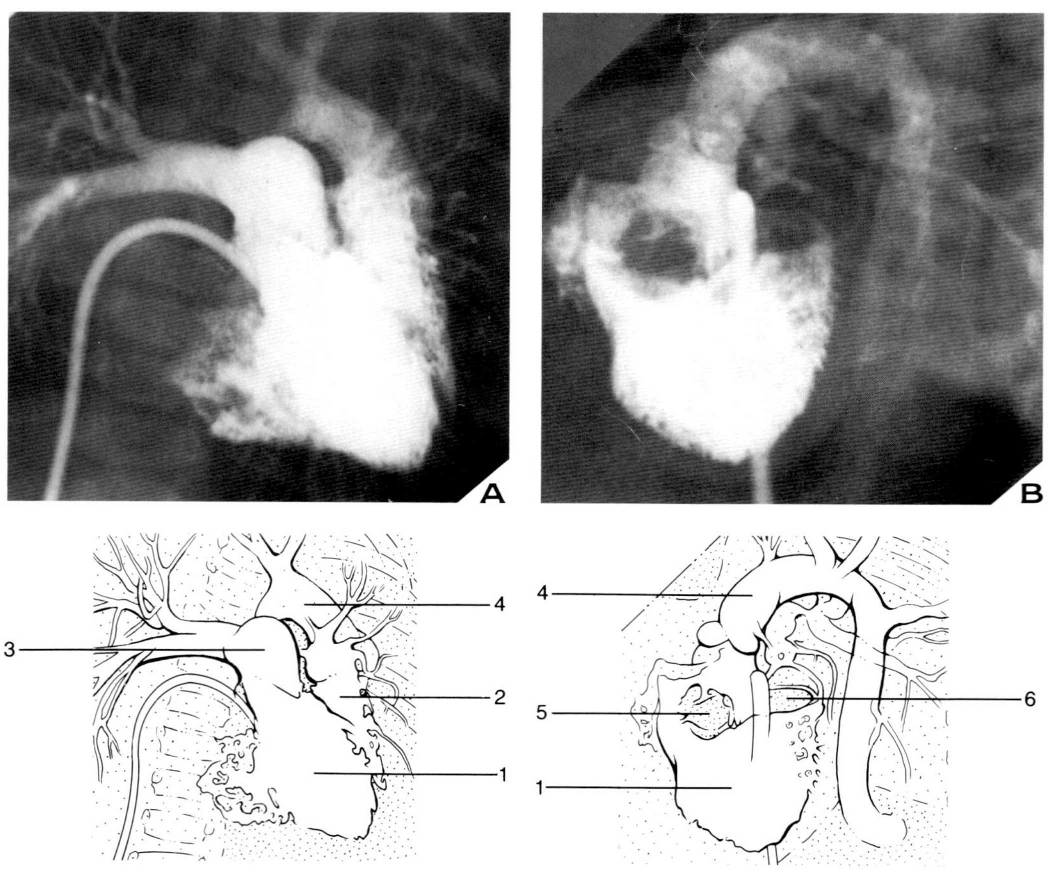

Fig. 10.10 Univentricular atrioventricular connection to a left ventricle. Frontal (A) and lateral (B) projections of ventricular injection (long-axis view). The catheter has been advanced from the inferior vena cava into the right atrium, and thence across the right atrioventricular valve into a large ventricular chamber with relatively smooth borders, which represents a left ventricle. The left atrioventricular valve connects with the left ventricle as well. The left ventricle supports the pulmonary trunk and the right ventricle supports the aorta.

1 left ventricle
2 right ventricle
3 pulmonary trunk
4 aorta
5 right atrioventricular valve
6 left atrioventricular valve

HEMODYNAMICS

In the various forms of tricuspid atresia, the left atrium acts as a mixing chamber in which the systemic and pulmonary venous return intermingle. The entire blood volume empties into the left ventricle, from which it is pumped into the pulmonary and systemic circulations.

In about 75 percent of hearts the ventriculoarterial connections are *concordant,* with the left ventricle supporting the aorta

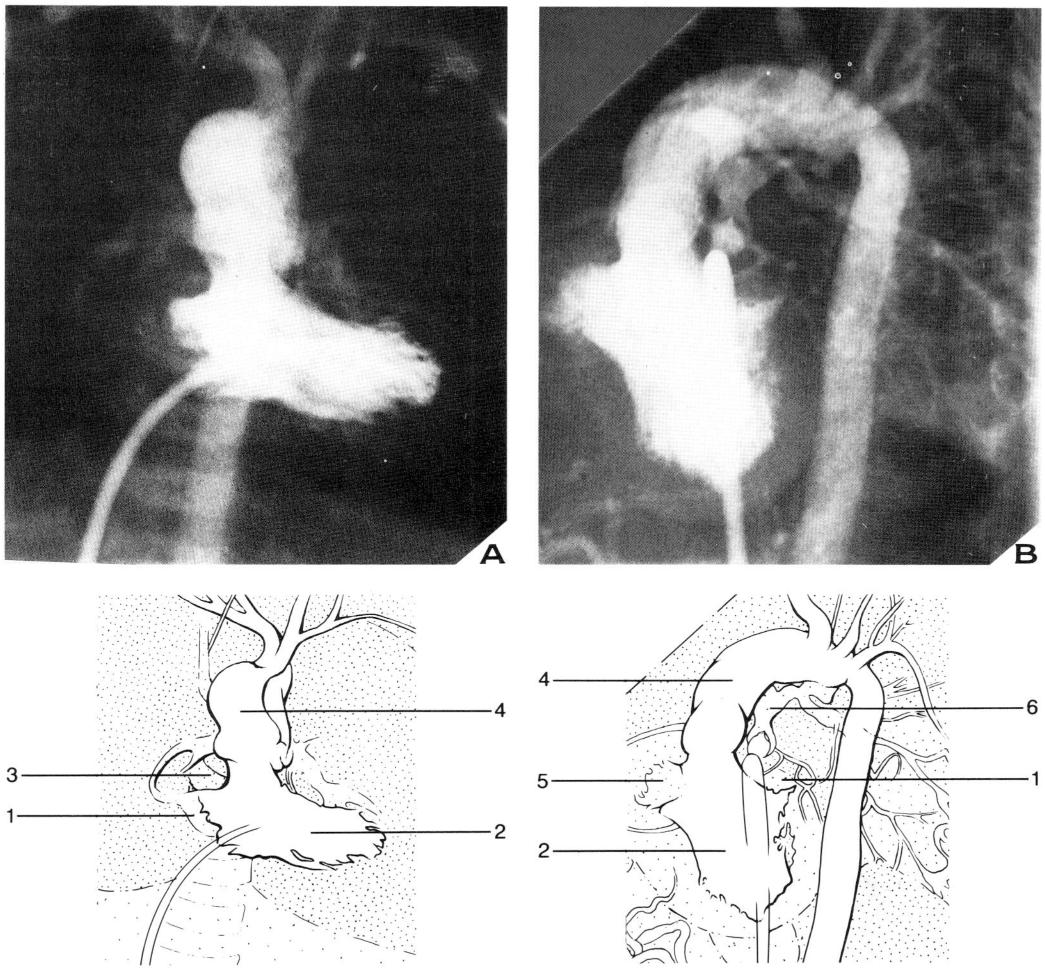

Fig. 10.11 Univentricular atrioventricular connection to a right ventricle (double-outlet right ventricle). Frontal (A) and left anterior oblique (B) projections. The catheter has crossed the left atrioventricular valve and has entered a ventricular chamber with a crista supraventricularis, indicating that it is the morphologic right ventricle. Both the aorta and the pulmonary trunk originate from the right ventricle. The pulmonary trunk, which lies posterior to the aorta, is severely hypoplastic.

1 left atrioventricular valve
2 right ventricle
3 crista supraventricularis
4 aorta
5 right atrioventricular valve
6 hypoplastic pulmonary trunk

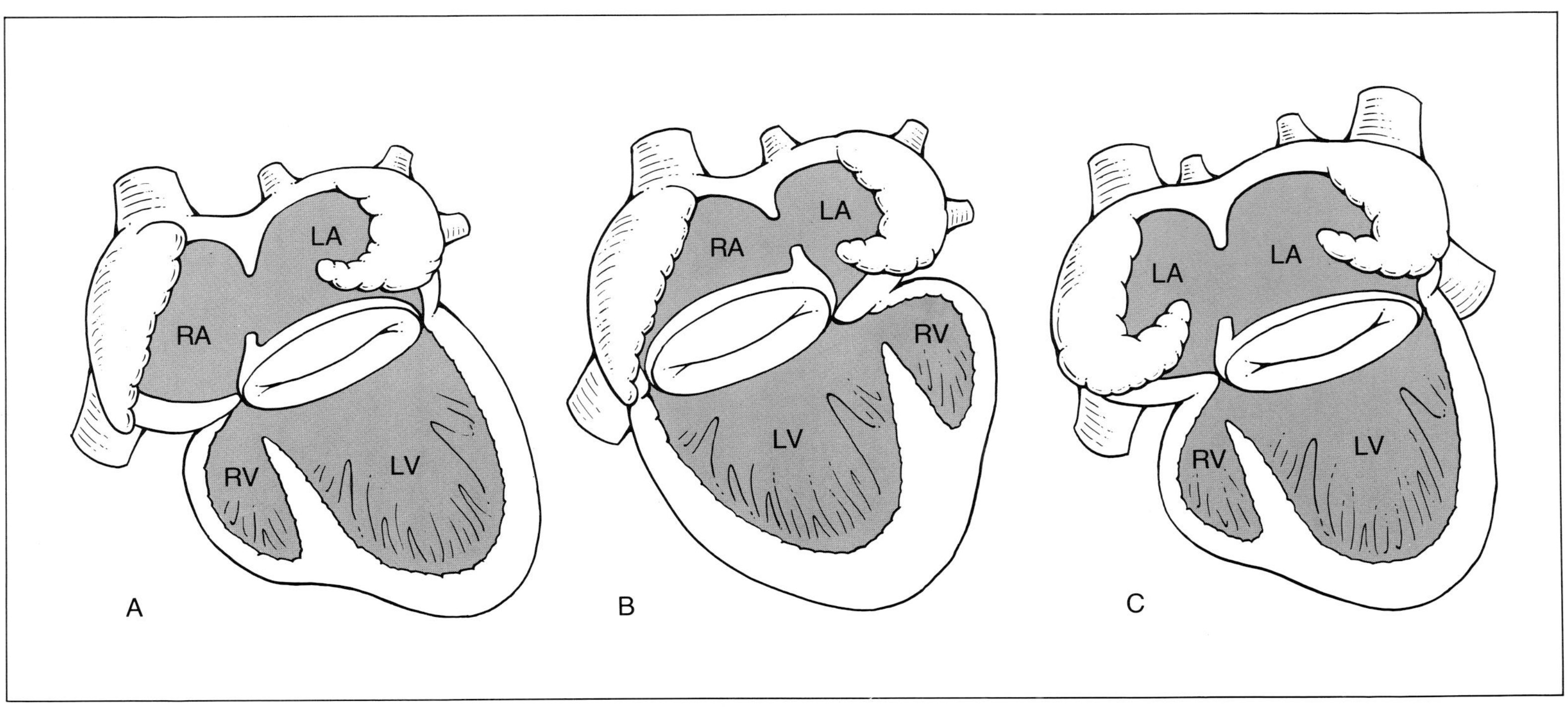

Fig. 10.12 Varieties of tricuspid atresia. (A) Right-sided tricuspid atresia in atrial situs solitus. (B) Left-sided tricuspid atresia in atrial situs solitus. (C) Right-sided tricuspid atresia in atrial isomerism.

and the right ventricle supporting the pulmonary trunk. The amount of blood that reaches the pulmonary circulation reflects the size of the VSD and the size of the right ventricle. In about 10 percent of patients with a concordant ventriculoarterial connection, the VSD is large enough to flood the lungs, resulting in pulmonary plethora.

In the remaining 25 percent of cases the ventriculoarterial connection is *discordant;* most of the left ventricular output enters the pulmonary artery and the remainder crosses the VSD to enter the aorta. The clinical and hemodynamic features in patients with this form of tricuspid atresia resemble those of patients with TGA.

IMAGING AND INVASIVE DIAGNOSIS

Plain Films

The plain film findings depend on the nature of the ventriculoarterial connections and the size of the VSD. Chest films of patients with classical tricuspid atresia show atrial situs solitus (ratio of left to right main bronchus $\geq$1.4:1), a left cardiac axis, and a left-sided aortic arch. Heart size is usually normal, and the left border of the ventricular mass usually resembles a normal left ventricle. The right atrial border is usually flat or displaced toward the midline. The hypoplastic pulmonary artery cannot be identified as a discrete structure. The right and left pulmonary arteries are small, and the pulmonary vascular markings are decreased in size and number. In a cyanotic patient this constellation of findings strongly suggests tricuspid atresia (Fig. 10.13). Although the plain film findings of classical tricuspid atresia may superficially resemble those of tetralogy of Fallot, the latter is not associated with a "left ventricular configuration" of the heart.

As noted above, a large VSD is present in about 10 percent of patients with tricuspid atresia and concordant ventriculoarterial connection. Patients with this malformation complex exhibit various degrees of cyanosis. Their plain films typically show left ventricular enlargement, a prominent pulmonary trunk, and pulmonary plethora. TGA, which may have very similar plain film findings, is the main differential diagnosis in a cyanotic patient.

Echocardiography

Tricuspid atresia and related malformations are clearly shown on the four-chamber projection, which demonstrates the absence of a connection between the right atrium and the sub-

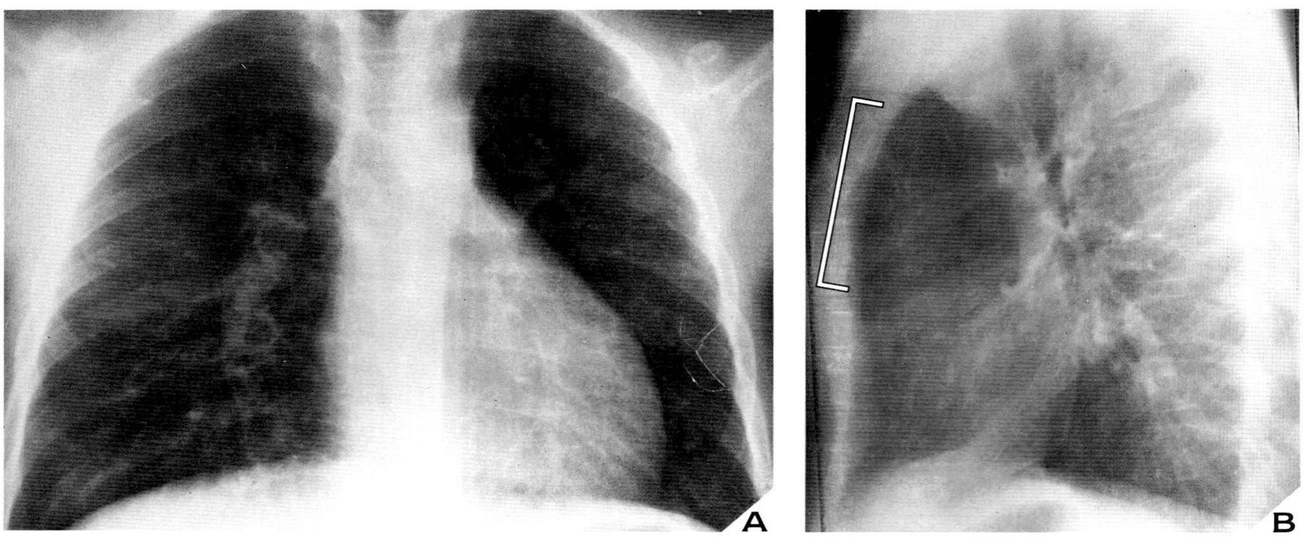

Fig. 10.13 Right tricuspid atresia. Frontal (A) and lateral (B) chest films in a patient with atrial situs solius show the typical radiographic features of classical tricuspid atresia. The heart is of normal size and the left lower heart border has a "left ventricular" configuration; the retrosternal space, normally occupied by the right ventricle, is empty (*brace* in B). The pulmonary trunk cannot be identified on the frontal projection. The left pulmonary artery is small in comparison with the right pulmonary artery, which has been enlarged by a previous surgical shunt. The pulmonary vascularity is diminished.

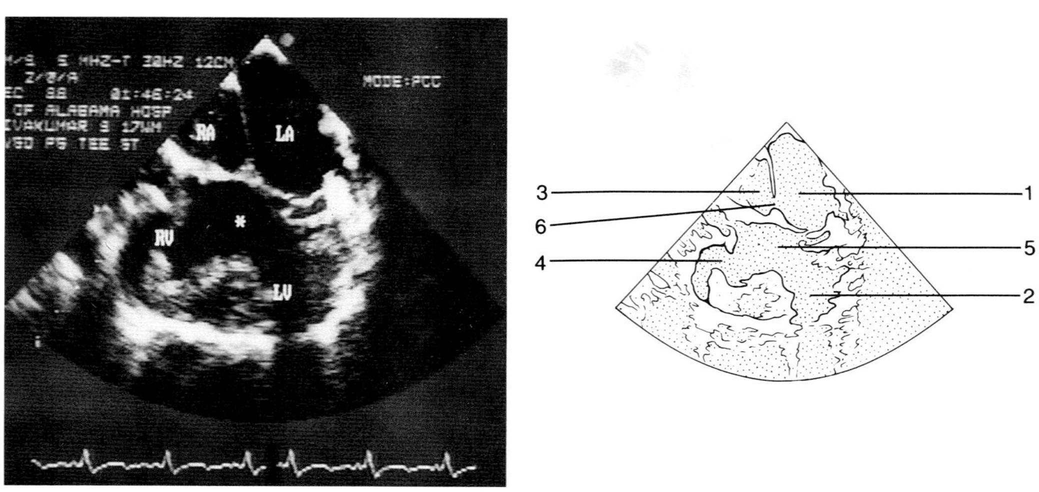

Fig. 10.14 Tricuspid atresia (echocardiographic features). Apical four-chamber view. The right and left ventricles are well depicted. The ventricles communicate via a large VSD. The right and atria communicate via a very small ASD. The left atrioventricular valve consists of two leaflets. The atretic right atrioventricular valve appears as an echogenic segment which represents fibrous and fatty tissue in the atrioventricular groove.

1 left atrium
2 left ventricle
3 right atrium
4 right ventricle
5 ventricular septal defect
6 atrial septal defect

jacent ventricle as well as patency of the left atrioventricular valve, the size and position of the right ventricle, and the VSD (Fig. 10.14).

MRI

Fletcher and his colleagues have analyzed the MRI findings in patients with various forms of right atrioventricular valve atresia (Fig. 10.15). In the common form of right atrioventricular valve atresia (classical tricuspid atresia), the right atrioventricular connection is absent and the muscular floor of the right atrium is separated from the ventricular mass by the atrioventricular sulcus. The fat-filled atrioventricular sulcus appears on ECG-gated axial MR images as a bright linear or roughly triangular structure in the expected location of the right atrioventricular valve (Fig. 10.16). Rarely, there is a potential atrioventricular connection; in these hearts the atrioventricular valve is represented by an imperforate membrane which is interposed between the right atrium and a dominant left ventricle (double-inlet left ventricle with an imperforate tricuspid valve) or a hypoplastic right ventricle. In such cases the atrioventricular sulcus appears shallow on MR images and the tricuspid valve appears as a thin, imperforate membrane (Fig. 10.17). Hence,

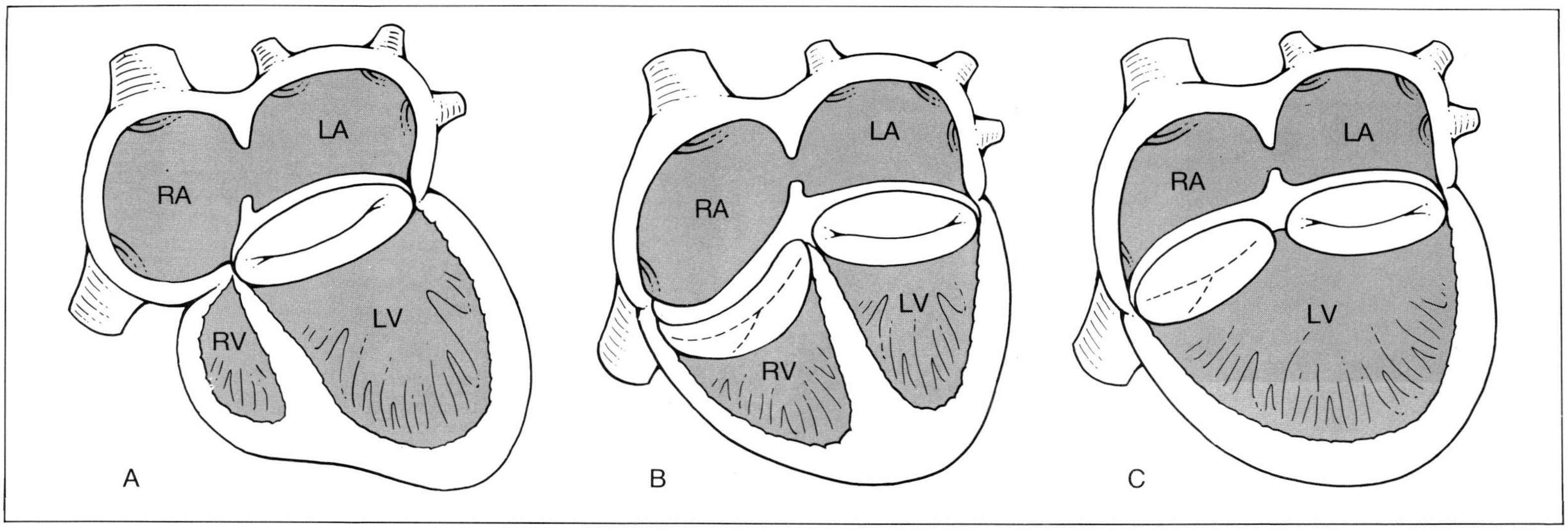

Fig. 10.15 Absent right atrioventricular connection and imperforate tricuspid valve. (A) Common type of tricuspid atresia. Atrioventricular sulcus is interposed between floor of right atrium and ventricular mass, including rudimentry right ventricle. (B) Imperforate atrioventricular valve with concordant atrioventricular connection. In this rare type of right atrioventricular atresia, which may exhibit features of Ebstein's malformation (see Chapter 14), there is potentially a direct communication between the right atrium and right ventricle. (C) Double-inlet left ventricle with potential connection between right atrium and dominant left ventricle, guarded by an imperforate valve. (Adapted by permission from Fletcher BD, et al. Right atrioventricular valve atresia: Anatomic evaluation with MR imaging. *AJR* 1987; 148:671)

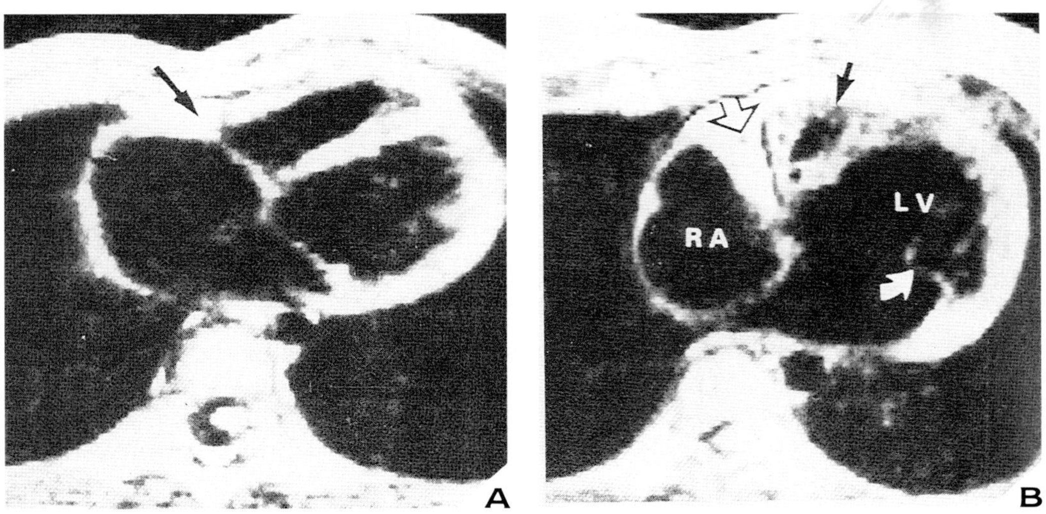

Fig. 10.16 Tricuspid atresia (MRI). Systolic axial ECG-gated MR images. (A) Normal heart. Fat occupies shallow atrioventricular sulcus (*arrow*). Closed mitral and tricuspid valves are normal. (B) Absent right atrioventricular connection. Elongated atrioventricular sulcus extends posteriorly between right atrium (RA) and rudimentary right ventricle (*black arrow*). Coronary artery (*open arrow*) is surrounded by fat within sulcus. No potential right atrioventricular valve orifice can be identified. A portion of the left atrioventricular (*white arrow*) between the left atrium posteriorly and the left ventricle (LV). Compare with Fig. 10.15A. (Reproduced by permission from Fletcher BD, et al. Right atrioventricular valve atresia: Anatomic evaluation with MR imaging. *AJR* 1987; 148:671)

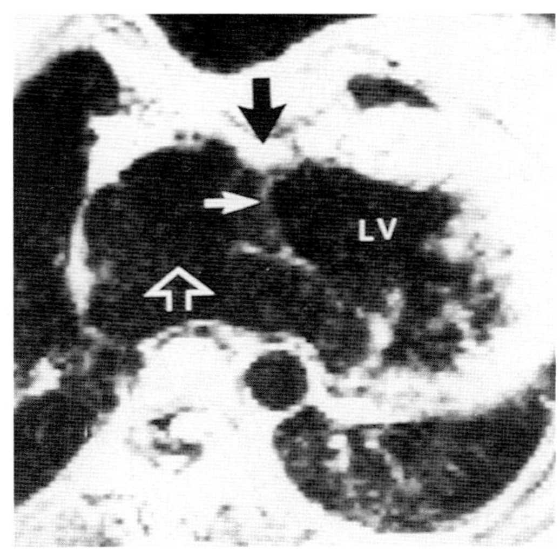

Fig. 10.17 Tricuspid atresia (MRI). Axial MR image in a patient with double-inlet left ventricle and an imperforate right atrioventricular valve (compare with Fig. 10.14C). The atrioventricular sulcus (*black arrow*) is shallow. A thin, imperforate atrioventricular valve (*white arrow*) obstructs the right atrioventricular orifice. The right atrium potentially communicates with the dominant left ventricle (LV). There is a large atrial septal defect (*open arrow*). (Reproduced by permission from Fletcher BD et al. Right atrioventricular valve atresia: Anatomic evaluation with MR imaging. *AJR* 1987; 148:671)

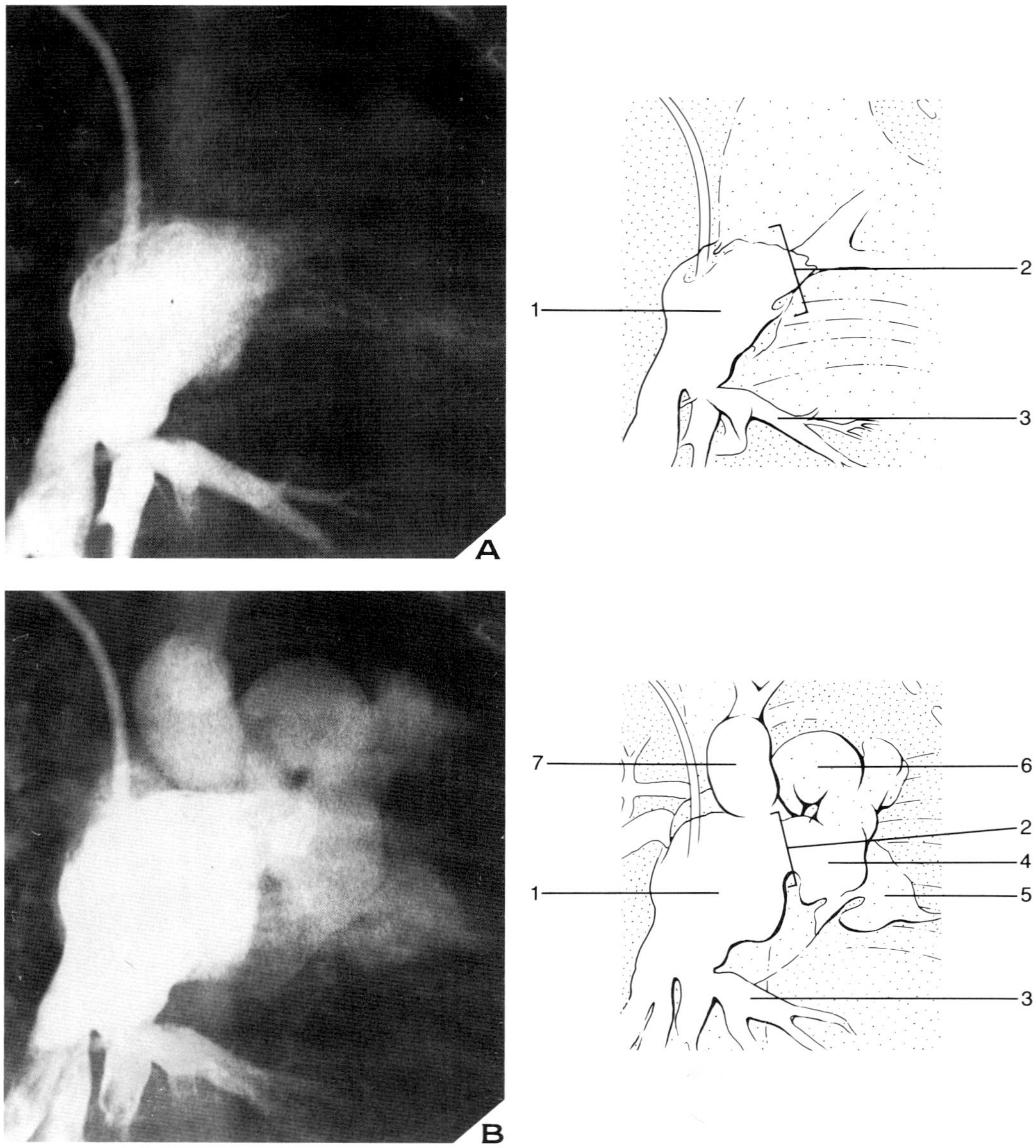

Fig. 10.18 Right tricuspid atresia. Early (A) and late (B) phases of right atrial angiogram. The right atrium is displaced to the left, resulting in flattening of the right heart border. The right and left atria communicate via a large ASD; the absence of a connection between the right atrium and right ventricle is well demonstrated in B. The left ventricle, pulmonary artery, and aorta are visualized on the late phase. Note reflux into hepatic veins, which persists into the late phase, indicating impaired drainage of the right atrium.

1	right atrium	5	left ventricle
2	ASD	6	pulmonary trunk
3	hepatic veins	7	aorta
4	left atrium		

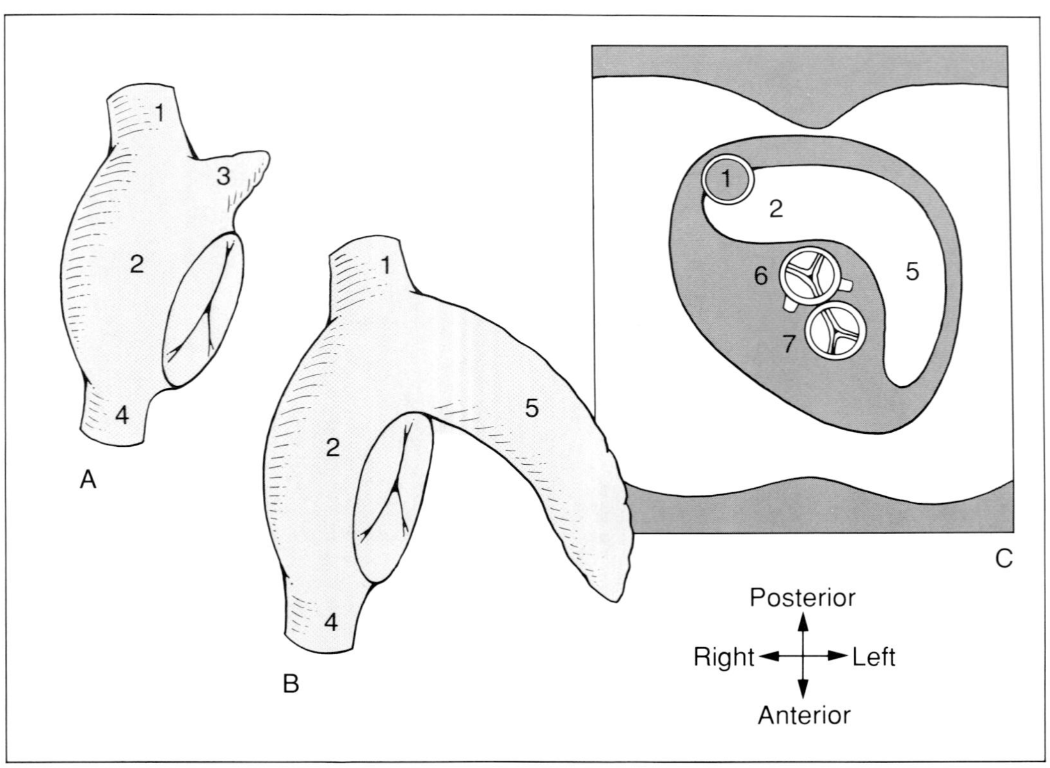

Fig. 10.19 Juxtaposition of atrial appendages. (A) Normal right atrium (frontal projection). (B, C) Right atrium with left juxtaposition of atrial appendage in frontal (B) and axial (C) projections. Two factors contribute to an apparent reduction in atrial capacity in this anomaly: 1, the right atrium is displaced to the left and lies behind the aorta; and 2, a considerable portion of the right atrial chamber has been assimilated into the enlarged atrial appendage, which lies to the left of the pulmonary trunk. The ascending aorta and pulmonary trunk are of equal size.

1	superior vena cava	5	enlarged, elongated right atrial appendage (extending to left of great arteries)
2	right atrium	6	aorta
3	normal right atrial appendage	7	pulmonary trunk
4	inferior vena cava		

the appearance of the atrioventricular sulcus can help to differentiate an absent atrioventricular connection from an imperforate valve through which normal circulation might be established.

Angiocardiography

A right atrial injection demonstrates a large ASD in patients with classical tricuspid atresia. The right atrium is displaced to the left, and the right atrial border is usually flat (Fig. 10.18). Not infrequently there is left juxtaposition of the atrial appendages, an anomaly that produces an apparent reduction in the capacity of the right atrial chamber (Fig. 10.19).

After a right atrial injection, the right ventricular chamber does not become opacified and there is a clear space in the position it normally occupies. The left atrium and left ventricle are both large and connect in the usual way.

In hearts with concordant ventriculoarterial connections, the aorta lies posterior and to the right of the pulmonary artery; the pulmonary trunk is small and usually does not form any part of the left upper mediastinal contour. If there is no VSD the right and left pulmonary arteries are small and their peripheral branches are decreased in size and number, although normally distributed. When there is a large VSD the pulmonary arteries are enlarged and the lungs plethoric, as with any other large left to right shunt (Fig. 10.20).

The right ventricle is demonstrated on the lateral projection of a left ventriculogram or the levophase of a right atrial injection. The right ventricle can be identified as a small anterior chamber which communicates, via a VSD, with the left ventricle; it lacks an inlet and does not contribute to the left upper cardiac border (as in a normal heart). The relations of the VSD to the subaortic and subpulmonic segments, as well as associated cardiac malformations, are best demonstrated on axial projections (Fig. 10.21).

MITRAL ATRESIA

In this malformation the left atrioventricular valve is absent and there is no direct connection between the left atrium and the left ventricle; the right atrium connects with the morphologic right

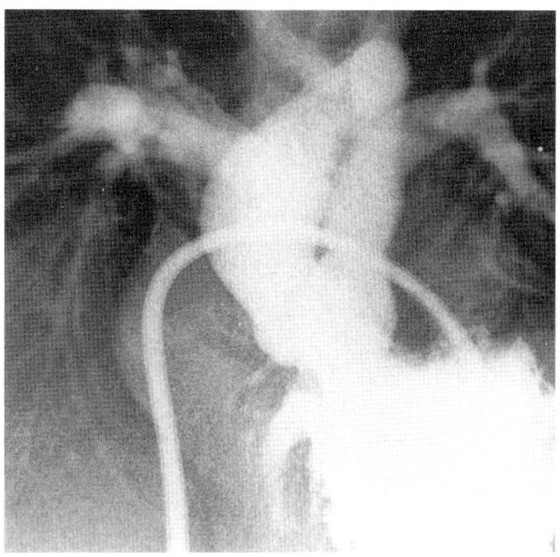

Fig. 10.20 Right tricuspid atresia. Long axis projection of left ventriculogram in a patient with right tricuspid atresia shows a large VSD and large pulmonary arteries. The trabecular portion of the hypoplastic right ventricle is situated anteriorly, indicating that the ventricles are normally related.

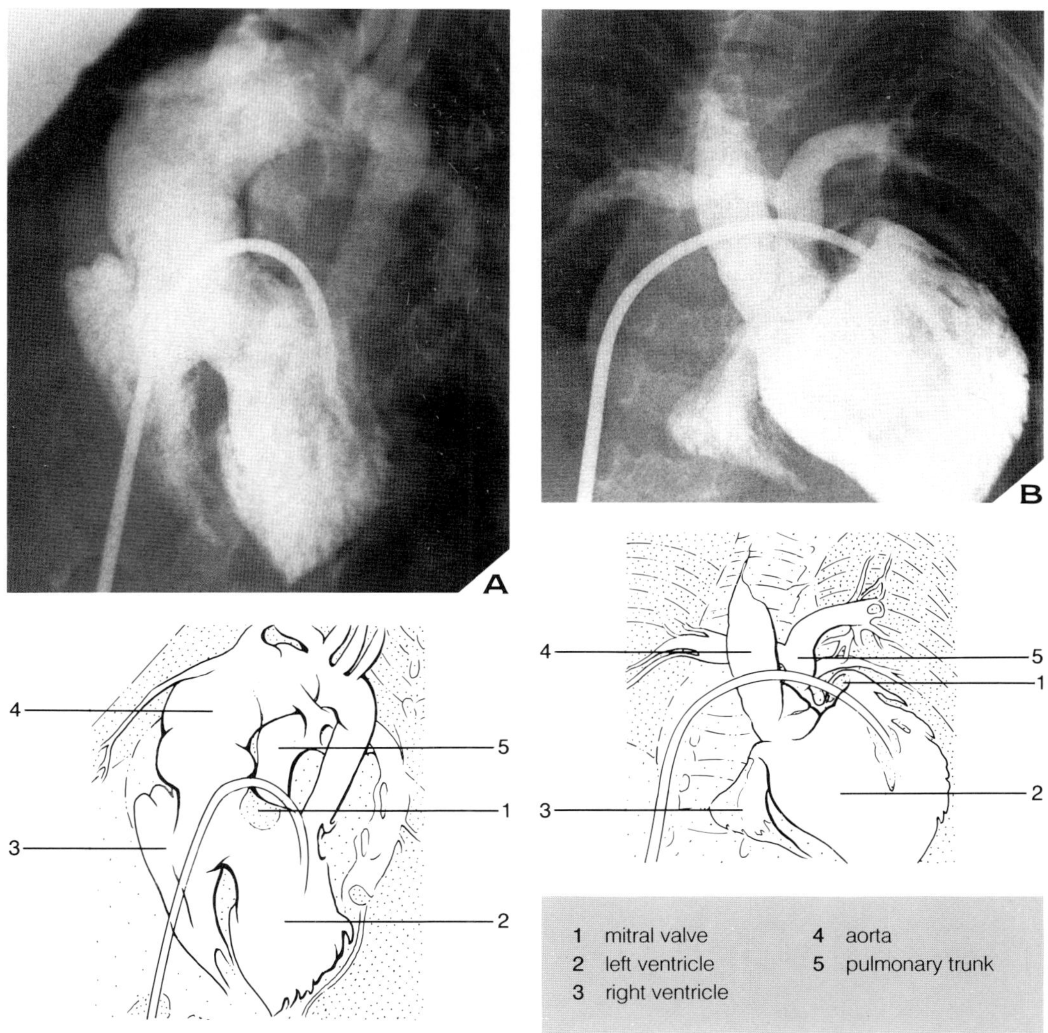

Fig. 10.21 Right tricuspid atresia. Frontal (A) and long-axis (B) projections of left ventriculograms obtained in two different patients. The catheter has been advanced from the inferior vena cava into the right atrium, across the foramen ovale into the left atrium, and across a large mitral valve into the ventricle. The ventricles are normally related but the right ventricle is incomplete owing to absence of the inlet segment. The ventriculoarterial connection is concordant in the patient shown in A and discordant in the patient shown in B. Severe subpulmonic stenosis is present in both patients.

ventricle via a tricuspid valve. In the great majority of cases, the left atrium is superior to the atretic mitral valve, although other atrioventricular arrangements can occur. The left atrium receives the pulmonic venous return and empties into the right atrium via an ASD. Severe pulmonary venous hypertension results if the ASD is restricted. In most instances, however, the ASD is large, in which case the right atrium serves as a mixing chamber and is larger than normal.

CLINICAL FEATURES

The clinical manifestations of mitral atresia are largely determined by the nature of the ventriculoarterial connections. The latter may be concordant (the most common arrangement) or discordant, or there may be a double-outlet right ventricle. In hearts with concordant ventriculoarterial connections, the morphologic right ventricle supports the pulmonary trunk and the morphologic left ventricle supports the aorta; a portion of the

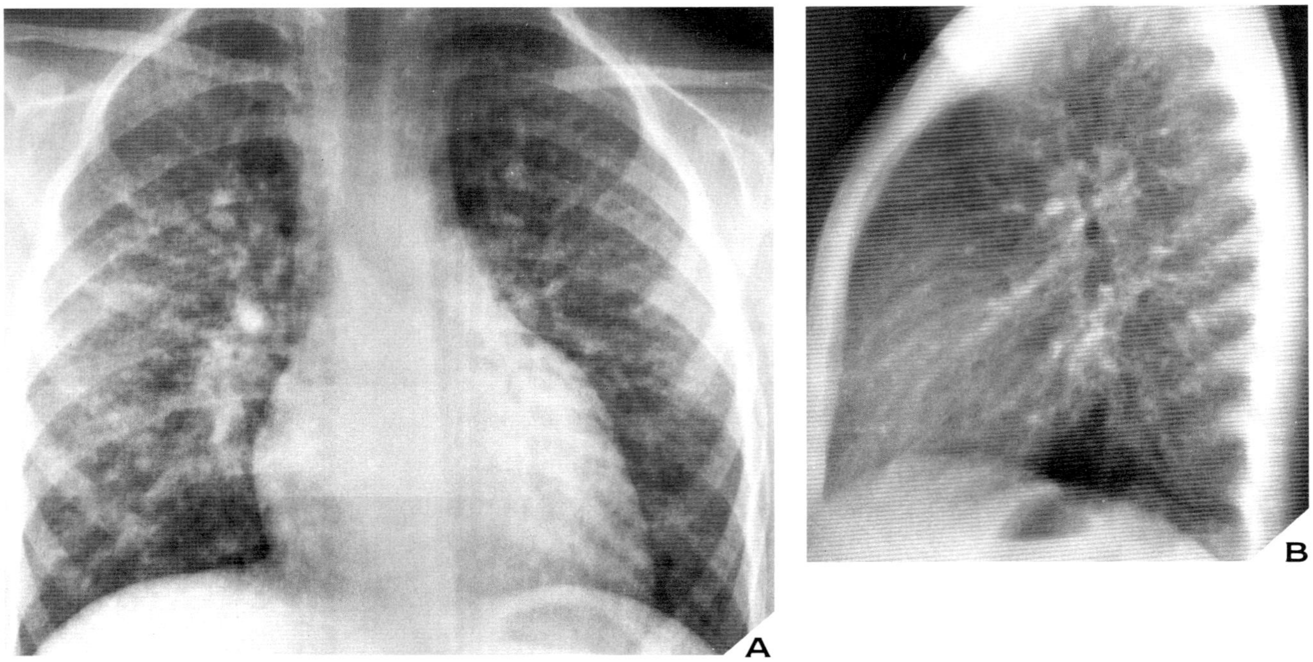

Fig. 10.22 Mitral atresia. Frontal and lateral chest films in a patient with mitral atresia and an unrestricted ASD show mild cardiomegaly with enlargement of the right atrium and right ventricle. There is marked pulmonary plethora, indicating the presence of a large left to right shunt at atrial level. The situs is solitus.

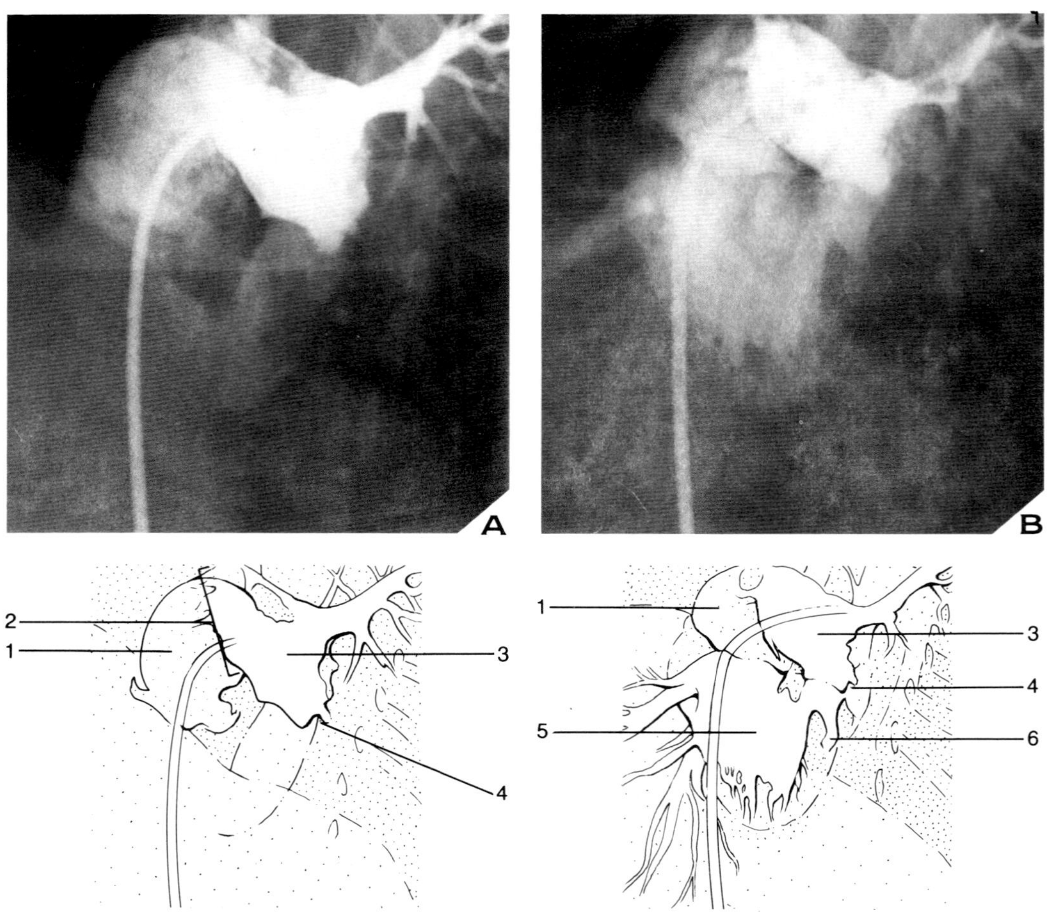

Fig. 10.23 Mitral atresia. Early (A) and late (B) phase of left atriogram (four-chamber view). The catheter has traversed an ASD of the sinus venosus type to enter a normal-sized left atrium. The site of the normal mitral valve is represented by a small dimple. There is a large left to right shunt across the ASD, resulting in opacification of the right atrium and right ventricle (B).

1 right atrium
2 ASD
3 left atrium
4 dimple at site of atretic mitral valve
5 right ventricle
6 left ventricle

right ventricular output is diverted (via a VSD) into the morphologic left ventricle and thence into the systemic circulation. Mitral atresia may also be associated with hypoplasia of the left ventricle and atresia of the aortic valve, the so-called hypoplastic left ventricle ("hypoplastic left heart") complex (see below).

IMAGING

Plain Films

In patients with isolated mitral atresia and a large ASD, plain films demonstrate cardiomegaly with marked right atrial and right ventricular enlargement, a dilated pulmonary trunk, and plethoric lungs (Fig. 10.22). The size of the aorta varies with the size of the VSD. In patients with a small VSD or an intact ventricular septum, the aorta is very small. This is also the case in patients with a hypoplastic left ventricle (see below).

Angiocardiography

Mitral atresia is best demonstrated on a left atrial injection. When the ASD is large, the size of the left atrium is normal or decreased in size; when the ASD is restricted, the left atrium is enlarged. A small dimple in the inferior border of the left atrium marks the site of the atretic mitral valve (Fig. 10.23).

HYPOPLASTIC LEFT VENTRICLE (HLV)

This malformation complex is characterized by atresia or hypoplasia of the mitral valve, hypoplasia of the left ventricle and/or aortic valve, and an intact ventricular septum. The right ventricle functions as an isolated ventricular pump; it receives the entire blood flow and pumps it into the pulmonary trunk and across a patent ductus arteriosus into the aorta. Because the ascending aorta and the aortic valve are hypoplastic, blood from the patent ductus arteriosus courses in retrograde fashion to supply the aortic arch and its branches, ascending aorta, and coronary arteries. Patients with HLV typically present in the neonatal period with congestive heart failure and cyanosis. Some infants present with a low-output syndrome, which may be of abrupt onset; owing to systemic hypoperfusion, these babies tend to be ashen rather than cyanotic.

IMAGING AND INVASIVE DIAGNOSIS

Plain Films

Although HLV is the most frequent cause of congestive heart failure during the first week of life, the plain film findings are generally nonspecific. A minority of infants present with a distinctive radiographic pattern which is virtually diagnostic of this malformation. These infants exhibit cardiomegaly with marked prominence of the right atrium, and prominence of the central pulmonary arteries, pulmonary plethora, and pulmonary edema. The right upper mediastinal border is flat, owing to the small size of the ascending aorta; the right side of the cardiovascular silhouette resembles a "flopped" or "mirror-image" numeral 5 (with the clavicle representing the horizontal-line portion, the flat upper mediastinal border the vertical-line portion, and the dilated right atrium the curved portion of the "5") (Fig. 10.24). More often, however, there is generalized cardiac enlargement, a prominent pulmonary trunk, pulmonary plethora, pulmonary edema, and dilatation of the superior vena cava and azygos vein; this constellation of findings strongly

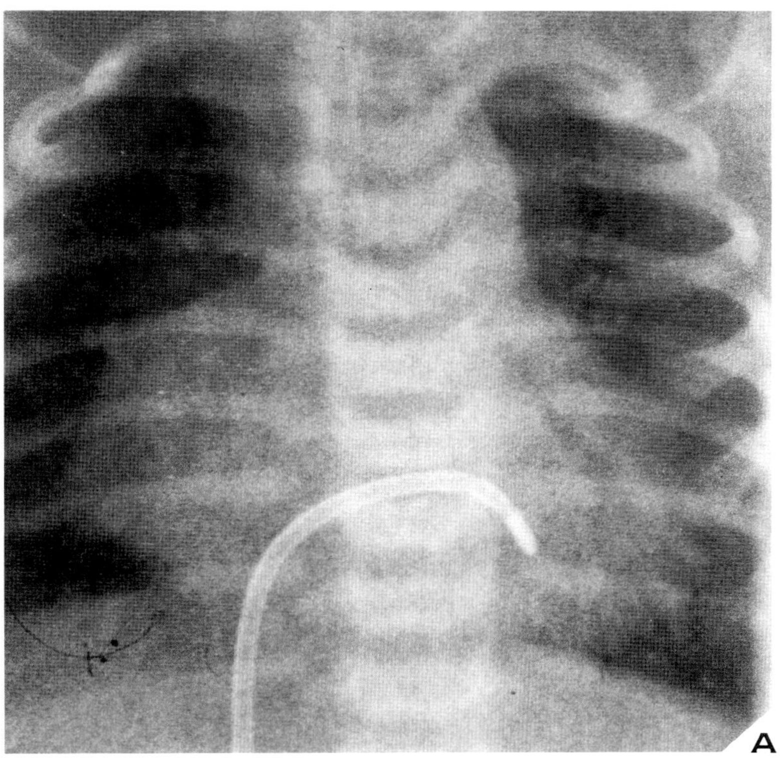
A

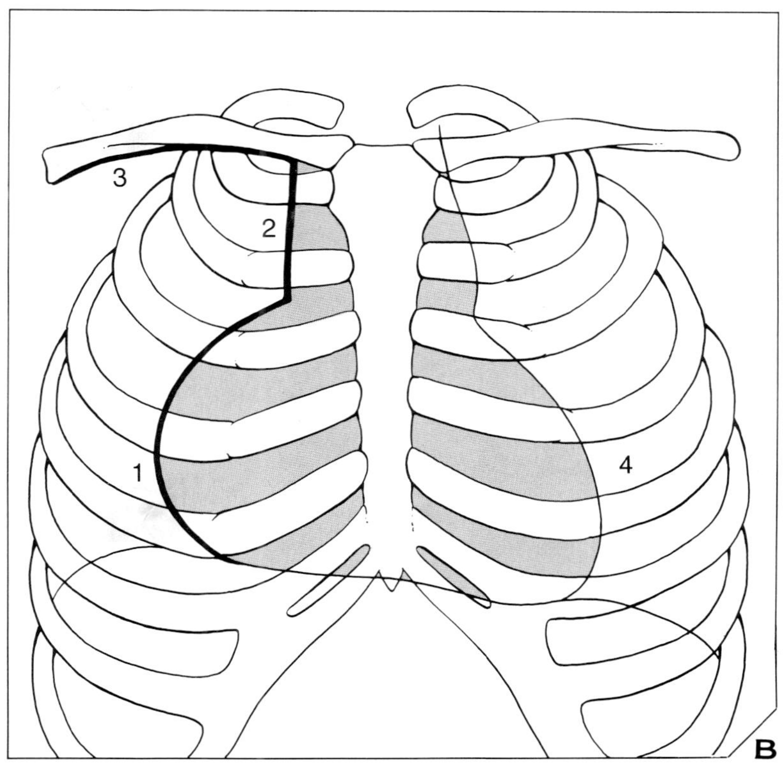

B

Fig. 10.24 Hypoplastic left ventricle. (A) Chest film in a neonate shows a slightly enlarged heart with elevation of the apex and marked prominence of the right atrium. The upper right mediastinal border is flat, owing to hypoplasia of the ascending aorta. The combination of the prominent right atrium, flat upper mediastinal border, and clavicle (not included in this image) gives the appearance of a "flopped" or "mirror-image" numeral 5. The vascular catheter has crossed from the right atrium to the right ventricle via the tricuspid valve. (B) Diagrammatic representation of the "flopped 5" sign.

1 dilated right atrium
2 flat right mediastinal border (hypoplastic ascending aorta)
3 right clavicle
4 upturned cardiac apex (dilated right ventricle)

suggests the diagnosis of HLV in an infant who is cyanotic in the first week of life. However, chest films are frequently normal or reveal only nonspecific cardiac enlargement (Fig. 10.25). Patients with this radiographic pattern usually are not severely cyanotic.

Echocardiography

Echocardiography shows a large right ventricle, a small left ventricular chamber, a diminutive aorta, and an atretic aortic valve (which may appear as a membrane) (Fig. 10.26). Color Doppler imaging reveals reversal of flow in the aortic arch, with retrograde perfusion of the coronary arteries.

Angiocardiography

Right ventriculography demonstrates a large right ventricle, large pulmonary arteries, and dilatation of the peripheral pulmonary arteries, with dilated pulmonary veins evident on the levophase. Late images show retrograde opacification of the aortic arch and ascending aorta (Fig. 10.27).

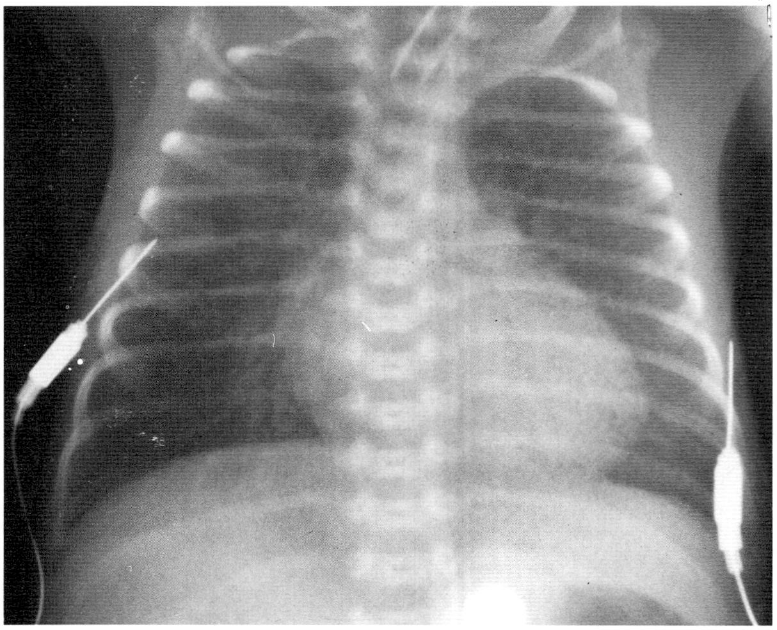

Fig. 10.25 Hypoplastic left ventricle. Chest film of a neonate who "crashed" on the third day of life shows a normal cardiac silhouette and vascular pedicle. There is minimal pulmonary edema.

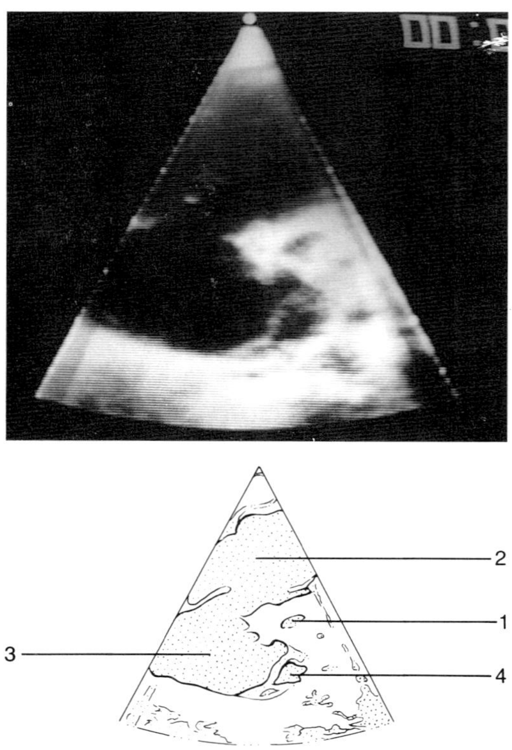

Fig. 10.26 Hypoplastic left ventricle (echocardiographic findings). Apical four-chamber section demonstrates enlargement of the right atrium and right ventricle and a diminutive left atrium and left ventricle. Note absence of left atrioventricular valve.

1 hypoplastic left ventricle
2 enlarged right ventricle
3 enlarged right atrium
4 small left atrium

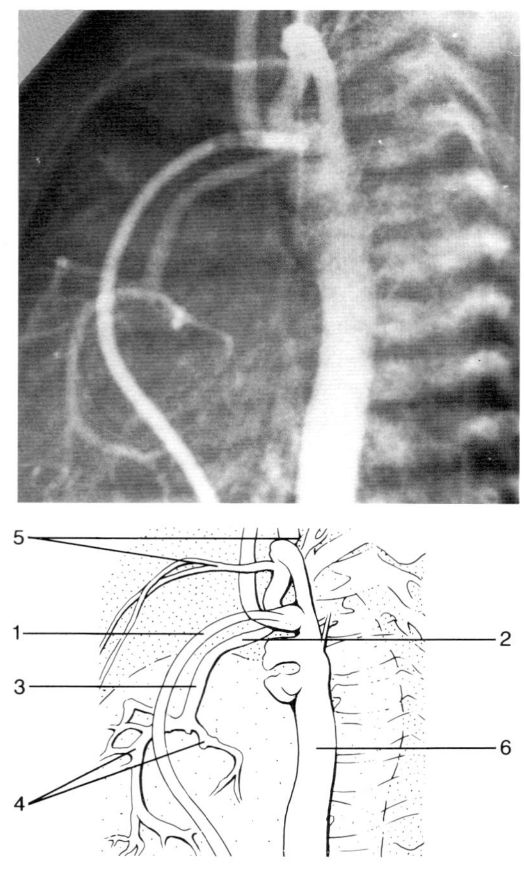

Fig. 10.27 Hypoplastic left ventricle. Late phase of pulmonary arteriogram (lateral projection) obtained after passing a catheter from the right ventricle into the pulmonary trunk. There is retrograde opacification of the hypoplastic aortic arch and ascending aorta, with retrograde filling of the branches of the aortic arch and the coronary arteries.

1 catheter
2 hypoplastic aortic arch
3 hypoplastic ascending aorta
4 coronary arteries
5 branches of aorta arch
6 descending aorta

CHAPTER 11

Abnormal Ventriculoarterial Connections

In this group of congenital malformations, the ventricular chambers connect with the great arteries in an abnormal manner.

CONCORDANT ATRIOVENTRICULAR CONNECTION

TETRALOGY OF FALLOT

Tetralogy of Fallot is the most common condition in this category. The underlying abnormality is an anteriorly displaced infundibular septum, which results in the three basic malformations that characterize the disorder: severe stenosis of the right ventricular outflow tract; a large infundibular VSD; and an overriding aorta which originates (to a greater or lesser degree) from both ventricles (Fig. 11.1). Hypertrophy of the right ventricle, the fourth element of the tetralogy, is a consequence of the three basic defects.

PATHOPHYSIOLOGY

Stenosis of the right ventricular outflow tract, accompanied by a large VSD, leads to increased right ventricular pressure. A portion of the right ventricular output enters the systemic circulation (*directly* via the overriding aorta and *indirectly* via the VSD) resulting in a right to left shunt. The stenotic right ventricular outflow tract further restricts pulmonary blood flow. Because of

CHAPTER LABELING KEY

RA	right atrium	LV	left ventricle
LA	left atrium	Ao	aorta
RV	right ventricle		

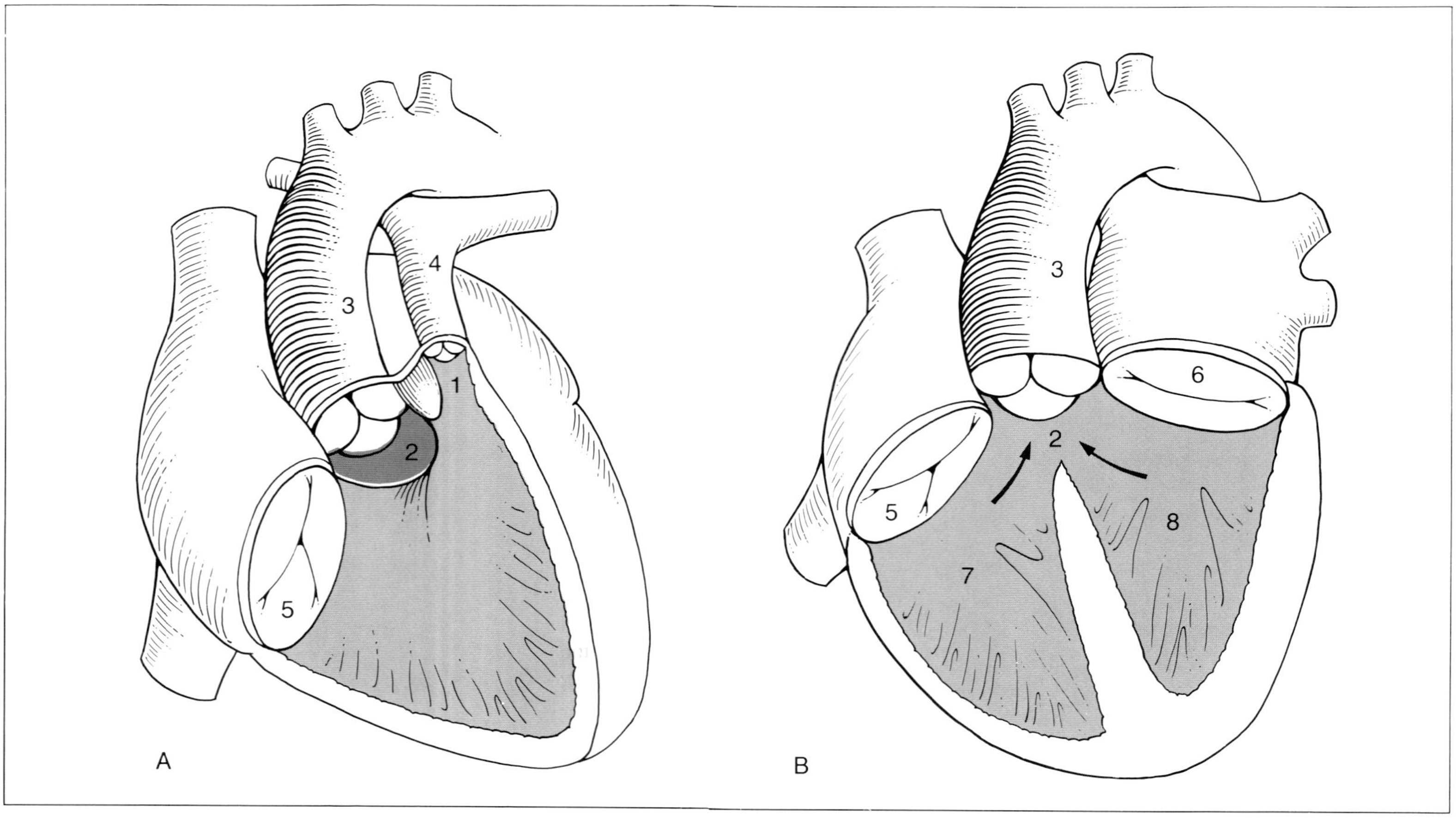

Fig. 11.1 Tetralogy of Fallot. (A) Classical tetralogy of Fallot as seen from the right ventricle. (B) Cross-section through ventricular septum demonstrating overriding of the aorta. Both ventricles connected with the aorta.

1 stenosis of right ventricular outflow tract produced by abnormal position of ventricular septum
2 VSD located immediately beneath aortic valve but related to tricuspid valve
3 aorta
4 pulmonary trunk
5 tricuspid valve
6 mitral valve
7 trabecular portion of right ventricle
8 left ventricle

the abnormal flow pattern, the pulmonary trunk and main pulmonary arteries are smaller than normal. The right ventricular pressure and the volume overload lead to right ventricular hypertrophy, with equalization of left and right ventricular pressure (Fig. 11.2). The left ventricle is usually normal in size and contractility. The atria are normal or slightly decreased in size.

In some patients the ventricular septum is displaced anteriorly and there is relatively little outflow obstruction; there is a net left to right shunt and peripheral saturation is almost normal. Because these patients are not overtly cyanotic, this disorder has been called "pink tetralogy" (Fig. 11.3).

IMAGING AND INVASIVE DIAGNOSIS

Plain Films

In most cases the heart is of normal size; however, there is evidence of right ventricular enlargement. The right ventricle forms the left lower portion of the cardiac silhouette, including the cardiac apex, which is separated from the diaphragm and

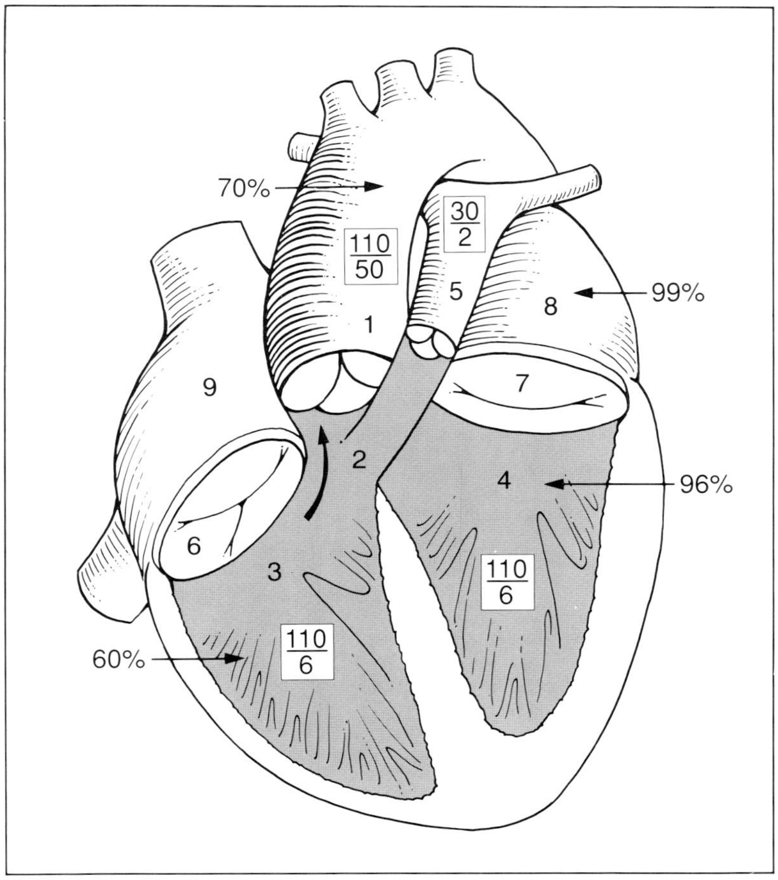

Fig. 11.2 Oxygen saturation and pressures in classical tetralogy of Fallot. Right and left ventricular pressures are equal. There is a significant pressure gradient between the right ventricle and the pulmonary trunk. The blood in the aorta is markedly desaturated.

1 aorta
2 right ventricular outflow tract
3 right ventricle
4 left ventricle
5 pulmonary trunk
6 tricuspid valve
7 mitral valve
8 left atrium
9 right atrium

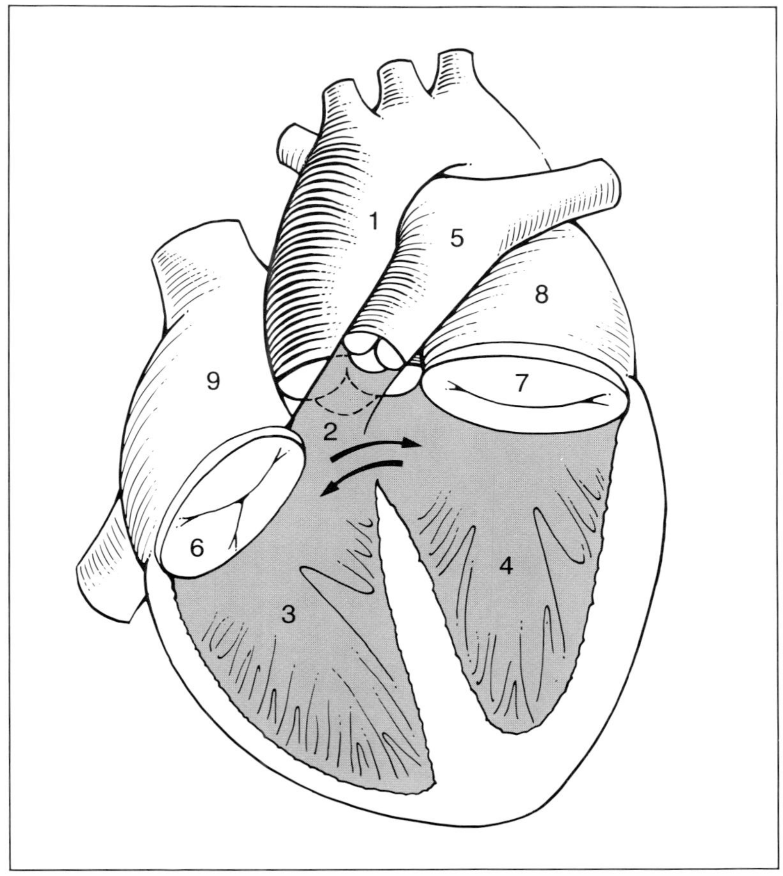

Fig. 11.3 "Pink tetralogy." So-called "pink tetralogy" is really a combination of a VSD and pulmonary valvar stenosis; hence it does not fit the definition of tetralogy of Fallot. However, patients with this combination of defects may present with peripheral desaturation.

1 aorta
2 right ventricular outflow tract
3 right ventricle
4 left ventricle
5 pulmonary trunk
6 tricuspid valve
7 mitral valve
8 left atrium
9 right atrium

points upward. On the lateral view, the zone of contact between the heart and the anterior chest wall is increased, reflecting right ventricular hypertrophy (Figs. 11.4 and 11.5). The appearance of the central and peripheral pulmonary vasculature is determined by the volume of blood entering the pulmonary artery, either directly (from the right ventricle) or indirectly (via systemic collaterals). The pulmonary trunk and the main pulmonary arteries are usually smaller than normal, and the pulmonary vascular markings are diminished in size and number. In the absence of significant right ventricular outflow obstruction ("pink tetralogy"), or after a palliative shunt, pulmonary perfusion may be normal or even increased (Fig. 11.5A).

To sum up, the classical radiographic findings in tetralogy of Fallot are: a normal-sized heart with an upturned apex; a diminutive or inapparent pulmonary trunk; increased contact between the heart and anterior chest wall, indicating right ventricular hypertrophy; and diminished pulmonary vascularity. The combination of an upturned apex and a diminutive pulmonary trunk produces a typical "boot-shaped" heart (Figs. 11.4 and 11.5). A right aortic arch is present in about 40 percent of patients with tetralogy of Fallot (Fig. 11.4A).

Tricuspid atresia and pulmonary atresia with VSD can simulate tetralogy of Fallot on plain films. However, tricuspid atresia is associated with left ventricular enlargement (see Fig. 10.11), whereas pulmonary atresia with VSD can be considered a severe form of tetralogy of Fallot.

Angiocardiography

On the right ventriculogram the right ventricle is seen to form most of the cardiac silhouette. The infundibular septum, which is deviated anteriorly and to the left, appears as a filling defect in the midportion of the right ventricular outflow tract (Fig. 11.6). The pulmonary trunk is hypoplastic and usually does not contribute to the left cardiac contour. The right and left pulmonary arteries, as well as their peripheral branches, are smaller than normal (Figs. 11.6B and 11.7). Branch stenoses of the pulmonary arteries are not uncommon.

Opacification of the aorta after a right ventricular injection indicates the presence of VSD (Fig. 11.6). The latter is most clearly seen on the lateral projection (Fig. 11.8). Owing to its biventricular origin, the aorta also receives opacified blood directly from the right ventricle.

The ascending aorta is in a normal position, posterior and to the right of the pulmonary artery, and is usually enlarged. Both the aortic arch and the descending thoracic aorta are on the right in 40 percent of patients with tetralogy of Fallot.

Echocardiography

All of the diagnostic features of tetralogy of Fallot are clearly shown by echocardiography (Fig. 11.9; see Appendix). However, echocardiography is less accurate than angiocardiography in detecting abnormalities of the pulmonary arteries (eg, branch stenoses).

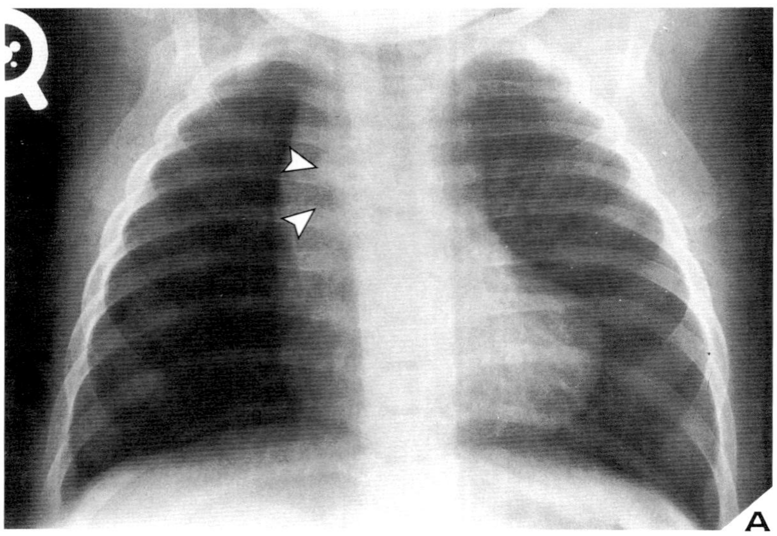

A

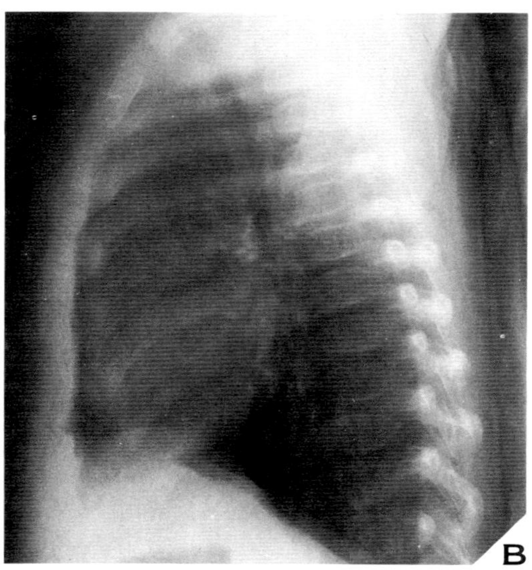

B

Fig. 11.4 Tetralogy of Fallot with right aortic arch (infant). (A) Frontal and (B) lateral chest films of a cyanotic infant show a normal-sized heart with an upturned apex. The pulmonary artery segment is concave, giving the heart a distinctive "boot-shaped" configuration. The pulmonary vasculature is diminished bilaterally. The zone of contact between the heart and the chest wall is increased on the lateral projection, indicating right ventricular enlargement. The aortic arch is on the right (*arrows* in A).

The most frequent arch anomaly in patients with tetralogy is right aortic arch with mirror image branching (RAA/MIB). Right aortic arch with aberrant left subclavian artery (RAA/ALS) also occurs in patients with tetralogy, though it is less common. Whereas RAA/MIB is almost invariably associated with congenital heart disease—tetralogy of Fallot and truncus arteriosus in particular—RAA/ALS is usually found in otherwise normal individuals. The barium esophagram is helpful in differentiating the two types of right aortic arch. Whereas the esophagram is normal in patients with RAA/MIB, there is a prominent impression on the posterior aspect of the esophagus in patients with RAA/ALS.

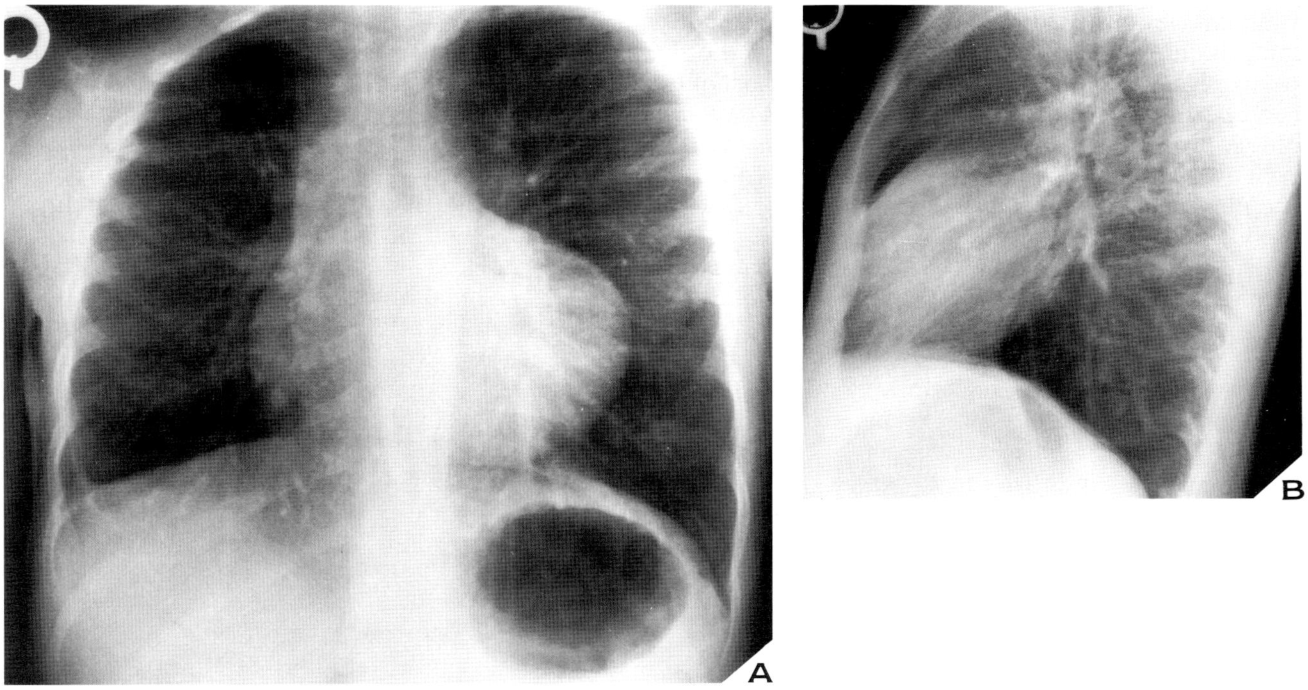

Fig. 11.5 Tetralogy of Fallot (child). (A) Frontal and (B) lateral chest films show moderate cardiomegaly with an upturned apex ("boot-shaped heart"). Note the increased contact of the heart with the chest wall on the lateral view, indicating right ventricular enlargement. The pulmonary vasculature is normal as a result of a palliative right-sided Blalock–Taussig anastomosis performed during infancy.

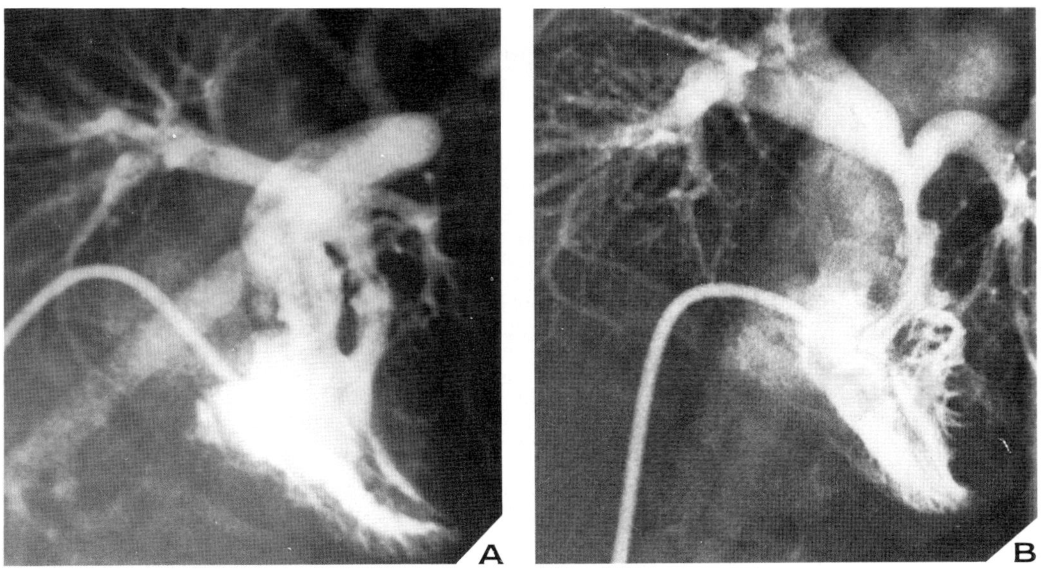

Fig. 11.6 Tetralogy of Fallot. Right ventriculograms (right anterior oblique projection) in two different patients. (A) Classical appearance of abnormal right ventricular outflow tract. The abnormally positioned infundibular septum appears as a filling defect in the outflow tract. The aortic root overrides the trabecular septum. The VSD is seen behind the infundibular septum. Opacified blood enters the aorta from the right ventricle directly and via the VSD. The pulmonic valve is stenotic. (B) A special angled view of the bifurcation demonstrates hypoplasia of the pulmonary trunk and left pulmonary artery. There is post-stenotic dilatation of the right pulmonary artery.

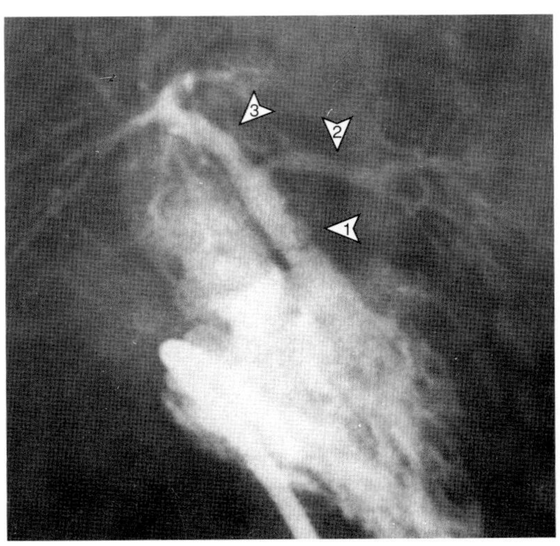

Fig. 11.7 Tetralogy of Fallot with severe hypoplasia of pulmonary arteries. Left anterior oblique projection of right ventriculogram shows a diminutive pulmonary trunk (*arrow* 1). The left (*arrow* 2) and right (*arrow* 3) pulmonary arteries are markedly hypoplastic.

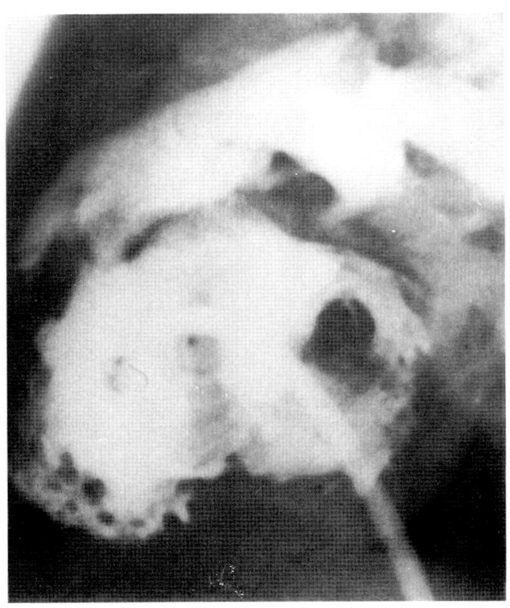

Fig. 11.8 Tetralogy of Fallot. Right ventriculogram (lateral projection) demonstrates stenosis of the right ventricular outflow tract and a VSD.

Magnetic Resonance Imaging

All of the key features of tetralogy of Fallot—VSD, stenosis of the right ventricular outflow tract, and overriding aorta—are clearly demonstrated by MRI (Figs. 11.10 and 11.11). However, the most important contribution of MRI is its ability to delineate the pulmonary trunk and main pulmonary arteries *noninvasively* with an accuracy comparable to that of angiography (Fig. 11.12). The multiplanar capability of MRI is helpful in characterizing the nature of the VSD. On axial and sagittal images, the perimembranous VSD characteristic of tetralogy of Fallot is closely related to the aortic and tricuspid valves, whereas a juxtaaortic muscular VSD is separated from the tricuspid valve by the posterior arm of the trabecular septum.

DISCORDANT VENTRICULO–ARTERIAL CONNECTION

COMPLETE TRANSPOSITION OF THE GREAT ARTERIES (TGA)

In this group of malformations, of which TGA is by far the most common, the right ventricle connects with the aorta and the left ventricle connects with the pulmonary artery. The systemic and pulmonary venous drainage patterns, as well as the atrioventricular connections, are normal (Fig. 11.13). The systemic and pulmonary circulations are parallel and separate, an arrangement that is incompatible with life unless a shunt exists

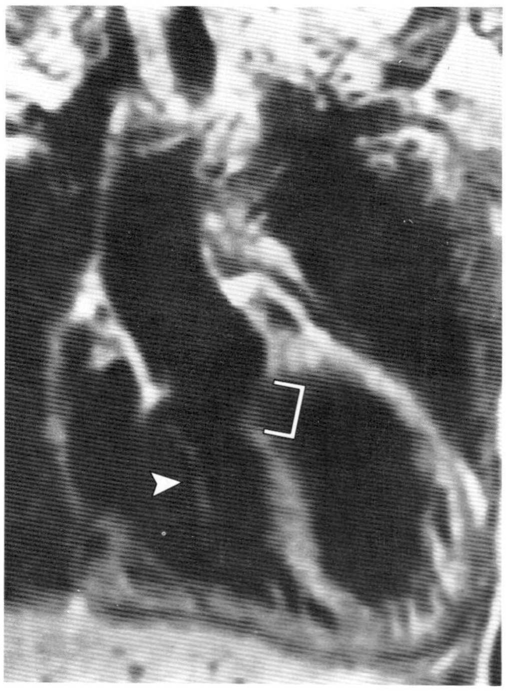

Fig. 11.10 Tetralogy of Fallot (MRI). Gated spin–echo image. Coronal section shows the right ventricle connecting with the aorta via a perimembranous VSD *(bracket)*. The septal leaflet of tricuspid valve *(arrow)* is adjacent to the VSD.

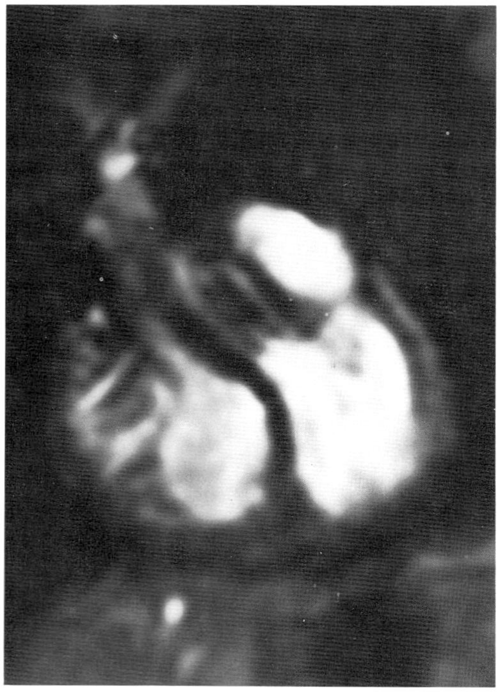

Fig. 11.11 Tetralogy of Fallot (cine MRI). Left anterior oblique projection shows the aorta overriding the ventricular septum. The connections between the left and right ventricles and the aorta are approximately the same size. The VSD is located beneath the aortic valve. Flowing blood has a bright signal on this pulse sequence.

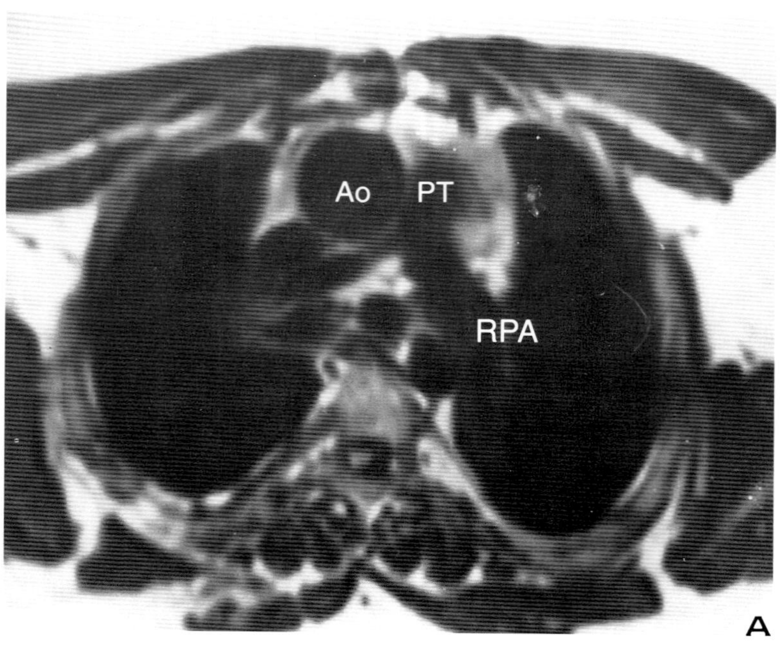

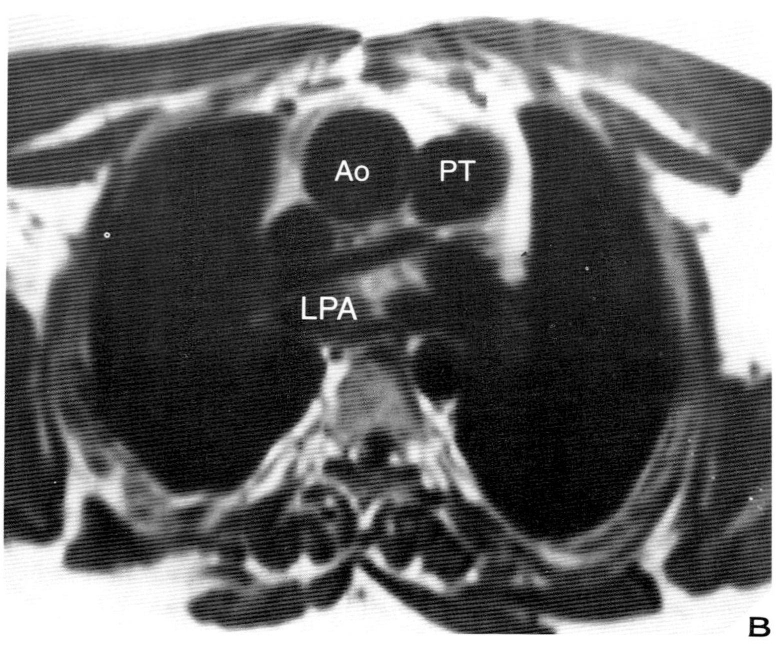

Fig. 11.12 Tetralogy of Fallot (MRI). Gated spin–echo images. (A) Axial section at the level of the right pulmonary artery shows a small pulmonary trunk and a normal-sized right pulmonary artery. (B) A more caudal section shows a hypoplastic left pulmonary artery.

(usually an ASD) that enables mixing to occur. An emergency balloon septotomy (Rashkind procedure) may be lifesaving in a newborn infant with an ASD that is too small to sustain life (see Chapter 16).

MORPHOLOGY

The right ventricle is in the usual position, ie, anterior and to the right of the left ventricle, which is also in normal position. The right ventricular outflow tract is deviated to the right; the left ventricular outflow tract is displaced to the left and is slightly more anterior than normal. Thus, the right and left ventricular outflow tracts are parallel to each other (Fig. 11.5B).

The proximal segments of the aorta and pulmonary trunk are also oriented in parallel fashion. The aorta usually lies anterior and to the right of the pulmonary trunk; however, the spatial orientation of the great arteries is quite variable (Fig. 11.14). Rarely, the ascending aorta is posterior to the pulmonary trunk. Ninety-four percent of patients with TGA have a left aortic arch.

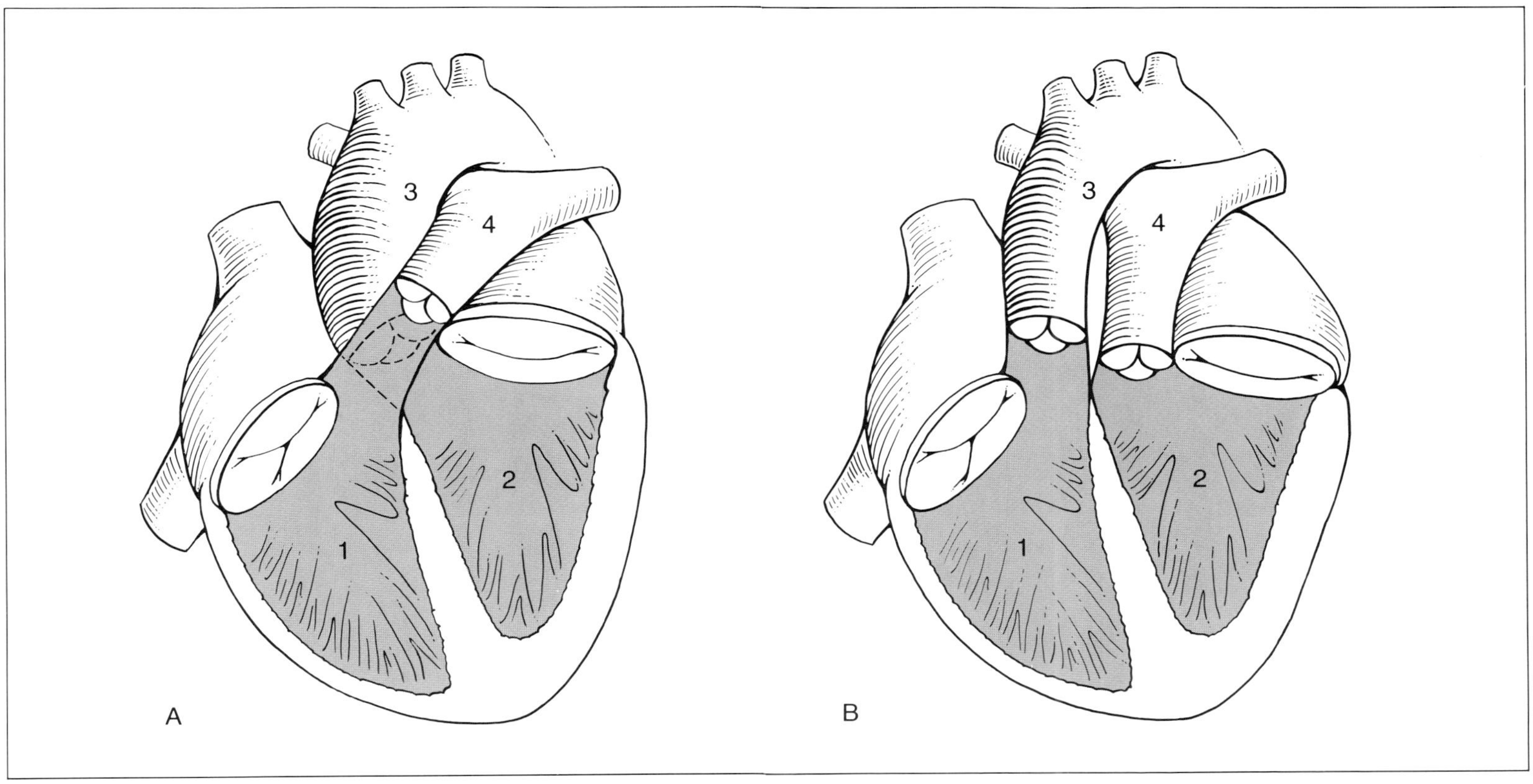

Fig. 11.13 Transposition of the great arteries. (A) Normal crossing ventriculoarterial relationship. (B) Parallel arrangement of ventricular outflow tracts.

1 right ventricle
2 left ventricle
3 aorta
4 pulmonary trunk

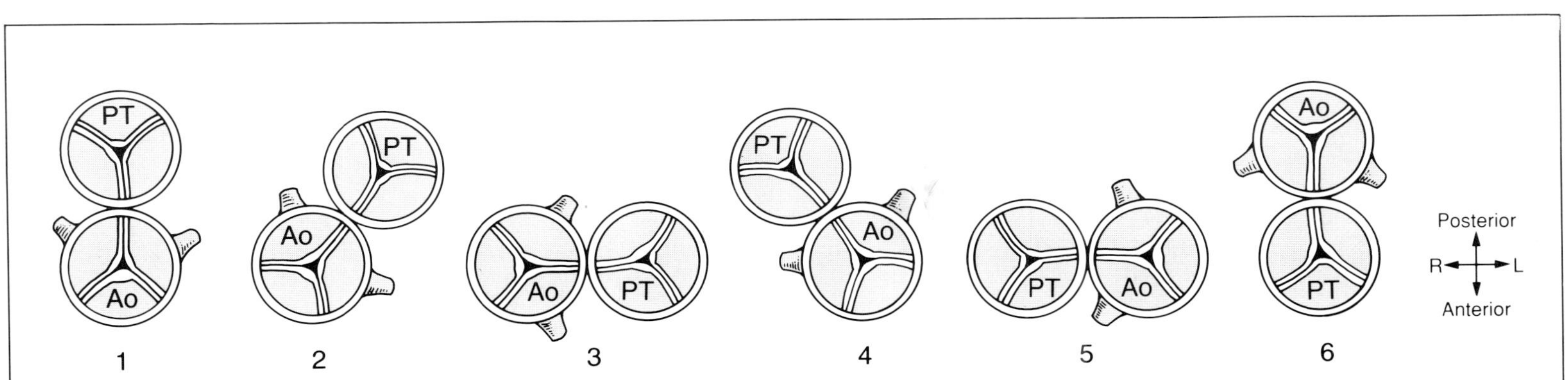

Fig. 11.14 Transposition of the great arteries: relationship of great arteries. Possible arrangements of the great arteries at the level of the sinuses of Valsalva (viewed from above).

1 anteroposterior relationship, aorta anterior to pulmonary trunk
2 right oblique relationship, aorta anterior and to the right of pulmonary trunk (most common)
3 side-by-side relationship, aorta to the right of pulmonary trunk
4 left oblique relationship, aorta anterior and to the left of pulmonary trunk
5 side-by-side relationship, aorta to the left of pulmonary trunk
6 anteroposterior relationship, aorta posterior to pulmonary trunk (least common)
Ao aorta
PT pulmonary trunk

PATHOPHYSIOLOGY

Typically, a bidrectional shunt is present at the atrial level, the magnitude of which is determined by the compliance of each ventricle. A portion of the oxygenated pulmonary venous blood entering the left atrium passes through the ASD into the right atrium, where it mixes with unoxygenated systemic venous blood. The mixed (ie, partially desaturated) blood passes through the tricuspid valve into the right ventricle and is pumped into the aorta (Fig. 11.15). The degree of systemic desaturation (and the severity of the cyanosis) depends on the volume of blood entering the pulmonary circulation and the magnitude of the left to right shunt across the ASD.

CLINICAL PICTURE

Patients with TGA and an intact ventricular septum or restricted VSD are typically cyanotic at birth and die from hypoxia and acidosis; balloon atrial septostomy (Rashkind procedure) may be lifesaving in such cases. Infants with TGA and a large VSD present with mild cyanosis during the second or third week of life; in such cases congestive failure, secondary to pulmonary venous hypertension and myocardial dysfunction, dominates the clinical picture.

Patients with TGA and a large VSD have a better prognosis than those with an intact ventricular septum. However, when all varieties of TGA are considered as a group, the survival rate is 55 percent at 1 month, 15 percent at 6 months, and only 10 percent at 1 year.

IMAGING AND INVASIVE DIAGNOSIS

Plain Films

In the neonate, chest films typically show mildly increased pulmonary blood flow (plethora), relatively normal-sized cardiac chambers, and a narrow vascular pedicle; the pulmonary trunk, which forms part of the left heart border in a normal neonate, is hidden behind the aorta (Fig. 11.16). These radiographic findings strongly suggest TGA in a cyanotic neonate.

When there is a large VSD, chest films show generalized cardiomegaly with biventricular enlargement. The vascular pedicle is typically narrow. Unless pulmonic stenosis is present, the pulmonary vasculature is plethoric (Fig. 11.17). When the great arteries are in a side-by-side relationship and the pulmonary trunk is on the left, the plain film findings are indistinguishable from those of a large VSD; in such cases the presence of cyanosis strongly favors TGA.

In an older child or teenager, the frontal chest film typically shows cardiomegaly with enlargement of the right ventricle and both atria; increased contact between the right ventricle and anterior chest wall is seen on the lateral projection. Medial displacement of the pulmonary trunk results in a narrow vascular pedicle, which may be obscured by the thymus. In the most common arrangement, the pulmonary trunk is located behind the aorta and cannot be identified as a discrete structure on the frontal projection (Fig. 11.18). The right and left pulmonary arteries lie at the same level. When pulmonary flow is significantly increased, the pulmonary arteries are enlarged and the

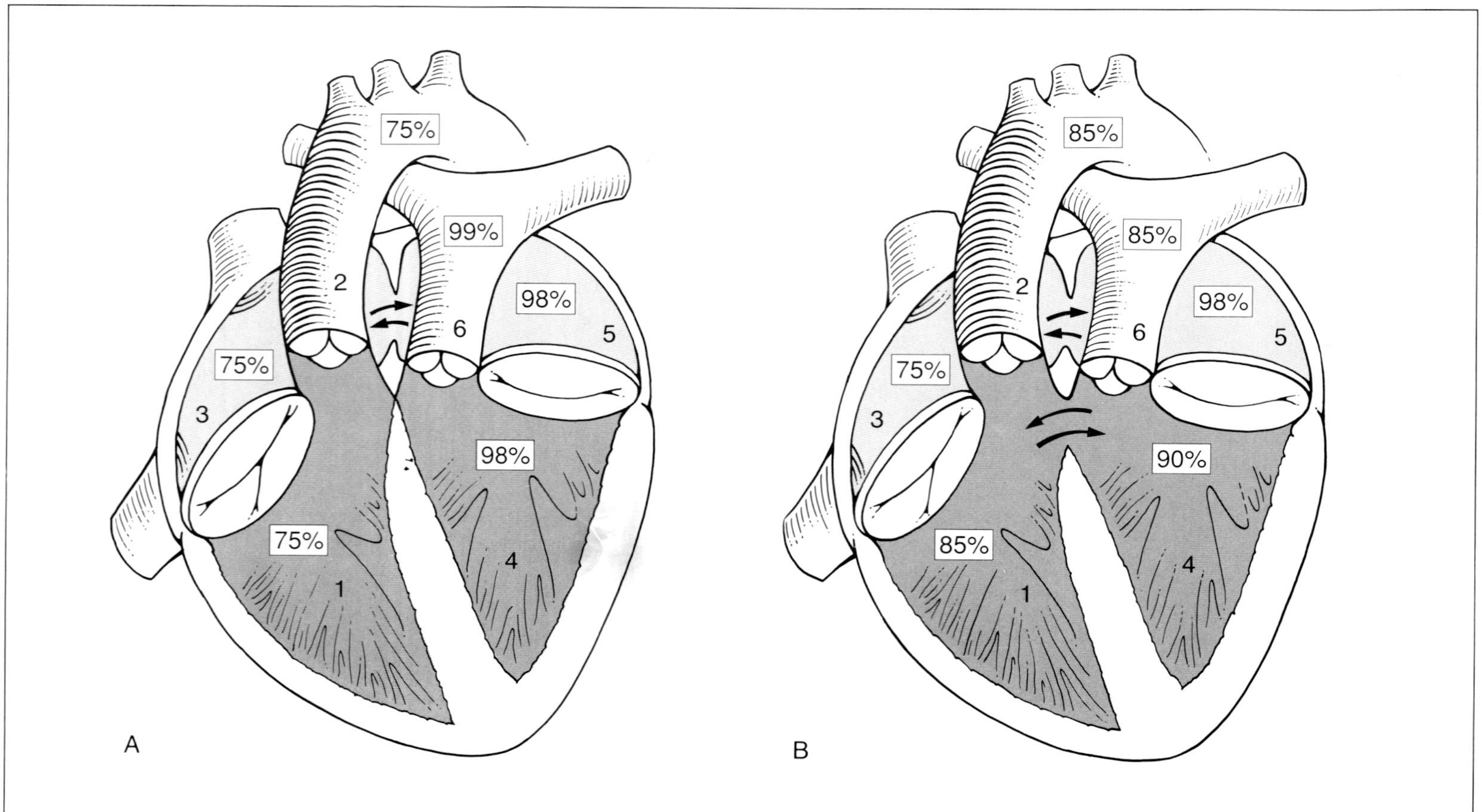

Fig. 11.15 Transposition of great arteries: hemodynamic features. (A) TGA with atrial septal defect and intact ventricular septum. (B) TGA with atrial septal defect and VSD. Note that saturation in the aorta is lower in patients with an intact ventricular septum.

1	right ventricle	4	left ventricle
2	aorta	5	left atrium
3	right atrium	6	pulmonary trunk

lung fields are plethoric. The medially displaced ascending aorta usually cannot be identified in the frontal projection. The aortic arch is usually on the left.

The narrow pedicle produces a distinctive "egg-shaped" heart, a finding that is helpful in differentiating TGA from other cardiac malformations (Figs. 11.16 to 11.18). It should be emphasized, however, that because of the variable spatial orientation of the great arteries, the vascular pedicle may appear normal or wide in some patients with TGA. Moreover, normal thymic tissue, which occupies the anterior mediastinum, may mask a narrow pedicle. (Although the vascular pedicle is typically very narrow in severely desaturated neonates with TGA, it may appear normal after balloon septostomy. Because this palliative procedure does not alter relationships of the great arteries, the apparent widening of the vascular pedicle can be explained by regrowth of the thymus coincident with clinical improvement.)

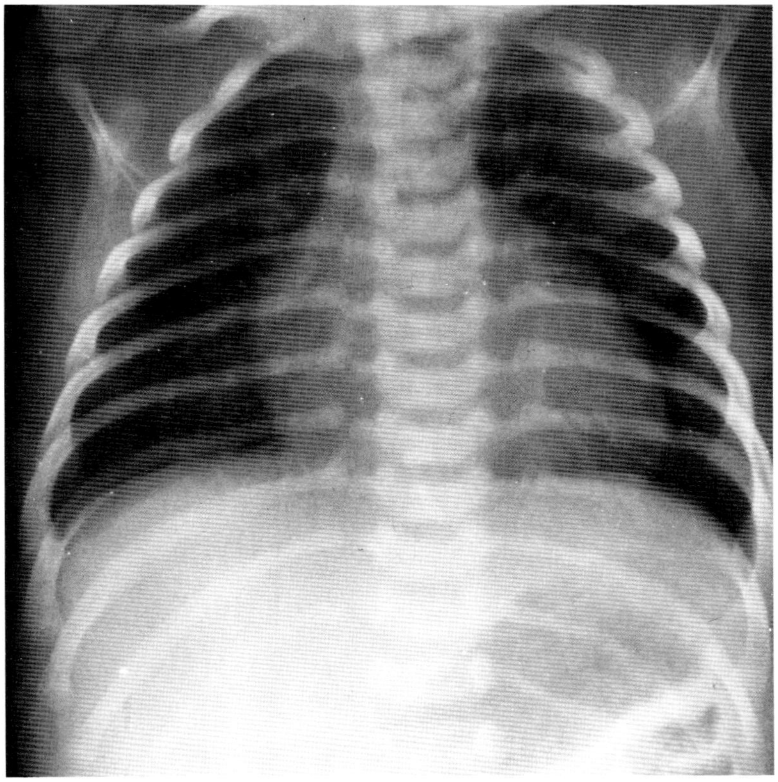

Fig. 11.16 Transposition of the great arteries with intact ventricular septum. Note prominence of the right atrium, narrow vascular pedicle, and decreased pulmonary vascularity in this cyanotic 3-week-old infant.

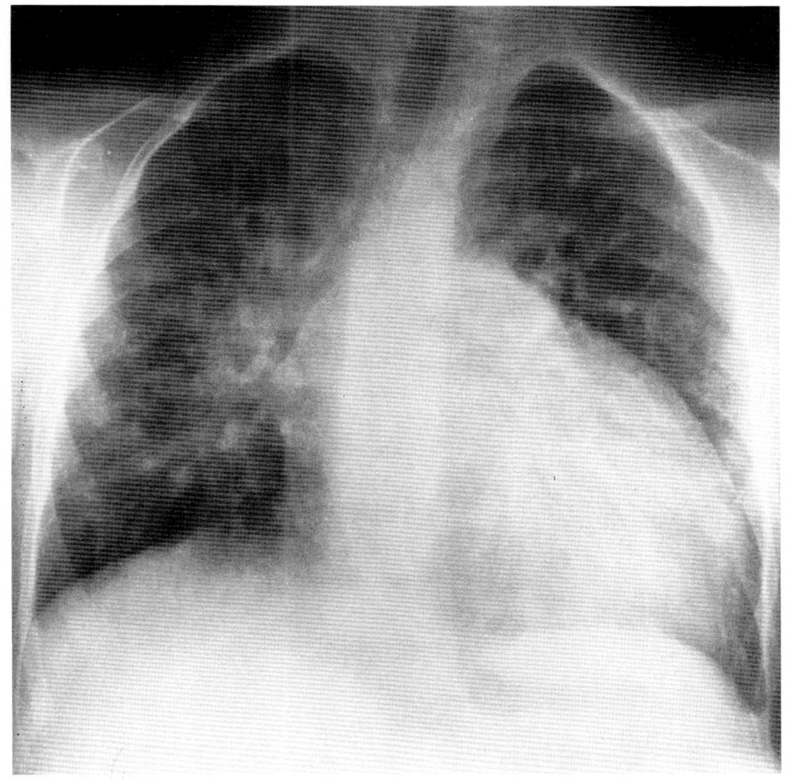

Fig. 11.17 Transposition of the great arteries with VSD. Cardiomegaly and marked pulmonary plethora are the prominent features in this patient with a large VSD.

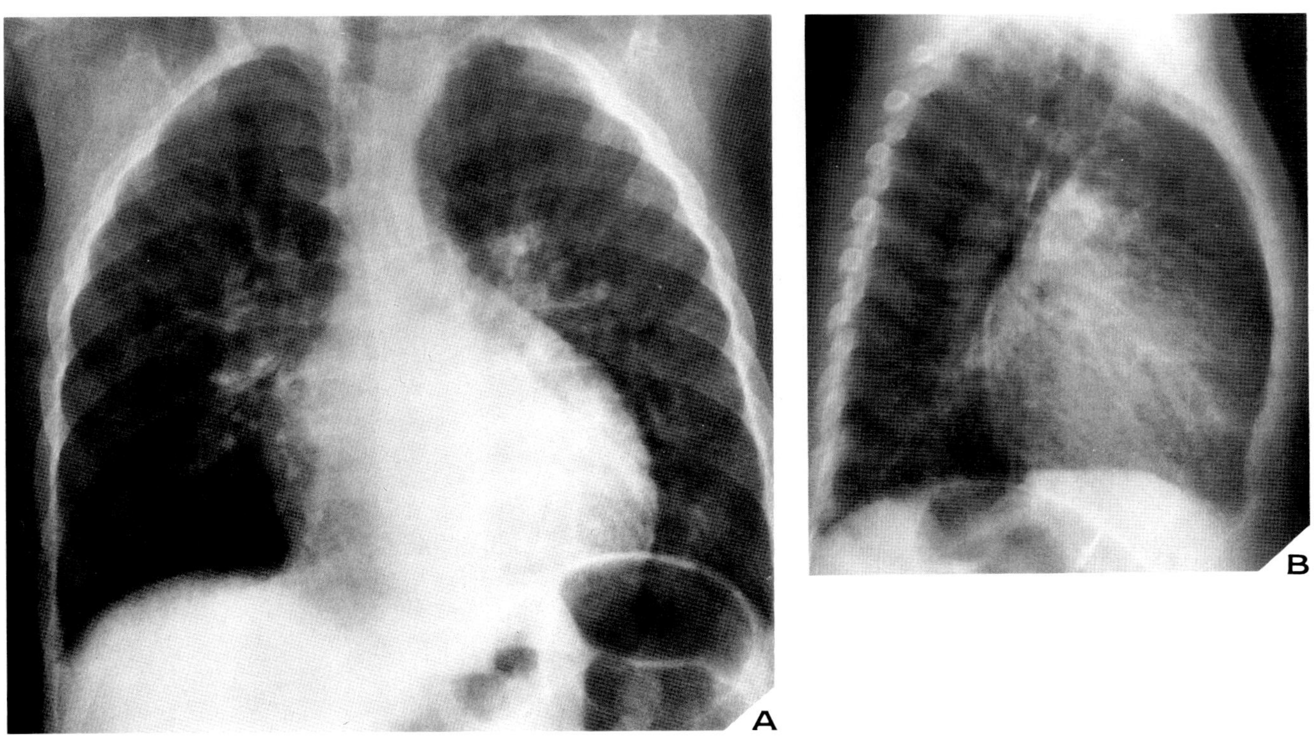

Fig. 11.18 Transposition of the great arteries with ASD. (A) Frontal and (B) lateral chest films show cardiomegaly with right ventricular and left atrial enlargement. The vascular pedicle is very narrow and the pulmonary trunk cannot be identified. The right and left pulmonary arteries are dilated. The small aortic arch is left-sided.

Angiocardiography

Both right and left ventriculography are necessary to depict the basic morphology of TGA as well as the associated malformations. In the classic arrangement, the relations of the right ventricle are normal but the right ventricular outflow tract is displaced to the right. The right ventricle connects with the aorta via a normally formed aortic valve. The aorta lies anterior and to the right of its normal position. The left ventricle is posterior and to the left of the right ventricle and connects with the pulmonary trunk via a normally formed pulmonic valve. The pulmonary trunk is posterior to the aorta, bifurcating immediately behind it (Fig. 11.19).

Most patients with TGA have additional cardiac malformations (eg, ASD, VSD, stenosis of the left ventricular outflow tract) (Fig. 11.20). These, as well as the degree of pulmonary resistance, can dramatically alter the hemodynamic pattern. For example, when pulmonary resistance rises to suprasystemic levels secondary to markedly increased pulmonary blood flow and pulmonary arterial hypertension, shunt reversal may occur.

Echocardiography

Complete TGA and associated intracardiac malformations are accurately depicted by echocardiography (Fig. 11.21). However, before definitive surgery, angiocardiography is usually performed to precisely delinate the pathologic anatomy.

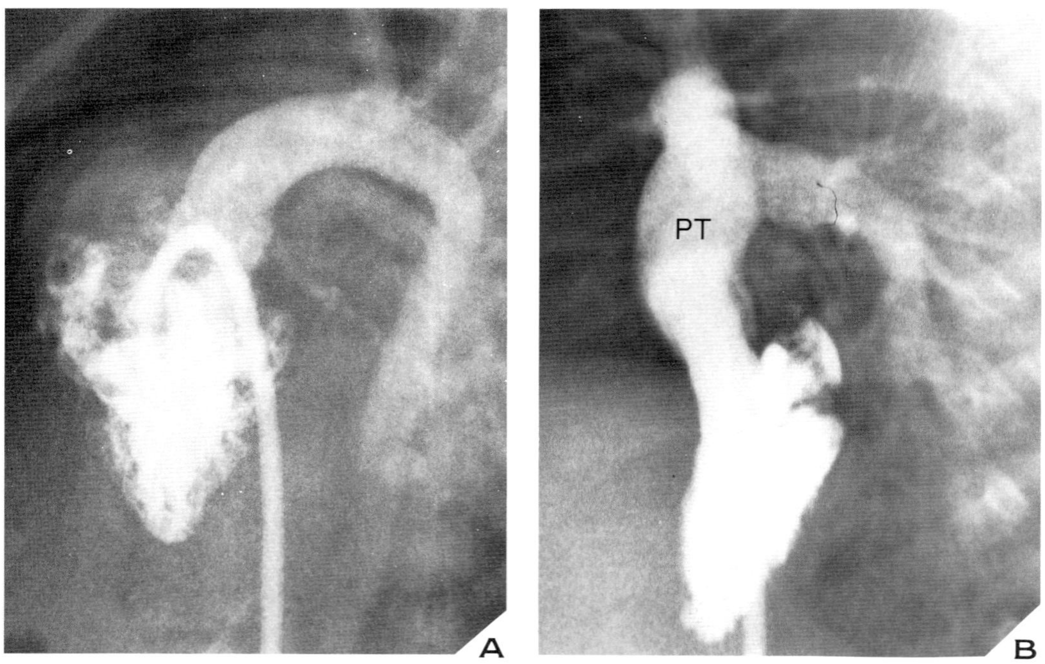

Fig. 11.19 Transposition of the great arteries. (A) Right and (B) left ventriculograms (long axis projection). The right ventricle is anterior and to the right of the left ventricle. The right ventricular outlet is displaced to the right and supports the aorta. The left ventricular outlet is displaced posteriorly and supports the pulmonary trunk (PT). The aorta is anterior to the pulmonary trunk.

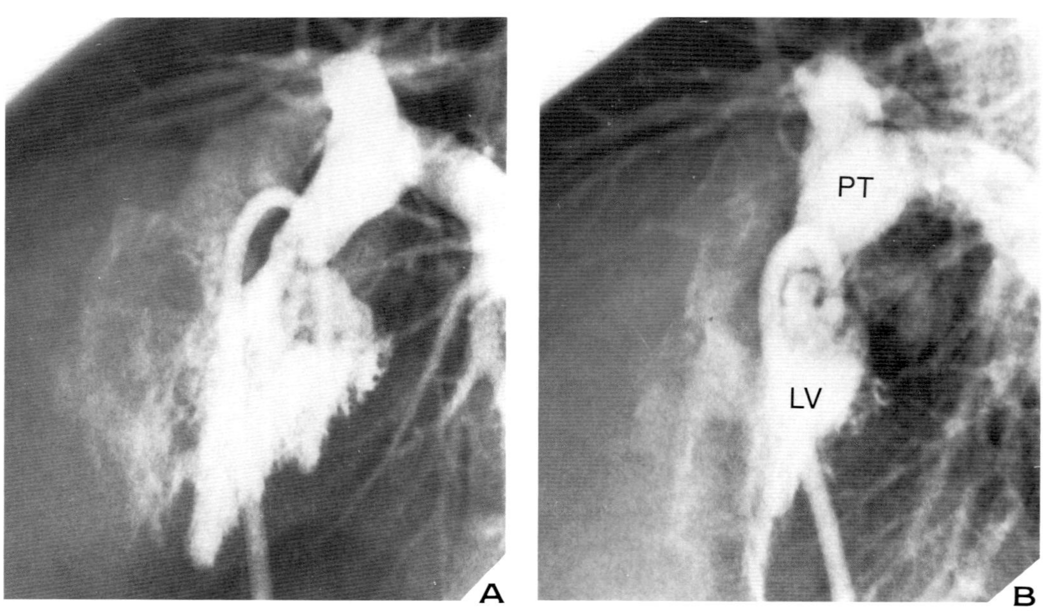

Fig. 11.20 Transposition of the great arteries with VSD and stenosis of the left ventricular outflow tract. Long axis projection of left ventriculogram in diastole (A) and systole (B). The left ventricle (LV) supports the pulmonary trunk (PT). There is a large muscular VSD in the trabecular portion of the septum. The left ventricular outflow tract is narrowed during systole (note the curvilinear filling defect in the left ventricular outflow tract in B).

VENTRICULOARTERIAL CONNECTION OF THE DOUBLE OUTLET TYPE ("DOUBLE-OUTLET VENTRICLE")

This category comprises malformations in which the aorta and pulmonary trunk arise entirely (or almost entirely) from a ventricular chamber. In the most common arrangement, both great arteries arise from the morphologic right ventricle (double-outlet right ventricle).

DOUBLE-OUTLET RIGHT VENTRICLE

Double-outlet right ventricle (DORV) denotes a group of malformations in which the aorta and pulmonary trunk both originate from the morphologic right ventricle. With rare exceptions, the only exit from the morphologic left ventricle is a VSD. DORV can occur either as an isolated malformation or in association with other cardiac defects.

In the most common arrangement, the atrioventricular connection is concordant and the great arteries arise from the morphologic right ventricle (Fig. 11.22). The relations of the aorta and pulmonary trunk are widely variable, however. In most instances the great arteries are normally related (pulmonary

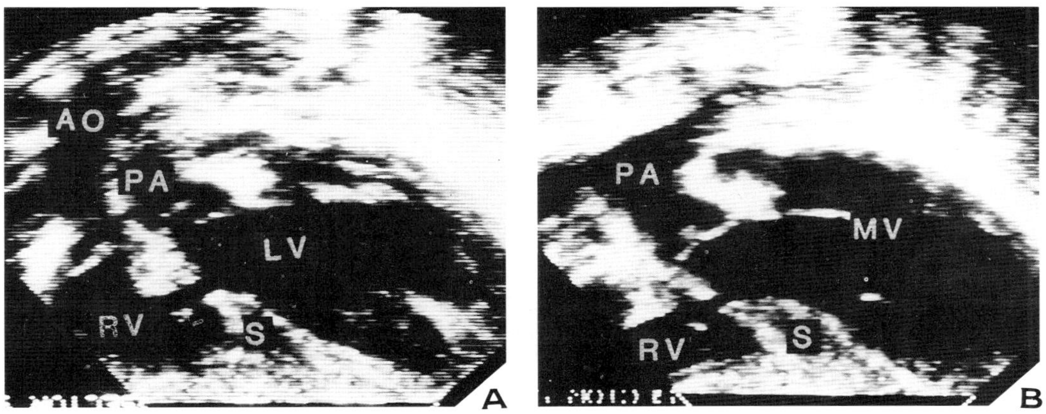

Fig. 11.21 Transposition of the great arteries (echocardiographic features). (A) In this long axis section the aorta connects with the morphologic right ventricle; the pulmonary trunk (PA) connects with the morphologic left ventricle. (B) Another long axis section shows the left ventricle supporting the pulmonary artery. The pulmonic valve is in a closed position.

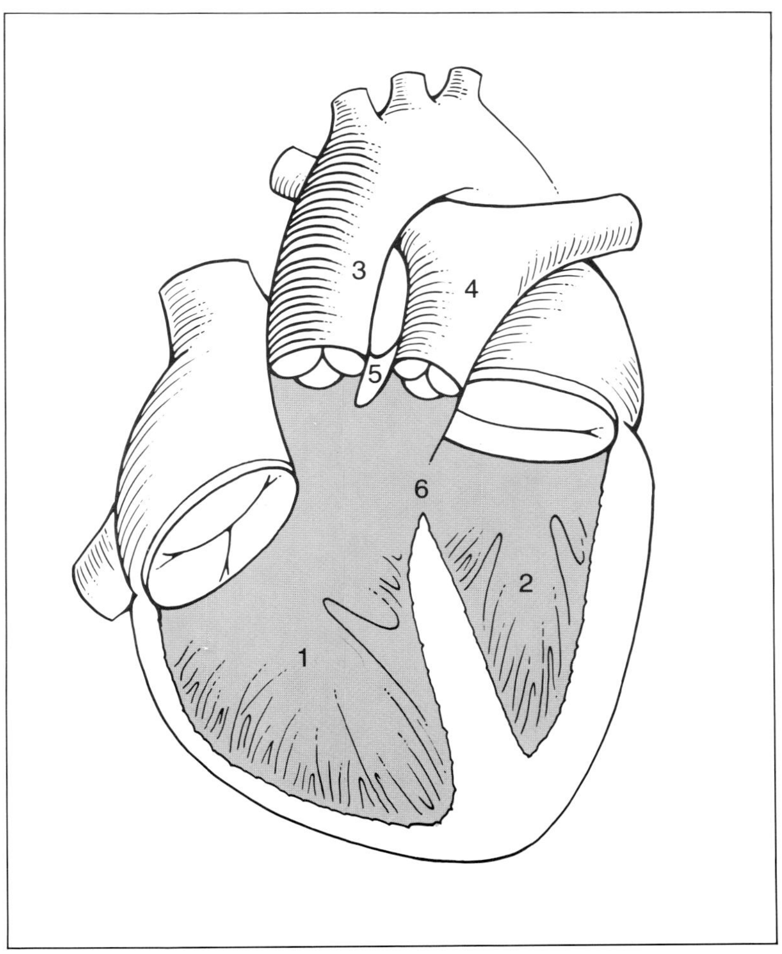

Fig. 11.22 Double-outlet right ventricle. In this example, the ventricular septum is related to the pulmonic valve. The left ventricle exits through a ventricular septal defect into the right ventricular outflow tract. The right ventricle has two exits: the aorta and the pulmonary trunk.

1 right ventricle
2 left ventricle
3 aorta
4 pulmonary trunk
5 infundibular septum
6 ventricular septal defect

trunk anterior and to the left of the aorta) (Fig. 11.23). Less often the aorta is anterior, lying to either the left or the right of the pulmonary trunk. Occasionally the great vessels are side by side, with the aorta located to the left or right of the pulmonary trunk.

PATHOPHYSIOLOGY

DORV is characterized by volume overload of the right ventricle with systemic pressures in the right ventricle; consequently, the right ventricle is both dilated and hypertrophied. The size of the left ventricle depends on the amount of blood it receives, which in turn is determined by the size of the connection between the right ventricle and the pulmonary trunk. When pulmonary blood flow is markedly increased, the left atrium and the left ventricle are also enlarged.

Because the mixing chamber is the morphologic right ventricle, which supports the aorta, peripheral desaturation is always present. However, most of the ventricular output flows into the low-resistance pulmonary circulation, which results in a significant increase in pulmonary blood flow and pulmonary arterial

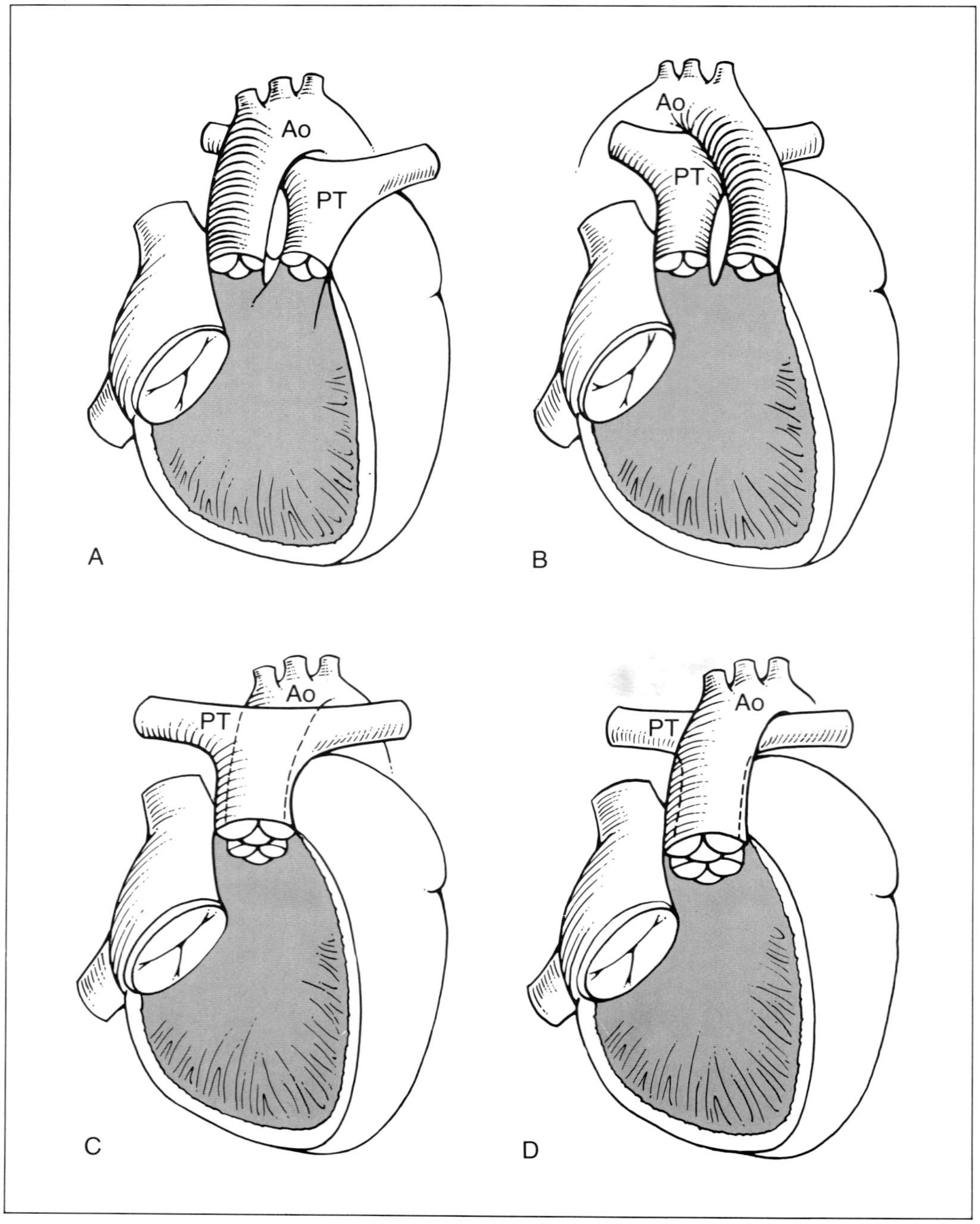

Fig. 11.23 Double-outlet right ventricle. The most common arrangements of the great arteries as they arise from the right ventricle in DORV are shown diagramatically. (A) Normally related great arteries with the pulmonary trunk anterior and to the left of the aorta. (B) Side-by-side relationship of the great arteries with the aorta to the left of the pulmonary trunk. (C) Anteroposterior relationship of the great arteries with the pulmonary trunk anterior to the aorta. (D) Anteroposterior relationship of the great arteries with the aorta anterior to the pulmonary trunk.

hypertension. This in turn leads to a progressive increase in pulmonary resistance similar to that seen in patients with a large VSD. The degree of desaturation depends on the relationship of the arterial valves with the VSD. When the VSD is mainly related to the aortic valve, the desaturation is relatively mild, because most of the left ventricular output (oxygenated blood) enters the aorta. When the VSD is related to the pulmonic valve, there is marked desaturation, as in TGA with an intact ventricular septum or a restricted VSD.

CLINICAL FEATURES

Patients with DORV typically present with cyanosis and with the signs and symptoms of a large left to right shunt. Right ventricular overload may result in tricuspid insufficiency and right ventricular failure.

The presence of additional malformations can modify the clinical presentation. For example, when DORV is associated with pulmonic stenosis and the VSD is related to the aortic valve, the clinical picture resembles that of tetralogy of Fallot.

IMAGING

Plain Films

In the classical form of DORV (atrial situs solitus and concordant atrioventricular connection), chest films show mild cardiomegaly with right ventricular hypertrophy. The radiographic appearance of the vascular pedicle varies. It can appear normal when the pulmonary artery is anterior and to the left of the aorta; it may be very narrow when the great vessels lie in front of the another (Fig. 11.24); or it may be wide when the great arteries lie side by side. In the latter arrangement, the pulmonary artery is usually on the left and forms the left upper mediastinal contour (Fig. 11.25). (When the aorta is on the left, the left upper mediastinal border is formed by the ascending aorta.)

The appearance of the pulmonary vasculature depends on whether the right ventricular outflow segment and the pulmonic valve are stenotic or widely patent. If there is no outflow obstruction, the pulmonary arteries, as well as their lobar and segmental branches, are enlarged and the lungs appear plethoric (Fig. 11.25). Pulmonary valvular or subvalvular stenosis is not uncommon, however, in which case the pulmonary trunk and main pulmonary arteries may be normal or decreased in size and the lungs may be normally perfused or oligenic.

To sum up: DORV is the most likely diagnosis in a cyanotic patient whose chest films show pulmonary plethora, cardiomegaly with right ventricular prominence, and a wide mediastinum with a prominent pulmonary trunk forming the left upper mediastinal border (Fig. 11.25). This combination of clinical and radiologic findings is not pathognomonic, however, because it may also occur in patients with double-outlet left ventricle (see below) and in some forms of complete TGA.

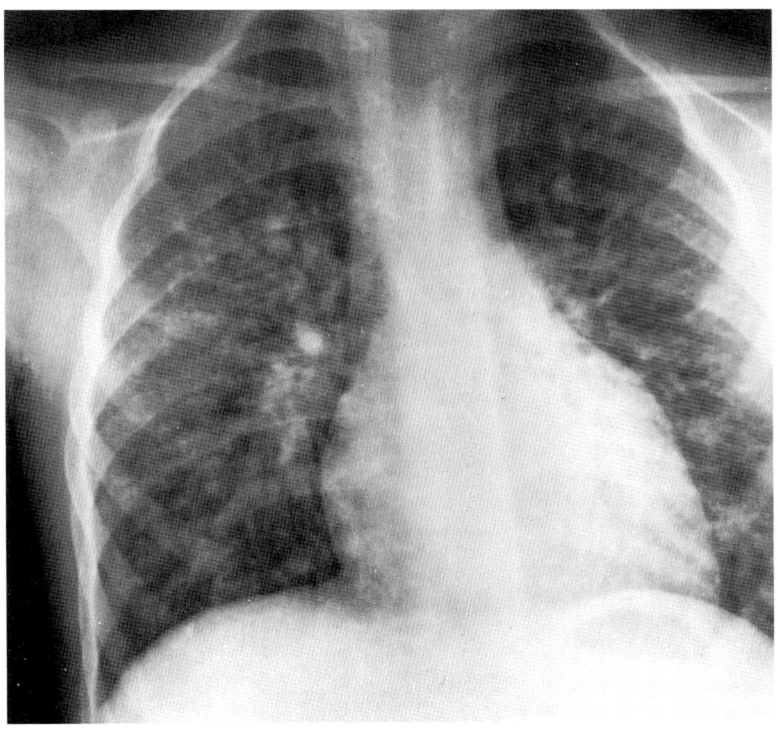

Fig. 11.24 Double-outlet right ventricle with narrow vascular pedicle. Posteroanterior chest film shows mild cardiomegaly with right ventricular enlargement. The atrial situs is solitus and the cardiac axis is to the left. The vascular pedicle is narrow owing to the medially displaced aorta and "missing" pulmonary trunk. The pulmonary vascularity is increased.

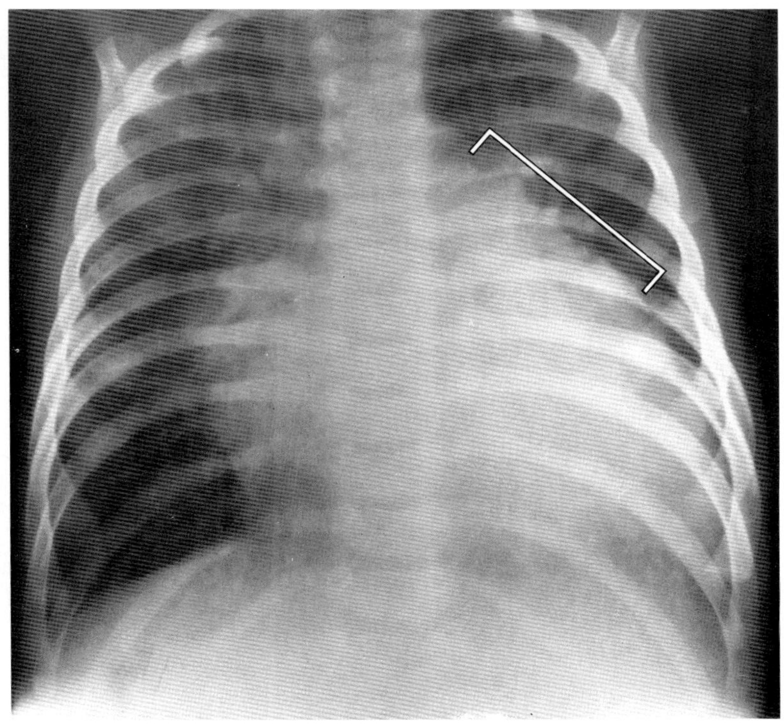

Fig. 11.25 Double-outlet right ventricle with wide vascular pedicle. Frontal chest film shows cardiomegaly with right ventricular enlargement. The vascular pedicle is wide, with the pulmonary trunk forming the left upper mediastinal border *(brace)*. The lung fields are plethoric, indicating increased pulmonary blood flow.

Angiocardiography

Right ventriculography demonstrates an enlarged right ventricle which supports both the aorta and the pulmonary trunk (Fig. 11.26). Axial projections demonstrate the morphology of the right ventricular outflow tract and the VSD, as well as the relationship of the latter to the aortic and pulmonic valves (Fig. 11.27). The VSD is usually of the perimembranous type, although occasionally it is located in the inlet or the trabecular muscle segment of the septum. (VSDs of the outlet segment, which is entirely derived from the right ventricle, are never found in patients with DORV.)

The right ventricular outflow tract typically consists of two channels separated by the muscular infundibular septum. One channel connects with the aortic valve and the other with the pulmonic valve (Fig. 11.27). The orientation of the infundibular septum determines the relations of the great arteries. When the infundibular septum is oriented in the *sagittal plane,* the aorta and pulmonary trunk lie side by side on the frontal projection (Fig. 11.26). When the infundibular septum is oriented in the *transverse plane,* the great arteries lie one in front of the other on the lateral projection (Fig. 11.27). When the right ventricular outflow tract is oriented *obliquely,* it is seen most clearly on oblique projections (either the right or left anterior oblique projection may be optimal for a given case). The VSD may be related to the aortic or pulmonic valve, or to both. Occasionally, the VSD may be at a considerable distance from the arterial valves ("noncommitted VSD"), or it may be committed to both the aortic and pulmonic valves ("double-committed VSD").

Echocardiography

All of the key features of DORV are clearly depicted on echocardiography (Fig. 11.28). Nevertheless, angiocardiography is usually performed before surgical correction is undertaken.

ATRESIA OF ONE ARTERY

In this group of malformations one great artery (either the pulmonary trunk or the aorta) is not connected to a ventricular chamber. There are three possible types of anomalous ventriculoarterial connections in this group: pulmonary atresia with a patent aortic valve; aortic atresia with a patent pulmonary trunk; and truncus arteriosus, a malformation in which a common trunk arising from the heart supplies the systemic, coronary, and pulmonary circulations.

PULMONARY ATRESIA

In this group of malformations the pulmonary arterial system is disconnected from the ventricular mass; consequently, the

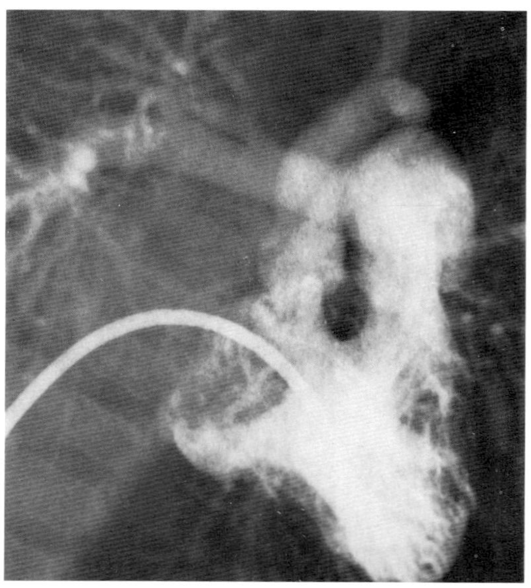

Fig. 11.26 Double-outlet right ventricle. Right ventriculogram (frontal projection) demonstrates right ventricular enlargement. The right ventricular outflow tract is divided into two channels (the filling defect between them represents the infundibular septum). The great arteries are in a side-by-side relationship, with the aorta situated on the right. The infundibular septum is oriented in the sagittal plane.

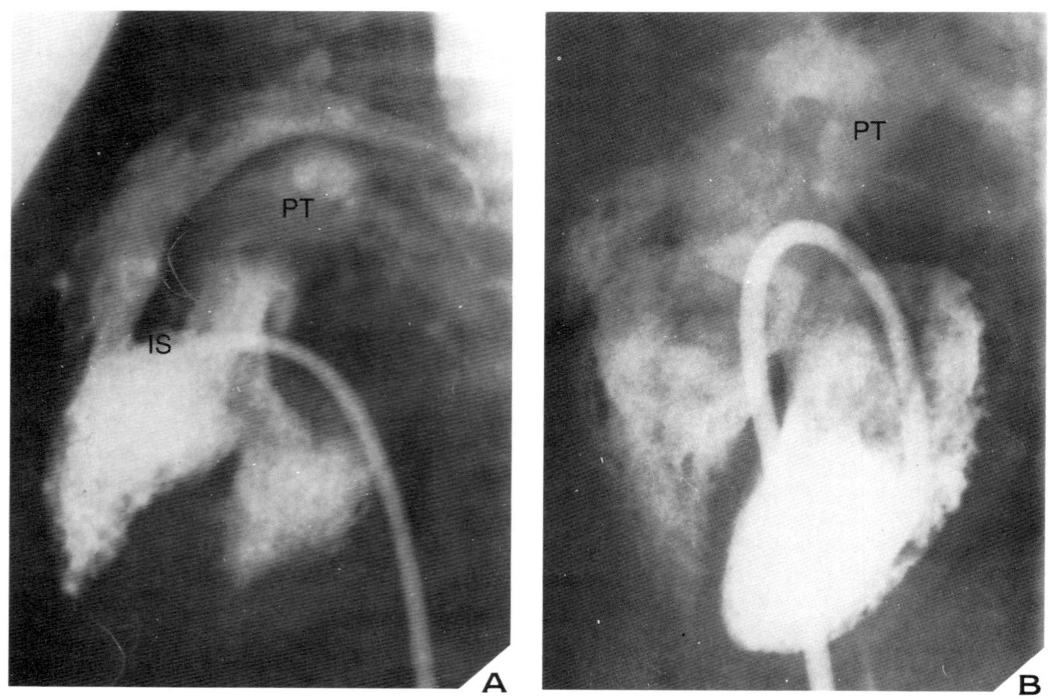

Fig. 11.27 Double-outlet right ventricle with subaortic stenosis. (A) Right ventriculogram (lateral projection) and (B) left ventriculogram (long axis projection). The left ventricle does not have an outlet; opacified blood exits from the left ventricle via a VSD and enters an enlarged right ventricle, which supports both the aorta and the pulmonary trunk (PT). The VSD is subpulmonic in location. The great arteries are in an anteroposterior relationship and the infundibular septum (IS) is oriented transversely. Note the relative narrowing of subaortic segment in (A). (The infundibular septum is obscured in B owing to the superimposition of the aorta and pulmonary trunk.)

entire cardiac output enters the aorta via a patent aortic valve. There may be an associated VSD, or the ventricular septum may be intact.

PULMONARY ATRESIA WITH VSD

In the most common arrangement, the aorta originates from both ventricles (ie, it overlies the VSD). Occasionally it arises exclusively from the right or left ventricle. Because the biventricular origin of the aorta is similar to that seen in tetralogy of Fallot, many authors consider pulmonary atresia with VSD to be a variety of tetralogy of Fallot. In most cases the aortic valve is normally formed. The pulmonary valve is absent, and the pulmonary trunk is either hypoplastic or absent. The left and right pulmonary arteries, as well as their intraparenchymal branches, are usually abnormal. They may be severely hypoplastic or atretic, or there may be an abnormal arborization pattern, with one or more segmental branches being absent.

Pathophysiology

As in a normal heart, the ventricles receive deoxygenated systemic venous blood from the right atrium and oxygenated pulmonary venous blood from the left atrium. Left and right atrial blood mixes in the ventricles and the entire cardiac output is pumped through the aortic valve into the aorta. The pressure is the same in both ventricles.

The pulmonary blood supply comes from several sources. In small infants, the lungs are perfused via a PDA and aortopulmonary collaterals. After infancy, most of the pulmonary blood flow comes from aortopulmonary collaterals which originate from the descending thoracic aorta and connect with the pulmonary arteries at the hila. Other potential collaterals include mediastinal arteries, branches of the subclavian arteries, and coronary–pulmonary artery fistulas.

Imaging and Invasive Diagnosis

Plain Films. The heart is usually of normal size, with right ventricular prominence (Figs. 11.29 to 11.31). On the frontal projection, the enlarged right ventricle forms the left border of the cardiac silhouette; on the lateral projection there is increased contact between the heart and the anterior chest wall. The pulmonary trunk is absent and the right and left pulmonary arteries are diminutive (Fig. 11.29). Because of the asymmetrical development of the right and left pulmonary arteries, the lungs may be unequally perfused. If the pulmonary blood supply is restricted, the lungs appear oligemic with sparse vascular markings (Figs. 11.29 and 11.30). The lungs may appear plethoric, however, in patients with large aortopulmonary collaterals.

It is usually possible to differentiate aortopulmonary collaterals from normal pulmonary artery branches. The collaterals appear on chest films as large channels superimposed on the hilar regions which often extend for a considerable distance

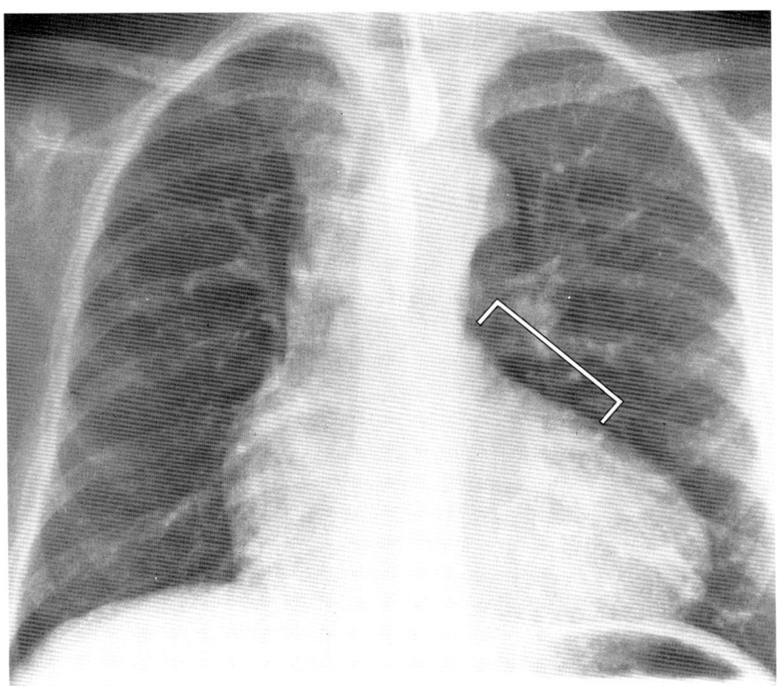

Fig. 11.29 Pulmonary atresia and VSD. Frontal chest film shows a slightly enlarged heart with an upturned apex indicating right ventricular hypertrophy. The left heart border is concave in the region of the pulmonary trunk *(brace)*. The main pulmonary arteries are small and the pulmonary vasculature is diminished. The aorta is prominent. The aortic arch and descending aorta are on the left.

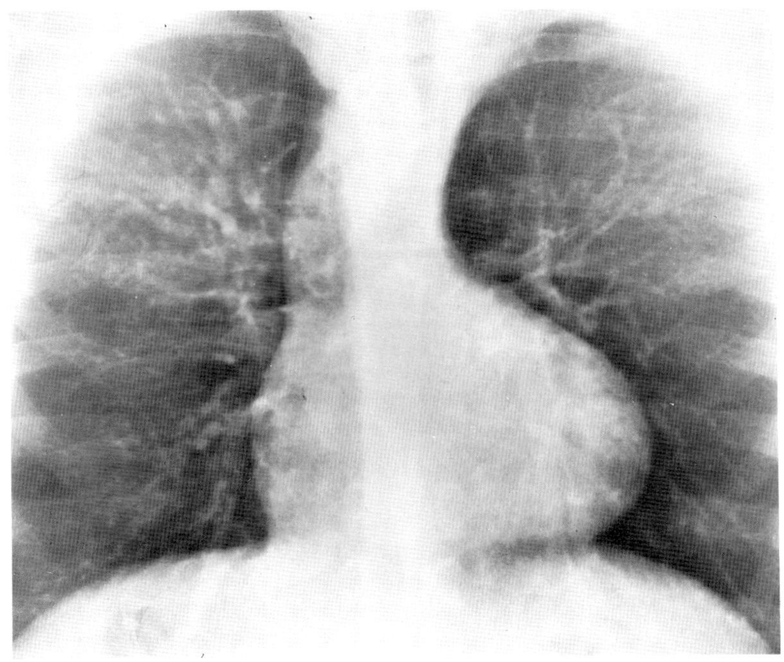

Fig. 11.30 Pulmonary atresia with VSD and right aortic arch. Frontal chest film shows a slightly enlarged heart with a prominent right ventricle. The pulmonary artery segment is flat and the pulmonary vasculature is decreased. The many abnormal vascular channels above and below the right hilum represent aortopulmonary collaterals. The aortic arch is on the right.

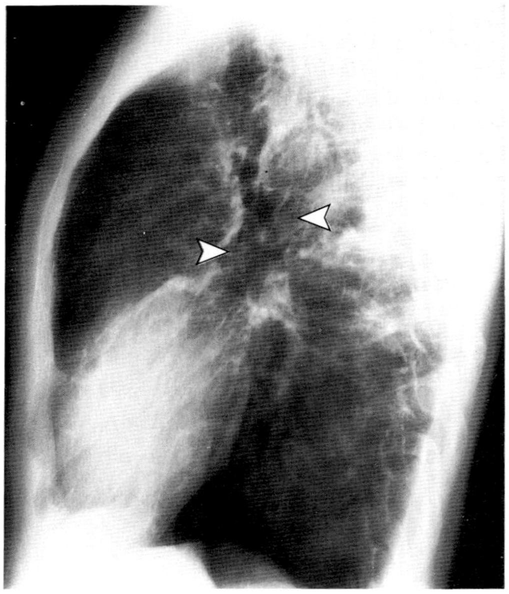

Fig. 11.31 Pulmonary atresia with VSD. Lateral chest film demonstrates absence of the left pulmonary artery *(arrows)*. There is increased contact between the heart and the anterior chest wall, indicating right ventricular hypertrophy.

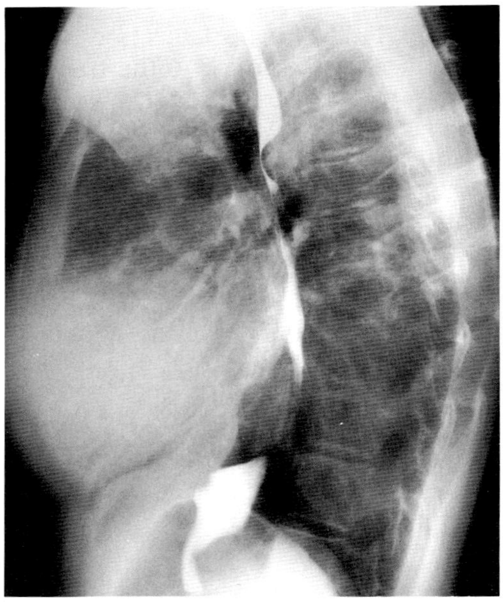

Fig. 11.32 Pulmonary atresia with VSD. Lateral chest film with barium-filled esophagus shows an impression on the posterior wall of the esophagus produced by a large aortopulmonary collateral.

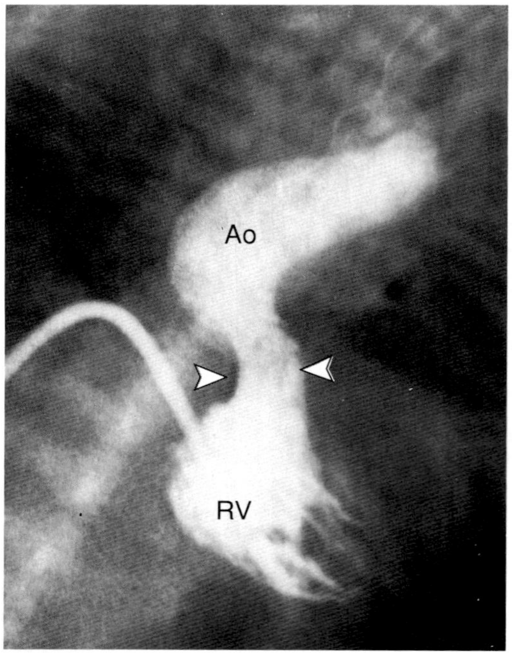

Fig. 11.33 Pulmonary atresia with VSD. Elongated right anterior oblique projection of right ventriculogram shows absence of the right ventricular outlet. The right ventricle (RV) communicates exclusively with the aorta (AO) through a VSD *(arrows)*.

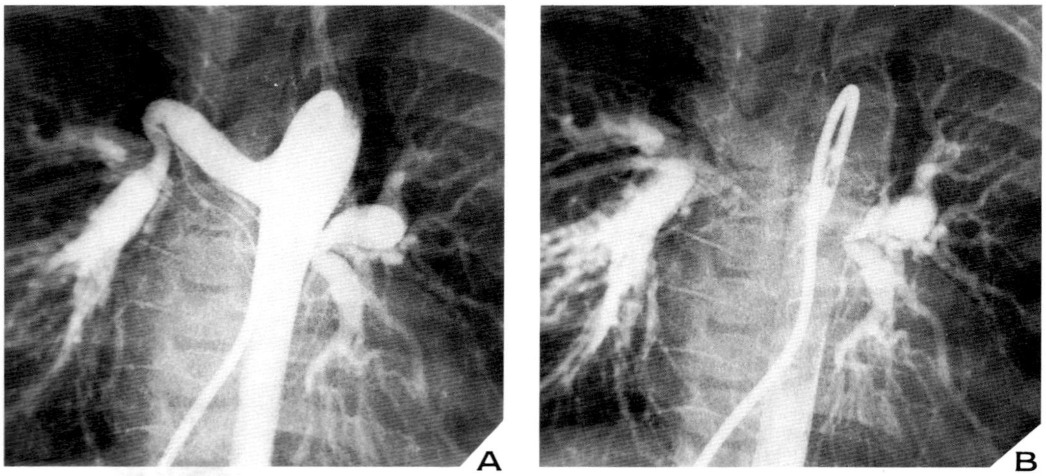

Fig. 11.34 Pulmonary atresia with VSD. (A) Early and (B) late phases of thoracic aortogram (frontal projection) demonstrate large aortopulmonary collaterals supplying the right and left pulmonary arteries. The collaterals connect distally to lobar arteries. The intrapericardial segments of the right and left pulmonary arteries are absent.

above and below the hilus (Fig. 11.30). On the lateral view, aortopulmonary collaterals are located posterior to the tracheobronchial tree; normal hilar vascular structures (ie, the right and left pulmonary arteries) are absent (Fig. 11.31). Aortopulmonary collaterals typically produce localized indentations on the anterior or posterior wall of the esophagus (Fig. 11.32).

The ascending aorta is prominent, forming the right border of the mediastinum on the frontal projection (Fig. 11.31) and protruding anteriorly on the lateral. A right aortic arch is present in about half the cases (Fig. 11.30).

Angiocardiography. Right ventriculograms obtained in the frontal or right anterior oblique projection demonstrate the ventricular morphology to best advantage. In the most common arrangement, the right ventricular outflow tract is atretic, the entire right ventricular output entering the aorta via a large juxtaaortic VSD. Angiograms show absence of the right ventricular outflow tract, with marked right ventricular hypertrophy (Fig. 11.33).

An important role of angiography is to ascertain the size and distribution of the pulmonary arteries and the aortopulmonary collaterals. This is usually accomplished by thoracic aortography or by selectively injecting one or more collaterals (Figs. 11.34 and 11.35). Pulmonary venography can be very informative in selected cases. For instance, an injection made with the catheter in a wedged position usually opacifies the entire pulmonary arterial tree in a patient with partial or complete occlusion of the intrapericardial segment of the pulmonary artery (Fig. 11.36).

Echocardiography. Echocardiography accurately demonstrates the intracardiac anatomy (Fig. 11.37 see appendix). However, angiocardiography is needed to evaluate the pulmonary circulation before surgical correction.

PULMONARY ATRESIA WITH INTACT VENTRICULAR SEPTUM (PA/IVS)

In this malformation there is no connection between the right ventricular chamber, which is very small, and the pulmonary artery. Because the ventricular septum is intact, there is an obligate atrial septal defect through which the systemic venous return reaches the left side of the heart. The left atrium, left ventricle, and aorta are connected in normal fashion. As in pulmonary atresia with VSD, the pulmonary blood supply is

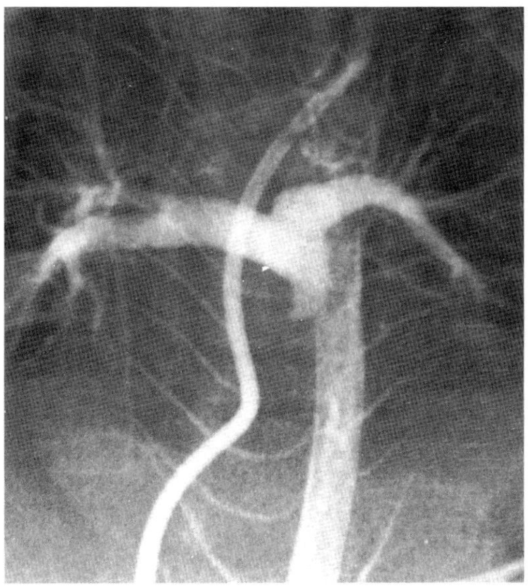

Fig. 11.35 Pulmonary atresia with VSD. Late phase of thoracic aortogram. Both lungs are perfused via a PDA. The right and left pulmonary arteries are confluent. The peripheral branches of both pulmonary arteries are distributed in normal fashion. The proximal portion of the hypoplastic pulmonary trunk is opacified.

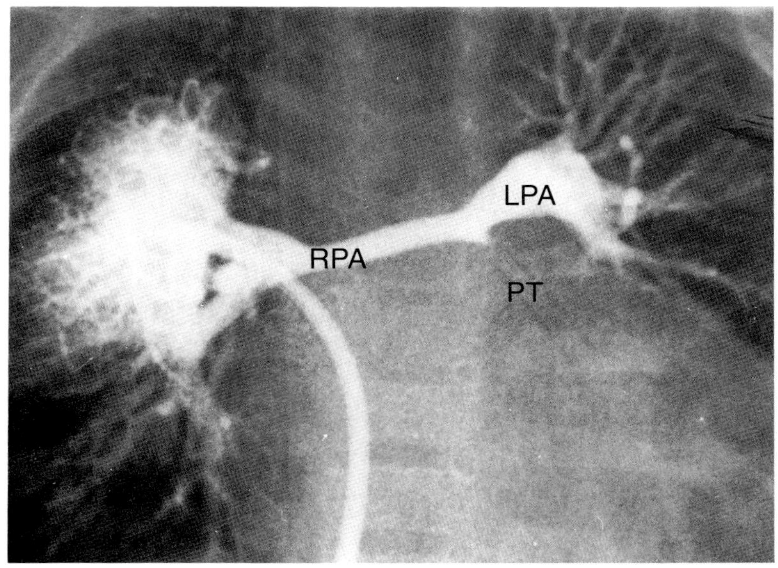

Fig. 11.36 Pulmonary atresia with VSD. The catheter has been passed from the right atrium into the left atrium and its tip advanced into a peripheral pulmonary vein in the right upper lobe. After injection of contrast material there is retrograde opacification of the right (RPA) and left (LPA) pulmonary arteries, which are confluent. The pulmonary trunk (PT) is atretic. The peripheral branches of the right and left pulmonary arteries are incompletely opacified.

derived from many sources, the most important of which is a patent ductus arteriosus (PDA) (Fig. 11.38).

Pathophysiology

Because the right ventricular chamber is very small, there is tricuspid insufficiency of varying degree; in patients with moderate to severe tricuspid insufficiency, the right atrium is enlarged as a result of volume overload. The right ventricular wall is markedly hypertrophied. In many patients the right ventricular wall contains prominent sinusoidal channels ("fistulas") which allow blood to flow between the right ventricular cavity and the coronary circulation. The magnitude of the shunt through these channels depends on the right ventricular pressure, which in turn is determined by the relative competence of the tricuspid valve. When right ventricular pressure is systemic or suprasystemic, blood flows into the coronary circulation and thence, in retrograde fashion, into the aorta (Fig. 11.39). Whereas normal (ie, antegrade) coronary artery blood flow occurs during diastole, retrograde flow through the sinusoidal channels occurs during systole.

Clinical Features

Patients with PA/IVS are cyanotic at birth. After spontaneous closure of the ductus arteriosus, which usually occurs soon after birth, the cyanosis becomes more intense. Infants with PA/IVS are characterized as "ductus dependent"; because the main systemic blood supply is via a PDA, they will die unless a systemic–pulmonary shunt is created before the ductus closes. If immediate surgery is not feasible, ductus closure can be delayed by intravenous infusion of prostaglandin E_1 or E_2.

Imaging

Plain Films. Chest films typically show cardiomegaly with right atrial enlargement, absence of the pulmonary artery, and pulmonary oligemia. The dominant left ventricle forms the left heart border (Fig. 11.40). The vascular pedicle is usually narrow, owing to the absence of the pulmonary artery. In some infants the aorta is markedly dilated, in which case the width of the pedicle may be normal. The pulmonary vasculature may appear normal or even plethoric in patients who have a large systemic to pulmonary shunt across the PDA.

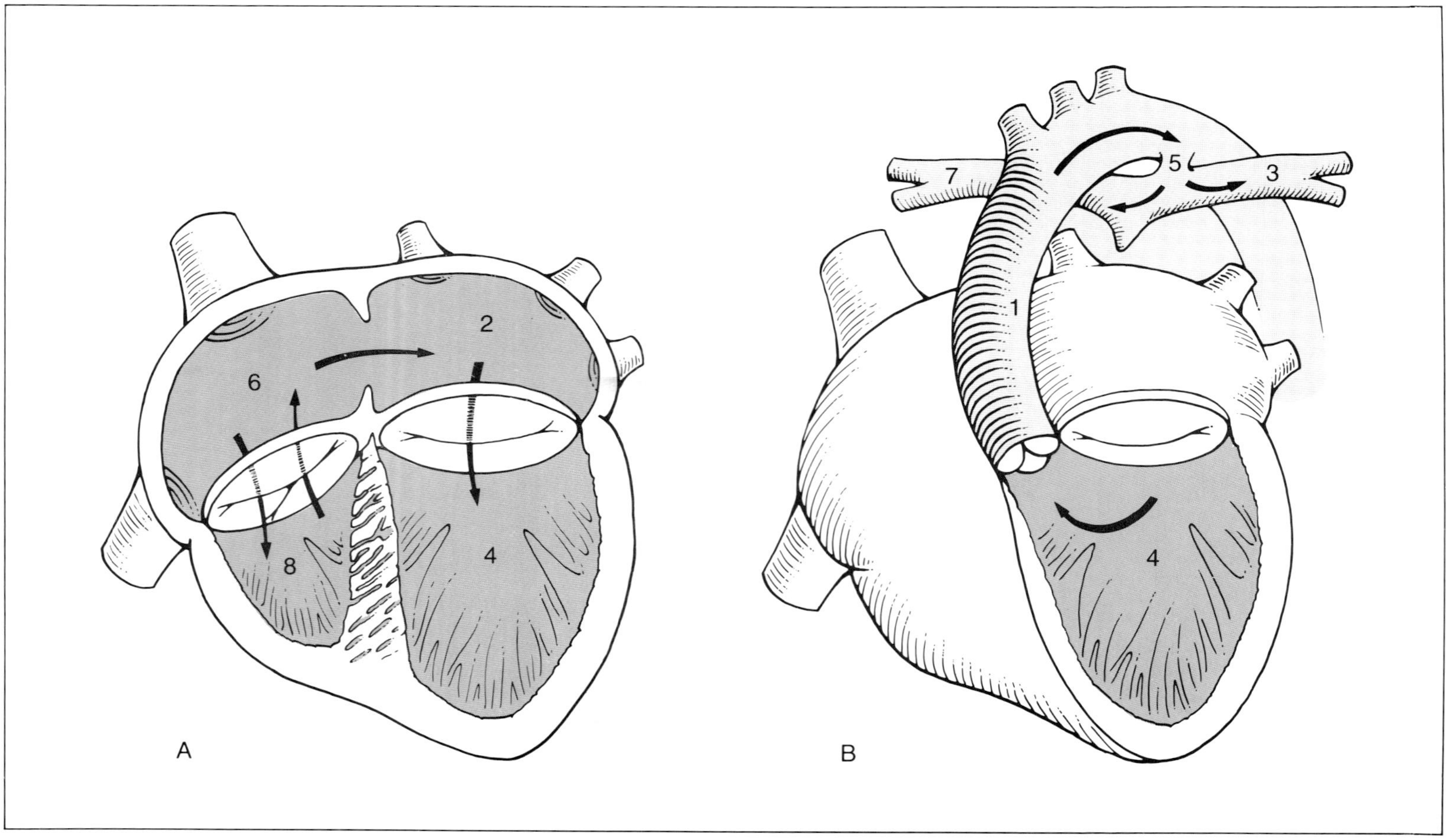

Fig. 11.38 Pulmonary atresia with intact ventricular septum. (A) Atrioventricular level. Some of the desaturated blood entering the right atrium passes through an ASD into the left atrium, mixes with oxygenated blood returning from the lungs, and enters the morphologic left ventricle from which it is pumped into the aorta. Some of the blood entering the right atrium enters the morphologic right ventricle and refluxes into the right ventricle via the tricuspid valve. Depending on the relative competence of the tricuspid valve, the right ventricular pressure may be normal or elevated. (B) Arterial level. Aortic blood passes through a patent ductus arteriosus into the pulmonary arteries. Thus the left atrium serves as the mixing chamber in this anomaly.

1	aorta	5	patent ductus arteriosus
2	left atrium	6	right atrium
3	left pulmonary artery	7	right pulmonary artery
4	left ventricle	8	right ventricle

Angiocardiography. Right atrial angiograms obtained in the lateral projection demonstrate the dilated right atrium and the diminutive right ventricle, as well as opacification of the left atrium via the ASD (Fig. 11.41). Selective right ventriculography demonstrates a small right ventricular chamber with marked mural hypertrophy. Patients with severe tricuspid insufficiency have massive reflux of contrast material onto the right atrium. If the tricuspid valve is relatively competent, con-

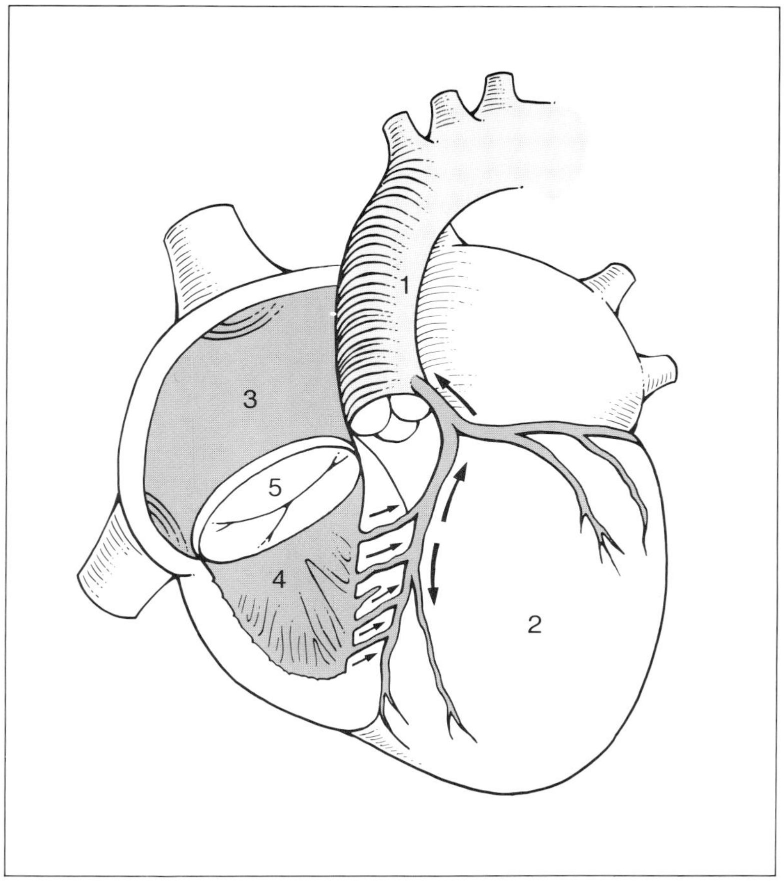

Fig. 11.39 Pulmonary atresia with intact ventricular septum: circulation through right ventricular–coronary artery fistulas. Cavitary–coronary artery fistulas traversing the myocardium of the small right ventricle are shown schematically. In this illustration the fistulas connect with the epicardial segment of the left coronary artery over the free wall of the left ventricle. Because right ventricular pressure is higher than systemic pressure, blood passes through the fistulas into the coronary circulation. Depending on hemodynamic conditions, it may be distributed to distal branches of the coronary arteries, or it may flow retrogradely into the aorta.

1 aorta
2 left ventricle
3 right atrium
4 right ventricle
5 tricuspid valve

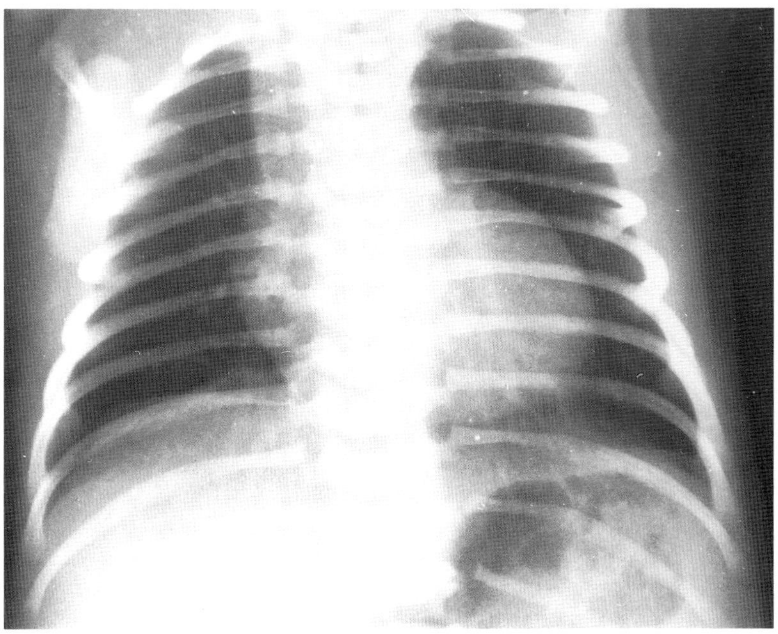

Fig. 11.40 Pulmonary atresia with intact ventricular septum. Chest film of a cyanotic newborn infant shows moderate cardiomegaly with prominence of the right atrial contour, sparse pulmonary vasculature, and absence of the pulmonary trunk. These findings in a patient who has been cyanotic since birth strongly suggest the diagnosis of pulmonary atresia with intact ventricular septum.

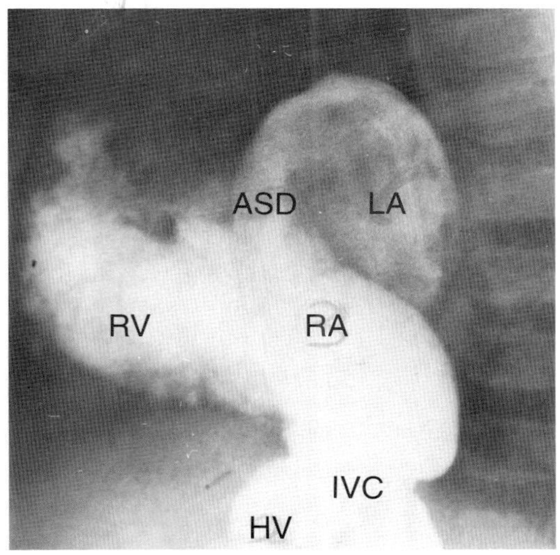

Fig. 11.41 Pulmonary atresia with intact ventricular septum. Lateral projection of right atriogram shows opacified blood passing across the tricuspid valve into the right ventricle, which lacks an outlet and ejects it back into the right atrium during ventricular systols. The entire right atrial output passes into the left atrium through a restricted atrial septal defect (ASD). Note the reflux into the inferior vena cava (IVC) and dilated hepatic veins. (HV)

trast material flows through the sinusoidal channels in the right ventricular wall and opacifies the coronary arteries (Fig. 11.42).

The left ventricle and pulmonary vasculature (opacified via the PDA) are evaluated by left ventriculography, which is performed by passing the catheter across the ASD. In most cases the left ventricle is both anatomically and functionally normal.

Echocardiography. The pertinent anatomic features are clearly shown by echocardiography (Fig. 11.43, Appendix).

TRUNCUS ARTERIOSUS

In this malformation all of the cardiac outflow passes through a single ventriculoarterial valve (the truncal valve) into a common channel (truncus arteriosus); the latter structure gives rise to the aorta and pulmonary arteries in various arrangements. With rare exceptions, truncus arteriosus is always associated with a VSD.

PATHOPHYSIOLOGY

Because most of the blood from the truncus enters the pulmonary circulation, the lungs are plethoric. Perfusion of the pulmonary circulation at high volume and high pressure leads to increased pulmonary resistance, eventually resulting in pulmonary hypertension.

CLINICAL PICTURE

Patients with truncus arteriosus typically present in early infancy with congestive heart failure. Although cyanosis is rarely

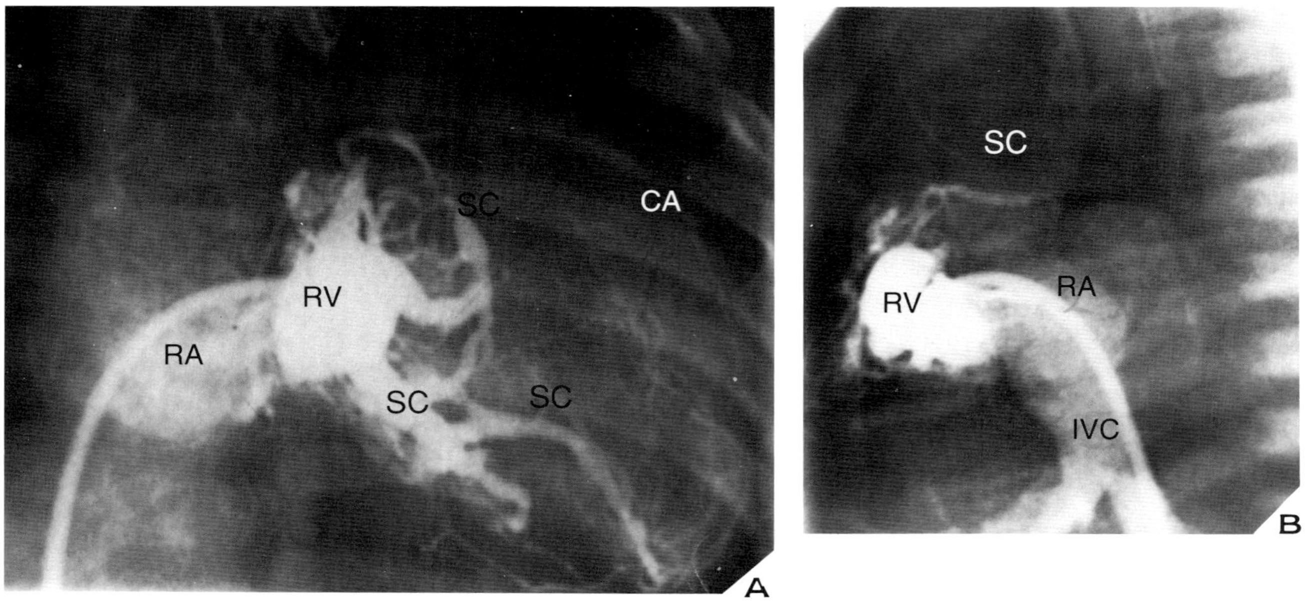

Fig. 11.42 Pulmonary atresia with intact ventricular septum. Frontal (A) and lateral (B) projections of selective right ventriculogram show a very small right ventricle with marked hypertrophy of the right ventricular wall. The tricuspid valve is incompetent, allowing reflux of opacified blood into the right atrium. Many sinusoidal channels (SC) ("fistulas") in the right ventricular wall connect the right ventricular chamber with branches of the coronary arteries (CA). (IVC = inferior vira cava)

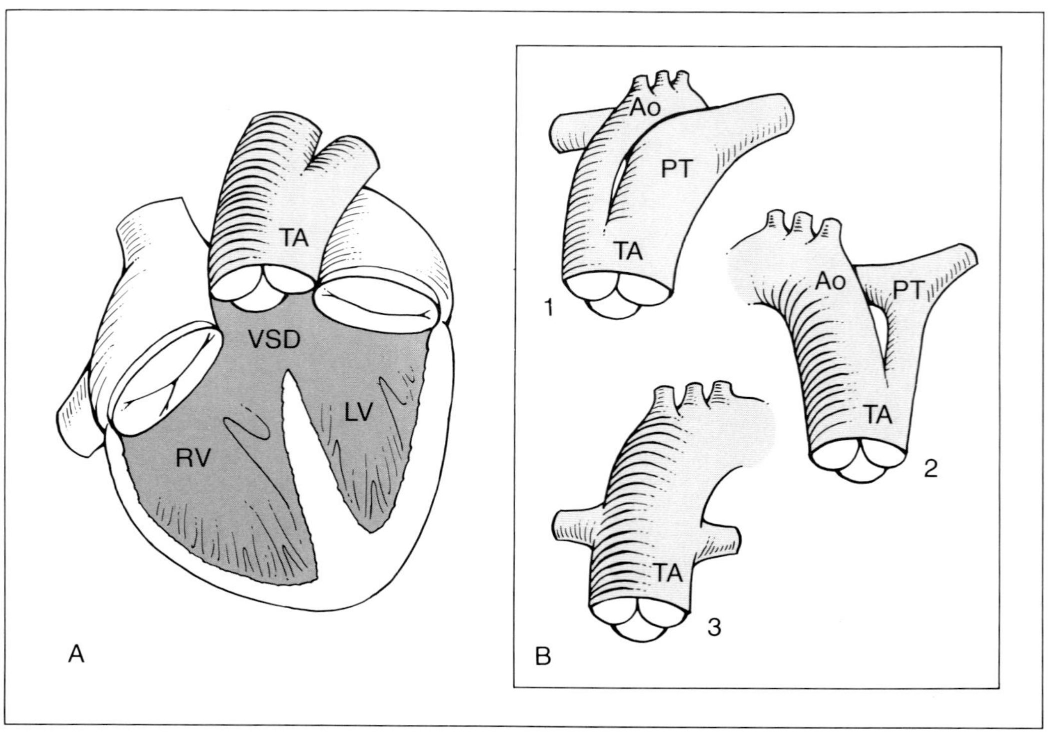

Fig. 11.44 Truncus arteriosus. (A) The right and left ventricles are connected via a large VSD. The truncal valve is derived from both ventricles. (B) Configuration of great arteries. (1) Truncus arteriosus with dominant pulmonary trunk. (2) Truncus arteriosus with dominant aorta. (3) Truncus arteriosus with absence of the pulmonary trunk (right and left pulmonary arteries arise directly from the aorta).

TA	truncus arteriosus	**Ao**	aorta
VSD	ventricular septal defect	**PT**	pulmonary trunk

present when the patient is first seen, it appears with the onset of pulmonary hypertension and progressively worsens.

Truncus arteriosus is usually fatal in infancy. About 50 percent of affected infants survive beyond the first month of life; 30 percent are alive at 3 months; 18 percent survive beyond 6 months; and only 12 percent are alive at 1 year of age. The latter group usually survive until the second decade, when the manifestations of pulmonary hypertension appear. The natural history of truncus arteriosus is modified by the presence of associated anomalies, such as insufficiency of the truncal valve or interruption of the aortic arch.

MORPHOLOGY

Classically, the atrioventricular connections are concordant (ie, the atria connect with the appropriate ventricles). The enlarged, hypertrophied right ventricle connects with the truncal valve through a large VSD. The left ventricle is slightly enlarged and connects with the truncal valve. The mitral and truncal valves are usually in fibrous continuity. The VSD is juxtaarterial, lying immediately beneath the truncal valve within the crista supraventricularis. In most instances the truncal valve is tricuspid, although on occasion it may have four or more cusps.

Although a wide variety of arrangements of the great arteries are theoretically possible, for practical purposes we need only consider two varieties: *pulmonary trunk present* and *pulmonary trunk absent*.

Pulmonary Trunk Present

(Figs. 11.44A and 11.44B). In this type an aortopulmonary septum is present but incomplete. The truncus is usually very short, dividing into the aorta and pulmonary artery just beyond the truncal valve. In the most common arrangement the pulmonary artery arises from the left posterior aspect of the truncus, runs superiorly, and divides into right and left pulmonary branches. The left pulmonary branch is usually in a higher position than normal. In the great majority of cases the aorta and pulmonary artery are similar in size. However, the pulmonary artery may be larger than the aorta if there is significant stenosis of the aortic arch.

Pulmonary Trunk Absent

(Fig. 11.44C) When the aortopulmonary septum is absent there is no main pulmonary artery; the right and left pulmonary arteries arise directly from the truncus. In these patients the aorta is much larger than the pulmonary arteries.

In both forms of truncus arteriosus, the proximal segment of the ascending aorta follows the usual course. In about 50 percent of cases, both the aortic arch and the descending thoracic aorta are on the right.

IMAGING AND INVASIVE DIAGNOSIS

Plain Films

The plain film findings vary with the morphology of the pulmonary arteries and the presence (or absence) of other malformations. In the classical form of truncus arteriosus, chest films show cardiomegaly, right ventricular hypertrophy, and pulmonary plethora (Fig. 11.45). Additional findings include a right aortic arch (in about 50 percent of cases) and an unusually high position of the left pulmonary artery. In older children and teenagers who develop pulmonary hypertension, pulmonary plethora is no longer evident; in these individuals the central pulmonary arteries are enlarged and the parenchymal vessels may be significantly decreased in size and number.

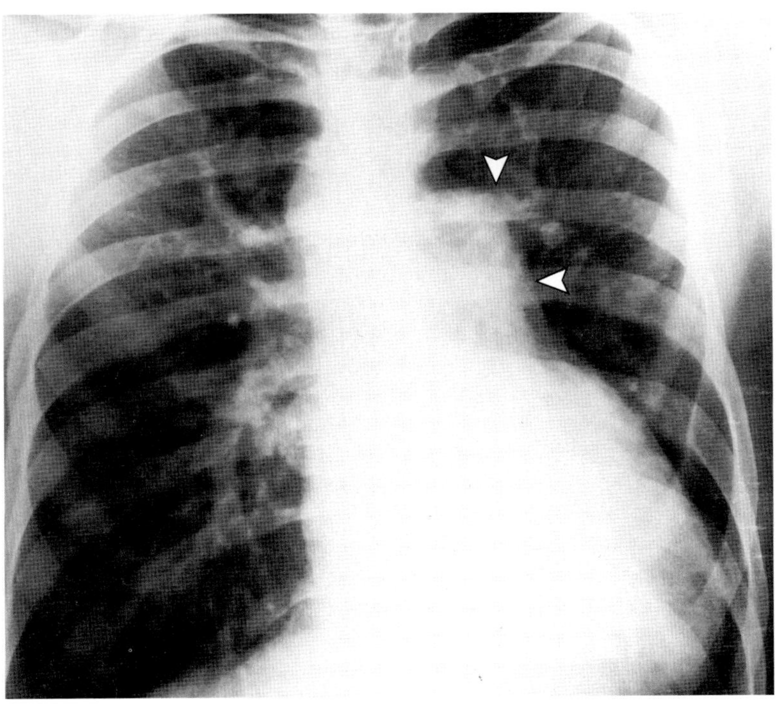

Fig. 11.45 Truncus arteriosus. Frontal chest film shows cardiomegaly with elevation of the apex indicating right ventricular hypertrophy. The pulmonary trunk cannot be identified and the left pulmonary artery *(arrows)* is in a higher position than normal. The pulmonary vasculature is plethoric. There is a right aortic arch. The combination of plethora, right aortic arch, and elevated left pulmonary artery in a cyanotic patient strongly suggests the diagnosis of truncus arteriosus.

Angiocardiography

Right ventriculography demonstrates enlargement and hypertrophy of the right ventricle. Although the main intra- and extracardiac features of truncus arteriosus can be identified on frontal and lateral views, the VSD and its relation to the truncal valve are more clearly visualized on the long axial projection (Fig. 11.46).

Pulmonary Trunk Present. When the aorta is the dominant vessel, it appears prominent on the frontal projection. The main pulmonary artery is inconspicuous; it is generally situated behind and to the left of the aorta (Fig. 11.47). The right and left pulmonary arteries are of unequal size; the left, which is usually the larger, is more cephalad. When the aorta is hypoplastic it is hidden in the mediastinum, behind the prominent pulmonary trunk.

Pulmonary Trunk Absent. In this arrangement, which is much less common, the position and size of the pulmonary branches vary according to their site of origin and the way they connect with the truncus (Fig. 11.48).

Echocardiography

Although the intracardiac features of truncus arteriosus are clearly depicted by echocardiography (Fig. 11.49, Appendix), angiography is necessary to demonstrate the great vessels and the pulmonary vasculature.

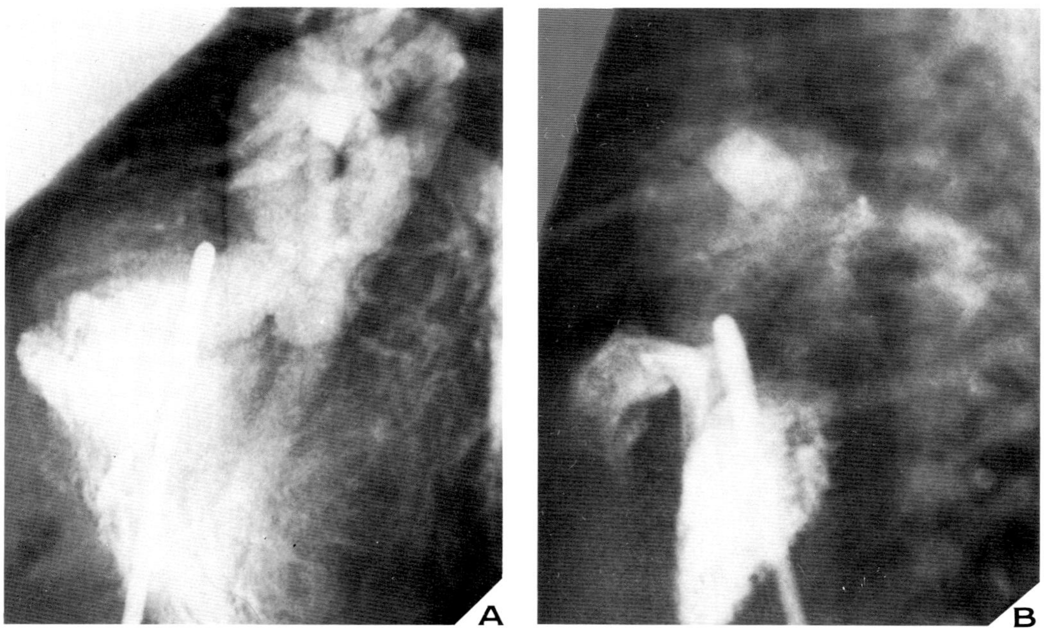

Fig. 11.46 Truncus arteriosus. (A) Right and (B) left ventriculograms (long axis projection) demonstrate right ventricular enlargement. The right ventricle communicates with the truncus via a VSD, which is located beneath the truncal valve. The left ventricle is normal and supports the truncal valve. The aorta is the dominant vessel. The pulmonary trunk lies to the left of the aorta.

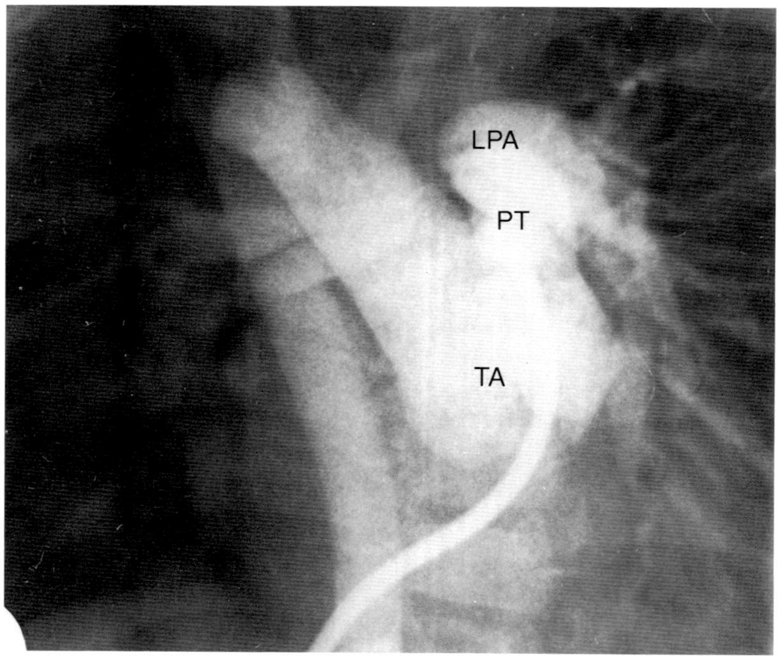

Fig. 11.47 Truncus arteriosus. Selective injection into the truncus arteriosus (TA) (frontal projection) shows it dividing into the aorta (on the right) and the pulmonary trunk (PT) (on the left). The aorta is the dominant vessel and there is a right aortic arch. The left pulmonary artery (LPA) is in a higher position than normal.

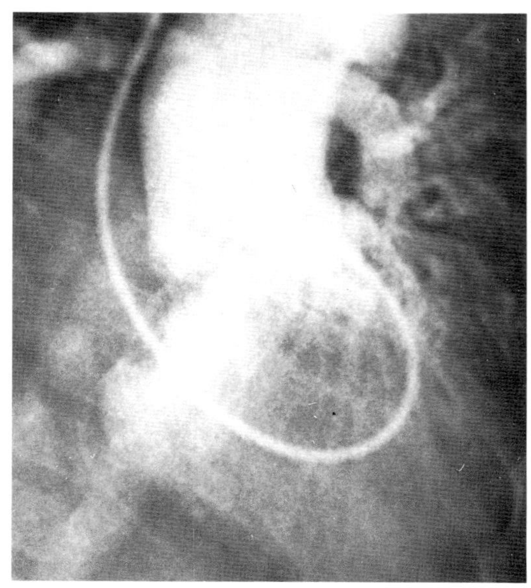

Fig. 11.48 Truncus arteriosus with absent pulmonary trunk. An angiogram obtained with the catheter in the truncus demonstrates small right and left pulmonary arteries arising directly from the truncus. A pulmonary trunk cannot be identified.

CHAPTER 12

Congenital Obstructing Lesions

OBSTRUCTIONS ON THE LEFT SIDE OF THE HEART

Congenital obstructions can be encountered at the level of the pulmonary veins (eg, pulmonary vein stenosis); the left atrium (eg, cor triatriatum sinister, supramitral ring); the mitral valve (mitral stenosis); left ventricular outflow tract (subvalvular stenosis); aortic valve; ascending aorta (supravalvular stenosis); or aortic arch (interrupted aortic arch, coarctation of the aorta) (Fig. 12.1).

PULMONARY VEIN STENOSIS

Pulmonary vein stenosis can be congenital or acquired. In infants and children it is almost always due to a congenital stenosis of the pulmonary veins, in which case it may be associated with other congenital malformations. Acquired pulmonary vein stenosis, seldom encountered in childhood, is usually secondary to mediastinitis or therapeutic irradiation.

Congenital stenosis of the pulmonary veins (SPV) usually occurs at the junction between the pulmonary vein and the left

CHAPTER LABELING KEY			
RA	right atrium	LV	left ventricle
LA	left atrium	Ao	aorta
RV	right ventricle		

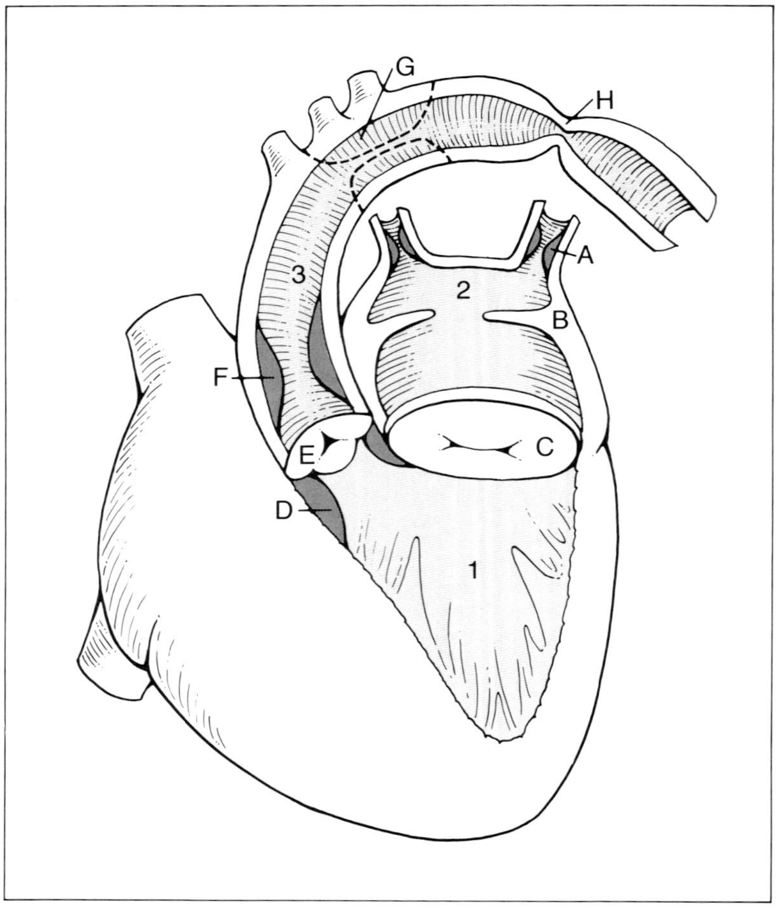

1 left ventricle	2 left atrium	3 aorta

Fig. 12.1 Obstructing lesions on the left side of the heart. (A) Stenosis of the pulmonary veins. (B) Cor triatriatum. (C) Mitral stenosis. (D) Subaortic stenosis. (E) Valvular aortic stenosis. (F) Supravalvular aortic stenosis. (G) Interrupted aortic arch. (H) Coarctation of the aorta.

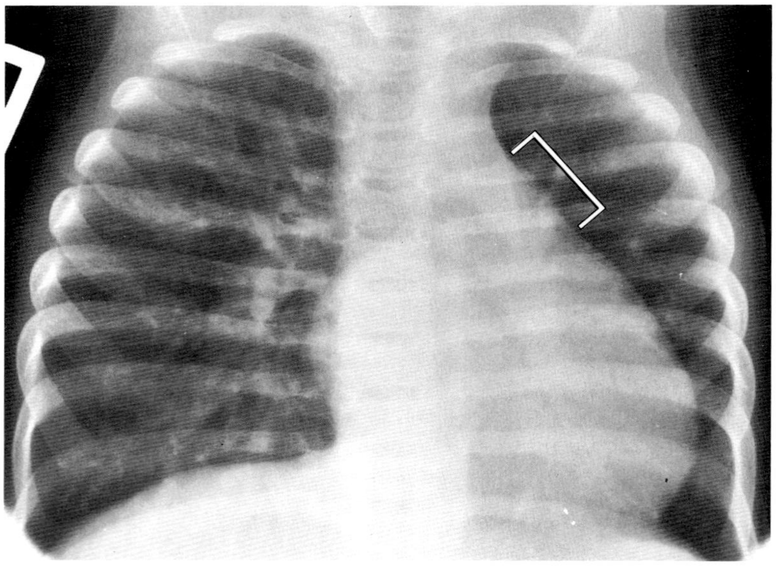

Fig. 12.2 Pulmonary vein stenosis. Frontal chest film shows mild cardiomegaly with right ventricular hypertrophy. The pulmonary trunk (*brace*) is prominent. The pulmonary vasculature is asymmetrical, being decreased on the left and plethoric on the right. In this child, both left pulmonary veins were severely stenotic at the level of the left atrium.

atrium, occasionally extending into the intraparenchymal segment of the affected pulmonary vein. All four pulmonary veins are generally involved to a variable extent.

HEMODYNAMIC AND CLINICAL FEATURES

Stenosis of the pulmonary veins, whether congenital or acquired, results in increased pulmonary resistance in the territory drained by the stenotic vein (or veins), with diversion of the blood to other territories. Pulmonary arterial and right ventricular pressures are usually increased as well.

Patients with congenital SPV typically present during the first month of life with failure to thrive and respiratory distress. Not infrequently, the clinical picture is dominated by an associated malformation (eg, VSD), in which case the existence of congenital SPV may not be suspected. Patients with acquired SPV have signs and symptoms of pulmonary venous hypertension.

IMAGING AND INVASIVE DIAGNOSIS

Plain Films

Chest films of patients with congenital SPV typically show moderate cardiomegaly with right ventricular enlargement and prominence of the pulmonary trunk and main pulmonary arteries. The pulmonary vasculature is irregularly and asymmetrically distributed. The portions of the lungs that are drained by the most severely obstructed veins exhibit diminished vascularity (hypoperfusion); elsewhere the lungs are plethoric (Fig. 12.2). In some instances there may be localized pulmonary edema. Patients with acquired SPV exhibit the typical radiographic findings of pulmonary venous hypertension (see Chapter 24).

Cardiac Catheterization and Angiocardiography

Cardiac catheterization demonstrates increased systolic pressure in the right ventricle and pulmonary trunk. The pulmonary arterial diastolic pressure and the wedge pressure are increased. The diagnosis is confirmed by selective catheterization of each pulmonary vein to verify the presence of a gradient between the pulmonary veins and the left atrium.

Pulmonary angiograms clearly demonstrate the uneven, asymmetrical distribution of the pulmonary vasculature which is the hallmark of this disorder (Fig. 12.3). There is dyssynchronous opacification of the pulmonary veins: the most markedly obstructed pulmonary veins are the last to opacify and retain contrast material for the longest time (Fig. 12.4). The stenosis is

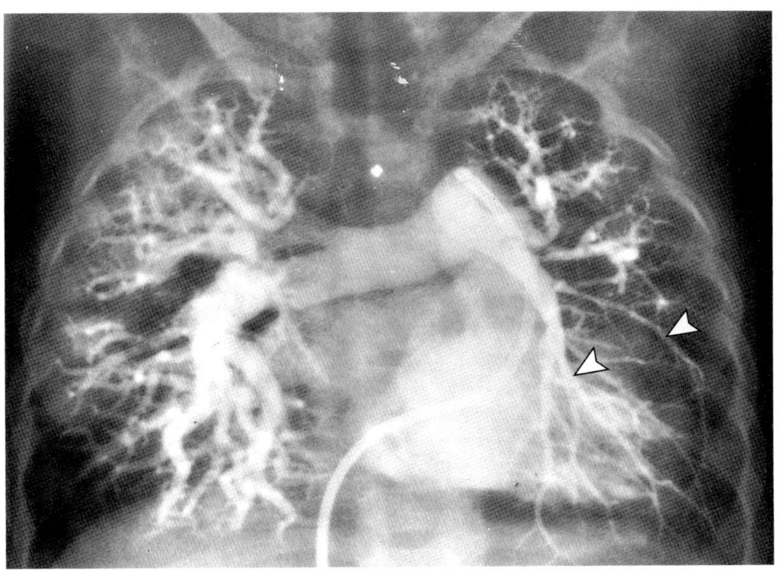

Fig. 12.3 Pulmonary vein stenosis. Pulmonary arteriogram demonstrates a large right pulmonary artery with dilated branches that extend into the periphery. The left pulmonary artery and the branches supplying the left lower lobe (*arrows*) are smaller than normal. The levophase (not illustrated) demonstrated severe stenosis of the left pulmonary veins.

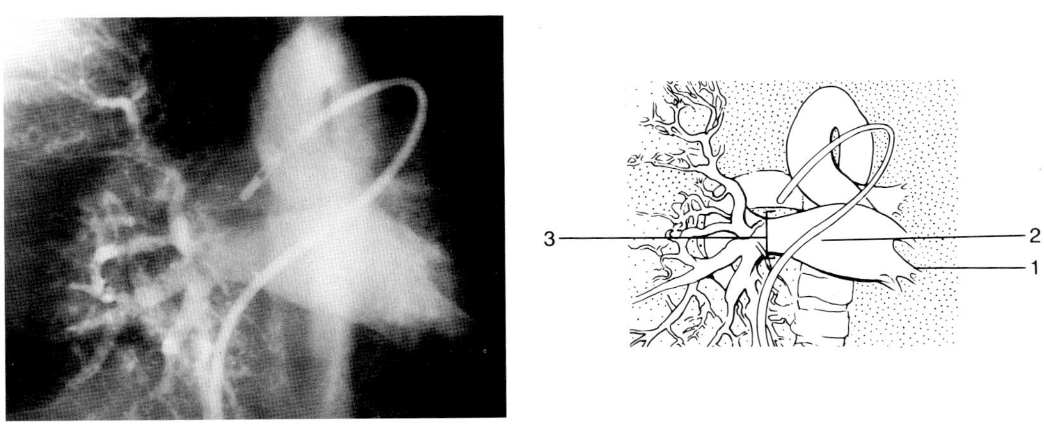

Fig. 12.4 Pulmonary vein stenosis. Levophase of selective right pulmonary arteriogram shows stasis of contrast material in the veins draining the right lung. The individual branches are tubular and dilated. Note stenosis of the upper and lower pulmonary veins, just proximal to the point at which they connect with the left atrium.

1 left ventricle
2 left atrium
3 stenosis

clearly demonstrated by selectively injecting contrast material into the affected pulmonary vein (Fig. 12.5).

COR TRIATRIATUM SINISTER

In this anomaly the left atrium is divided by a fibromuscular septum, or membrane, into two compartments ("chambers"): the *inferior chamber* (true left atrium), which contains the left atrial appendage and the mitral valve, and a *superior chamber* (common pulmonary venous chamber), which receives all four pulmonary veins (Fig. 12.6). The two compartments communicate via a narrow opening in the fibromuscular septum.

Cor triatriatum is commonly associated with an ASD. The ASD usually connects the inferior chamber with the right atrium (Fig. 12.6B). Less often, it connects the superior chamber with the right atrium (Fig. 12.6C).

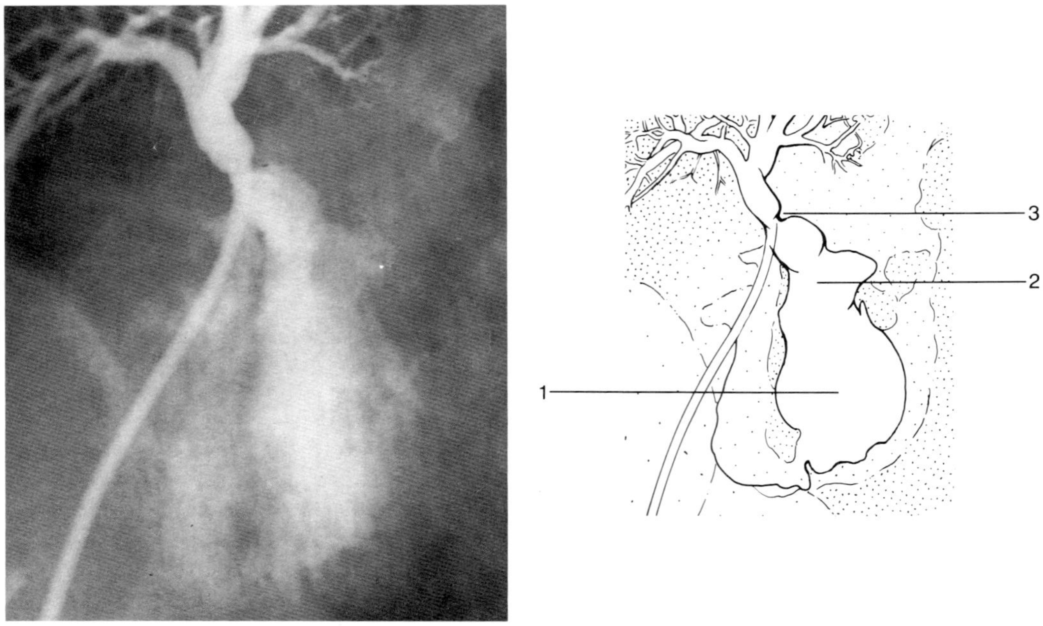

Fig. 12.5 Pulmonary vein stenosis. Selective injection of the right upper pulmonary vein (four-chamber view) shows a stenotic segment. Pressure measurements demonstrated a significant gradient. This patient had an ASD of the sinus venosus type.

1 left ventricle
2 left atrium
3 stenotic segment

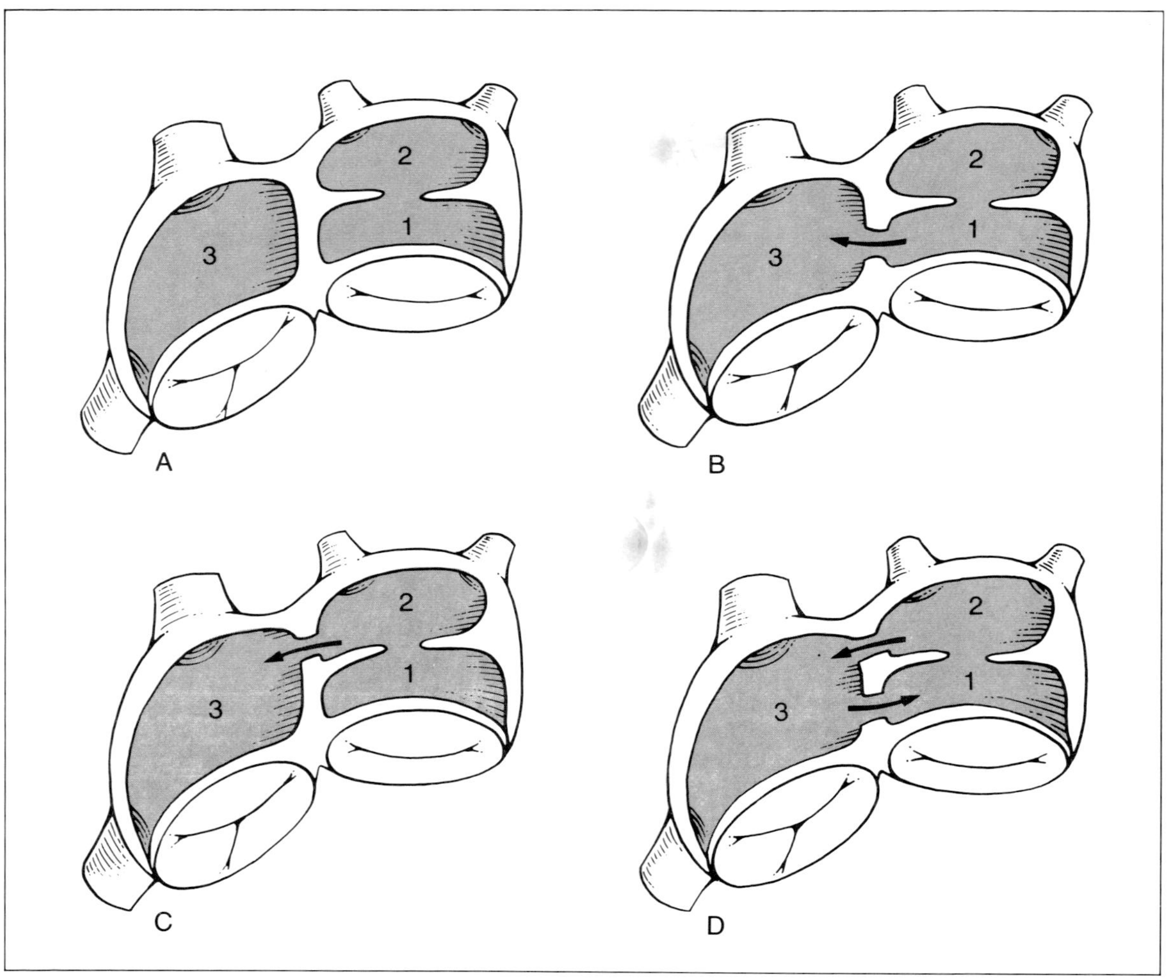

Fig. 12.6 Cor triatriatum. (A) Septation of left atrium without ASD. (B) Cor triatriatum with ASD connecting the inferior chamber of the left atrium with the right atrium. (C) Cor triatriatum with ASD connecting common pulmonary vein chamber of left atrium with the right atrium. C is hemodynamically equivalent to total anomalous pulmonary venous connection to the right atrium. (D) Double connection to right atrium.

1 inferior chamber of left atrium
2 common pulmonary vein chamber
3 right atrium

HEMODYNAMIC FEATURES

Impaired emptying of the left atrium results in increased pulmonary venous pressure and pulmonary arterial hypertension. When the superior (common pulmonary venous) chamber and right atrium communicate via a large ASD, the hemodynamic pattern is similar to anomalous pulmonary venous connection to the right atrium. Because of the obstruction within the left atrium, pressure in the inferior chamber (true left atrium) is less than right atrial pressure; therefore, when there is an associated ASD, there is a right to left shunt at the atrial level and cyanosis is present. The magnitude of the right to left shunt depends on the pressure in the inferior chamber (true left atrium), which in turn depends on the size of the aperture in the membrane separating the superior and inferior compartments.

CLINICAL FEATURES

Patients with cor triatriatum typically present in infancy with congestive heart failure. Patients with a large ASD between the inferior chamber (true left atrium) and right atrium are cyanotic. In the absence of an ASD, the clinical and radiologic features are those of pulmonary venous hypertension, the severity depending on the tightness of the aperture in the fibromuscular septum. Older children and adults typically present with clinical and radiographic features of pulmonary arterial hypertension secondary to the chronic pulmonary venous obstruction. Often, the clinical impression in such cases is "primary pulmonary hypertension." This subject will be further discussed in Chapter 17.

IMAGING AND INVASIVE DIAGNOSIS

Plain Films

In infants and young children, plain films show evidence of pulmonary venous hypertension, dilatation of the pulmonary trunk, and right ventricular enlargement; the left atrium is not enlarged (Fig. 12.7). Older children and adults typically exhibit right ventricular enlargement and evidence of pulmonary venous hypertension (cephalization) without left atrial enlargement. Some patients exhibit interstitial or airspace pulmonary edema (Fig. 12.8). The pulmonary trunk and main pulmonary arteries are usually enlarged secondary to pulmonary arterial

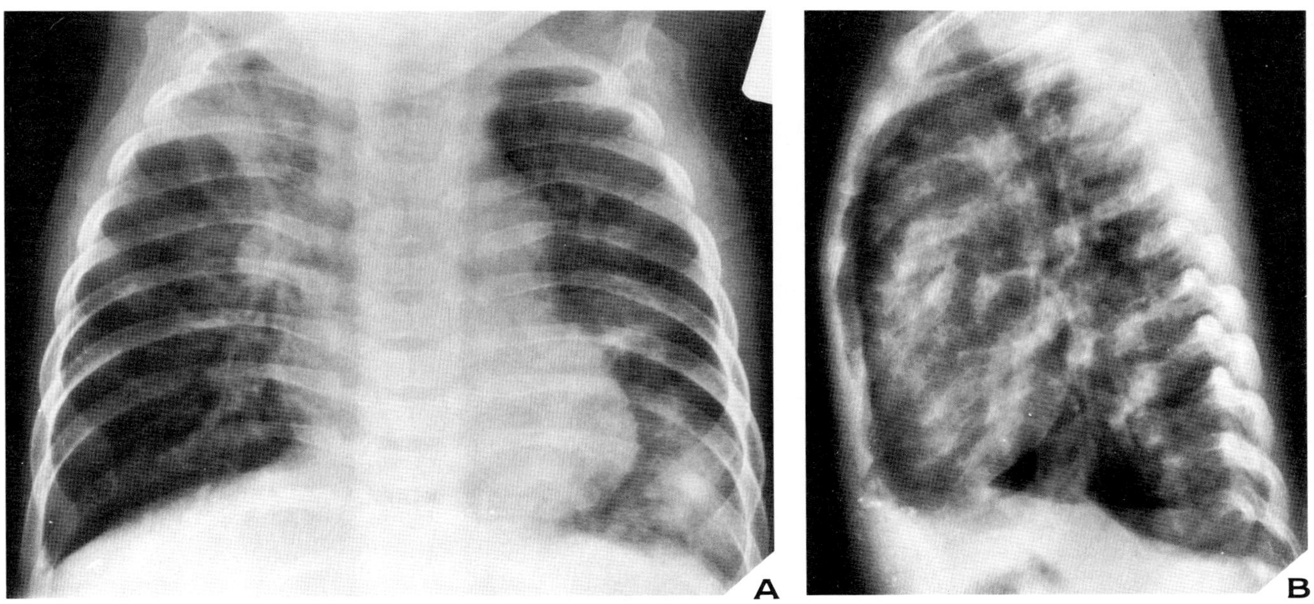

Fig. 12.7 Cor triatriatum sinister. (A) Frontal and (B) lateral chest films show right ventricular enlargement, a prominent pulmonary trunk, and diffuse interstitial pulmonary edema. In addition, there is atelectasis of the right upper lobe.

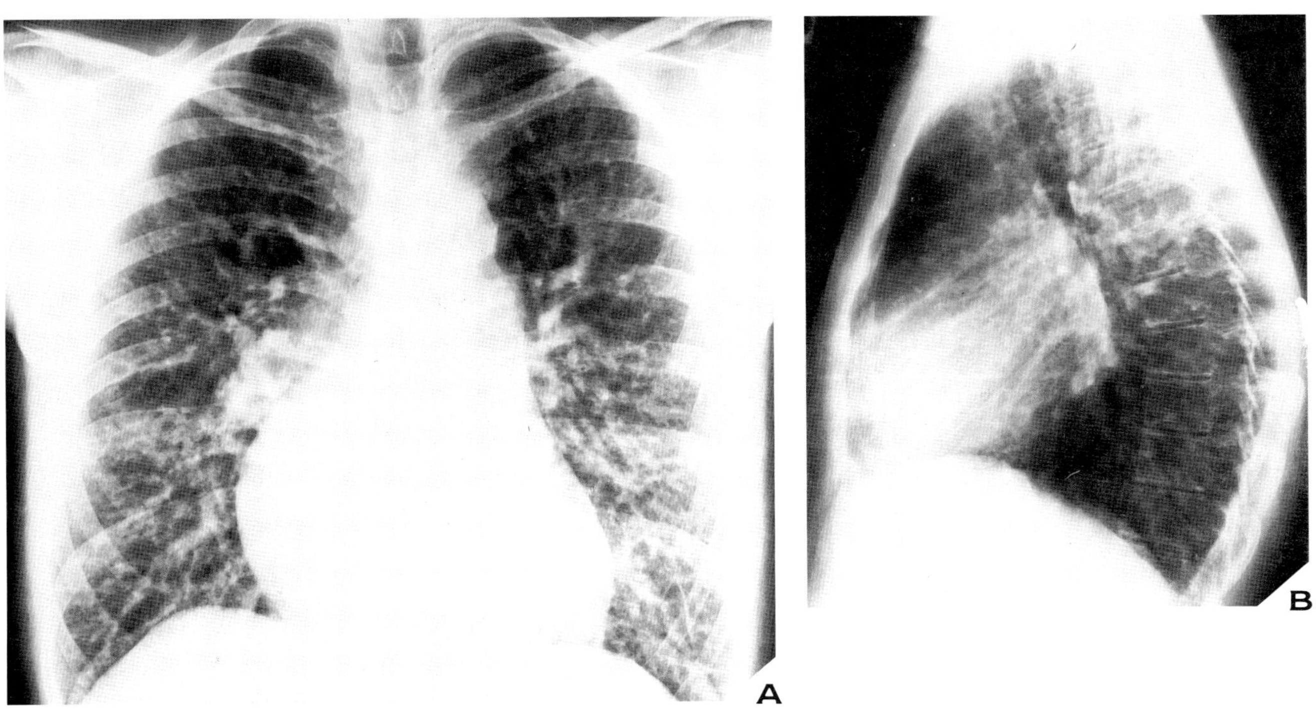

Fig. 12.8 Cor triatriatum sinister. (A) Frontal and (B) lateral chest films of a 30-year-old man show cardiomegaly with right ventricular enlargement, a dilated pulmonary trunk, and interstitial pulmonary edema. There is evidence of pulmonary venous hypertension (note Kerley B lines at both costophrenic angles).

hypertension. The peripheral pulmonary arterial branches are usually small and constricted, although they can be normal in patients with mild pulmonary hypertension.

This radiographic pattern strongly suggests the diagnosis of cor triatriatum; however, it is not specific, because similar findings are also present in patients with pulmonary vein stenosis or left atrial myxoma (see Chapter 26).

Echocardiography

Echocardiography accurately depicts the malformation and can obviate the need for cardiac catheterization and angiocardiography (Fig. 12.9). The echocardiographic diagnosis of cor triatriatum is based on demonstration of the fibromuscular membrane separating the superior (common venous) compartment from the inferior compartment (true left atrium) (Fig. 12.9).

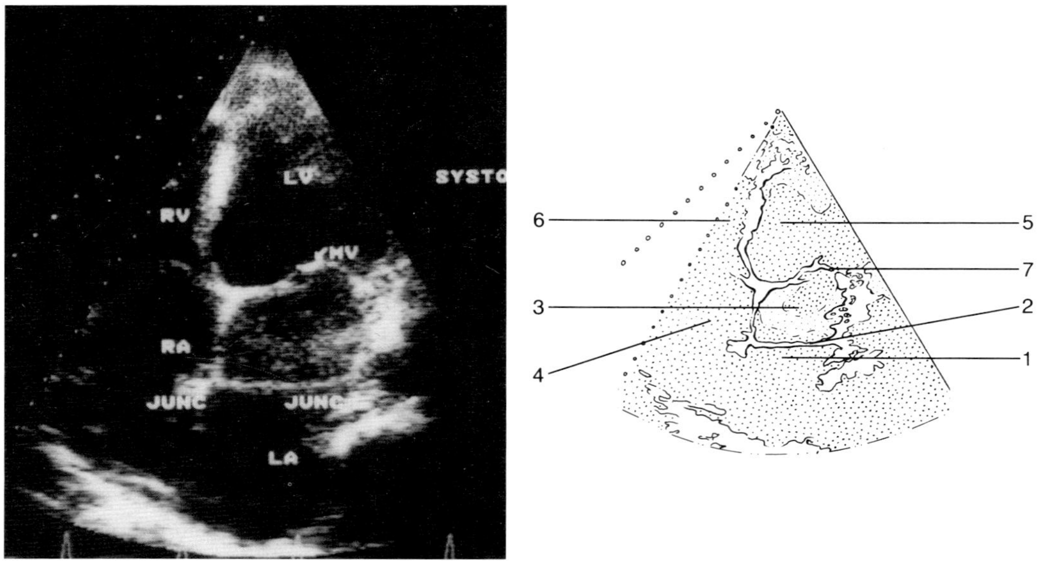

Fig. 12.9 Cor triatriatum sinister. Two-dimensional echocardiogram (four-chamber section) shows the left atrium divided into two compartments by a fibromuscular septum. The posterior (superior) compartment is the junction chamber, which receives the pulmonary veins. The inferior chamber (true left atrium) is related to the mitral valve.

1 posterior (superior) chamber
2 fibromuscular septum
3 inferior chamber (true left atrium)
4 right atrium
5 left ventricle
6 right ventricle
7 mitral valve

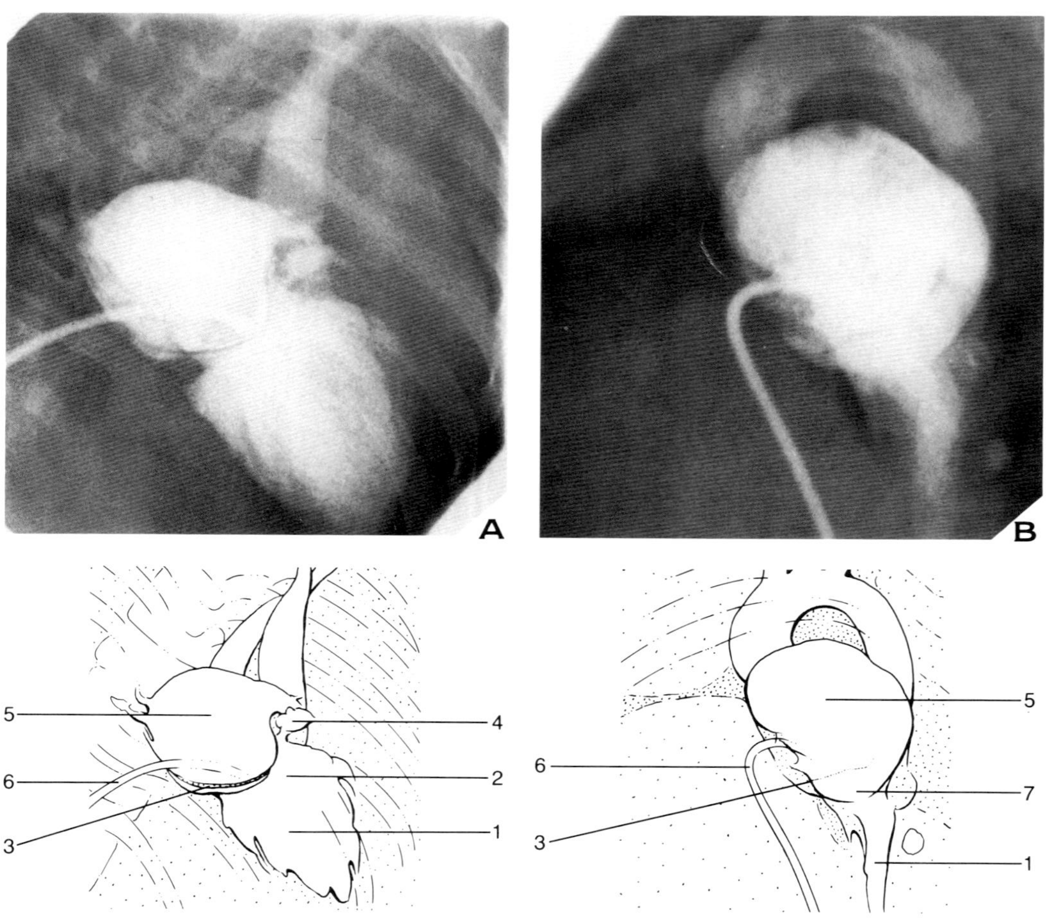

Fig. 12.10 Cor triatriatum sinister. Right (A) and left (B) anterior oblique projections of a left atrial injection. The linear filling defect in the inferior portion of the left atrium represents the fibromuscular septum that divides the left atrium into inferior and superior chambers. The inferior chamber connects with a normal mitral valve and includes the left atrial appendage. The superior chamber receives all four pulmonary veins. The atrial septum is intact.

1 left ventricle
2 mitral valve
3 septum
4 left atrial appendage
5 common pulmonary vein chamber of left atrium
6 catheter in left atrium (passed across foramen ovale)
7 inferior chamber of left atrium

Echocardiography is also the modality of choice for nonobstructive cor triatriatum; sections through the atria in the four-chamber view clearly depict this malformation.

Cardiac Catheterization and Angiocardiography

Cardiac catheterization confirms the presence of pulmonary venous hypertension, the severity of which depends on the tightness of the stenosis. The wedge pressure is elevated to a variable degree. The ratio between the wedge pressure and the end diastolic left ventricular pressure reflects the severity of the narrowing between the common pulmonary venous chamber and the true left atrium.

Compartmentalization of the left atrium is seen on the venous phase of a pulmonary arteriogram, although a selective left atrial injection may show it more clearly (Fig. 12.10). The superior (common pulmonary venous) chamber opacifies first, followed by the inferior chamber (true left atrium). Although the fibromuscular septum (membrane) is relatively thick in older children and adults, it may be quite delicate in young patients.

CONGENITAL MITRAL STENOSIS

MORPHOLOGY

Congenital mitral stenosis results from dysgenesis of one or more components of the mitral valve (including the adjacent portion of the left atrium). Although it can occur as an isolated malformation, it is frequently associated with other congenital defects, particularly anomalies of the left-sided ventricle and aorta. The stenosis is caused by narrowing of the supravalvular, annular, and/or valvular components of the mitral valve apparatus. There may be an additional subvalvular obstruction caused by a hypertrophied or misplaced papillary muscle or by fusion of the chordae tendinae. In most instances, developmental abnormalities are present at several levels. The echocardiographic diagnosis of cor triatriatum is based on demonstration of the fibromuscular membrane separating the superior (common venous) compartment from the inferior compartment (true left atrium) (Fig. 12.9). Echocardiography is also the modality of choice for nonobstructive cor triatriatum; sections through the atria in the four-chamber view clearly depict this malformation.

CLINICAL FEATURES

The signs and symptoms of isolated congenital mitral stenosis are similar to those of the acquired type (see Chapter 18). However, the early presentation and the absence of a history of rheumatic heart disease favor the diagnosis of congenital mitral stenosis. Typical symptoms include the manifestations of pulmonary venous hypertension (eg, dyspnea, orthopnea, paroxysmal noctural dyspnea) and recurrent pulmonary infection. In the later stages there are more dramatic manifestations of pulmonary venous hypertension, including congestive heart failure and peripheral and central cyanosis.

When congenital mitral stenosis occurs as an isolated malformation, diagnosis usually presents no problem. Diagnosis may be difficult, however, when it is associated with ASD, severe aortic stenosis, or a tight coarctation of the aorta.

IMAGING AND INVASIVE DIAGNOSIS

Plain Films

As in acquired mitral stenosis, the most striking plain film finding is left atrial dilatation. The heart is usually enlarged, and the classical signs of pulmonary venous hypertension are ordinarily present (Fig. 12.11).

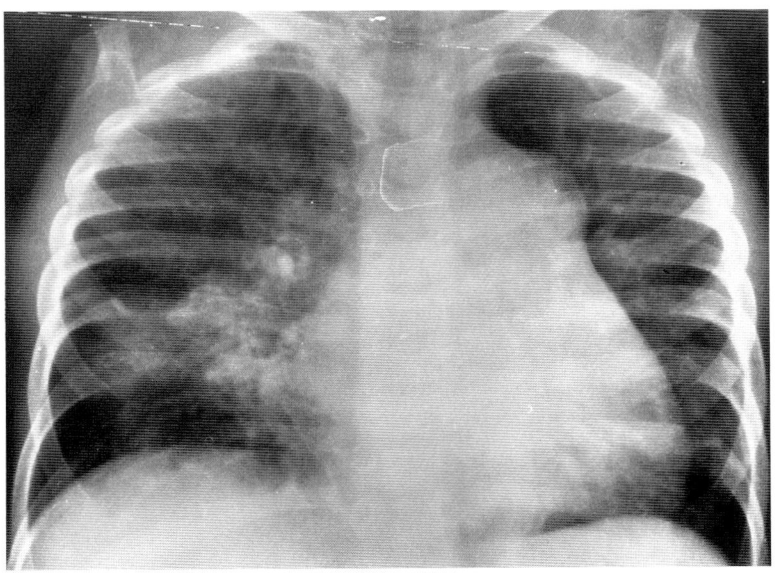

Fig. 12.11 Congenital mitral stenosis. Frontal chest film of a child shows cardiomegaly with left atrial (note the double density within the cardiac silhouette) and right ventricular enlargement (note the upturned apex). The pulmonary trunk and the left and right main pulmonary arteries are dilated. Note the interstitial pulmonary edema, which reflects the severe pulmonary venous hypertension.

Echocardiography

Two-dimensional echocardiography, augmented by color Doppler imaging, clearly demonstrates the abnormal morphology of the valvular apparatus, as well as any associated lesions, and is the diagnostic modality of choice (Fig. 12.12).

Cardiac Catheterization and Angiocardiography

Cardiac catheterization demonstrates both increased wedge pressure and increased pulmonary trunk pressure. Increased right ventricular pressure is frequently present also, reflecting right ventricular hypertrophy. The severity of the mitral stenosis is indicated by the difference between the wedge pressure and the left ventricular end diastolic pressure.

Oblique projections obtained after selective injection of contrast material into the left atrium are usually needed for diagnosis. The valve ring (annulus) usually appears small. In patients with a parachute mitral valve, the valvular apparatus, which ends in an isolated papillary muscle, appears funnel-shaped during diastole. Together with the negative shadow produced by the isolated papillary muscle, this produces a distinctive hourglass appearance (Fig. 12.13). In patients with a hammock mitral valve, the valve leaflets appear as a low-lying hammock-shaped membrane during diastole. The valve is usually tethered to abnormally short and malformed papillary muscles. The latter are attached to the left ventricular wall in an abnormal position.

In patients with supravalvular mitral stenosis, angiograms demonstrate a thin, linear filling defect just above the mitral valve (Fig. 12.14). The degree of obstruction varies. In some instances the stenosis is so severe as to suggest cor triatriatum; however, the fact that the filling defect is *below* the level of the left atrial appendage should suggest the correct diagnosis.

AORTIC STENOSIS

MORPHOLOGY

Aortic stenosis (AS) may involve the aortic valve itself or may be above or below it (Fig. 12.15). *Subvalvular AS* may be caused by an obstructing membrane, a fibromuscular tunnel, or septal hypertrophy. *Valvular AS* is usually due to malformed valve leaflets. In most instances the stenotic valve is bicuspid; however, stenosis of a trileaflet aortic valve secondary to fusion of the commissures may also occur. In infants with valvu-

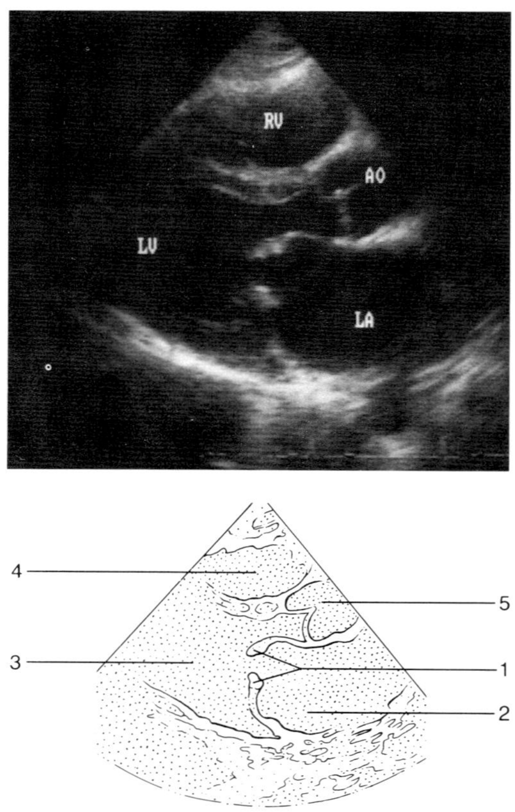

1 thickened mitral valve leaflets
2 left atrium
3 left ventricle
4 right ventricle
5 aorta

Fig. 12.12 Congenital mitral stenosis. Two-dimensional echocardiogram (parasternal long axis section, in diastole) demonstrates restricted opening of mitral valve leaflets. The leaflets are abnormally thick.

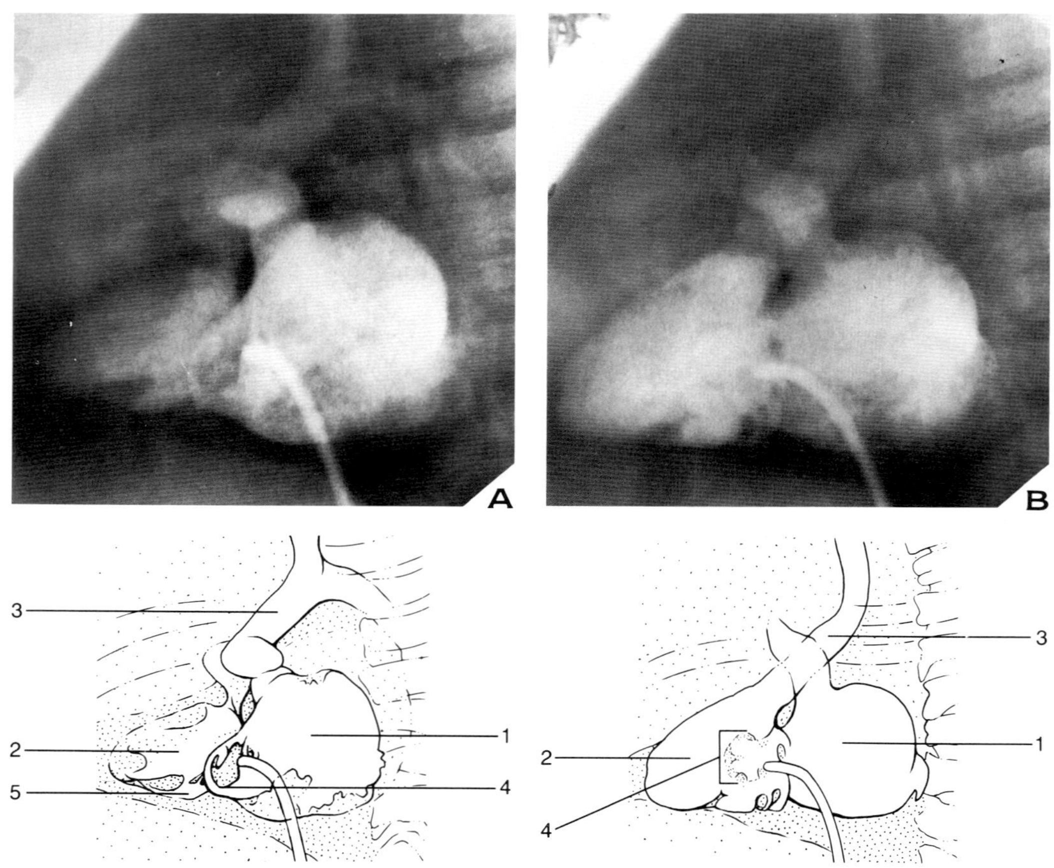

1 left atrium
2 left ventricle
3 aorta
4 stenotic mitral valve (parachute type)
5 papillary muscle

Fig. 12.13 Congenital mitral stenosis (parachute mitral valve). Lateral projection of left atriogram in early (A) and late (B) diastole in a patient with severe mitral stenosis demonstrates a small mitral annulus. The fused mitral leaflets form a funnel that resembles a parachute. There is a single papillary muscle close to the mitral leaflets. The head of the papillary muscle is directed towards the more apical portion of the mitral valve.

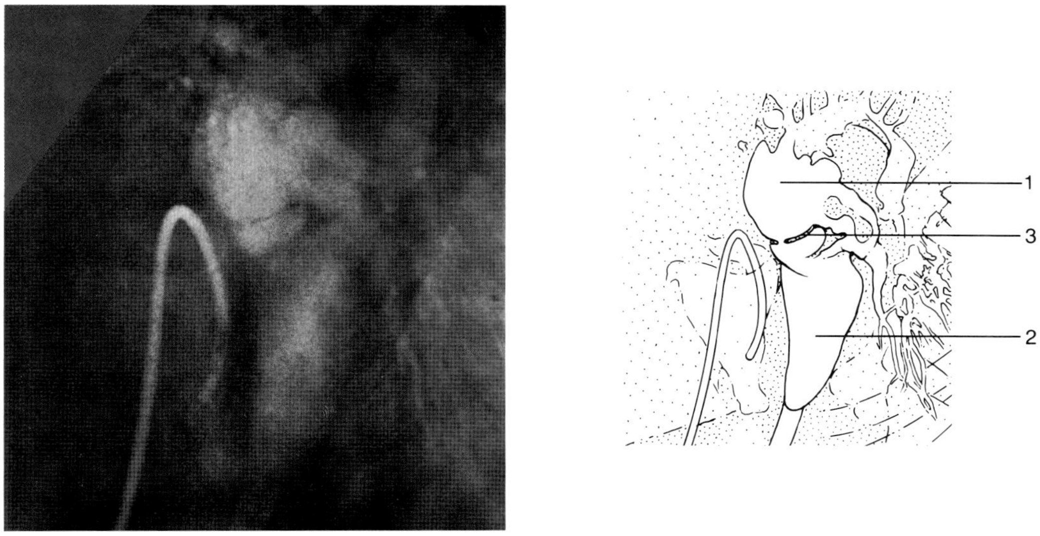

Fig. 12.14 Supravalvular mitral stenosis (supramitral ring). Venous phase of right ventriculogram (long axial projection) demonstrates a lucent line (which represents the supramitral ring) in the left atrium, close to the mitral valve.

1 right atrium	3 supramitral ring
2 left ventricle	

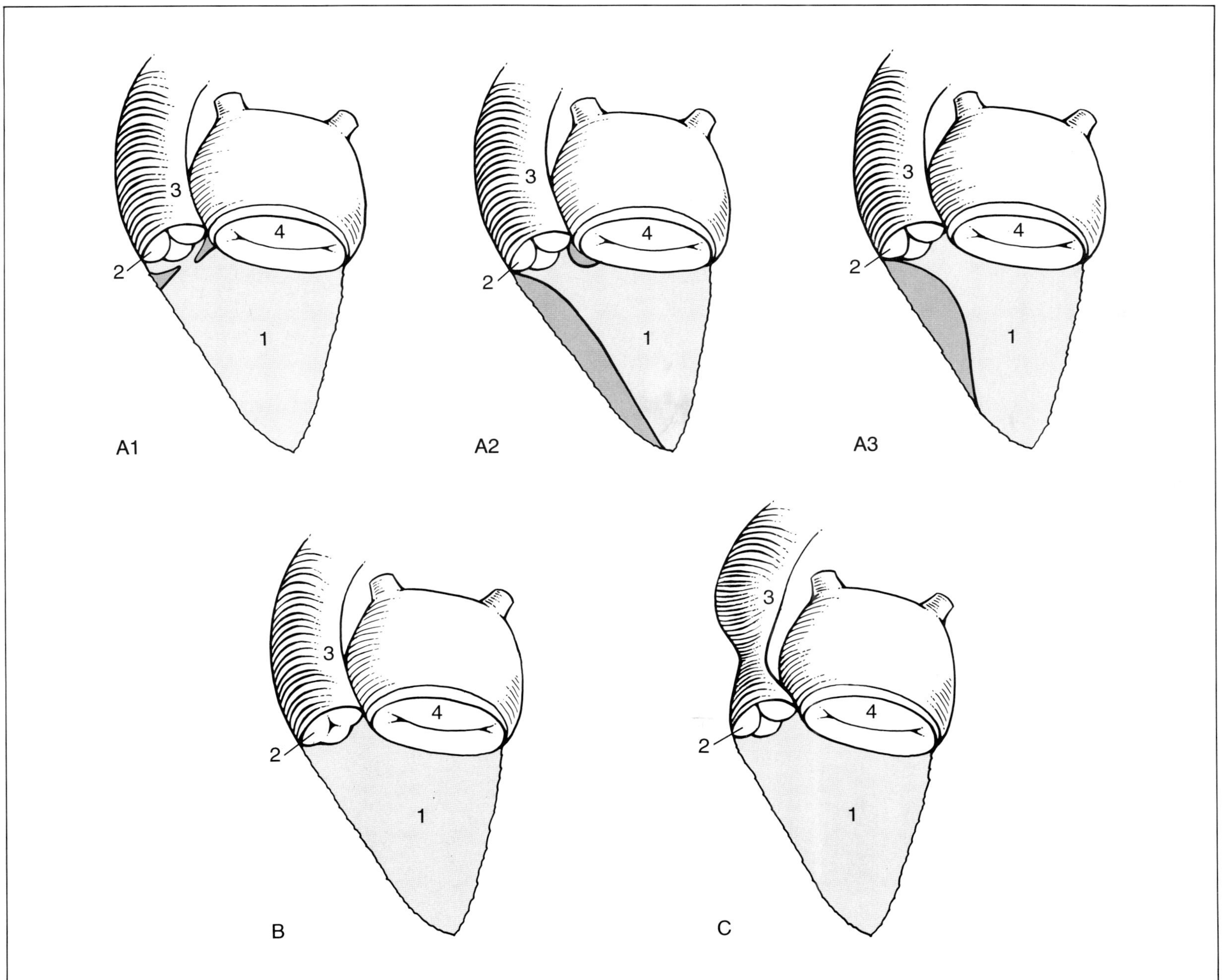

Fig. 12.15 Types of aortic stenosis. Viewed from the left ventricle. (A) Subaortic stenosis: (A1) discrete subaortic (diaphragmatic) type; (A2) fibromuscular type; (A3) muscular type (septal hypertrophy). (B) Valvular stenosis. (C) Supravalvular stenosis.

1 left ventricle	3 aorta	4 mitral valve
2 aortic valve		

lar AS the leaflets are thick, with rolled edges, and the commissures are fused. *Supravalvular AS* can take two forms: a circumscribed ring just above the sinuses of Valsalva, or a tubular narrowing beginning just above the sinuses of Valsalva. The latter may extend into the aortic arch, in which case it may involve the branches to the head and/or upper extremities. In patients with supravalvular AS, the opening of the coronary cusps is restricted, resulting in decreased coronary arterial flow and myocardial hypoperfusion.

CLINICAL FEATURES

The neonate with severe congenital AS typically presents with pallor, perspiration, and feeding difficulty; physical examination reveals a small pulse volume. Older children and young adults with hemodynamically significant AS are often asymptomatic, in which case the onset of exertional dyspnea, angina, or effort syncope is the first clue to the underlying malformation. Auscultation reveals a systolic ejection murmur radiating to the carotid vessels. Electrocardiography demonstrates left ventricular hypertrophy.

IMAGING AND INVASIVE DIAGNOSIS

Plain Films

The hallmark of *valvular AS* in the older child or teenager is left ventricular hypertrophy. During infancy and early childhood, however, the radiologic findings are nonspecific. At this age, chest films of patients with severe valvular AS typically show generalized cardiac enlargement and pulmonary edema. Downward displacement of the apex, which is characteristic of left ventricular enlargement in older patients, is not seen until two or three years of age. In older children and teenagers, poststenotic dilatation of the ascending aorta can usually be identified on the frontal film as a discrete bulge of the right mediastinal border (Fig. 12.16). The pulmonary trunk, main pulmonary arteries, and pulmonary vascularity are normal. The plain film findings in older children and teenagers with congenital AS are similar to those in adults with acquired AS (see Chapter 18).

In most instances, the plain film findings in patients with *supravalvular AS* are similar to the findings in those with valvular AS. In an occasional patient the combination of left ventricular hypertrophy and a diminutive aortic arch will suggest the correct diagnosis (Fig. 12.17). Supravalvular AS is occasionally associated with mental retardation and a distinctive elfin facies (Williams syndrome); many of these patients also have peripheral pulmonic stenosis (see below). Although some patients with Williams syndrome have an elevated serum calcium level, or were hypercalcemic in the past, it is not clear whether hypercalcemia is a constant feature of this disorder.

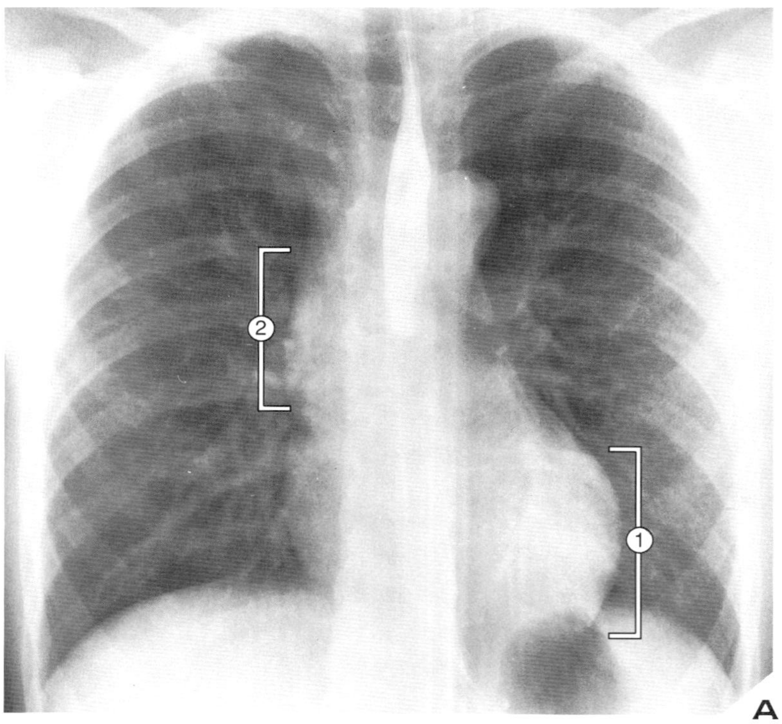

A

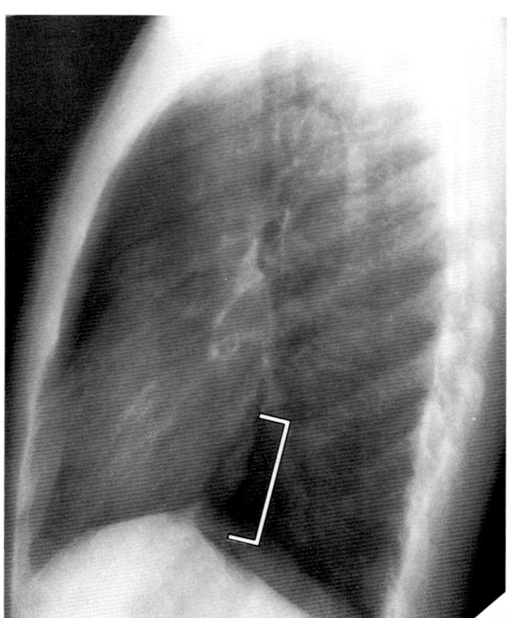

B

Fig. 12.16 Valvular aortic stenosis. (A) Frontal and (B) lateral chest films in a 5-year-old boy demonstrate prominence of the left lower heart border (*brace* 1 in A) and posteroinferior displacement of the posterior heart border (*brace* in B), indicating left ventricular enlargement. The dilated ascending aorta forms a prominent bulge along the right mediastinal border (*brace* 2 in A). The aortic arch is also dilated (note the prominent aortic "knob" in A).

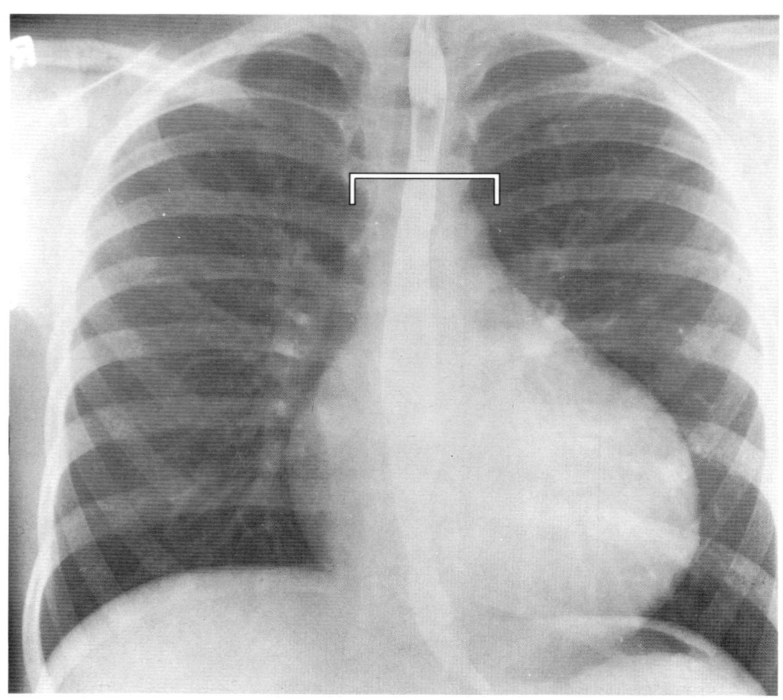

Fig. 12.17 Supravalvular aortic stenosis associated with peripheral pulmonic stenosis (Williams syndrome). Frontal chest film shows biventricular hypertrophy and a narrow vascular pedicle *(brace)*. The aortic arch and pulmonary trunk are diminutive in this patient with obstructing lesions on both sides of the heart. The pulmonary vasculature is decreased secondary to widespread peripheral pulmonary stenosis.

The plain film findings in patients with *subvalvular AS* (subvalvular ring or septal hypertrophy) are similar to those in patients with valvular AS; however, dilatation of the ascending aorta is less common in the former.

Cardiac Catheterization and Angiocardiography

Cardiac catheterization typically demonstrates increased systolic and diastolic pressures in the left ventricle. A gradient across the aortic valve of greater than 75 mm Hg, or a cross-sectional area of the aortic valve of less than 0.5 cm^2/square meter of body surface, indicates severe aortic stenosis. Left ventricular end diastolic pressure is elevated in patients with left ventricular failure; with more severe left ventricular decompensation, left atrial and pulmonary venous pressure are also elevated.

Left ventriculograms obtained in the long axial or elongated right anterior oblique projection clearly depict the various types of AS. The diaphragmatic form of subvalvular AS appears as a linear negative ring or shelf-like defect (Fig. 12.18), whereas the fibromuscular form appears as a tubular narrowing of the left ventricular outflow tract (Fig. 12.19). In patients with

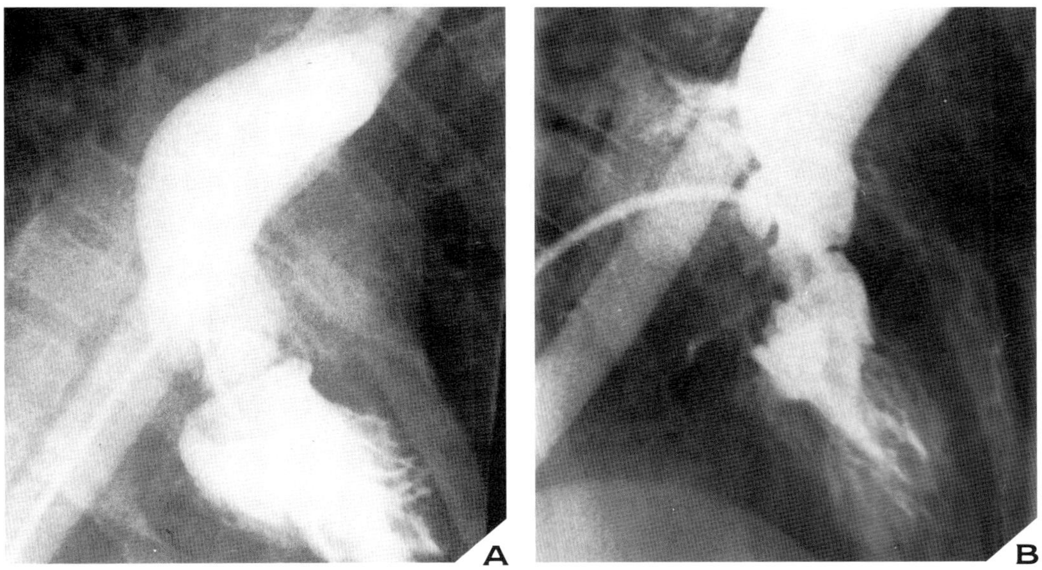

Fig. 12.18 Subvalvular aortic stenosis (ring type). Left ventriculograms in two patients. (A) In this child a linear defect is seen beneath the aortic valve during diastole. At operation this proved to be a complete ring of fibrous tissue (diaphragmatic type of subvalvular aortic stenosis). (B) In a second patient, a shelf-like deformity of the anterolateral aspect of the left ventricular outflow tract is seen during systole. At operation this proved to be an incomplete subvalvular ring.

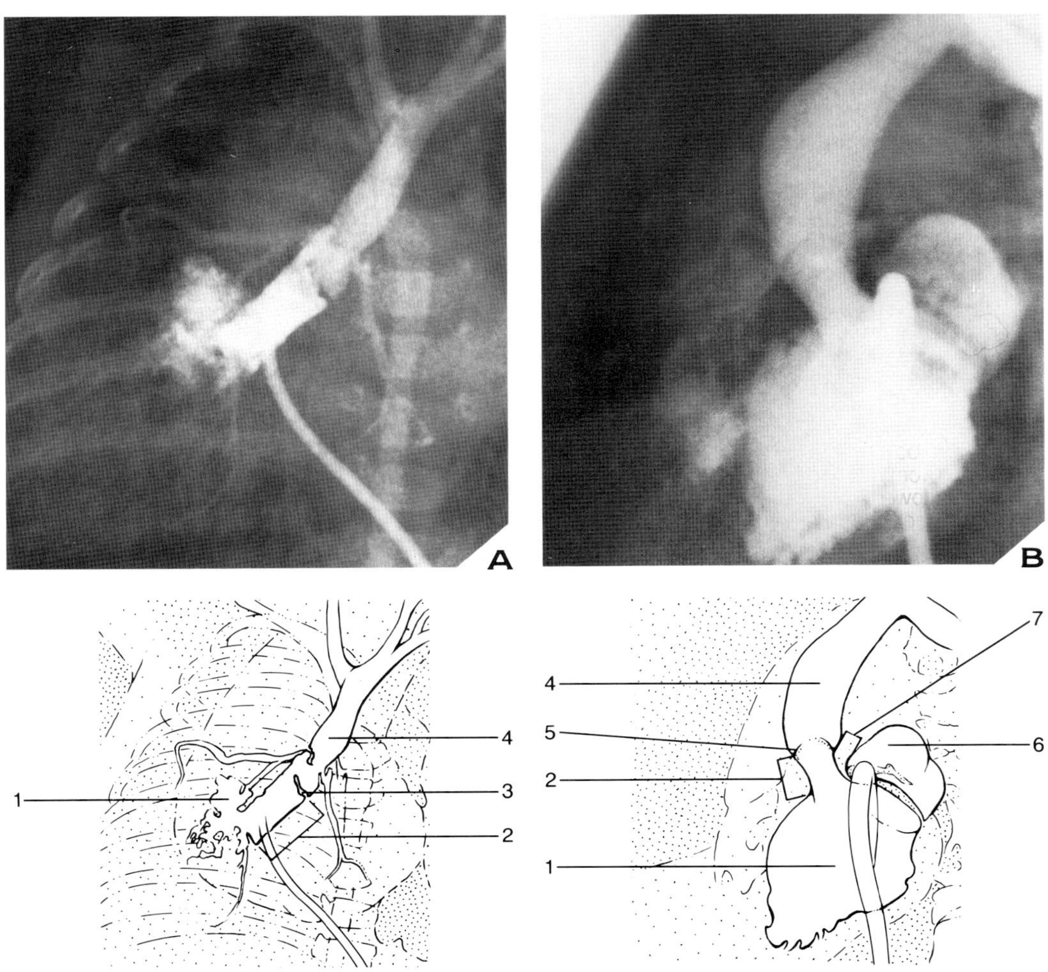

Fig. 12.19 Subaortic stenosis (tubular type). Angiographic findings in two patients. (A) Selective injection of the subaortic segment of the left ventricle in an infant with situs inversus, dextrocardia, and coarctation of the aorta. The left ventricular outflow tract is represented by a narrow, tubular channel. (B) Left ventriculogram in another patient demonstrates a mild tubular stenosis of the left ventricular outflow tract. Additional findings include valvular stenosis of the aortic valve and absence of continuity between the mitral and aortic valves.

valvular AS, movement of the leaflets is restricted during systole, the stenotic valve resembling a dome with a small central aperture (Fig. 12.20).

Bicuspid aortic valve is well demonstrated by thoracic aortography. Contrast material outlines the noncoronary cusp on one side and the fused right and left cusps on the other, which produces a distinctive "fish mouth" appearance during systole. If the bicuspid valve is stenotic, the leaflets do not retract completely during systole (Fig. 12.21) (see also Chapter 18).

Angiograms demonstrate a ring-like constriction or tubular narrowing of the ascending aorta in patients with supravalvular AS. The narrowing begins just above the sinuses of Valsalva and may involve the entire ascending aorta, even extending into the aortic arch and its branches (Fig. 12.22).

INTERRUPTION OF THE AORTIC ARCH

MORPHOLOGY

In this malformation, which may be associated with a left or right arch, there is a discontinuity between two segments of the aortic arch. In 55 percent of cases there is a gap in the arch between the origins of the left common carotid and left subclavian arteries; in 40 percent the arch is interrupted distal to the origin of the left subclavian artery; and in 5 percent the gap is proximal to the origin of the left common carotid artery. Interruption of the aortic arch is frequently associated with valvular and/or subvalvular aortic stenosis.

HEMODYNAMIC AND CLINICAL FEATURES

Patients with interruption of the aortic arch present in the neonatal period with severe congestive heart failure owing to the volume overload imposed by the left to right intracardiac shunt across the foramen ovale, which increases precipitously after the ductus closes. The trunk and lower extremities are perfused (via the ductus) by unsaturated blood. Before ductus closure there may be differential cyanosis between the upper and lower extremities. The femoral pulses are diminished at birth and disappear after the ductus closes.

IMAGING AND INVASIVE DIAGNOSIS

Plain films show an enlarged heart with pulmonary plethora and pulmonary venous hypertension. Echocardiography, cine CT, and MRI show the major features of the anomaly; however, angiocardiography is usually necessary to completely define the malformation before surgery. Left ventriculography demon-

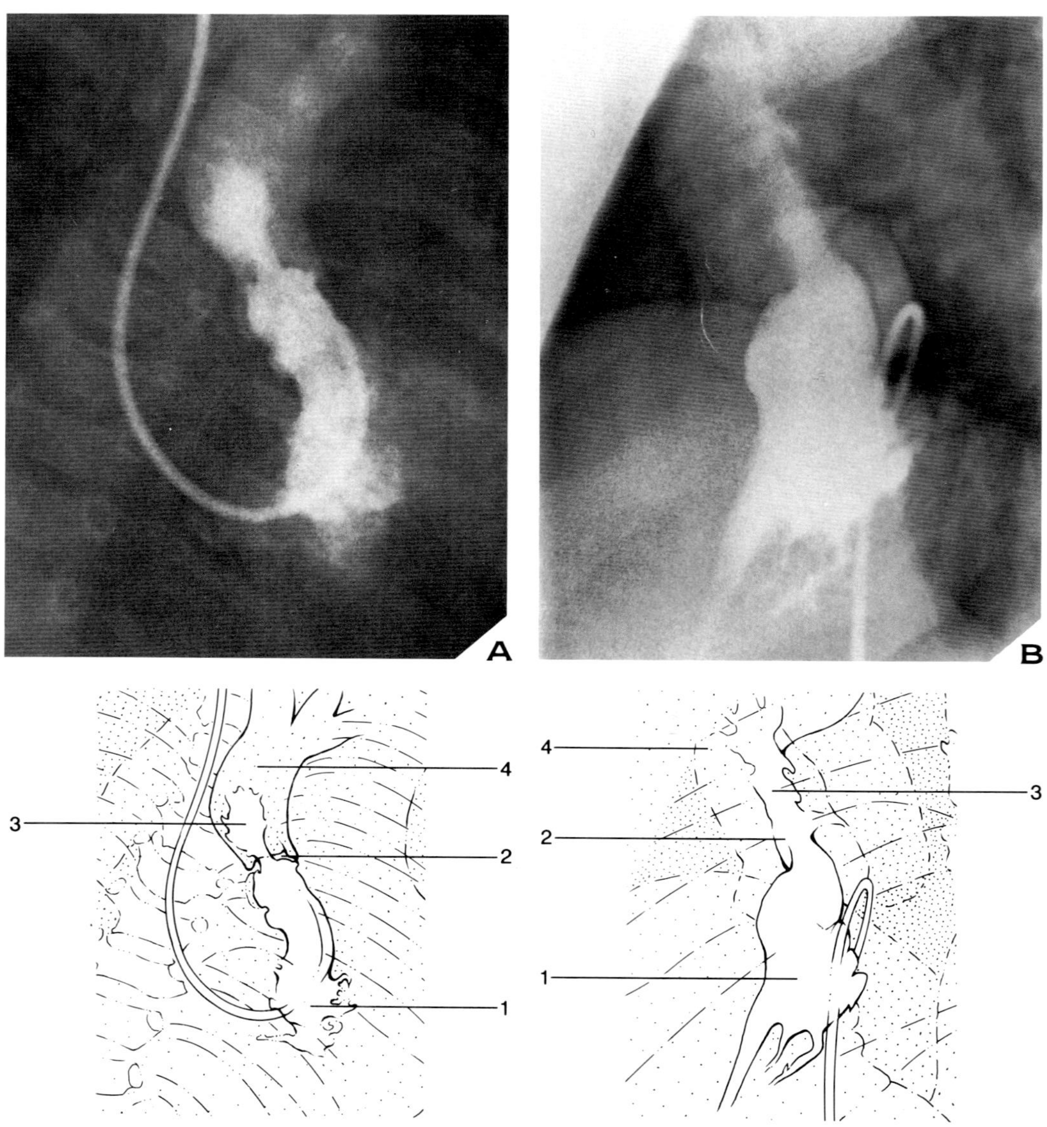

Fig. 12.20 Valvular aortic stenosis. Left ventriculograms in two children. (A) Right anterior oblique projection. Note the domed appearance of the aortic valve leaflets and the central jet of contrast material. (B) Left anterior oblique projection. The aortic valve is domed-shaped and the contrast jet is eccentric.

1 left ventricle
2 dome-shaped aortic valve
3 jet of contrast material
4 aorta

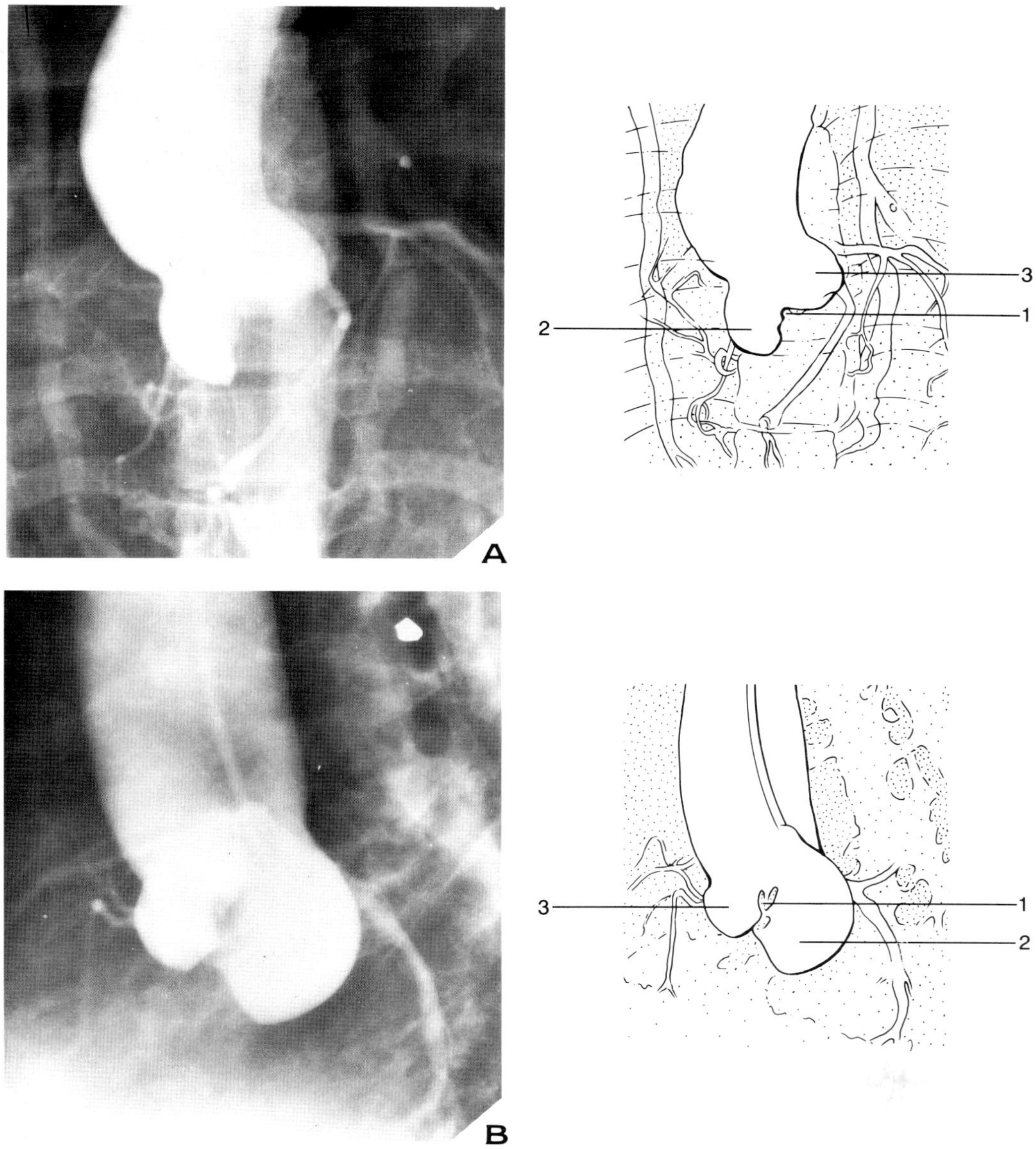

Fig. 12.21 Stenotic bicuspid aortic valve. (A) Frontal and (B) lateral projections of thoracic aortogram show restricted movement of the aortic valve during systole. The right (posterior) leaflet is the noncoronary cusp; the left (anterior) leaflet is the coronary cusp. The stenotic aperture of the aortic valve appears as a filling defect in A and B.

1 stenotic aperture of aortic valve
2 noncoronary cusp
3 coronary cusp

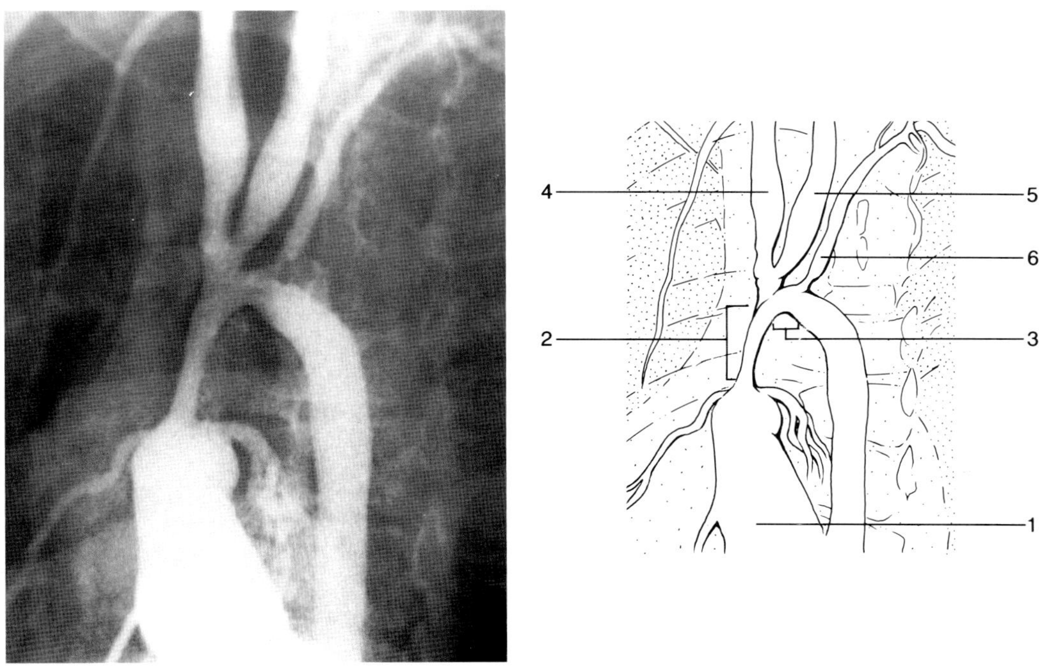

Fig. 12.22 Supravalvular aortic stenosis. Left ventriculogram (left anterior oblique projection) demonstrates tubular narrowing of the entire ascending aorta. The proximal portion of the aortic arch and the origins of the carotid, innominate, and subclavian arteries are also involved.

1 left ventricle
2 stenotic ascending aorta
3 stenotic aortic arch
4 innominate artery
5 left carotid artery
6 left subclavian artery

strates the stenosis (if present) of the left ventricular outflow tract and/or aortic valve and the gap in the aortic arch. Right ventriculography demonstrates a large right ventricle with massive dilatation of the pulmonary trunk. Before ductus closure, opacified blood flows across the ductus from the left pulmonary artery to the descending thoracic aorta. In patients in whom the arch is interrupted between the origin of the left common carotid and left subclavian arteries (the most common arrangement), the left subclavian artery is seen to arise from the descending thoracic aorta (Figs. 12.23 and 12.24).

COARCTATION OF THE AORTA

Coarctation of the aorta is a congenital stenosis of the proximal descending thoracic aorta at the level of its connection with the ductus arteriosus. The coarctation typically takes the form of a shelf-like narrowing along the left posterolateral aspect of the aorta. The ascending aorta and the proximal portion of the aortic arch are usually dilated. Distal to the origin of the left subclavian artery, the aortic arch is narrowed and displaced medially. Collaterals derived from branches of the subclavian arteries

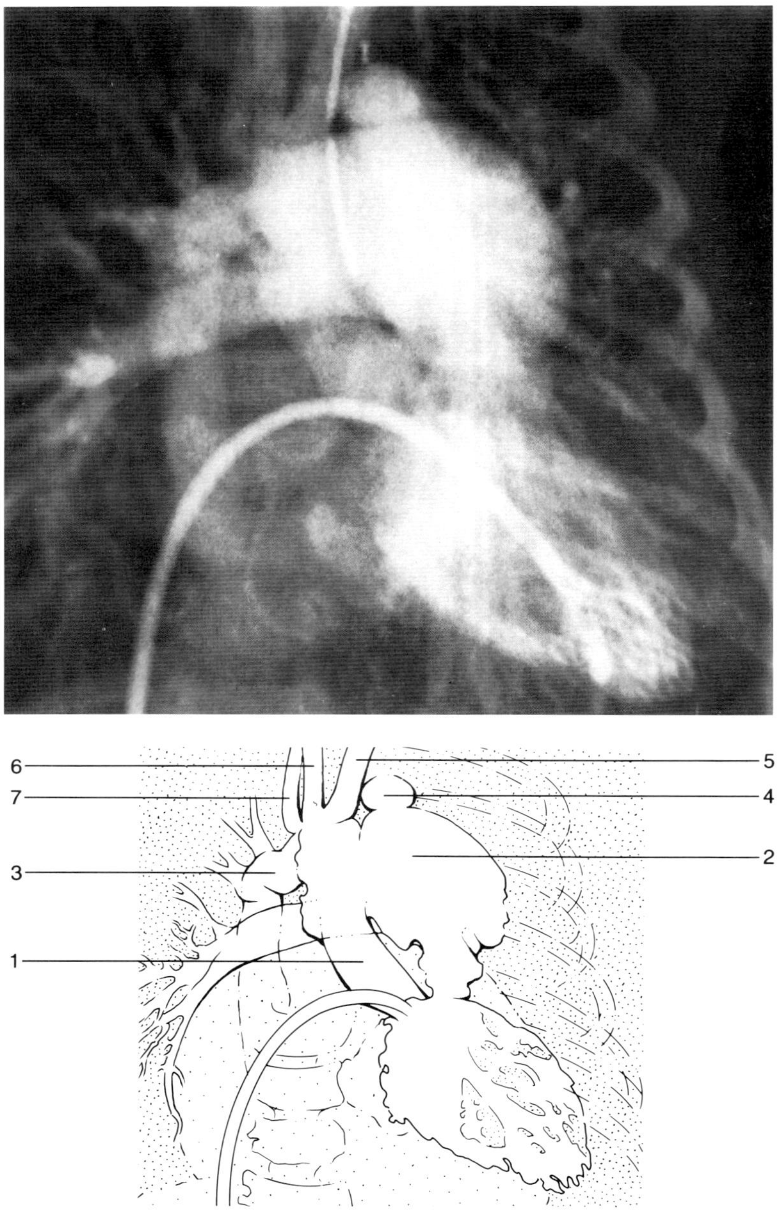

1	ascending aorta	5	left innominate artery
2	pulmonary trunk	6	right common carotid artery
3	patent ductus arteriosus	7	right subclavian artery
4	left pulmonary artery		

Fig. 12.23 Interruption of the aortic arch. Frontal projection of left ventriculogram demonstrates a right-sided ascending aorta and a right aortic arch. A large patent ductus arteriosus connects the right pulmonary artery with the upper descending thoracic aorta. The aortic arch is interrupted beyond the origin of the right subclavian artery.

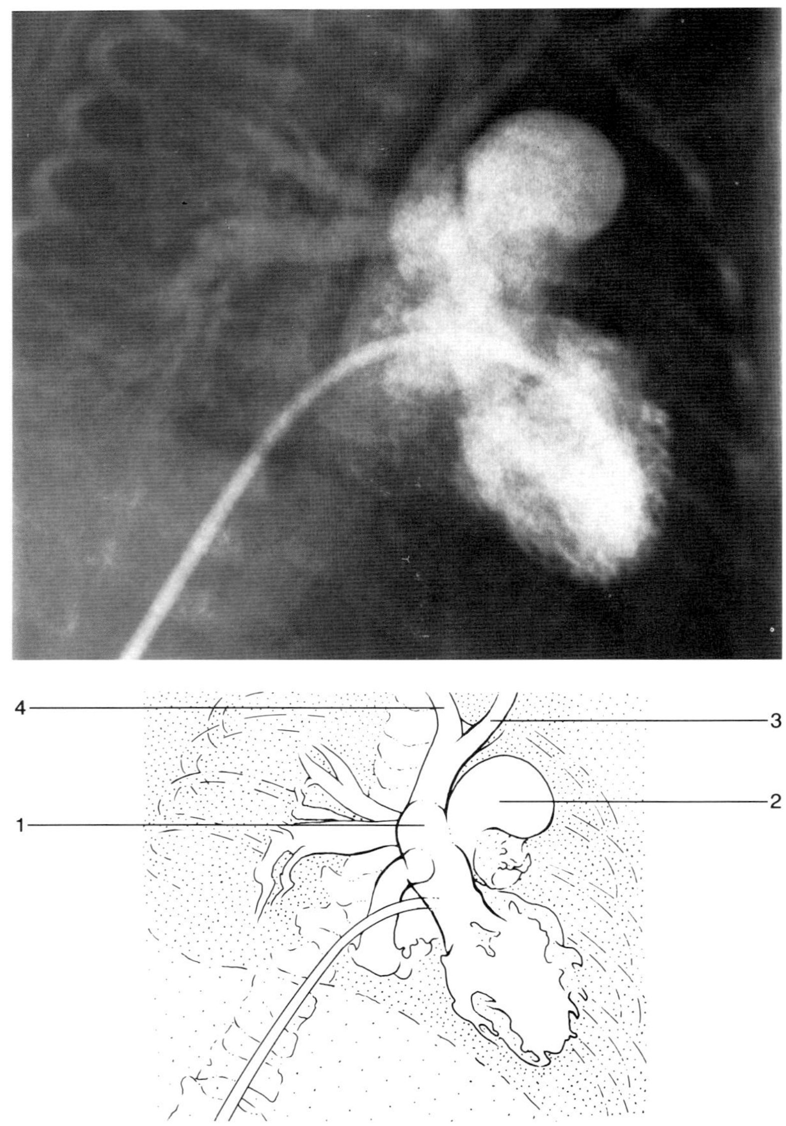

1	ascending aorta	3	left common carotid artery
2	pulmonary trunk	4	right innominate artery

Fig. 12.24 Interruption of the aortic arch. Frontal projection of left ventriculogram. The ascending aorta terminates in the innominate and left carotid arteries. The left subclavian artery is not opacified, indicating that the aortic arch ends after the origin of the left common carotid artery. The aortic arch is left-sided.

supply the descending thoracic aorta and its branches (Fig. 12.25). The commonest collateral pathway is the internal mammary–intercostal artery pathway. The rib notching typically seen in teenagers and adults results from the enlarged intercostal arteries associated with this pathway. Other collateral pathways include small mediastinal and aberrant arteries. Five percent of patients with coarctation of the aorta do not have collaterals.

Coarctation of the aorta may exist as an isolated lesion or in association with subvalvular AS, valvular AS, or a bicuspid aortic valve. The latter may become stenotic or incompetent in later life. Occasionally coarctation of the aorta is one component of a complex cardiac malformation.

HEMODYNAMIC AND CLINICAL FEATURES

Systolic pressure is increased in the aortic segment proximal to the stenotic segment and decreased distal to it. The left ventricle hypertrophies and eventually fails.

Approximately 10 percent of patients with isolated coarctation of the aorta present with signs and symptoms of congestive heart failure (tachypnea, feeding difficulties, and sweating) during the neonatal period. (Congestive heart failure is more common when coarctation is associated with a VSD or other left to right shunt.) The femoral pulses are absent or significantly decreased when compared with the radial and brachial pulses. The blood pressure in the arms is significantly greater than in the lower extremities (a difference of 20 mm Hg or more). When the coarctation is proximal to the ductus there is usually a right to left shunt at the level of the ductus, in which case the upper part of the body may be pink and the lower part of the body will appear cyanotic.

Isolated coarctation of the aorta is usually asymptomatic during infancy, although the abnormal pulses and the blood pressure differential can be detected on careful physical examination. ECG may show evidence of left ventricular hypertrophy.

Isolated coarctation is usually asymptomatic in older children, although it may present at this age with congestive heart failure secondary to left ventricular dysfunction.

Isolated coarctation is usually asymptomatic in adolescents and young adults, and is usually suggested by the findings on physical examination or chest films. Hypertension is the rule at this age and, unless treated, congestive heart failure will usually develop by 30 years of age.

IMAGING AND INVASIVE DIAGNOSIS

Plain Films

The typical plain film findings in the neonate are nonspecific cardiac enlargement and congestive heart failure. Cardiomegaly with left ventricular enlargement and normal pulmonary vasculature suggests the possibility of coarctation in an older infant. Characteristic plain film findings are usually present by 6 years of age. These include cardiomegaly with left ventricular hypertrophy, an inconspicuous or inapparent aortic arch, prominence of the left subclavian artery, and poststenotic dila-

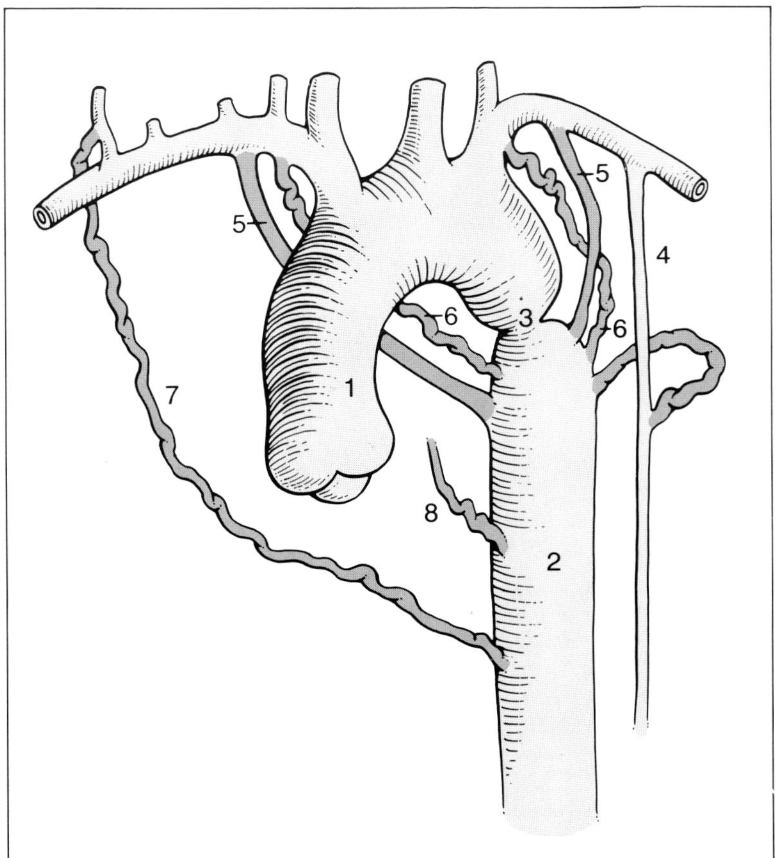

Fig. 12.25 Collateral circulation in coarctation of the aorta. The most common collateral pathways are shown schematically. The great majority of the large collateral channels originate from the subclavian arteries and connect with the descending thoracic aorta. Only a few collateral pathways have a different origin (eg, the spinal artery, which originates from the ipsilateral vertebral artery).

1 ascending aorta
2 descending thoracic aorta
3 coarctation of the aorta
4 left mammary artery (connected to descending thoracic aorta via intercostal arteries)
5 aberrant artery originating from right subclavian artery and connecting with descending thoracic aorta
6 mediastinal arteries connecting left subclavian artery and descending thoracic aorta
7 collaterals from scapular arteries to descending thoracic aorta
8 collaterals from spinal artery to descending thoracic aorta

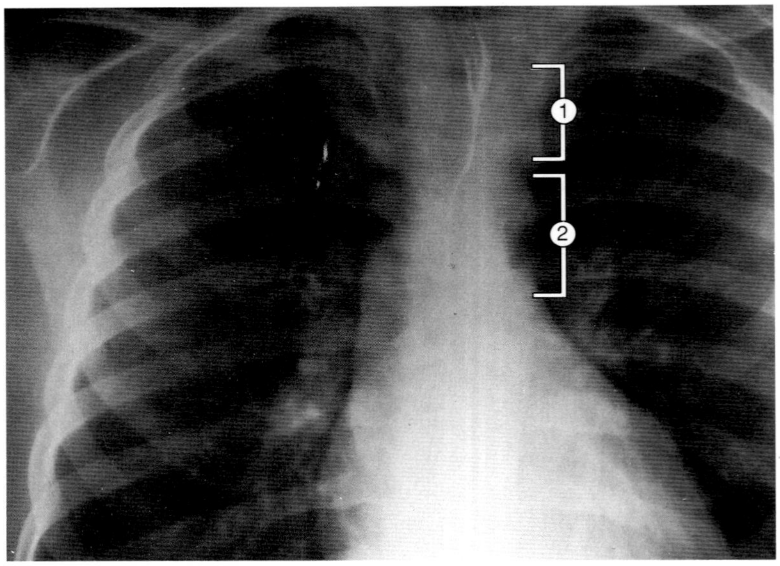

Fig. 12.26 Coarctation of the aorta. Frontal chest film of an adult with coarctation of the aorta shows an enlarged heart with prominence of the left lower heart border, indicating left ventricular enlargement. The aortic arch cannot be identified. However, both the left subclavian artery (*brace* 1) and the poststenotic segment of the descending thoracic aorta (*brace* 2) are prominent, producing a contour which resembles a "3" (see Fig. 12.29). Note the absence of rib notching, which indicates that intercostal arteries are not an important pathway in this patient.

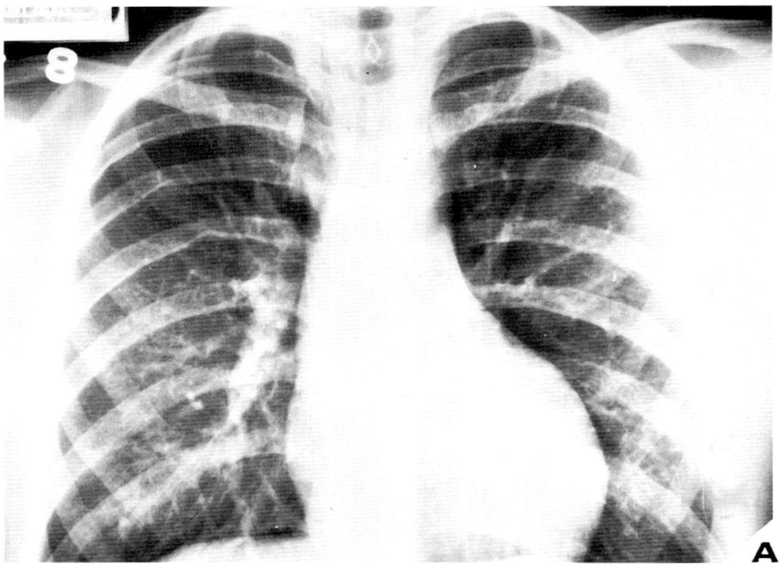

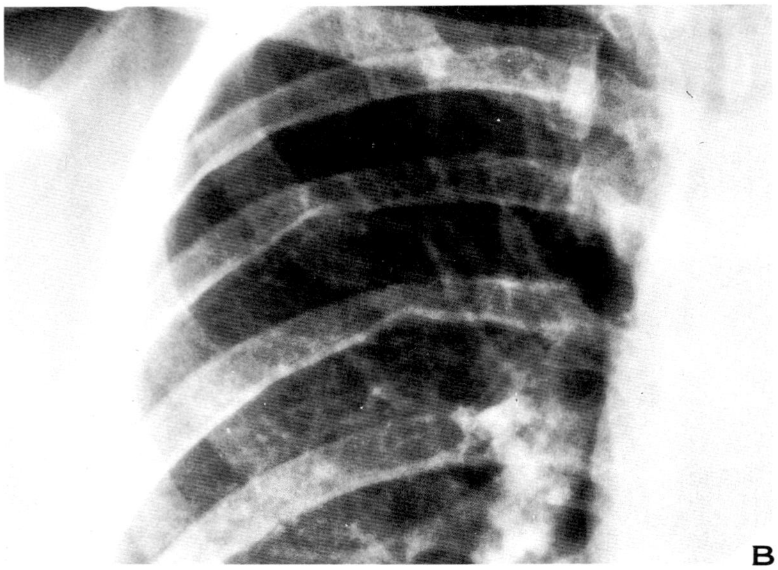

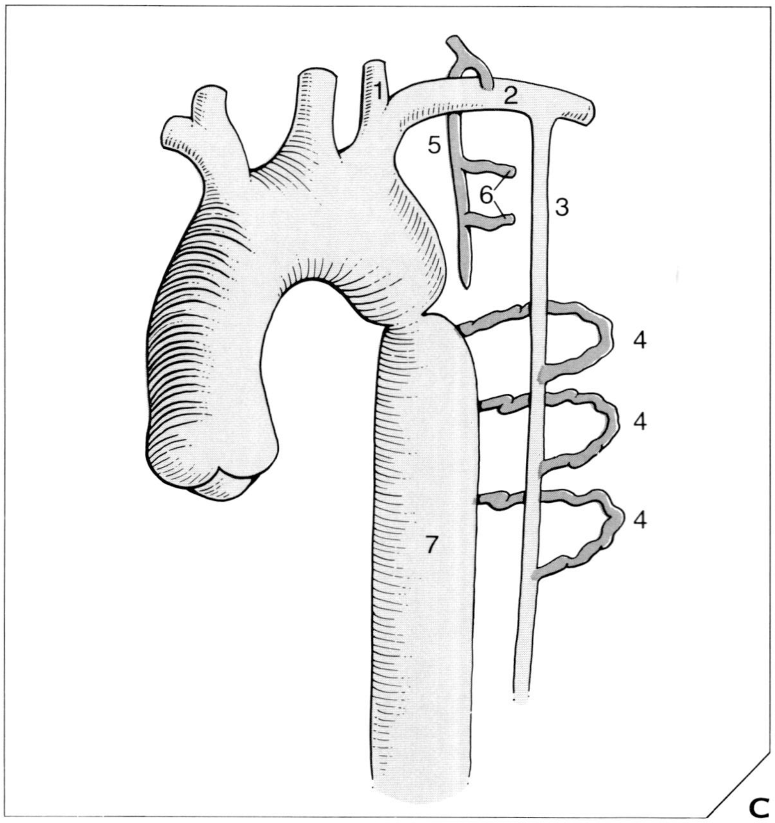

Fig. 12.27 Coarctation of the aorta. (A) Frontal chest film in an adult patient demonstrates prominence of the left lower heart border, indicating left ventricular enlargement. The aortic arch is diminutive. Note erosion ("notching") of the undersurface of the third and fourth ribs. (B) Detail of right upper ribs. The sclerotic margins of the erosions differentiate notching, which is caused by enlarged intercostal arteries, from the normal subcostal groove. (C) Rib notching associated with coarctation of the aorta is usually limited to the proximal third of the affected rib. It is rarely seen above the third or below the ninth rib. The sparing of the first and second ribs can be explained as follows: the first and second intercostal arteries arise from the so-called superior intercostal artery, which originates from the proximal segment of the subclavian artery (via the costocervical trunk); they do not connect with the distal aorta. Therefore, unlike the third through eighth intercostal arteries, which arise from the mammary arteries and connect with the descending thoracic aorta, the first and second intercostal arteries are not subjected to a high pressure gradient.

1 left vertebral artery
2 left subclavian artery
3 internal mammary artery
4 3rd, 4th, and 5th intercostal arteries
5 superior intercostal artery
6 1st and 2nd intercostal arteries
7 descending thoracic aorta

tation of the descending thoracic aorta. Even when rib notching is absent this constellation of findings strongly suggests the diagnosis of coarctation (in our experience, rib notching can seldom be appreciated before 8 years of age).

In teenagers and adults, the plain film findings are usually diagnostic (Figs. 12.26 and 12.27). The heart is typically enlarged,with prominence of the left lower heart border secondary to left ventricular hypertrophy. The ascending aorta is usually dilated and projects anteriorly and to the right. On the frontal projection, the dilated left subclavian artery forms a prominent bulge along the left upper mediastinal border. The hypoplastic distal aortic arch is inconspicuous or invisible on both frontal and lateral views (Fig. 12.28). The "3," or "reversed E," sign is usually evident, the dilated subclavian artery forming the upper part of the "3" and the dilated descending aorta the lower part of the "3." The mirror image ("reversed 3" sign) is seen on the frontal esophagram. The superior indentation of the barium column is produced by the distal aortic arch and the inferior indentation by the poststenotically dilated segment distal to the coarctation (Fig. 12.29).

Rib notching (caused by internal mammary–intercostal collaterals) is seen on plain films in 70 to 75 percent of adults with coarctation of the aorta (Fig. 12.27). In the remainder, collaterals are absent (about 5 percent) or the descending thoracic aorta is supplied by other collateral pathways (see Fig. 12.25).

Echocardiography

The anatomic features of the coarctation and the adjacent portions of the aorta are clearly demonstrated by two-dimensional echocardiography. Multiple projections are necessary for full evaluation of the aortic arch. The ascending and transverse segments and the proximal aortic isthmus are best seen on standard suprasternal notch, long axis, or high right parasternal views. The distal aortic isthmus and the proximal descending thoracic aorta are best seen on high left parasagittal images. Color Doppler imaging demonstrates turbulent flow through the stenotic segment.

MRI

Initial experience suggests that MRI is almost as accurate as cineangiography in the pretreatment evaluation of children with coarctation of the aorta. The site and characteristics of the coarcted segment, as well as associated cardiac abnormalities, are best demonstrated on spin–echo images obtained in the sagittal plane. Thin (5 mm) contiguous sections, using cardiac gating with acquisition at selected points in the cardiac cycle (usually mid to end systole), are usually the most informative, especially in young children in whom the area of coarctation is usually only a few millimeters in diameter. The aortic arch is optimally visualized on direct left anterior oblique images, which are particularly useful in excluding arch hypoplasia or a

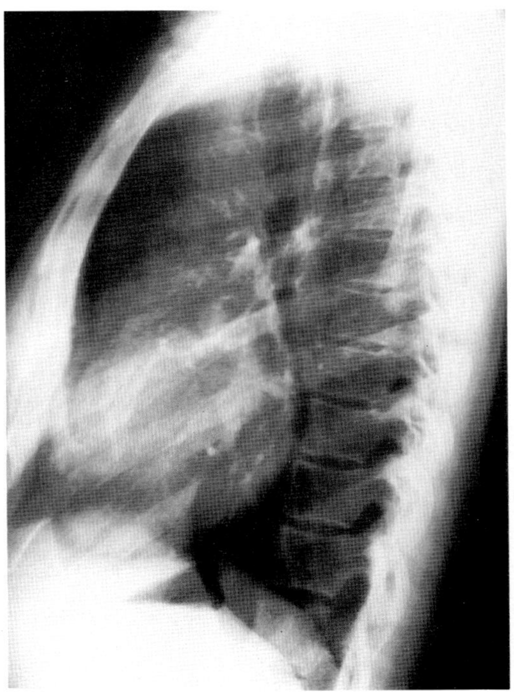

Fig. 12.28 Coarctation of the aorta. The aortic arch cannot be identified on the lateral film. The apparent absence of the aortic arch on the lateral projection should suggest the diagnosis of coarctation of the aorta.

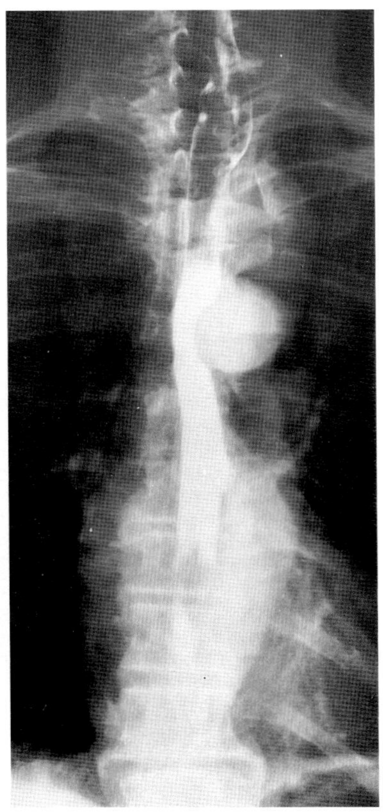

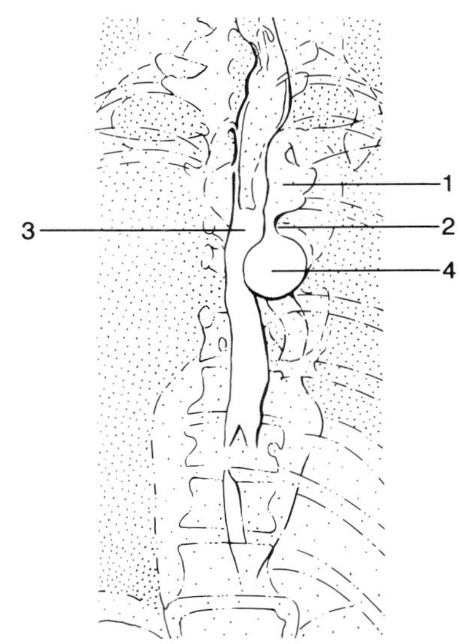

1 distal aortic arch
2 coarctation
3 esophagus
4 post stenotic dilatation

Fig. 12.29 Coarctation of the aorta. Frontal chest film with barium in the esophagus demonstrates the "reverse 3" or "E" sign. There are two discrete impressions of the esophagus: a proximal indentation (caused by the aortic arch and dilated subclavian artery) and a distal indentation (caused by the dilated poststenotic segment of the descending aorta).

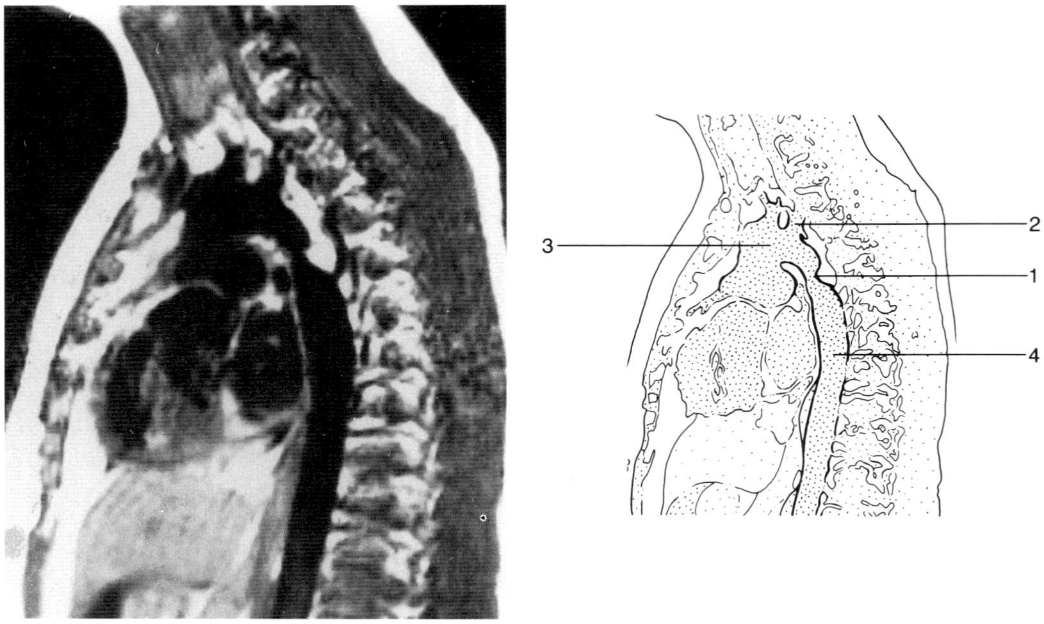

Fig. 12.30 Coarctation of the aorta. Left anterior oblique section of spin–echo MRI demonstrates the entire thoracic aorta. The coarcted segment appears as a narrowing at the junction between the aortic arch and the descending thoracic aorta. The left subclavian artery is dilated. The descending thoracic aorta is normal.

1	coarctation	3	aortic arch
2	left subclavian artery	4	descending thoracic aorta

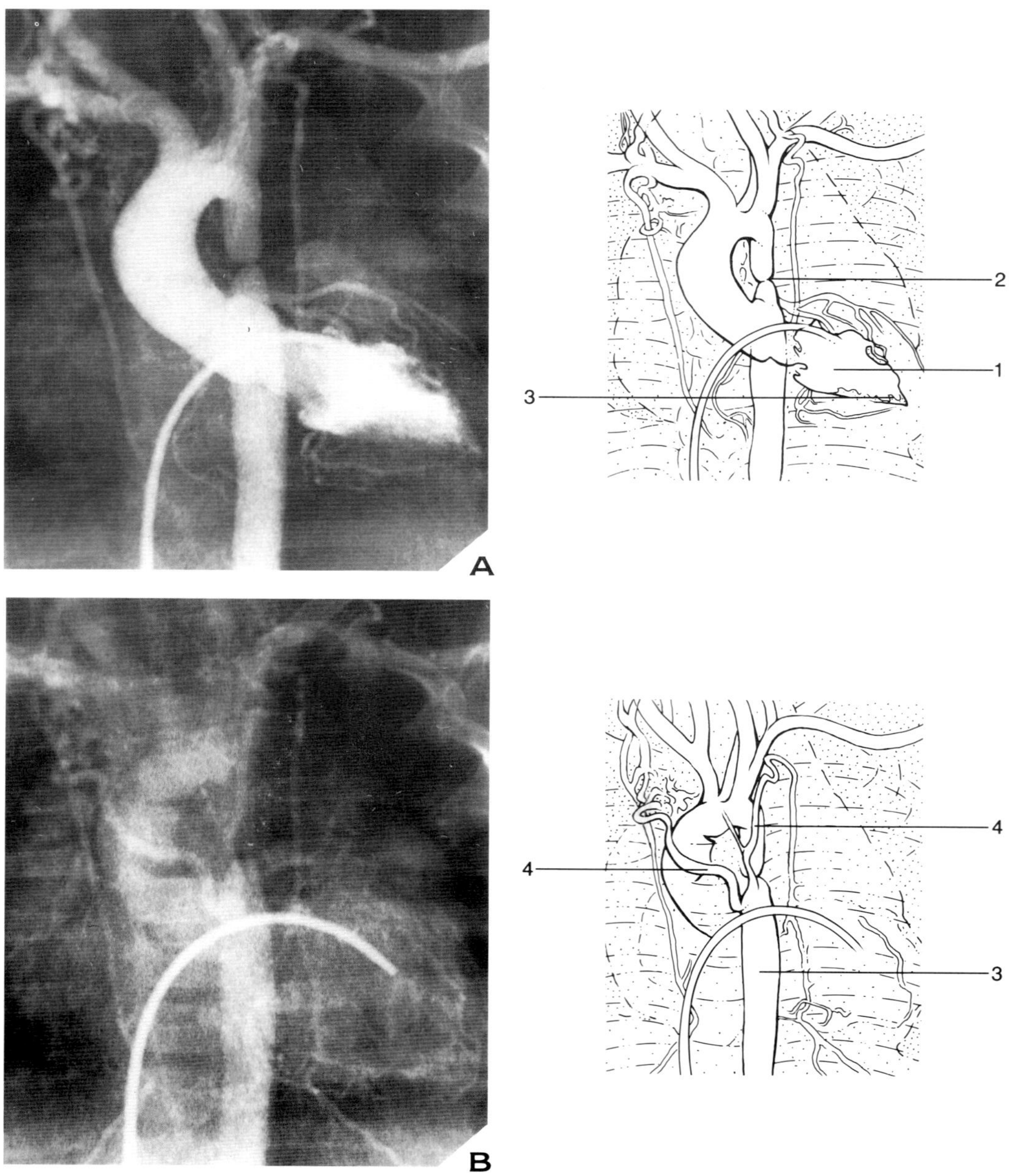

Fig. 12.31 Coarctation of the aorta. (A) Early phase of left ventriculogram in a 1-year-old child demonstrates a coarctation just beyond the origin of the left subclavian artery. Note the flat contour of the aortic arch and the dilated ascending aorta. (B) Late phase. Aberrant arteries arising from the subclavian arteries supply the descending thoracic aorta.

1	left ventricle	4	collaterals arising from right subclavian artery
2	coarctation		
3	descending thoracic aorta		

proximal coarctation. Collateral channels can frequently be identified on MRI; however, these vessels are much better studied by cineangiography (Fig. 12.30).

MRI has been used to identify candidates for balloon angioplasty (the results are poor in patients with long segments of hypoplasia) and to evaluate the coarctation site after surgery or angioplasty (see Chapter 16).

Cardiac Catheterization and Angiocardiography

Cardiac catheterization demonstrates elevated left ventricular systolic pressure and a pressure gradient across the coarcted segment. A gradient across the left ventricular outflow tract is occasionally present.

Thoracic aortography (aortic root or left ventricular injection) demonstrates the coarctation and the collateral blood supply (Fig. 12.31A). The coarcted segment is most clearly seen on the lateral projection (Fig. 12.32). The collateral channels (which arise from the subclavian arteries) are seen on the late phase. The most common collateral pathway consists of channels that connect the internal mammary arteries with the intercostals and the descending thoracic aorta (internal mammary–intercostal pathway). So-called aberrant arteries are not uncommon and may be visualized in such patients (Figs. 12.31B and 12.32B).

NONOBSTRUCTIVE COARCTATION OF THE AORTA

In some patients with coarctation, pressure measurements do not demonstrate a gradient across the narrow segment. Surgical repair is usually unwarranted, because these patients are ordinarily normotensive and do not have clinical or radiologic evidence of left ventricular overload. Nonobstructive coarctation is not innocuous, however, because turbulent flow may lead to thrombus formation or dissection. In addition, a bicuspid aortic valve may be present, which may become stenotic or incompetent.

Imaging

Plain films show a normal-sized heart and a prominent aortic arch. The descending aorta is usually prominent, and there may be marked angulation of the descending aorta (Fig. 12.33). The

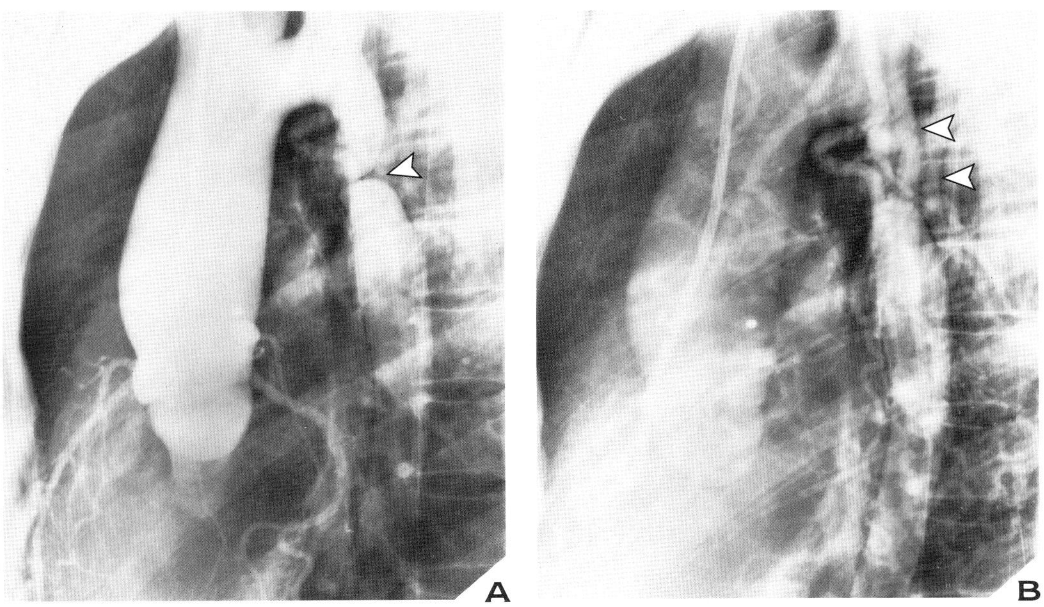

Fig. 12.32 Coarctation of the aorta. (A) Early phase of thoracic aortogram (lateral projection) demonstrates a severe coarctation *(arrow).* (B) Late phase demonstrates aberrant arteries *(arrows)* which provide collateral circulation to the descending thoracic aorta.

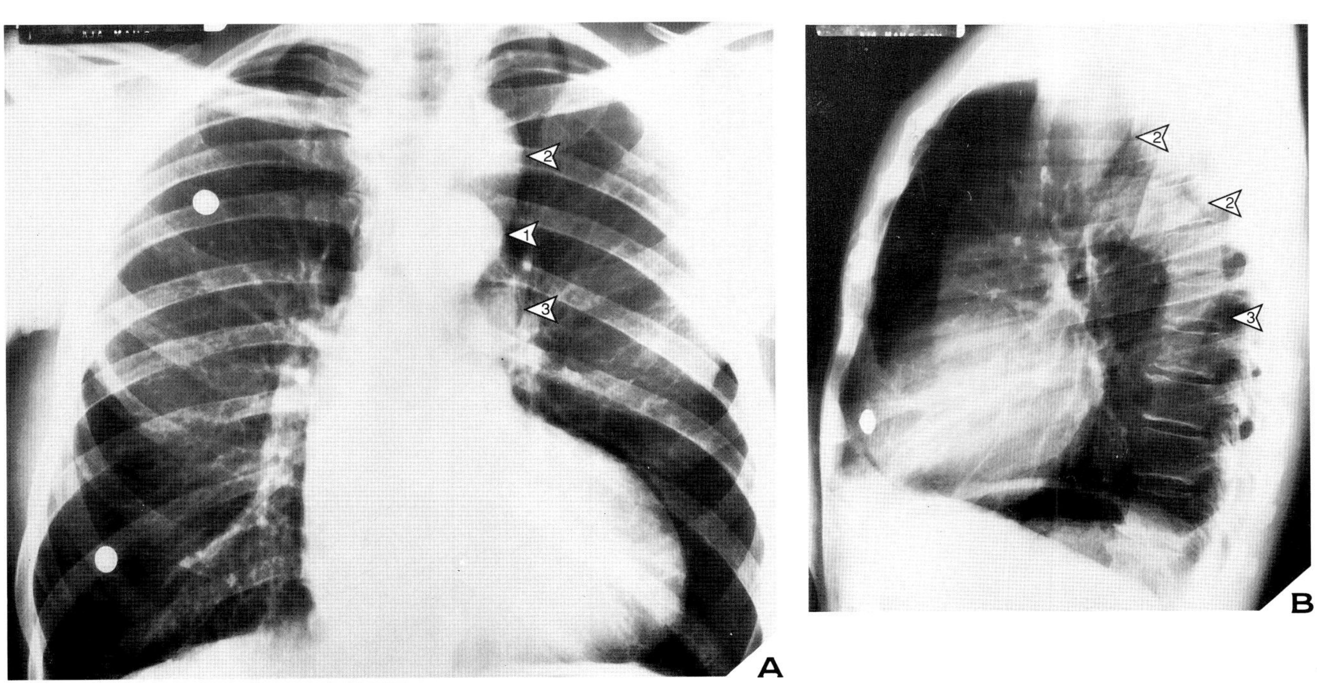

Fig. 12.33 Nonobstructive coarctation of the aorta. (A) Frontal and (B) lateral chest films in a patient with nonobstructive coarctation and valvular aortic stenosis demonstrate a prominent aortic arch (*arrow* 1 in A), marked dilatation of the left subclavian artery (*arrows* 2 in A and B), and angulation of the descending thoracic aorta (*arrows* 3 in A and B).

characteristic angulation of the descending aorta is clearly seen on thoracic aortograms obtained in the lateral or left anterior oblique projection (Fig. 12.34).

OBSTRUCTIONS ON THE RIGHT SIDE OF THE HEART

Obstructing lesions of the right side of the heart include congenital tricuspid stenosis, valvular pulmonic stenosis, and stenosis of the peripheral pulmonary arteries (peripheral pulmonary stenosis).

CONGENITAL TRICUSPID STENOSIS

Congenital tricuspid stenosis is rare. When tricuspid stenosis is encountered in childhood it is usually secondary to another disorder, either acquired (eg, rhematic heart disease) or congenital (eg, atrioventricular septal defect or hypoplastic right ventricle). The clinical picture is of systemic venous hypertension (dilated jugular veins, hepatomagaly, peripheral edema).

IMAGING AND INVASIVE DIAGNOSIS

Chest films in patients with severe tricuspid stenosis demonstrate enlargement of the right atrium and dilatation of the superior vena cava and azygos vein. Two-dimensional echocardiography demonstrates thickened tricuspid valve leaflets which do not open widely during diastole. Color Doppler imaging demonstrates high-velocity flow through the tricuspid valve in diastole. Cardiac catheterization, which can usually be omitted in patients with characteristic echocardiographic findings, demonstrates a diastolic gradient (greater than 4 mm Hg) between the right atrium and the right ventricle.

VALVULAR PULMONIC STENOSIS (PS)

MORPHOLOGY

In the most common type of valvular PS, the valve is normally formed; however, the leaflets are fused at the commissures, which prevents them from retracting completely during systole. Less often, the pulmonic valve is bicuspid; the deformed leaflets are fused at the commissures, resulting in PS of varying severity. In patients who present in infancy (''critical PS'') the

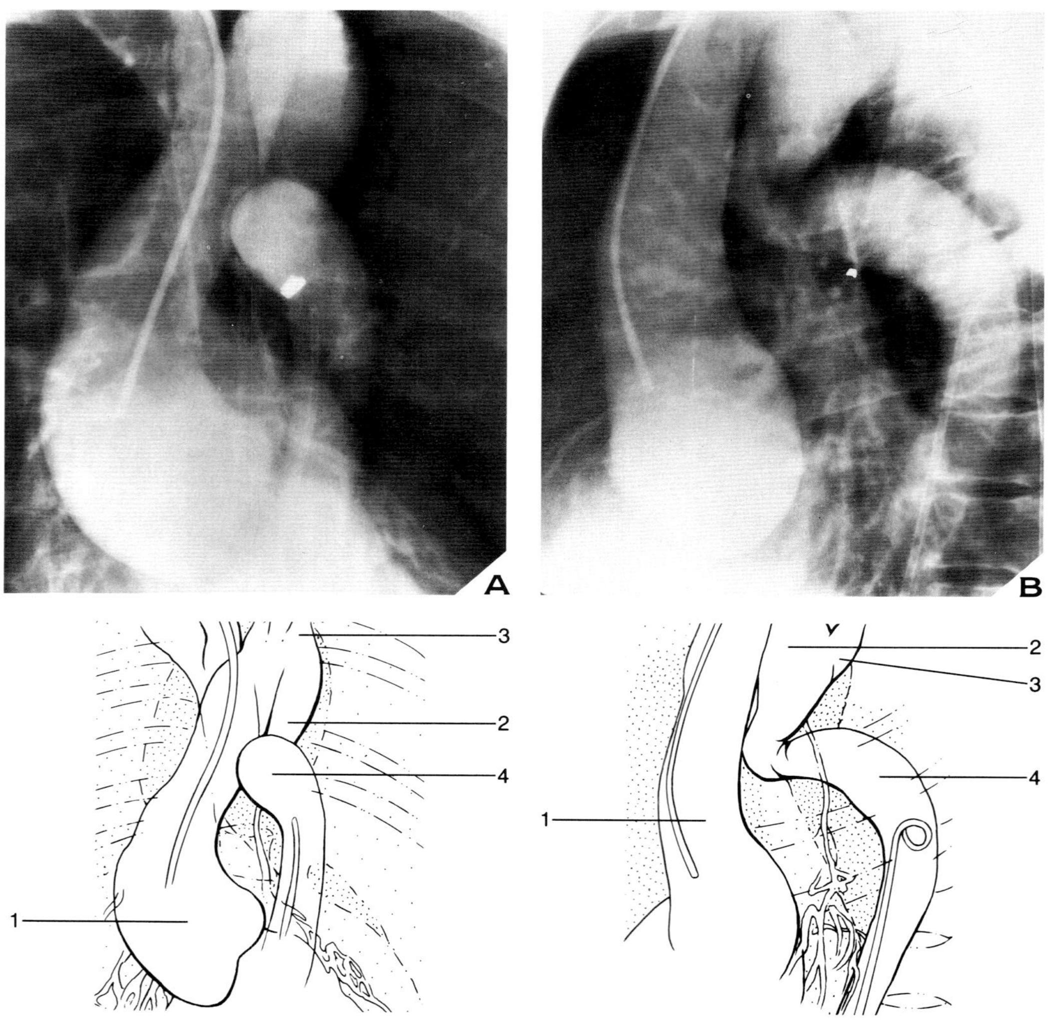

Fig. 12.34 Nonobstructive coarctation of the aorta. (A) Frontal and (B) lateral projections of thoracic aortogram demonstrate dilatation of the aortic arch and angulation of the descending thoracic aorta.

1 ascending aorta
2 aortic arch
3 dilated subclavian artery
4 descending thoracic aorta

pulmonic valve is usually dyplastic; the leaflets are thick, with rolled edges, and are fused at their free borders. This form of PS is often accompanied by right ventricular hypoplasia.

HEMODYNAMIC FEATURES

The pulmonary trunk and the left pulmonary artery are usually enlarged, owing to the jet effect produced by turbulent blood flow beyond the stenotic valve. The right pulmonary artery, which does not receive the full impact of the turbulent flow, is smaller than the left (Fig. 12.35). Blood flow to both lungs is normal, and the pulmonary vascular bed is normally developed.

Valvular PS leads to right ventricular outflow obstruction, which causes an increase in right ventricular pressure, which in turn may lead to tricuspid insufficiency. Pulmonary blood flow is severely reduced in infants with high-grade outflow obstruction (critical PS) (see below).

CLINICAL FEATURES

Neonates with high-grade outflow obstruction (critical PS) are critically ill, presenting with tachypnea and severe desaturation owing to right to left shunting at the atrial level. Cyanosis is usually absent if the atrial septum is intact.

After the neonatal period, infants with severe PS present with similar symptoms but are not as acutely ill. After the first year of life, children with severe PS are usually asymptomatic; most often the diagnosis is made when the characteristic murmur is detected on routine physical examination. Teenagers

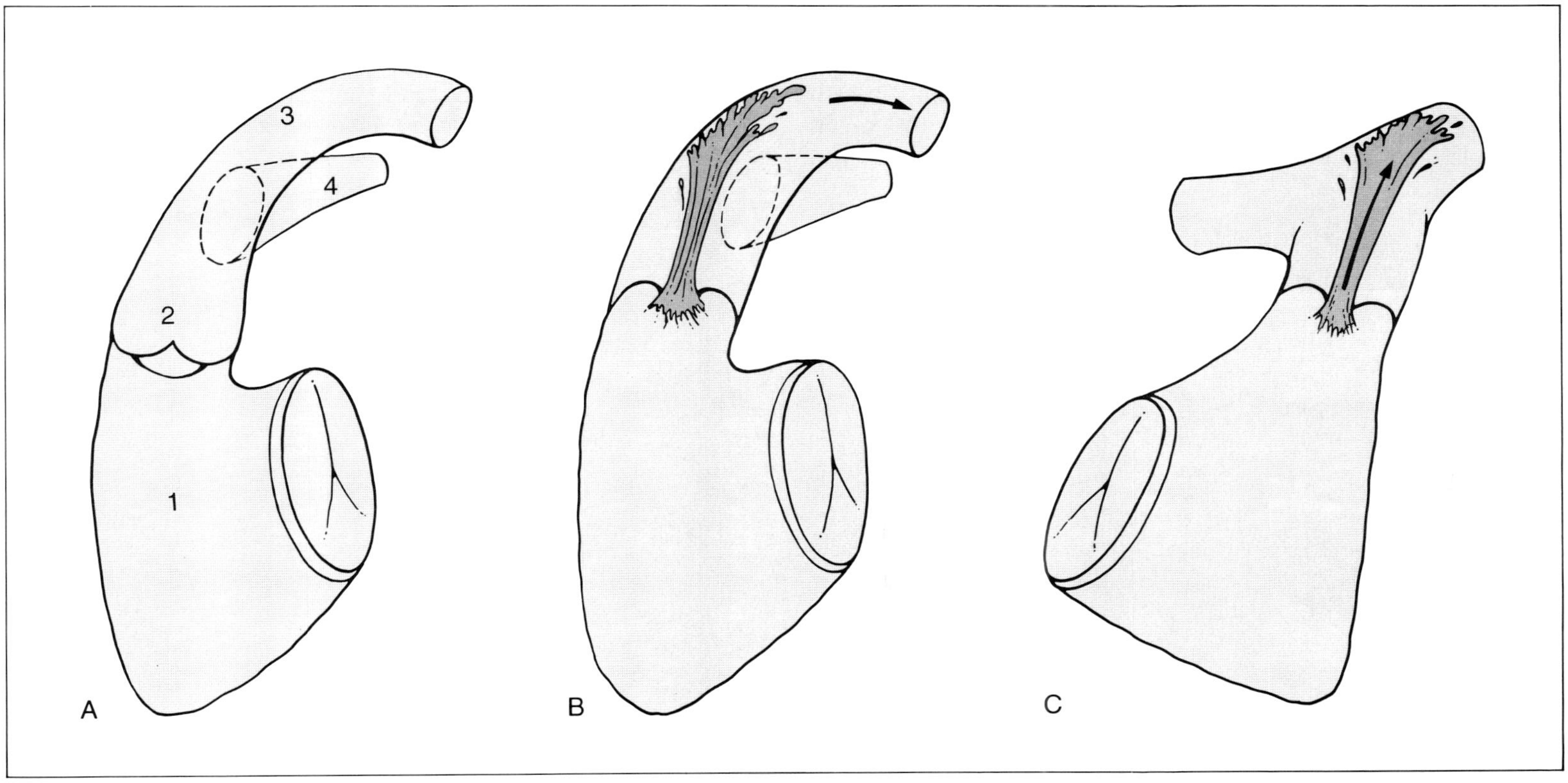

A *Normal* Lateral projection of right ventriculogram in systole.
B *Valvular pulmonic stenosis.* Lateral projection of right ventriculogram in systole
C *Valvular pulmonic stenosis.* Frontal projection of right ventriculogram in systole

1 right ventricle
2 pulmonary trunk
3 left pulmonary artery
4 right pulmonary artery

Fig. 12.35 Jet effect in valvular pulmonic stenosis. The jet caused by blood passing through the stenotic valve is directed towards the upper part of the pulmonary trunk and the left pulmonary artery, both of which receive its full impact. The right pulmonary artery arises at a right angle to the pulmonary trunk and does not receive the full impact of the jet. This explains why the left pulmonary artery is larger than the right pulmonary artery in patients with valvular pulmonic stenosis.

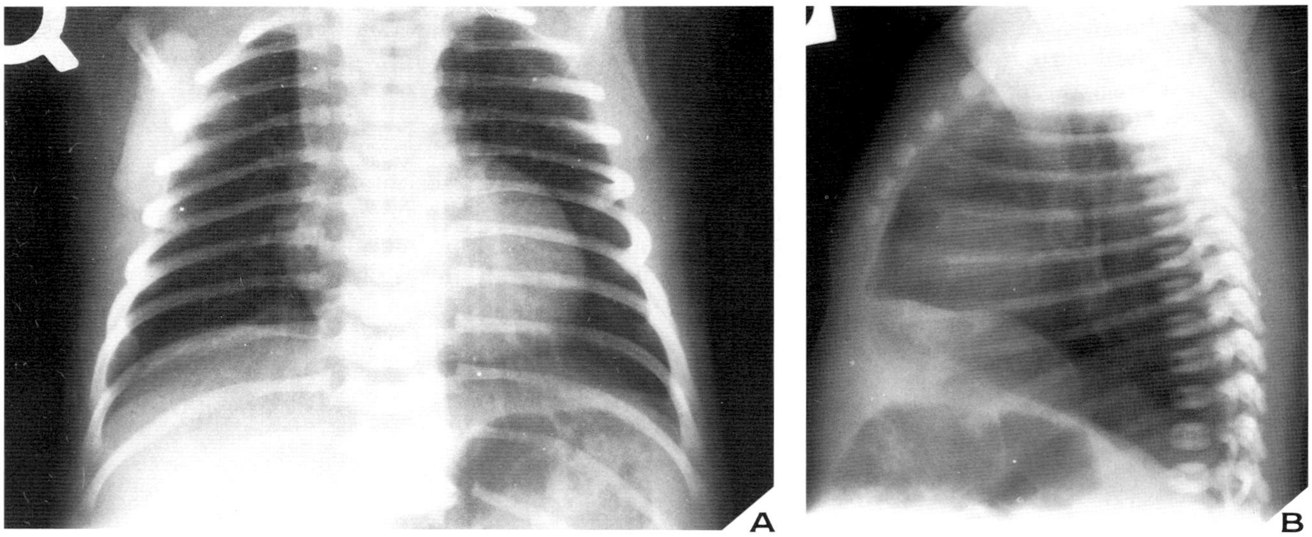

Fig. 12.36 Critical pulmonic stenosis. (A) Frontal and (B) lateral chest films of a cyanotic neonate show mild cardiac enlargement with prominence of the right ventricle. The pulmonary vasculature is diminished, and the pulmonary trunk cannot be identified. The right atrial contour is rounded, indicating right atrial enlargement secondary to tricuspid insufficiency.

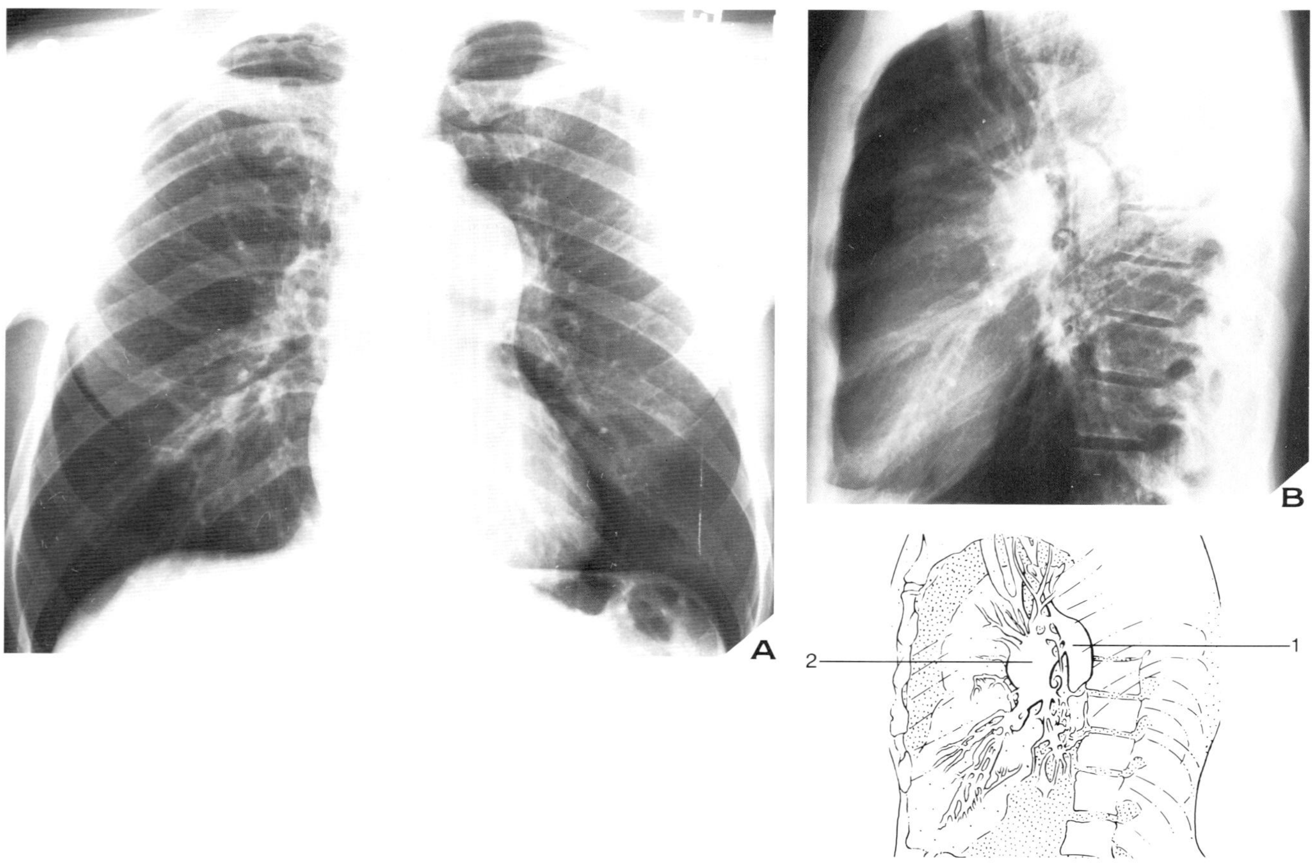

Fig. 12.37 Pulmonic valvular stenosis. (A) Frontal and (B) lateral chest films show marked dilatation of the pulmonic trunk and left pulmonary artery. Note the disparity in the size of the right and left pulmonary arteries in B.

1 left pulmonary artery
2 right pulmonary artery

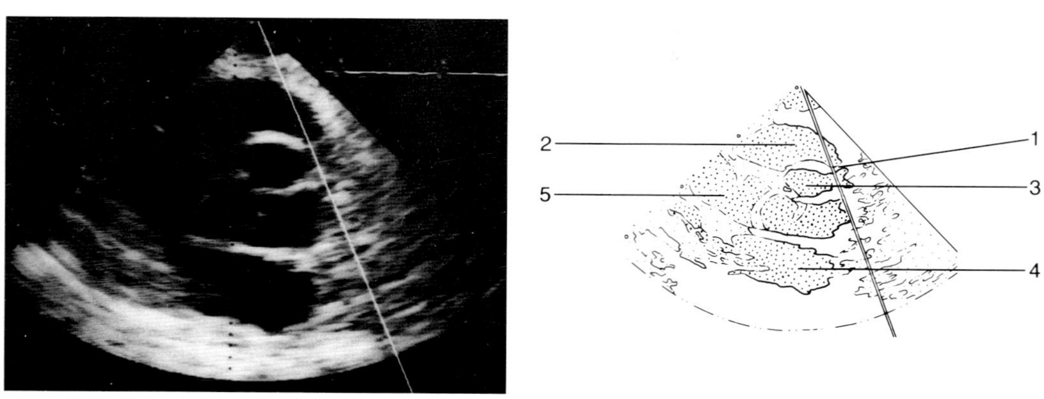

Fig. 12.38 Critical pulmonic stenosis. Two-dimensional echocardiogram. Short axis section at the level of the aortic valve shows severe stenosis of the pulmonic valve. The right ventricular outflow tract is slightly dilated.

1 stenotic pulmonic valve
2 dilated right ventricular outflow tract
3 aorta
4 left atrium
5 right atrium

and adults with severe valvular PS present with signs and symptoms of chronic right ventricular failure.

Infants with PS associated with severe ventricular hypoplasia are often asymptomatic, presenting later with progressive symptoms similar to those seen in tricuspid atresia.

IMAGING

Plain Films

Chest films of an infant with critical PS show an enlarged heart with dilatation of the right atrium secondary to tricuspid incompetence. The pulmonary vasculature is usually diminished (Fig. 12.36).

In older children and teenagers with pulmonic stenosis, chest films typically show right ventricular enlargement and prominence of the pulmonary trunk and main pulmonary arteries. Although both pulmonary arteries are prominent, the left is usually larger; this disparity is best appreciated on the lateral projection (Fig. 12.37).

Echocardiography

Two-dimensional echocardiography is diagnostic in an infant with critical PS. The valve leaflets are thick (they are usually fused), and their motion is restricted. The tricuspid valve is usually incompetent and the right ventricle may be hypoplastic (Fig. 12.38).

MRI

Transverse spin–echo images obtained at the level of the pulmonic annulus demonstrate a small annulus (as compared with that of the aortic valve). Cine images demonstrate turbulence in the pulmonary trunk during systole.

Cardiac Catheterization and Angiocardiography

In patients with severe pulmonic stenosis, cardiac catheterization demonstrates increased right ventricular systolic pressure and a significant gradient across the pulmonic valve.

The pertinent anatomic features are clearly shown by right ventriculography. During systole, the stenotic valve appears as a dome with a central aperture (Figs. 12.39 and 12.40); partial collapse of the sinuses of Valsalva may be evident on the lateral projection (Fig. 12.39B). A jet of opacified blood can be seen just beyond the valve. The size of the jet roughly corresponds to the cross-sectional area of the stenotic orifice, which may be

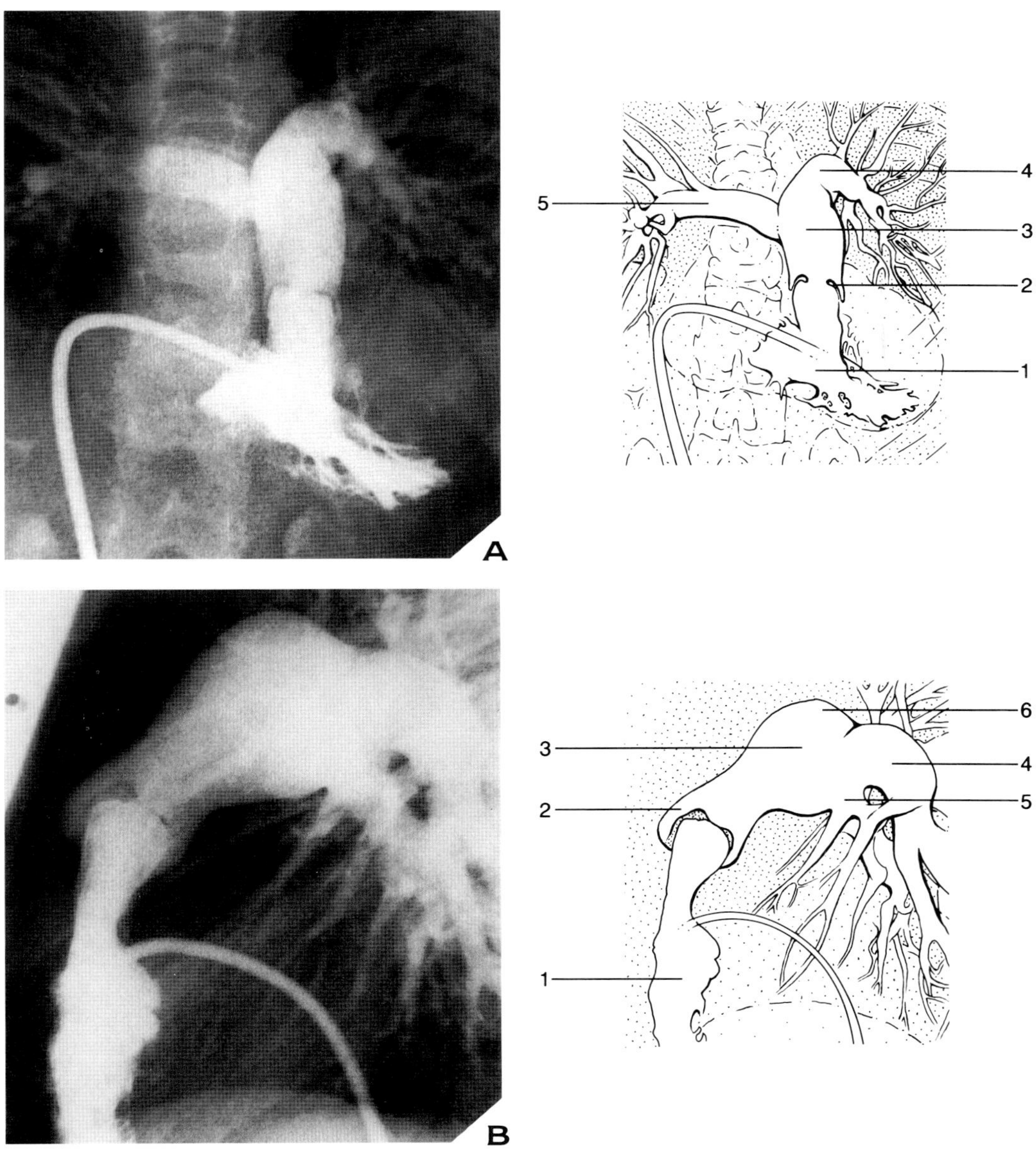

Fig. 12.39 Pulmonic valvular stenosis. (A) Frontal and (B) lateral projections of right ventriculogram show "doming" of the stenotic pulmonic valve during systole. There is post-stenotic dilatation of the pulmonary trunk with a dilated ductus diverticulum. The left pulmonary artery is larger than the right.

1 right ventricle
2 dome-shaped pulmonic valve
3 pulmonary trunk
4 left pulmonary artery
5 right pulmonary artery
6 dilated ductus diverticulum

markedly restricted in patients with severe PS (Fig. 12.40). Both the dilated pulmonary trunk and the disproportionate enlargement of the main pulmonary arteries, characteristic features of valvular PS, are well demonstrated on the frontal projection (Fig. 12.39A). Patients with severe PS frequently have a prominent ductus diverticulum (Fig. 12.39).

PERIPHERAL PULMONARY STENOSIS

Peripheral pulmonary stenosis (PPS) is characterized by narrowing of the major pulmonary arteries. It may involve the pulmonary trunk, the bifurcation, the right or left pulmonary arteries, or the lobar and/or segmental branches. The stenotic lesions are usually multiple and bilateral, varying in severity from minimal narrowing to almost complete occlusion of the affected artery. PPS may occur as an isolated lesion, although it is most often associated with Williams syndrome (supravalvular aortic stenosis, hypercalcemia during infancy, a peculiar elfin facies, and mental retardation). PPS is relatively common in patients who contracted transplacental rubella infection early in gestation (rubella embryopathy).

HEMODYNAMIC AND CLINICAL FEATURES

The clinical picture varies widely: mildly affected individuals are asymptomatic, whereas those with widespread involvement may develop severe congestive heart failure. Exertional dyspnea and excessive fatigability are the usual manifestations in childhood. Severely affected individuals have clinical signs of right ventricular failure (eg, distended jugular veins) with ECG evidence of severe right ventricular overload. Clubbing and hemoptysis occur late in the course of disease and are associated with an ominous prognosis.

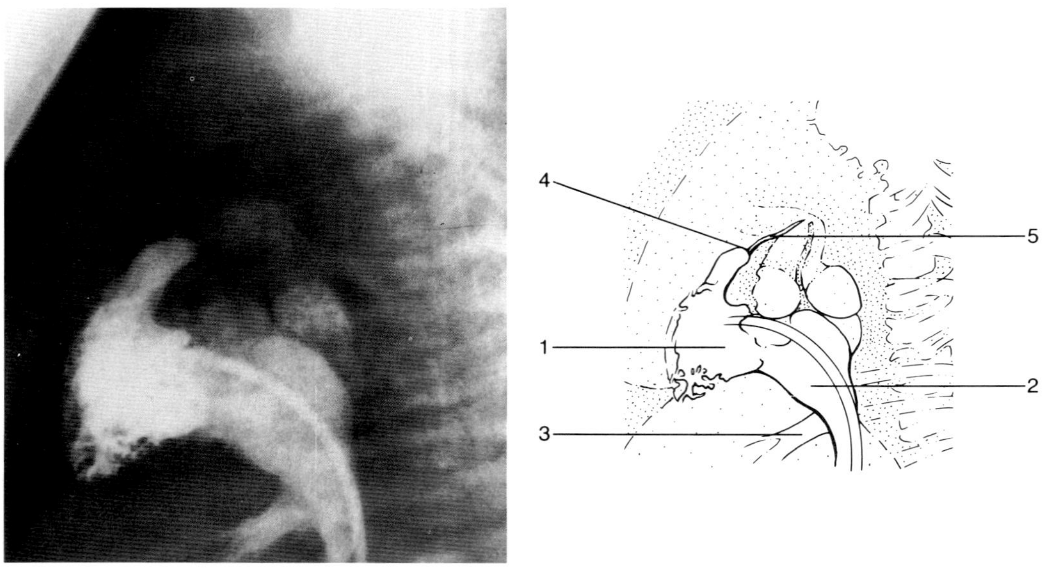

Fig. 12.40 Critical pulmonic valvular stenosis in a neonate. Lateral projection of right ventriculogram shows severe pulmonic stenosis with marked tricuspid regurgitation (note dense opacification of right atrium, inferior vena cava, and dilated hepatic veins). At operation (pulmonic valvulotomy), the pulmonic valve was found to consist of a membrane with a small central aperture.

1 right ventricle
2 right atrium
3 hepatic veins
4 stenotic pulmonic valve
5 jet of opacified blood

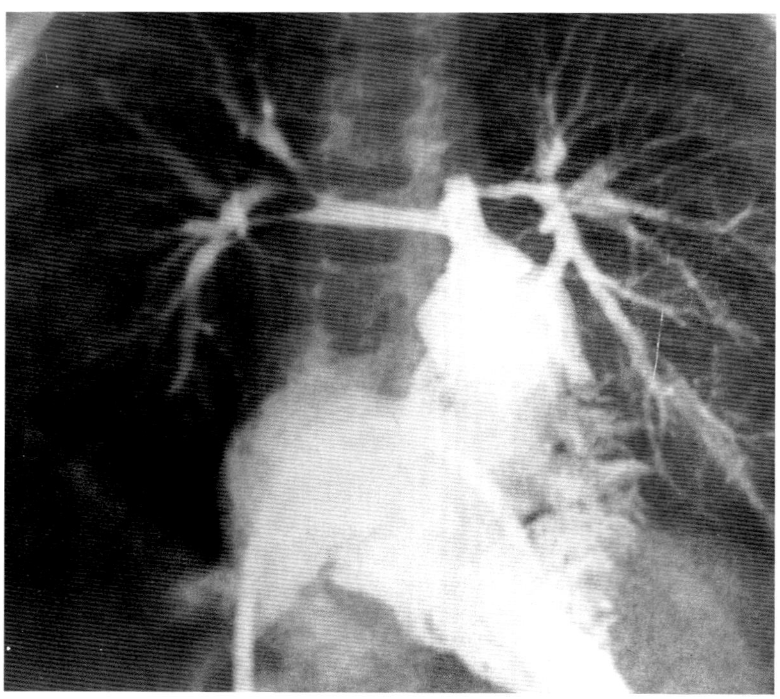

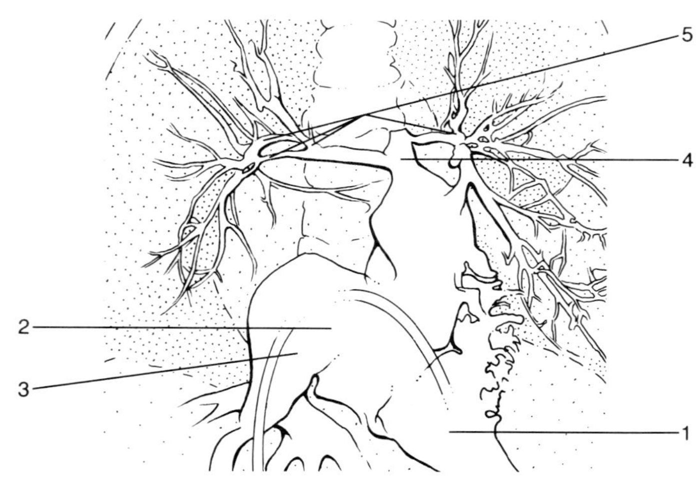

1 right ventricle
2 right atrium
3 inferior vena cava
4 small pulmonary trunk
5 stenotic pulmonary arteries

Fig. 12.41 Peripheral pulmonary stenosis. Frontal projection of right ventriculogram demonstrates a large right ventricle with a wide outflow tract and a small pulmonary trunk. The right and left pulmonary arteries are very small and tubular, and there is focal narrowing of the lobar and segmental branches. Note opacification of the right atrium and inferior vena cava, indicating the presence of moderate tricuspid insufficiency. This patient also had supravalvular aortic stenosis (not illustrated).

IMAGING AND INVASIVE DIAGNOSIS

Plain Films

The plain chest film findings are not diagnostic. If the pulmonary trunk is involved, it will be smaller than normal; the pulmonary trunk will be enlarged, however, if the stenosis is more peripheral. Pulmonary perfusion is usually normal, although localized or generalized pulmonary oligemia may be seen in some instances.

Cardiac Catheterization and Angiocardiography

Cardiac catheterization demonstrates increased pressure in the right ventricle, pulmonary trunk, and main pulmonary arteries.

On right ventriculography (Fig. 12.40) or pulmonary arteriography, the affected arteries appear as narrow, tubular channels which do not taper normally; distal to the stenotic segments the affected arteries are dilated (poststenotic dilatation) (Fig. 12.41). Although extensive bilateral involvement is the rule, on occasion only a single lobar or segmental branch is affected. The right ventricle is usually enlarged and hypertrophied, and tricuspid insufficiency may be present. Thoracic aortography is routinely performed to exclude coexistent supravalvular aortic stenosis.

CHAPTER 13

Valvular Insufficiency

Congenital cardiac malformations may lead to incompetence of the valves on the right or the left side of the heart. The most common cause of congenital tricuspid incompetence is Ebstein's malformation; less frequent causes include congenital tricuspid insufficiency and Uhl's anomaly. (The latter is a malformation of the inlet portion of the right ventricle in which the ventricle is fibrotic owing to congenital absence of the myocardium, resulting in dilatation of the tricuspid annulus and tricuspid incompetence.) Pulmonic valvular insufficiency may result from congenital absence of the pulmonic valve leaflets; the pulmonic valve may also become incompetent in patients with pulmonary arterial hypertension. The most common cause of congenital mitral insufficiency is prolapse of one or both mitral leaflets. Dysplasia of the mitral leaflets is a rare cause of congenital mitral insufficiency. Although isolated congenital aortic valvular insufficiency is rare, the aortic valve may be incompetent in patients with VSD or sinus of Valsalva aneurysm.

CHAPTER LABELING KEY

RA	right atrium	LV	left ventricle
LA	left atrium	Ao	aorta
RV	right ventricle	PT	pulmonary trunk

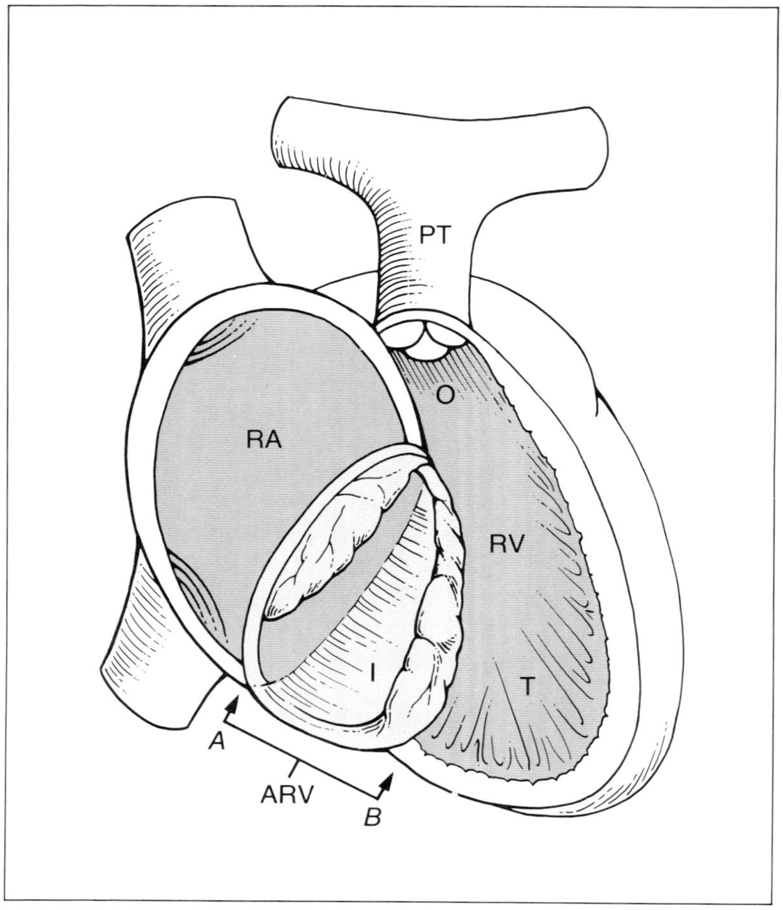

A	annulus of the tricuspid valve	T	trabecular portion of right ventricle
ARV	atrialized (smooth) portion of right ventricle	O	outlet portion of right ventricle
B	point beyond which septal leaflet is no longer plastered to right ventricular wall	I	inlet portion of right ventricle

Fig. 13.1 Ebstein's malformation. The tricuspid annulus *(A)* is in its normal position; between *A* and *B* the septal leaflet of the tricuspid valve is plastered against the right ventricular wall. The region between *A* and *B* represents the atrialized (smooth) portion of the right ventricle.

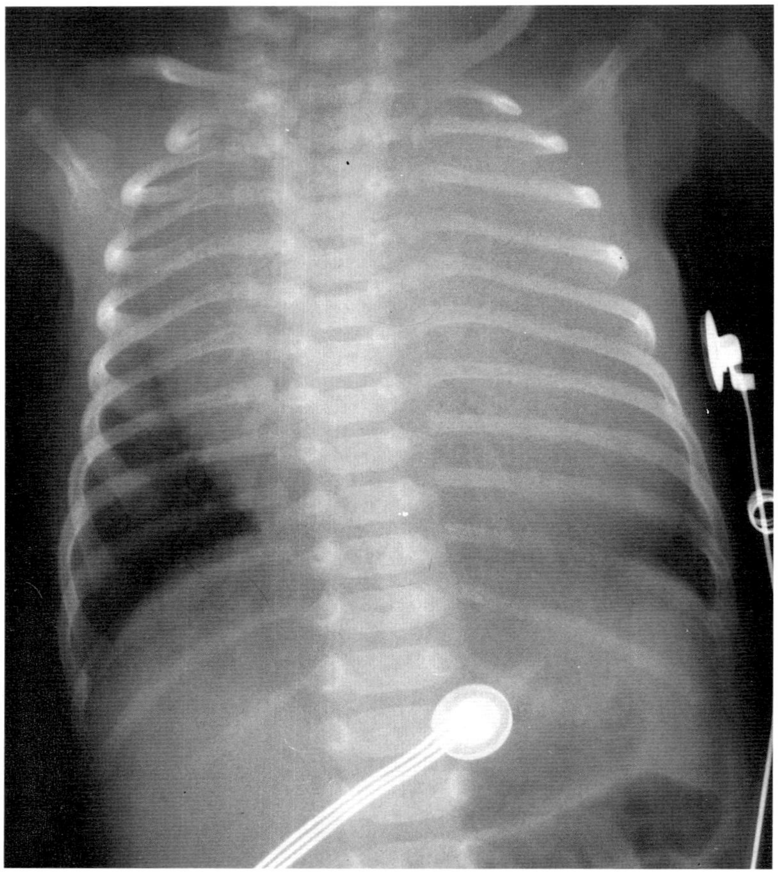

Fig. 13.2 Ebstein's malformation. Chest film of a cyanotic newborn infant shows massive cardiomegaly and markedly diminished pulmonary vascularity. Echocardiography revealed Ebstein's malformation with fusion of the tricuspid valve leaflets and a large atrial septal defect.

VALVULAR INSUFFICIENCY ON THE RIGHT SIDE OF THE HEART

EBSTEIN'S MALFORMATION

MORPHOLOGY

In Ebstein's malformation, one or more tricuspid valve leaflets are plastered to the right ventricular wall (Fig. 13.1). The septal leaflet is invariably involved, and the inferior leaflet is occasionally involved; the anterior leaflet is only rarely affected. In the most severely affected hearts, all three tricuspid leaflets are involved (in some instances the leaflets are fused distally). The malformed leaflets separate from the ventricular wall at the junction between the inlet and trabeculated portions of the right ventricle. The thin-walled inlet region, which has relatively few muscle fibers and contracts poorly, has been termed the "atrialized" portion of the right ventricle. The right ventricular outflow tract is usually displaced to the left of the pulmonic valve. Ebstein's malformation is frequently found in association with an ASD of the fossa ovalis type or with a dilated patent foramen ovale.

HEMODYNAMIC FEATURES

Ebstein's malformation of the nonobstructive type leads to severe tricuspid insufficiency, which in turn results in right to left shunting through a patent foramen ovale or ASD. The pulmonary trunk and the main right pulmonary arteries, as well as their lobar and segmental branches, are usually decreased in size owing to the decreased pulmonary blood flow.

In the less common obstructive form of Ebstein's malformation, in which the fused leaflets form a membranous barrier between the atrialized and functional portions of the right ventricle, the hemodynamic manifestations are similar to those of tricuspid atresia.

CLINICAL FEATURES

Infants with the obstructive form of Ebstein's malformation typically present during the first week of life with cyanosis secondary to right to left shunting, severe cardiomegaly, and congestive heart failure.

In patients with the more common nonobstructive form of Ebstein's malformation, the clinical manifestations depend on the degree of right ventricular malfunction, the severity of the tricuspid insufficiency, and the magnitude of the right to left shunt. Signs and symptoms may be absent in patients with mild tricuspid insufficiency and minimal right ventricular dysfunction. Patients with severe tricuspid insufficiency exhibit signs of systemic venous hypertension (ascites, peripheral edema). The degree of cyanosis depends on the magnitude of the right to left shunt at the atrial level. Older children typically present with mild dyspnea and fatigue. Exercise tolerance decreases with the onset of congestive heart failure. About one third of patients with Ebstein's malformation exhibit severe cyanosis, whereas mild desaturation is the rule in the rest. Physical examination reveals marked cardiomegaly with a quiet precordium and apex, reflecting the large size and increased compliance of the right atrium and the atrialized portion of the right ventricle. A pansystolic murmur of tricuspid insufficiency, maximal at the lower left sternal border, is usually present.

IMAGING AND INVASIVE DIAGNOSIS

Plain Films

The chest films of neonates and young infants with the obstructive form of Ebstein's malformation show marked cardiac enlargement, often with a giant right atrium, and diminished pulmonary circulation (Fig. 13.2). In patients with the nonobstructive form, the frontal projection typically shows a large heart with a globular configuration reflecting right ventricular and right atrial enlargement; the lateral projection (Fig. 13.3)

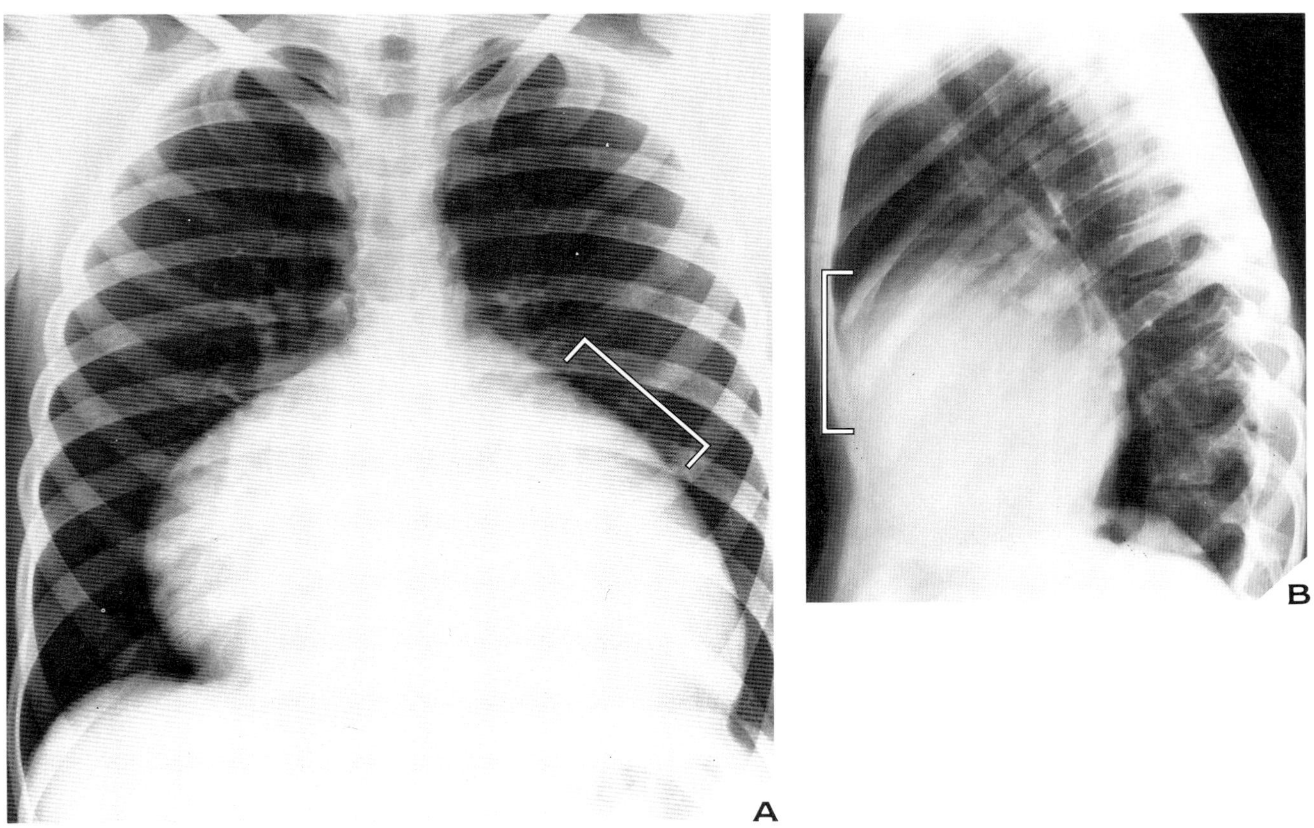

Fig. 13.3 Ebstein's malformation. (A) Frontal and (B) lateral chest films in a patient with tricuspid insufficiency caused by an Ebstein's malformation show marked cardiac enlargement. On the frontal projection, the right atrium bulges to the right; on the lateral, it projects anteriorly and superiorly, filling in the retrosternal space (*brace* in B). The right ventricular outflow tract is displaced to the left, producing a localized deformity of the left upper heart border (*brace* in A). The vascular pedicle is small. The pulmonary vasculature is diminished owing to the right to left shunt at atrial level.

shows an increased zone of contact between the heart and the anterior chest wall. The enlarged right atrial appendage encroaches on the retrosternal space. The vascular pedicle is usually narrow owing to the hypoplasia of the main pulmonary artery. The left atrium and left ventricle are usually normal. (When the right atrium and right ventricle are markedly enlarged, the left-side chambers are displaced posteriorly, and therefore may appear enlarged on plain films.) The pulmonary vascularity may be normal or decreased, depending on the size of the right to left shunt.

Echocardiography

Echocardiography accurately depicts the characteristic features of Ebstein's malformation, ie, the abnormal attachment of the septal leaflet of the tricuspid valve and the paradoxical motion of the ventricular septum (Fig. 13.4).

MRI

The characteristic features of Ebstein's malformation are well seen on axial and coronal ECG-gated spin–echo images (Figs. 13.5 and 13.6).

Cardiac Catheterization and Angiocardiography

Cardiac catheterization and angiocardiography, in conjunction with echocardiography, accurately depict the functional and morphological features of the disorder. In most patients with Ebstein's malformation the right atrial pressure is elevated, and the venous pulse contours show a dominant "V" wave with a steep "Y" descent. The atrial pressure pulse may be normal, despite severe tricuspid insufficiency, in patients with marked right atrial dilatation. The right ventricular and pulmonary artery pressures are usually normal. The right ventricular end diastolic pres-

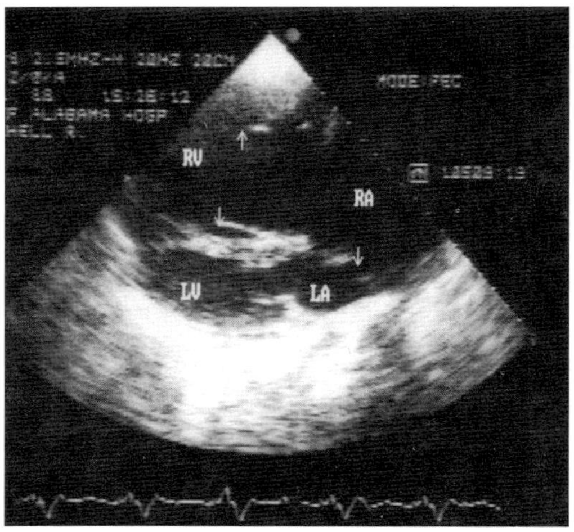

Fig. 13.4 Ebstein's malformation. Long axial parasternal section of 2-D echocardiogram shows right ventricular and right atrial enlargement. The septal leaflet of the tricuspid valve is plastered to the ventricular septum, preventing normal closure of the tricuspid orifice. The ventricular septum is intact. There is an atrial septal defect.

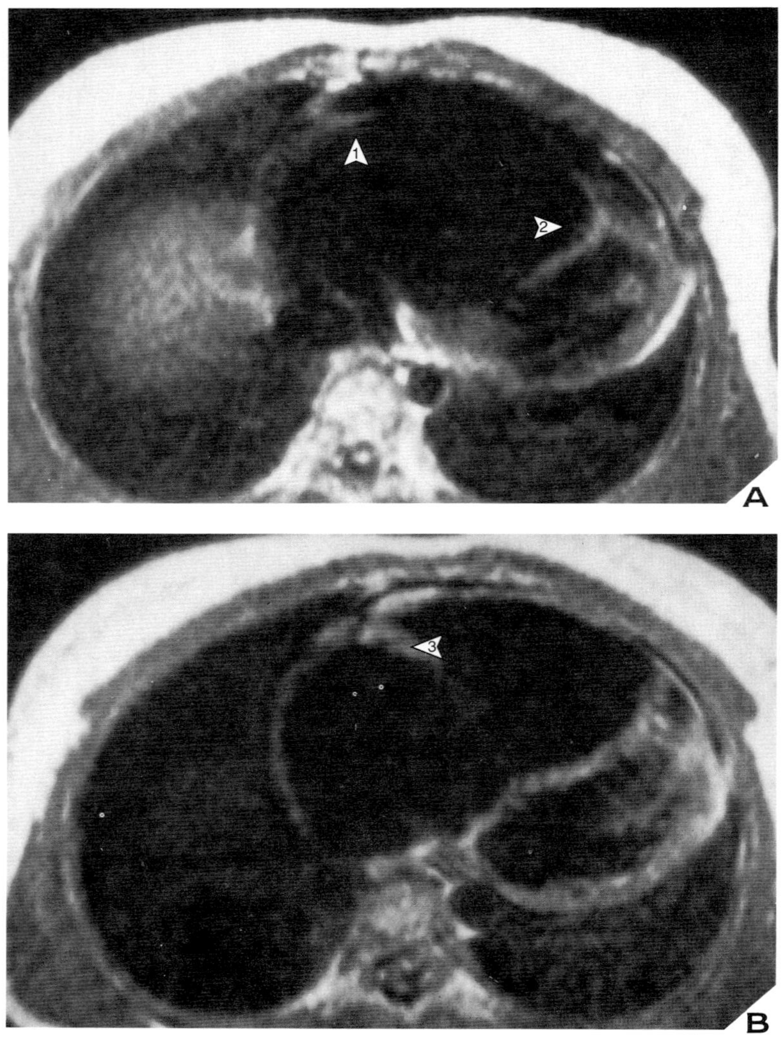

Fig. 13.5 Ebstein's malformation, (A, B) Axial MR images in a 12-year-old boy with Ebstein's malformation shows a markedly enlarged right atrium and the atrialized portion of the right ventricle. The proximal attachment of the anterior tricuspid leaflet to the atrioventricular junction (arrow 1) and its distal attachment to the ventricular septum (arrow 2) are well seen in A. The septal leaflet is plastered against the ventricular septum. The muscular ridge separating the compressed trabecular portion of the right ventricle from its atrialized portion is seen in A and B. The triangular structure in B (arrow 3) is adipose tissue between the right atrium and the dilated right ventricular outflow tract. The ventricular septum bulges towards the left ventricle. (Reproduced with permission from Link KM et al: MR Imaging of Ebstein anomaly; Results in four cases. *AJR* 1988; 150:363. ©American Roentgen Society)

sure may be elevated in some patients with severe tricuspid insufficiency; it may be decreased or normal if there is a large right to left shunt at atrial level. The great majority of patients with Ebstein's malformation have systemic arterial desaturation secondary to right to left shunting at the atrial level.

When the catheter is pulled back from the functional portion of the right ventricle into the atrialized portion, the intracardiac electrocardiogram demonstrates continuous right ventricular electrical potentials while the pressure pulse changes from a ventricular to an atrial pattern.

The morphologic features of Ebstein's malformation are best seen on right ventriculograms obtained in the elongated right anterior oblique projection, which demonstrate the atrialized and trabecular portions of the right ventricle, the normal position of the tricuspid annulus, and the point at which the plastered tricuspid leaflets separate from the right ventricular wall.

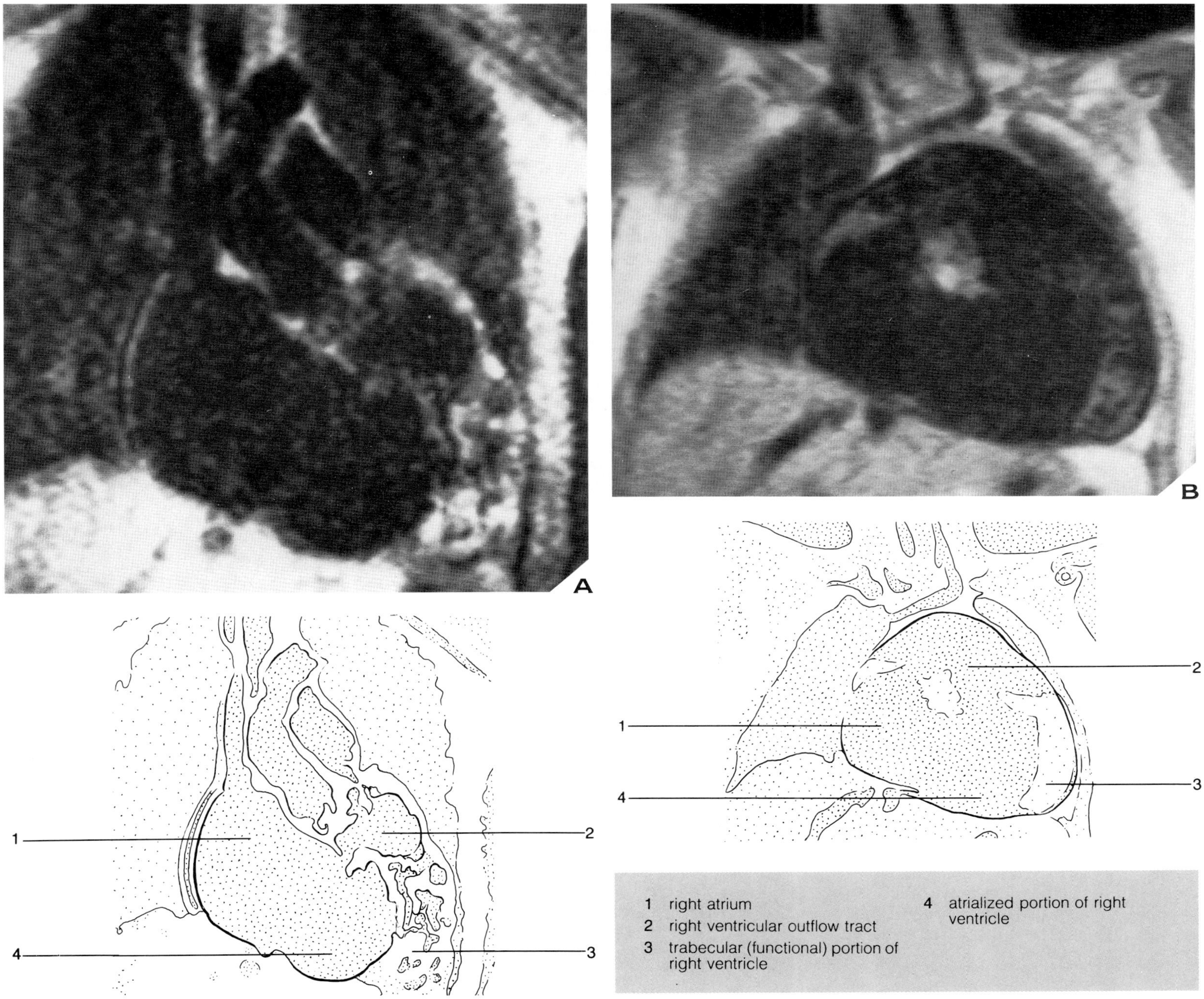

Fig. 13.6 Ebstein's malformation. Coronal MR scans in a 15-year-old boy (A) and a 10-year-old boy (B) with Ebstein's malformation show the characteristic features of this anomaly. The atrialized and compressed trabecular portions of the right ventricle are separated by a leftward convex vertical structure, which represents the junction between the atrialized and the functional portion of the right ventricle. The functional portion of the right ventricle extends cephalad into the right ventricular outflow tract. (Reproduced with permission from Link KM et al: MR imaging of Ebstein anomaly: Results in four cases. *AJR* 1988; 150:363. ©American Roentgen Society)

On the frontal projection, the right ventricular outflow tract is displaced to the left and forms the left cardiac contour (Fig. 13.7).

ABSENCE OF THE PULMONIC VALVE LEAFLETS

In this malformation the leaflets of the pulmonic valve are absent; the pulmonic valve is represented by a fibrous ring or diaphragm. Although this anomaly may exist as an isolated lesion, it is usually associated with tetralogy of Fallot. In such cases the VSD is usually very large, encompassing the entire outlet portion of the right ventricle. The pulmonic valve leaflets are absent in 3 to 5 percent of patients with tetralogy of Fallot.

HEMODYNAMIC AND CLINICAL FEATURES

The hemodynamic manifestations are those of pulmonic insufficiency with right ventricular volume overload. The pulmonary arteries arteries dilate during systole and collapse during diastole. The tricuspid valve is usually incompetent. The pulmonary trunk and the right and left pulmonary arteries are massively dilated, becoming progressively larger with increasing age. Although the lobar and segmental arteries are relatively small, they are normal.

Infants with absence of the pulmonic valve leaflets typically present with respiratory symptoms (eg, pneumonia, bronchospasm, respiratory failure). Children typically present with a history of recurrent respiratory infections, limited exercise tolerance, and growth retardation. Physical examination reveals both a systolic and a diastolic murmur.

IMAGING AND INVASIVE DIAGNOSIS

Plain Films

Infants with isolated absence of the pulmonic valve leaflets exhibit cardiomegaly with massive right ventricular and right atrial enlargement. The pulmonary trunk and main pulmonary arteries are markedly dilated, and the peripheral vascular markings are sparse. Compression of the main bronchi by the massively dilated central pulmonary arteries may cause obstructive emphysema of one or more lobes.

The plain film findings in infants in whom the anomaly is associated with tetralogy of Fallot are very similar to those in infants with isolated absence of the pulmonic valve leaflets. A right aortic arch strongly suggests an associated tetralogy.

In older children and teenagers, plain films show right ventricular enlargement and posterior displacement of the left ventricle. The pulmonary trunk and the right and left pulmonary arteries are massively enlarged, whereas the peripheral vascular markings are relatively inconspicuous (Fig. 13.7). The discrepancy in the size of the central and peripheral vessels is most dramatic on films obtained during diastole. This discrepancy is less conspicuous during systole; indeed, the pulmonary vasculature may appear relatively normal on a film exposed during systole. (The marked moment-

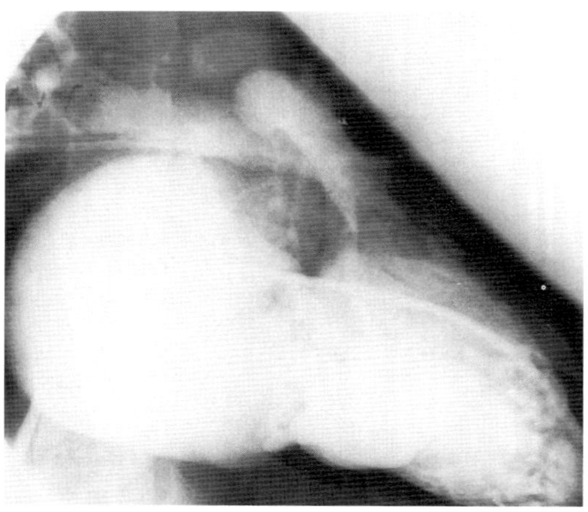

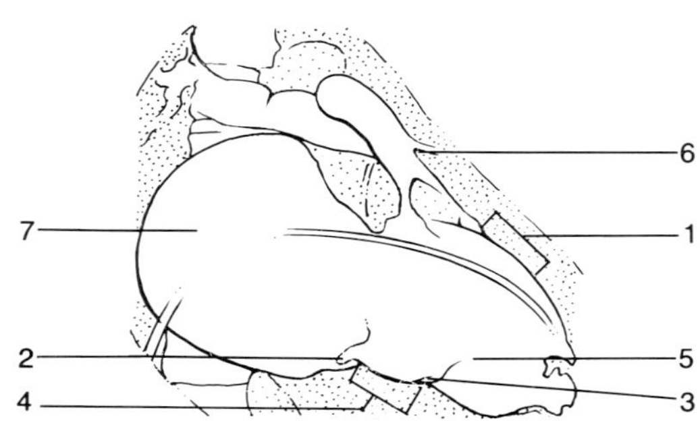

Fig. 13.7 Ebstein's malformation. Frontal projection of right ventriculogram shows displacement of the right ventricular outflow tract to the left (it forms the left heart border). The tricuspid annulus is in normal position. The abnormal attachment of the adherent septal leaflet of the tricuspid valve defines the extent of the atrialized portion of the right ventricle. Note the dense opacification of the right atrium, indicating severe tricuspid insufficiency.

1 right ventricular outflow tract (displaced to left)
2 tricuspid annulus
3 abnormal attachment of adherent septal leaflet
4 atrialized portion of right ventricle
5 trabecular portion of right ventricle
6 pulmonic valve
7 right atrium

to-moment changeability of the pulmonary vasculature is most obvious on fluoroscopy. However, because chest films are randomly exposed at different points in the cardiac cycle, it can usually be appreciated on serial films.) The discrepancy between the central and peripheral vessels is especially striking in patients with tetralogy of Fallot, whose lungs are underperfused owing to the coexistent right to left shunt and right ventricular outflow tract stenosis.

Echocardiography

The right ventricular outflow tract, pulmonary annulus, abnormal valve leaflets, pulmonary trunk, and main pulmonary arteries are best seen on short-axis sections. When conventional 2-D echocardiograms are augmented with color Doppler imaging, the severity of the pulmonary valvular insufficiency can also be assessed (Fig. 13.9; see Appendix).

MRI

The morphologic features and functional disturbances can be demonstrated by MRI. The enlargment of the right ventricle, pulmonary trunk, and main pulmonary arteries is clearly seen on spin–echo images, although the abnormalities of the leaflets usually cannot be appreciated owing to the limited resolution. Cine images demonstrate the pulmonic and tricuspid valvular insufficiency.

Cardiac Catheterization and Angiocardiography

In patients with isolated absence of the pulmonic valve leaflets, cardiac catheterization demonstrates elevated systolic pressure in the right ventricle and pulmonary trunk. In patients with right ventricular failure, the right ventricular end diastolic pressure and right atrial pressure are elevated. (The latter is transmitted to the caval veins and their tributaries.) At this stage, angiocardiography demonstrates tricuspid incompetence with right atrial and right ventricular dilatation.

When absence of the pulmonic leaflets is associated with tetralogy of Fallot, the intracardiac morphology is the same as that in ordinary tetralogy. However, the infundibular and valvular stenoses are minimal, resulting in a small gradient between the right ventricle and the pulmonary trunk, and pulmonic insufficiency is present. Angiocardiography demon-

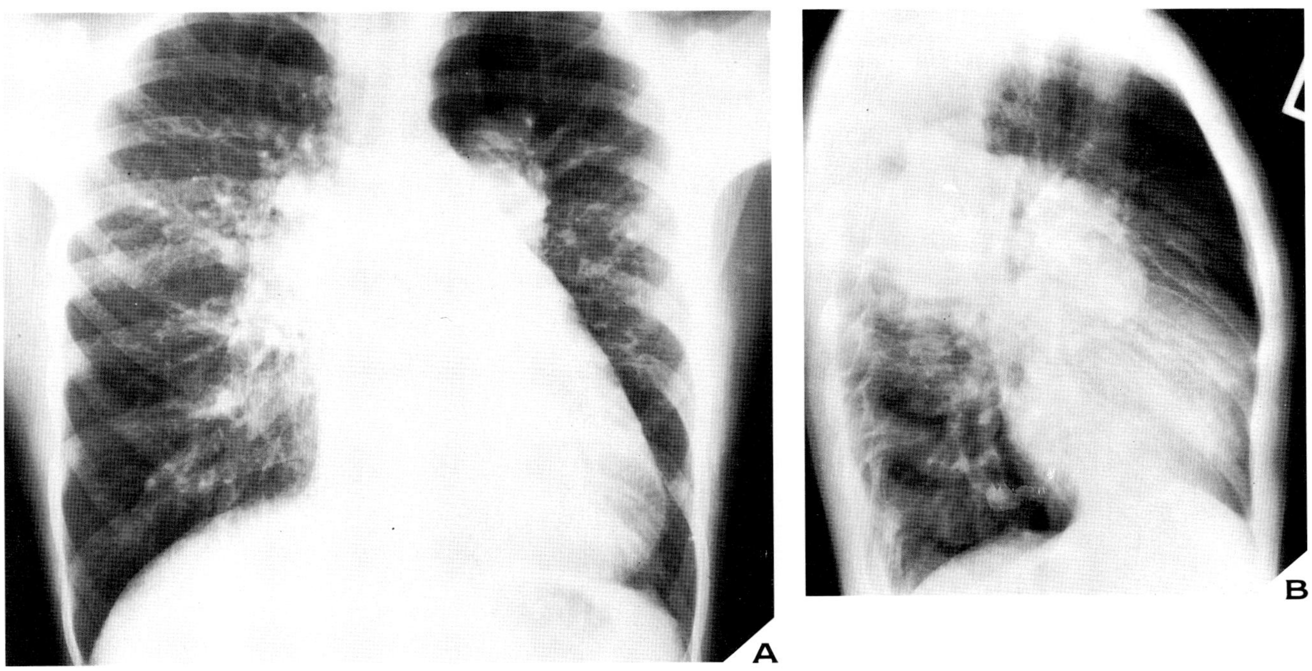

Fig. 13.8 Isolated absence of the pulmonic valve leaflets. (A) Frontal and (B) lateral chest films show right ventricular enlargement and marked dilatation of the pulmonary trunk and central pulmonary arteries. The septal and lobar branches are also prominent. Although the peripheral branches are of average size, they are relatively small when compared with the markedly enlarged central vessels.

strates marked enlargement of the pulmonary trunk and its branches.

Right ventriculography demonstrates enlargement of the right ventricle and pulmonary trunk. The pulmonic valve is not visualized even on high-speed cineangiocardiograms (60 frames per second); instead, a ring-like filling defect is seen in the position of the pulmonic valve (Fig. 13.10). Right to left shunting (across the VSD and via the overriding aorta) is seen in patients with an associated tetralogy of Fallot (Fig. 13.11).

VALVULAR INSUFFICIENCY ON THE LEFT SIDE OF THE HEART

CONGENITAL MITRAL INSUFFICIENCY

Congenital mitral insufficiency may result from dilatation of the mitral annulus, prolapse of the anterior or posterior leaflets, hypoplasia of the posterior leaflet with shortening of the chordae tendinae, or malformation (cleft or shortening) of the leaflets. (Late-onset mitral insufficiency secondary to valve dysplasia is discussed more extensively in Chapter 18).

CLINICAL FEATURES

The clinical manifestations of congenital mitral insufficiency are similar to those of mitral insufficiency caused by rheumatic heart disease: congestive heart disease, dyspnea, orthopnea, and recurrent pulmonary infection. Auscultation typically reveals an apical pansystolic murmur radiating to the axilla.

IMAGING AND INVASIVE DIAGNOSIS

Plain Films

Plain films demonstrate cardiomegaly with left ventricular and left atrial enlargement. When the left atrium is markedly enlarged, it may form part of the right heart border. In patients with congestive heart failure, chest films show typical features of pulmonary venous hypertension (Fig. 13.12). In the absence of congestive failure the pulmonary vasculature appears normal.

Echocardiology

The diagnostic features of congenital mitral insufficiency are clearly seen on long axial views, which demonstrate left atrial enlargement, dilatation of the mitral annulus, and abnormal motion of the leaflets. (The abnormal motion is most evident when there is prolapse of one or both leaflets.) The regurgitant jet from the left ventricle is readily identified on color Doppler images (Fig. 13.13; see Appendix).

Cardiac Catheterization and Angiocardiography

Cardiac catheterization is performed to assess the severity of left ventricular dysfunction. The left ventricular end diastolic pressure is increased in patients with left ventricular failure (the capillary wedge pressure, which reflects the end diastolic pres-

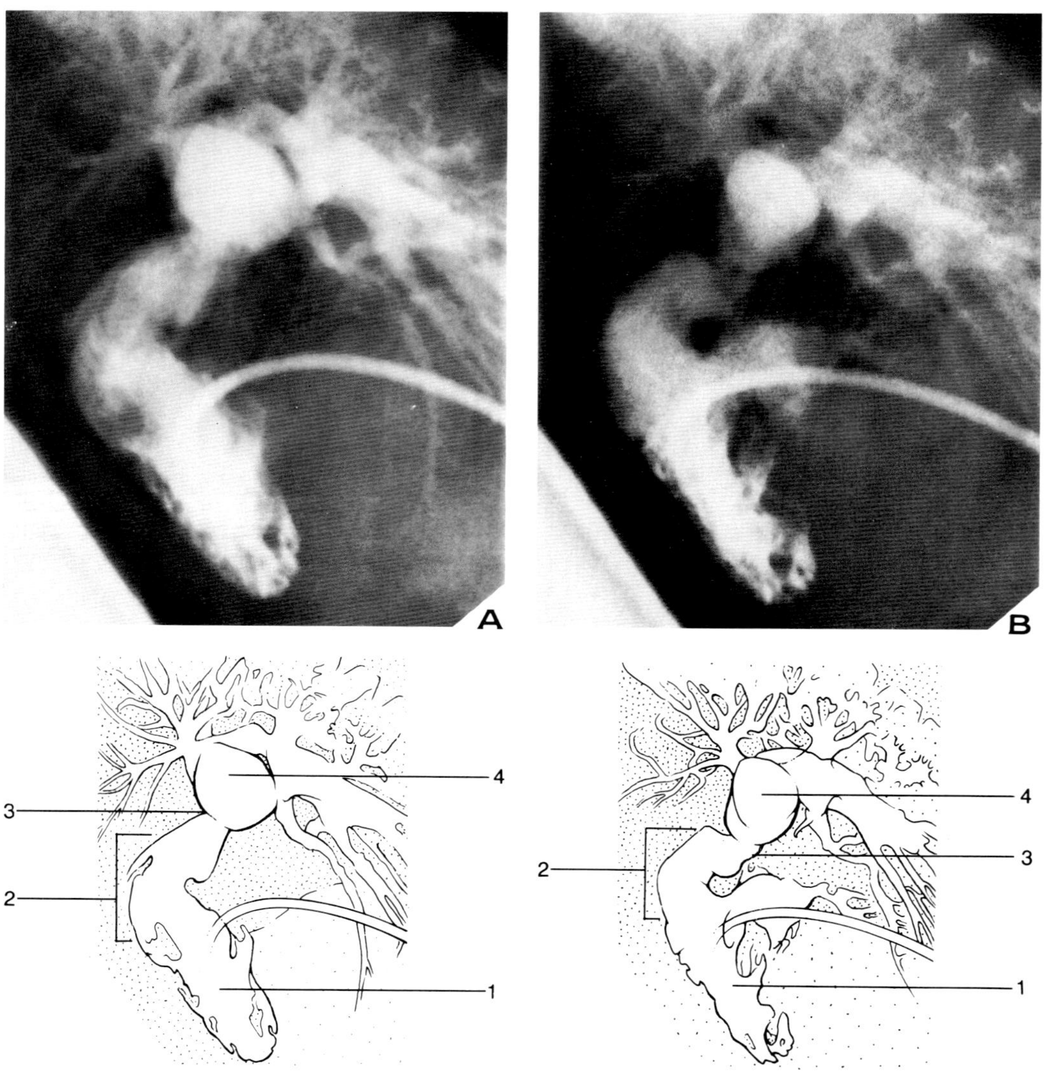

Fig. 13.10 Isolated absence of pulmonic valve leaflets. Lateral projections of right ventriculogram in systole (A) and diastole (B) demonstrate anterior prominence of the outlet segment. The outlet segment is not stenotic; however, the pulmonary trunk is dilated. The annulus of the dysplastic pulmonic valve is represented by the narrowed segment in A and B.

1 trabecular segment of right ventricle
2 outflow segment of right ventricle
3 annulus of dysplastic pulmonic valve
4 pulmonary trunk

sure, is also elevated). However, many patients with congenital mitral insufficiency have normal left ventricular function.

Mitral insufficiency is best demonstrated on left ventriculograms obtained in the long axial and lateral projections. Passing the catheter into the left ventricle from the left atrium, across the mitral valve, may cause artifactual ("catheter-induced") mitral incompetence; therefore, the catheter should be passed from the aorta into the left ventricle. The regurgitant jet is seen during systole; it can be anterior, posterior, or medial in location (Fig. 13.14). The severity of the mitral insufficiency is graded according to the degree of opacification of the left atrium.

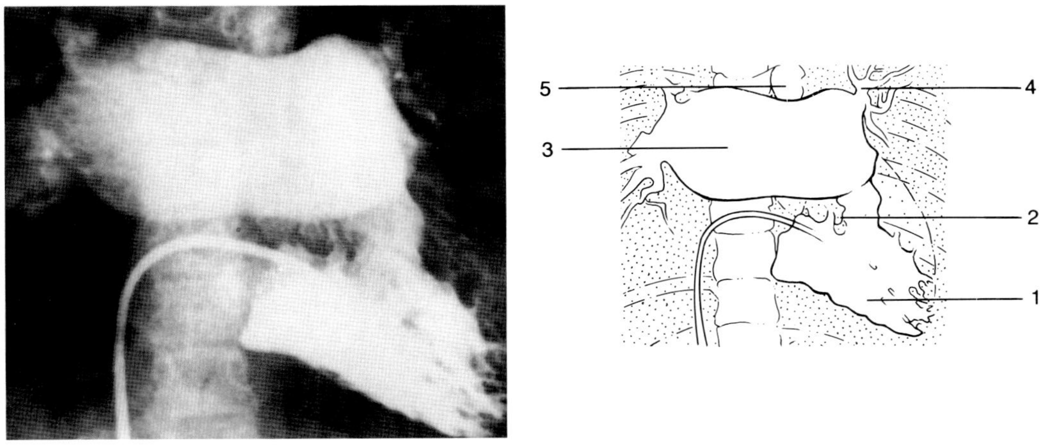

Fig. 13.11 Absence of pulmonic valve leaflets associated with tetralogy of Fallot. Frontal projection of right ventriculogram demonstrates displacement of the infundibular septum to the left and narrowing of the right ventricular outflow tract. The right ventricle connects with the aorta through a VSD. The right and left pulmonary arteries are markedly dilated. The lobar and segmental arteries are much smaller than normal.

1 right ventricle
2 infundibular septum (displaced to left)
3 right pulmonary artery
4 left pulmonary artery
5 aorta

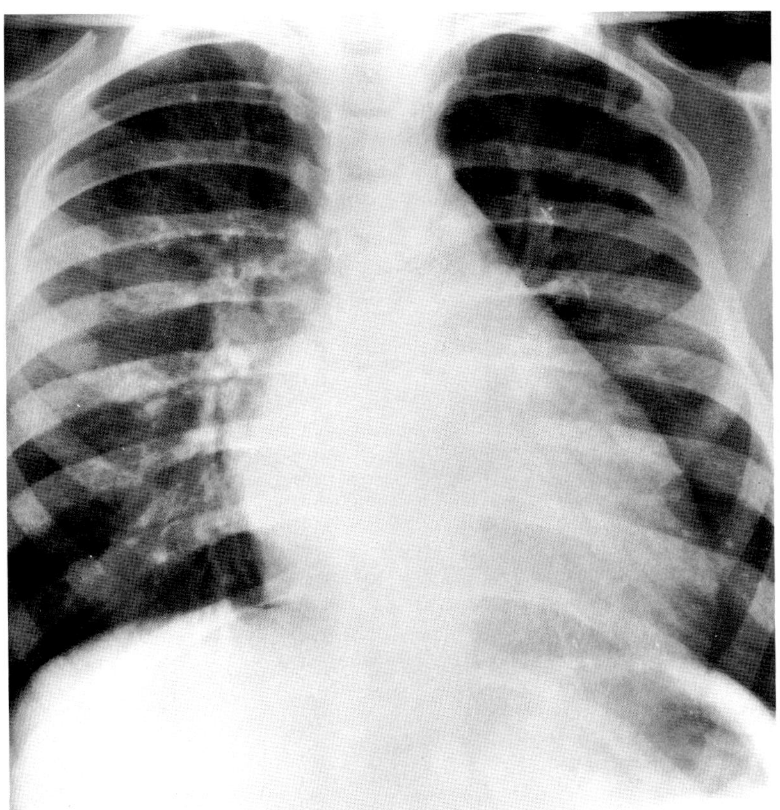

Fig. 13.12 Congenital mitral insufficiency. Posteroanterior chest film shows marked cardiomegaly with left ventricular and left atrial enlargement. The right border of the left atrium forms the right heart border. There is evidence of both pulmonary venous hypertension (note pulmonary venous engorgement) and pulmonary arterial hypertension (note dilated pulmonary trunk).

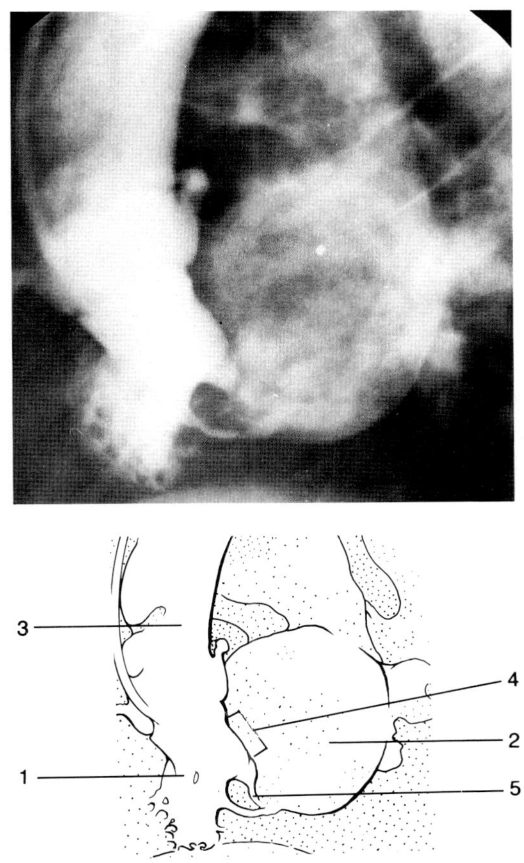

Fig. 13.14 Congenital mitral insufficiency. Lateral projection of left ventriculogram demonstrates reflux of contrast material into the left atrium during systole. The left atrium is markedly enlarged. The regurgitant jet of contrast material originates from the posterior portion of the mitral orifice, indicating malfunction of the anterior leaflet (see Chapter 18). The size and contractility of the left ventricle are normal.

1 left ventricle
2 left atrium
3 aorta
4 mitral valve
5 regurgitant jet

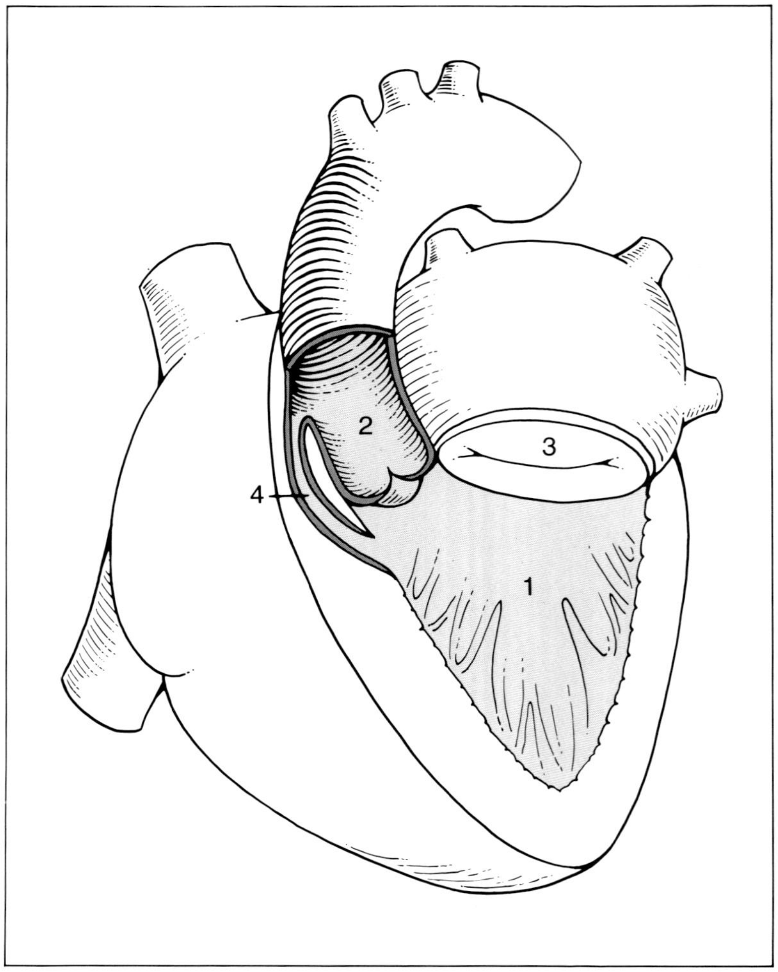

Fig. 13.15 Aortic–left ventricular tunnel. A congenital channel, originating from the aorta above the sinuses of Valsalva, has excavated the left ventricular wall and enters the left ventricle beneath the aortic valve. The hemodynamic, clinical, and radiologic features of this anomaly, which allows a large volume of blood to reflux into the left ventricle during diastole, closely resemble those of aortic insufficiency.

1 left ventricle
2 aorta
3 mitral valve
4 aortic-left ventricular tunnel

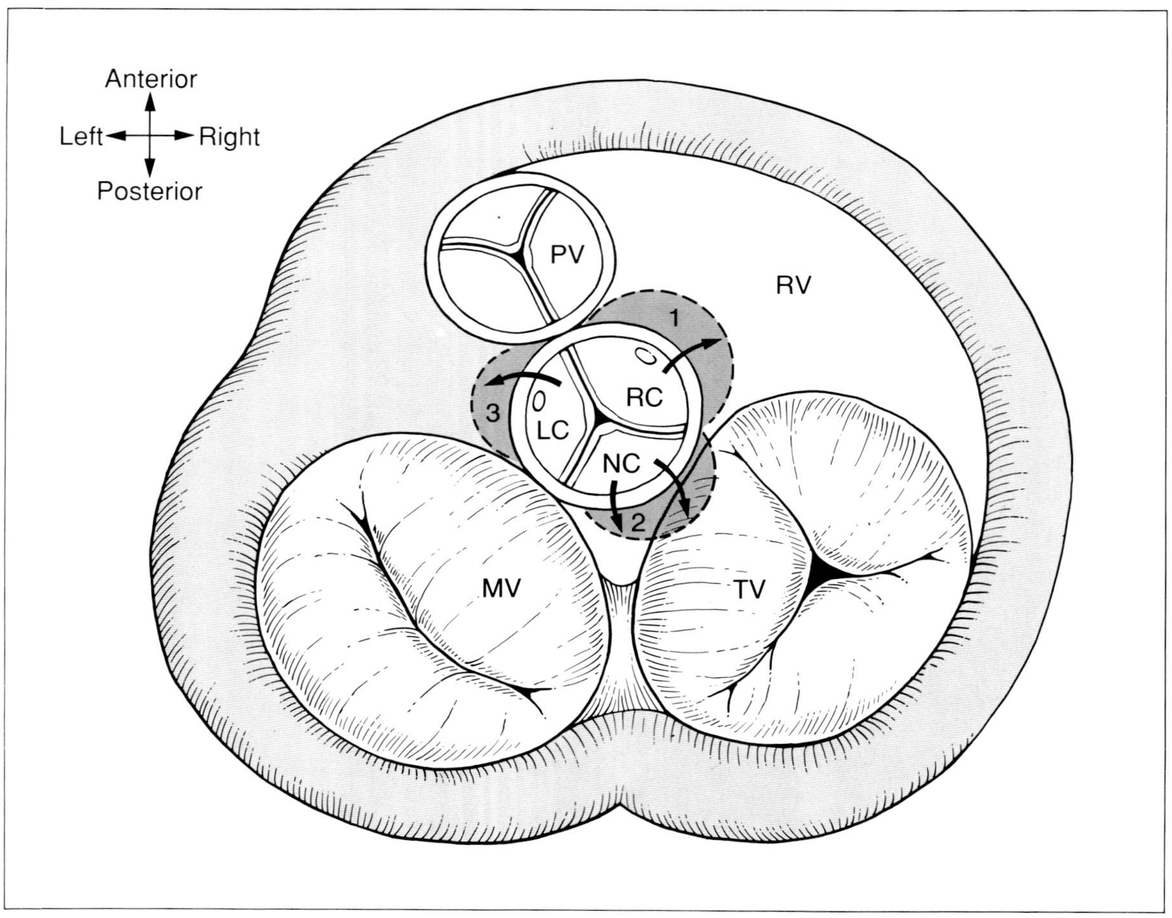

Fig. 13.16 Aneurysms of the sinuses of Valsalva. Relations of aortic sinuses of Valsalva at the base of the heart, as seen from above. Aneurysms of the right sinus of Valsalva protrude into or rupture into the right ventricular outflow tract (*arrow* 1). Aneurysms of the posterior (noncoronary) sinus of Valsalva protrude into or rupture into the right or left atrium (*arrows* 2). Aneurysms of the left sinus of Valsalva protrude into or rupture into the pericardial space (*arrows* 3).

TV tricuspid valve
LC left coronary cusp
PV pulmonic valve
MV mitral valve
RC right coronary cusp
NC noncoronary cusp

AORTIC VALVULAR INSUFFICIENCY

Although isolated congenital aortic valvular insufficiency is rare, the aortic valve is incompetent in some patients with aneurysms of the sinuses of Valsalva or with VSDs. The so-called aortic–left ventricular tunnel is a rare congenital malformation which can simulate aortic insufficiency (Fig. 13.15).

CONGENITAL ANEURYSM OF THE SINUSES OF VALSALVA

MORPHOLOGY AND PATHOGENESIS

Each of the three sinuses of Valsalva comprises a portion of the aortic wall and the adjacent cusp (leaflet). In a classic sinus of Valsalva aneurysm, both the aortic wall and the adjacent leaflet are dilated and protrude into adjacent structures. (Only rarely does the parietal portion of the sinus enlarge while its cusp remains intact.) Eventually the aneurysm may rupture.

Aneurysms of the right (coronary) sinus are the most common, followed in frequency by aneurysms of the noncoronary and the left coronary sinus (Fig. 13.16). Aneurysms of the right (coronary) sinus protrude into the right ventricular outflow tract or right atrium and may rupture into these structures. Aneurysms arising from the noncoronary sinus protrude, and may rupture, into the right or left atrium. Aneurysms of the left coronary sinus protrude into the pericardium and may rupture into it.

"Congenital" and "acquired" sinus of Valsalva aneurysms are both believed to have the same pathogenesis, ie, a congenital localized weakness of the aortic wall. Sinus of Valsalva aneurysms are found in 10 to 15 percent of patients with isolated VSD. Aneurysms of the right coronary cusp are particularly likely to develop in patients with a juxtaarterial VSD.

HEMODYNAMIC AND CLINICAL FEATURES

Individuals with unruptured sinus of Valsalva aneurysms usually have few hemodynamic or clinical manifestations, and the lesion is often discovered incidentally at autopsy. Occasionally an unruptured aneurysm interferes with the function of the aortic valve, resulting in aortic insufficiency and left ventricular volume overload. In patients with an associated VSD, the clinical manifestations are those of the VSD. The latter may go unrecognized, however, because the prolapsed leaflet frequently restricts the VSD and may occlude it completely.

Rupture of the aneurysm into the right atrium or right ventricle results in a left to right shunt. Rupture of the aneurysm into the left atrium leads to left ventricular and left atrial volume overload, which may progress to left ventricular failure; in such cases the elevated left ventricular end diastolic pressure results in pulmonary venous hypertension. Rupture into the pericardial space leads to acute cardiac tamponade, which is usually fatal.

IMAGING AND INVASIVE DIAGNOSIS

Plain Films

After rupture of a right sinus of Valsalva aneurysm into the right ventricle, chest films typically show biventricular enlargement and pulmonary plethora (Fig. 13.17). The right ventricular enlargement and pulmonary plethora are manifestations of the left to right shunt, and the degree of left ventricular enlargement correlates with the severity of the aortic insufficiency.

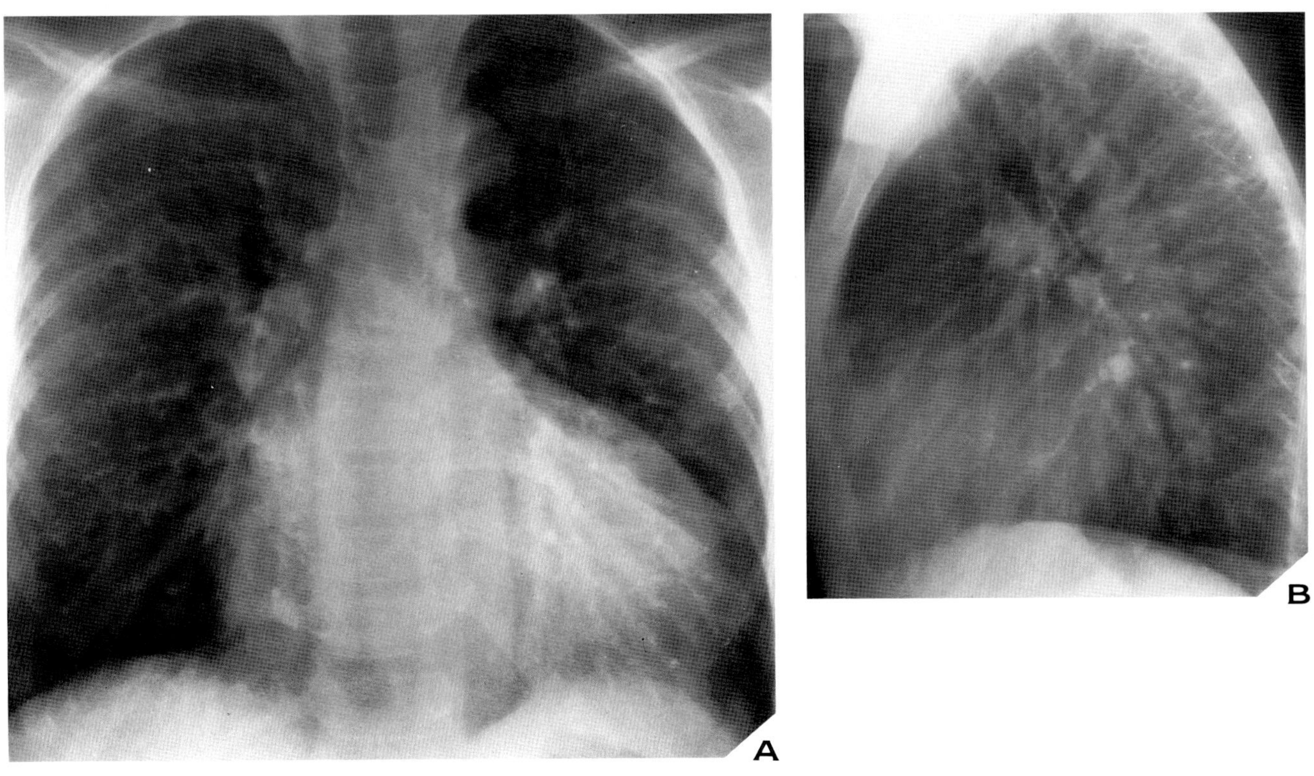

Fig. 13.17 Ruptured right sinus of Valsalva aneurysm. (A) Frontal and (B) lateral chest films of a 10-year-old boy show biventricular enlargement and plethoric pulmonary vasculature. The pulmonary trunk and aortic arch are normal. In a noncyanotic patient this combination of findings suggests a right sinus of Valsalva aneurysm which has ruptured into the right ventricle. (The left ventricular enlargement is presumably due to preexisting aortic insufficiency.) A ruptured right sinus of Valsalva aneurysm was confirmed by angiocardiography.

Echocardiography

Two-dimensional echocardiograms are very helpful in diagnosis. By the use of various scanning planes it is possible to demonstrate the size of the affected sinus of Valsalva and its relations with surrounding structures. Most of the pertinent features are demonstrated in short axis and long axis views. Short axis views at the level of the aorta demonstrate the morphology of all the three cusps and the abnormal motion of the wall and cusp in the affected sinus. The relationship of the right coronary cusp to the crista supraventricularis and the right ventricular outflow tract is clearly seen in this projection. In patients with aneurysms of the noncoronary sinus of Valsalva, the coronary cusp is seen to protrude into the right atrium (it also protrudes for a short distance into the left atrium). The long axial view demonstrates the leaflets. The right and left coronary cusps are demonstrated in one scanning plane; with greater angulation, one can demonstrate the noncoronary cusp as well. In patients with aneurysms of the right sinus of Valsalva, the four-chamber view may demonstrate a "mass" at the junction of the right atrium and the right ventricle, close to the medial commissure of the tricuspid valve. This apparent mass represents the right coronary cusp protruding into the right ventricle (Figs. 13.18 and 13.19).

Angiocardiography

Both left ventriculography and thoracic aortography are necessary to completely delineate the aneurysm and its sequelae. Aneurysms of the right sinus of Valsalva are best demonstrated on thoracic aortograms in frontal, lateral, and oblique projections. Rupture of the right sinus of Valsalva into the right ventricle results in opacification of the right ventricular outflow tract (Fig. 13.20). Long axis views are optimal for demonstrating the VSD that is commonly associated with a right sinus of Valsalva aneurysm. The prolapsed aortic cusp may partially occlude the VSD, in which case the latter will appear smaller than it actually is (Fig. 13.21).

The regurgitant right ventricular jet associated with a ruptured right sinus of Valsalva aneurysm is clearly seen in the lateral projection. When the rupture is close to the commissure between the right and left coronary cusps, the jet is close to the

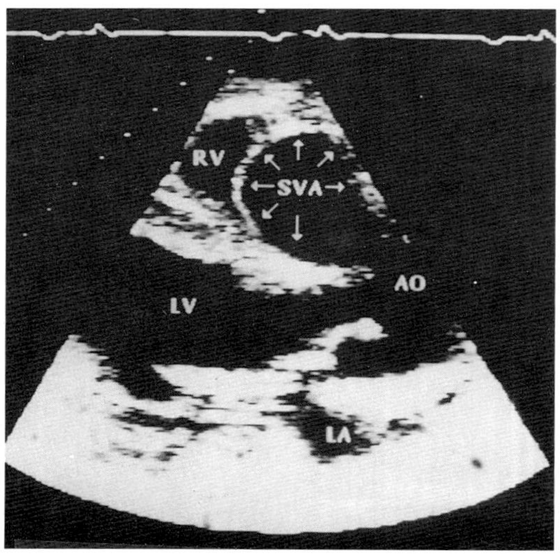

Fig. 13.18 Right coronary sinus of Valsalva aneurysm. Echocardiogram (parasternal long axial view) demonstrates marked enlargement of right coronary sinus of Valsalva, which protrudes into the right ventricular outflow tract. (Reproduced by permission from Jain SP, et al: Doppler color flow mapping in the diagnosis of sinus of Valsalva aneurysm. *Echocardiography* 1989; 6:532)

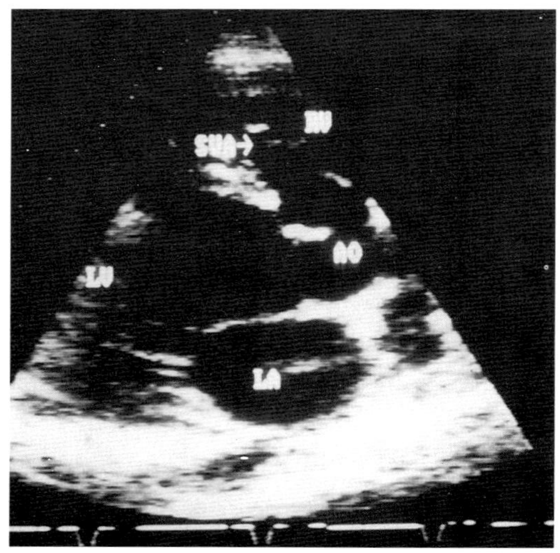

Fig. 13.19 Rupture of right sinus of Valsalva aneurysm into right ventricular outflow tract. Echocardiogram (parasternal long axial view) demonstrates a tubular structure connecting the right coronary sinus of Valsalva with the right ventricular outflow tract. Note multiple areas of echo "drop-out" within the aneurysm. (Reproduced by permission from Jain SP, et al: Echocardiography 6:534)

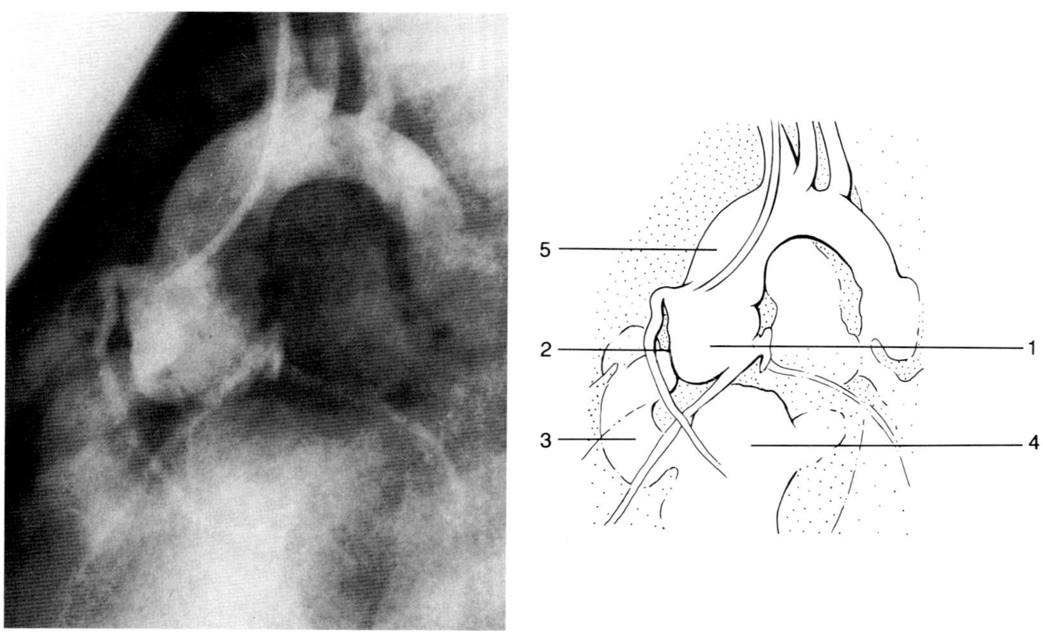

Fig. 13.20 Ruptured right sinus of Valsalva aneurysm. Left anterior oblique projection of thoracic aortogram. The dilated right coronary cusp communicates with the right ventricle, indicating that the aneurysm has ruptured. Note opacification of the left ventricle caused by aortic valvular insufficiency.

1 dilated right coronary cusp
2 site of rupture
3 right ventricle
4 left ventricle
5 aorta

pulmonic valve. When the rupture is at the junction between the right and noncoronary cusps the jet is directed into the inlet portion of the right ventricle. In some patients the jet is directed towards the midportion of the crista supraventricularis. In the elongated right anterior oblique projection, the aneurysm is seen to form the anteroinferior margin of the left side of the aorta. Depending on the site of the rupture, the regurgitant jet may be directed anterosuperiorly, anteriorly, or anteroinferiorly (Fig. 13.22).

Aneurysms of the noncoronary sinus of Valsalva are best seen on thoracic aortograms obtained in the elongated right anterior oblique and lateral projections. In the elongated right anterior oblique projection the noncoronary cusp is projected posteriorly and inferiorly; it is completely separate from the coronary cusps, both of which project anteriorly and to the left. Aneurysms of the noncoronary cusp project posteriorly and inferiorly into the right atrium or right ventricle. The regurgitant jet associated with rupture of the noncoronary cusp may be directed into the right atrium (ie, above the tricuspid valve) or into the right ventricle (ie, below the tricuspid valve). In the left anterior oblique projection the non-

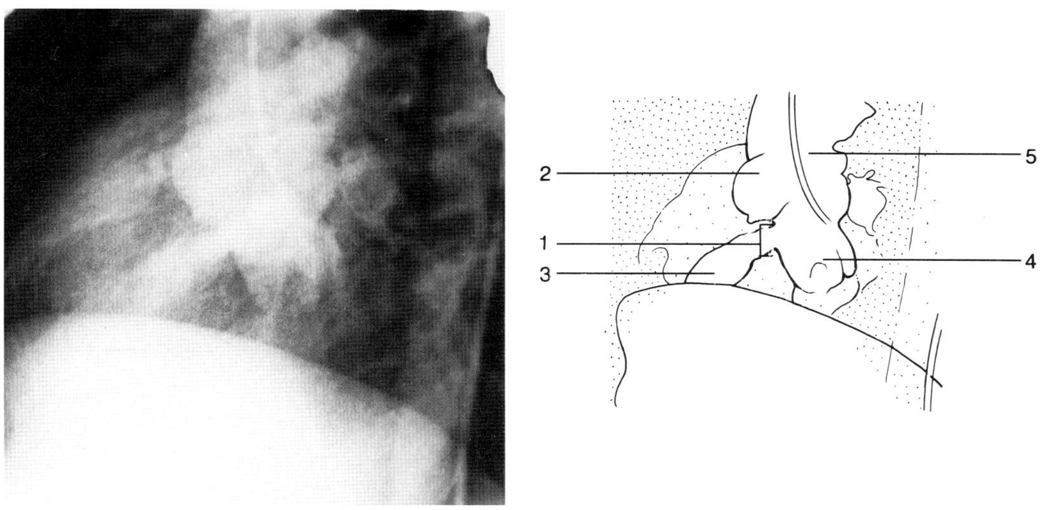

Fig. 13.21 Sinus of Valsalva aneurysm associated with VSD. Long axial projection of left ventriculogram demonstrates a restricted VSD which is partially occluded by the protruding right coronary cusp.

1 VSD
2 dilated right coronary cusp
3 right ventricle
4 left ventricle
5 aorta

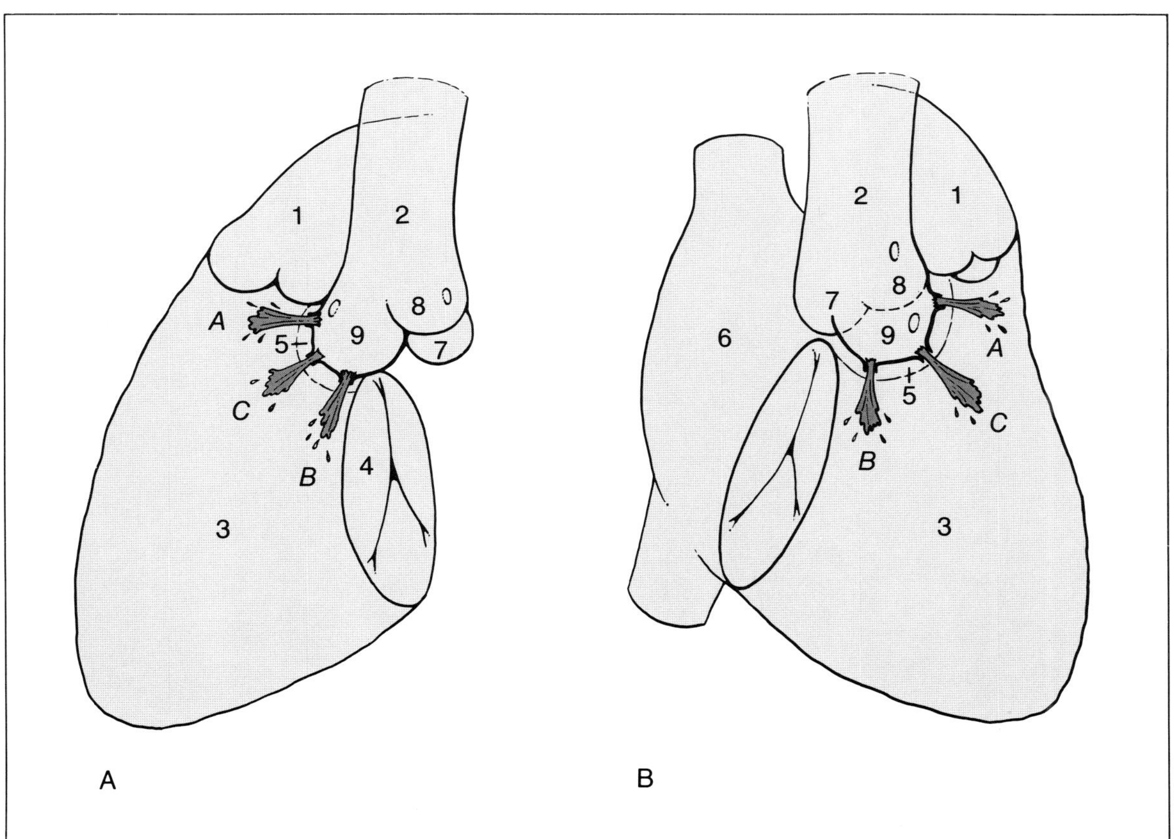

1 pulmonary trunk
2 aorta
3 right ventricle
4 tricuspid valve
5 crista supraventricularis
6 right atrium
7 noncoronary cusp and sinus of Valsalva
8 left coronary cusp and sinus of Valsalva
9 right coronary cusp and sinus of Valsalva
A, B, C regurgitant jet

Fig. 13.22 Angiographic features of ruptured aneurysm of the right sinus of Valsalva. (A) Lateral and (B) right anterior oblique projections of thoracic aortogram (diagrammatic). The sites of rupture are indicated by the position and direction of the regurgitant jet. *A* When the rupture is close to the commissure between the right and left coronary cusps, the jet enters the right ventricular outflow tract close to the pulmonic valve (ie, the most cephalic portion of the right ventricular outflow tract). *B* When the rupture occurs at the junction between the right and noncoronary cusps, the jet is directed towards the inlet portion of the right ventricle, close to the septal leaflet of the tricuspid valve. *C* When the rupture is in the middle of the right coronary cusp, the jet is directed towards the middle portion of the crista supraventricularis.

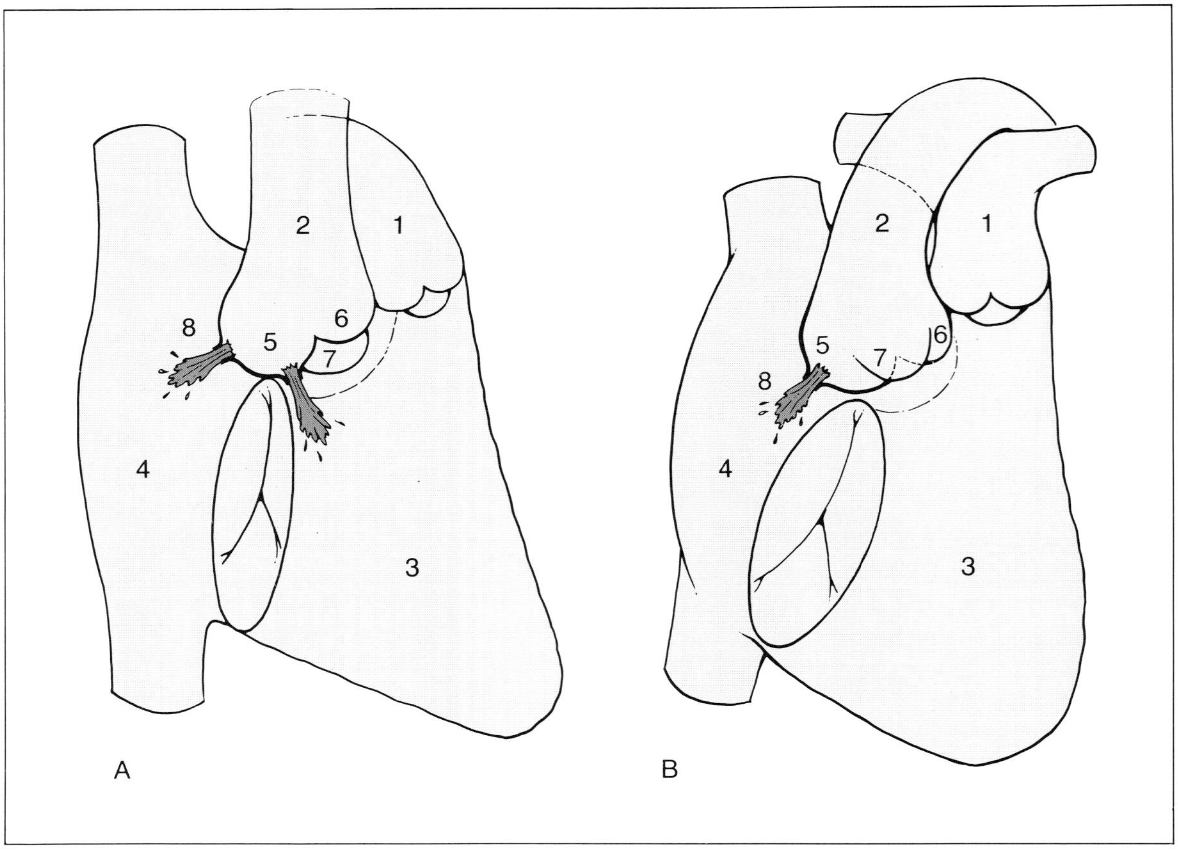

1 pulmonary trunk
2 aorta
3 right ventricle
4 right atrium
5 noncoronary cusp and sinus of Valsalva
6 left coronary cusp and sinus of Valsalva
7 right coronary cusp and sinus of Valsalva
8 regurgitant jet

Fig. 13.23 Angiographic features of aneurysms of the noncoronary sinus of Valsalva. (A) Right anterior oblique and (B) frontal projections of thoracic aortogram (diagrammatic). Aneurysms of the noncoronary cusp enlarge posteriorly and inferiorly, extending into the right atrium or right ventricle. When the rupture occurs in the midportion of the noncoronary sinus, or in the posterior portion (close to its junction with the left coronary cusp), the regurgitant flow enters the right atrium (ie, above the tricuspid valve). When the rupture occurs in the area close to the commissure with the right coronary cusp, the regurgitant jet enters the right ventricle (ie, below the tricuspid valve).

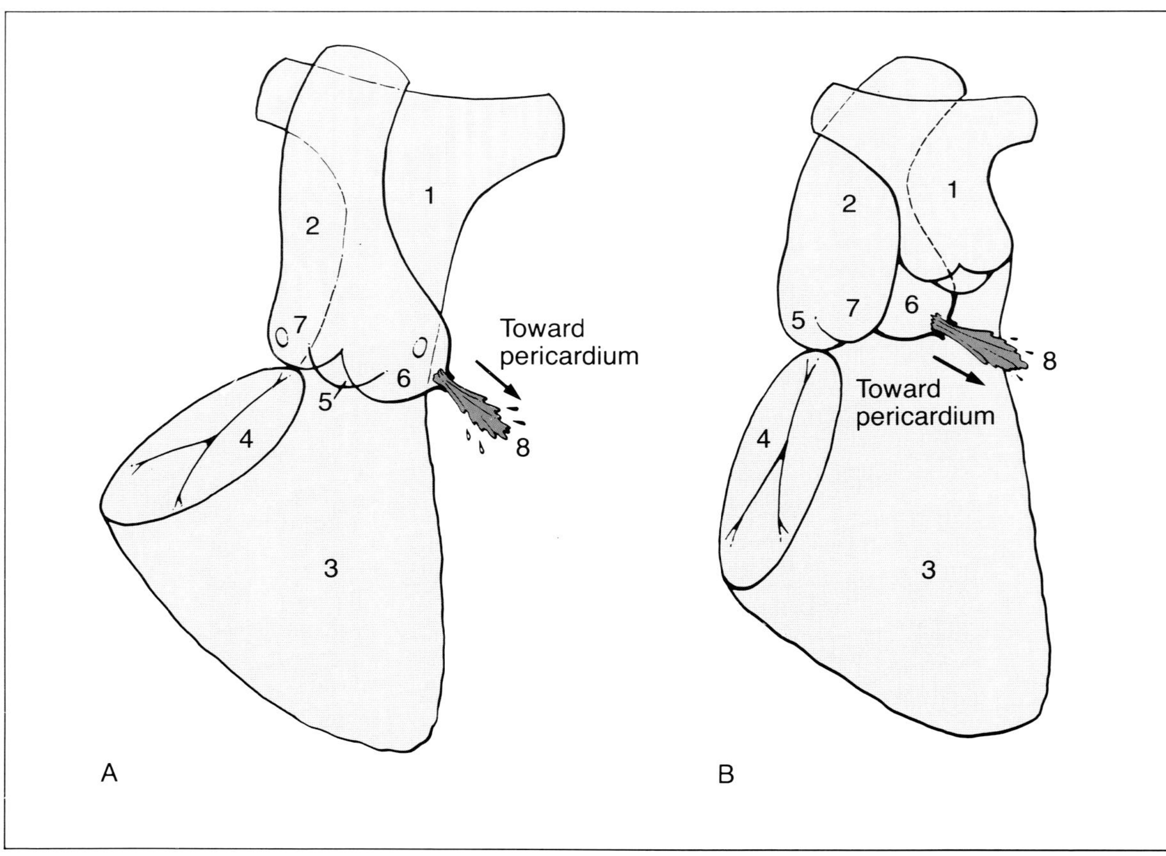

1 pulmonary trunk
2 aorta
3 right ventricle
4 tricuspid valve
5 noncoronary cusp and sinus of Valsalva
6 left coronary cusp and sinus of Valsalva
7 right coronary cusp and sinus of Valsalva
8 jet entering pericardial space

Fig. 13.24 Angiographic features of aneurysms of the left sinus of Valsalva. (A) Left anterior oblique and (B) Anteroposterior projection of thoracic aortogram. The relations of the aneurysm are clearly seen in A; the enlarged left coronary cusp projects posteriorly and is well separated from the other cusps. When the aneurysm ruptures, opacified blood enters the pericardium. Rupture of an aneurysm of the left sinus of Valsalva leads to acute hemopericardium and cardiac tamponade; therefore, this complication is seldom demonstrated angiographically.

coronary cusp is usually projected between the right and left cusps and is easy to identify when it is enlarged. When the noncoronary cusp ruptures, the regurgitant jet passes into the right atrium or right ventricle; when the sinus ruptures, the jet enters the right atrium. The jet is best demonstrated in the left anterior oblique projection (Fig. 13.23).

Aneurysms of the left sinus of Valsalva are very rare. On aortograms obtained in the left anterior oblique projection, the left cusp is projected posteriorly and is almost entirely separate from the other two cusps (Fig. 13.24). Rupture of the left cusp is seldom demonstrated angiographically, as most patients with this complication quickly develop a hemopericardium and pericardial tamponade, and are therefore too ill to undergo angiographic studies.

CHAPTER 14

Extracardiac Shunts

In addition to intracardiac shunts at the atrial and ventricular level (see Chapters 8 and 9), an abnormal communication at the level of the great arteries (eg, patent ductus arteriosus or aortopulmonary window) can result in a systemic to pulmonary arterial shunt. Arteriovenous shunting secondary to a vascular tumor (eg, hemangioendothelioma) or to an arteriovenous malformation or fistula is a rare cause of high-output heart failure in infants. Anomalous origin of the left coronary artery from the pulmonary artery can result in myocardial ischemia (see Chapters 20 and 21).

SYSTEMIC TO PULMONARY ARTERY SHUNTS

Three types of extracardiac malformation are associated with systemic to pulmonary shunts: aortopulmonary window, anomalous origin of the pulmonary artery from the ascending aorta, and patent ductus arteriosus (PDA).

AORTOPULMONARY WINDOW

In this anomaly, which results from a defect in the formation of the aortopulmonary septum early in fetal development, the ascending aorta and pulmonary trunk communicate above the sinuses of Valsalva. The aortic and pulmonic valves are usually normal.

HEMODYNAMICS AND CLINICAL FEATURES

Owing to the relatively low pulmonary resistance, blood flows from the aorta into the main pulmonary artery, flooding the pulmonary circulation. Like infants with a large VSD, patients with an aortopulmonary window typically present early in life with signs and symptoms of congestive heart failure. Infants with an aortopulmonary window are usually small, underdeveloped, and have repeated respiratory infections. Physical examination reveals marked cardiomegaly, accentuation of the second heart sound at the base, and a systolic murmur of variable intensity. Patients with a very large left to right shunt typically have jerky or collapsing peripheral pulses, reflecting the rapid aortic run-off. This finding may not be evident in patients with severe congestive failure or elevated pulmonary vascular resistance; in such cases the differential diagnosis must include PDA, truncus arteriosus, and VSD with aortic valvular insufficiency.

IMAGING AND INVASIVE DIAGNOSIS

Plain Films

Plain films show cardiomegaly and marked pulmonary plethora, ie, findings typical of any large left to right shunt.

Echocardiography

Sequential short-axis sections through the aorta and pulmonary trunk, progressing cephalad from the level of the arterial valves, demonstrates the abnormal connection of the great arteries. Color Doppler imaging confirms the presence of a left to right shunt at this level.

MRI

The abnormal connection between the aorta and pulmonary trunk can be demonstrated on transverse spin–echo images and on long axial projections in which the great arteries are seen in profile. The latter will also confirm the presence of separate aortic and pulmonary valves, ruling out truncus arteriosus. Cine MRI reveals a left to right shunt at the level of the aortopulmonary window.

Cardiac Catheterization

Oxygen saturation is higher in the pulmonary trunk than in the right atrium or right ventricle. In an occasional patient, oxygen saturation is greater in the right ventricle than in the right atrium, in which case differentiation from VSD or truncus arteriosus is not possible on the catheterization findings alone.

Angiocardiography

Thoracic aortography and left ventriculography are necessary for definitive diagnosis of aortopulmonary window. (The latter demonstrates the VSD that is commonly associated with this anomaly.) An aortic root injection will opacify the pulmonary trunk and demonstrate the window, which usually lies along the left posterolateral aspect of the aorta (Fig. 14.1). The pulmonary trunk and the main pulmonary arteries are usually enlarged. The pulmonary arteries have a normal branching pattern.

Differentiation from truncus arteriosus can be difficult in patients in whom the defect in the aortopulmonary septum is just above the sinuses of Valsalva (see Chapter 11). Angiographic demonstration of two separate, normally formed arterial valves and an intact ventricular septum will exclude truncus arteriosus in such cases.

ANOMALOUS ORIGIN OF ONE PULMONARY ARTERY FROM THE ASCENDING AORTA

In this rare malformation, either the left or the right pulmonary artery arises from the ascending aorta. Although this is usually an isolated anomaly, it can be associated with VSD or PDA.

HEMODYNAMICS AND CLINICAL FEATURES

Although only the ipsilateral pulmonary artery is subjected directly to increased flow at systemic pressures, vascular resistance in the contralateral lung is low, so that blood is shunted to this lung as well. Consequently, both lungs are overperfused.

The patient typically presents in early infancy with respiratory distress and congestive heart failure. Cyanosis may be present, either as a result of venous admixture in the lungs or right to left shunting (via the foramen ovale or a PDA) secondary to right ventricular failure. Physical examination usually reveals a systolic murmur along the left sternal border. The peripheral pulses are jerky or bounding, reflecting the rapid run-off from the aorta into the pulmonary circulation. Patients who survive beyond the first week of life later develop pulmonary hypertension, which characteristically involves both lungs.

IMAGING AND INVASIVE DIAGNOSIS

Plain Films

Chest films typically show cardiomegaly with left ventricular prominence and symmetrical overperfusion (plethora) of both lungs.

Echocardiography

The malformation can be demonstrated on short axial and long axial views obtained via a parasternal or, preferably, a transesophageal approach. The right or left pulmonary artery can be seen to arise from the pulmonary trunk in normal fashion, while its mate arises from the posterior aspect of the ascending aorta.

Cardiac Catheterization

Typically the pressure is elevated in the pulmonary artery that arises from the aorta (it may be normal in the rare patient in whom the ostium of the anomalous artery is stenotic). The pressure in the normally connected pulmonary artery is usually elevated to systemic or suprasystemic levels. The pulmonary vascular resistance in the lung supplied by the normally connected pulmonary artery has considerable prognostic significance, especially in older patients.

Angiocardiography

The morphology of the pulmonary arteries is clearly shown by angiocardiography; both left and right ventricular injections are needed to completely delineate the anomaly and to detect associated malformations. In the most common arrangement, the right pulmonary artery originates from the ascending aorta, in which case the right pulmonary artery is opacified after a left ventricular injection (Fig. 14.2), and the left pulmonary artery, which originates from the main pulmonary artery, is opacified after a right ventricular injection.

PERSISTENT PATENT DUCTUS ARTERIOSUS (PDA)

In this anomaly, which results from persistence of the fetal ductus arteriosus, there is a connection between the upper descending thoracic aorta and the pulmonary artery. PDA is one of the most common malformations of the cardiovascular system. It may be isolated or may occur in association with other congenital cardiovascular malformations. It may be unilateral, occurring either on the left or right side, or bilateral.

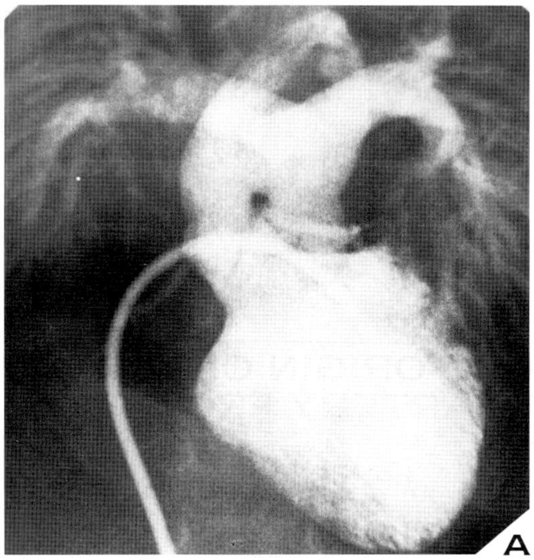

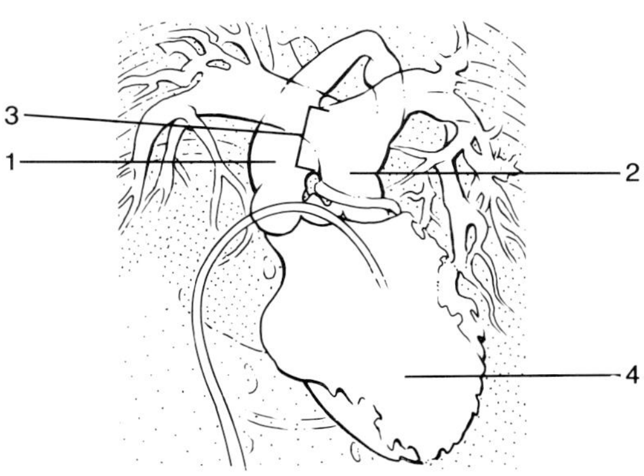

1 aorta	3 aortopulmonary window (brace indicates margins of defect)
2 pulmonary trunk	4 left ventricle

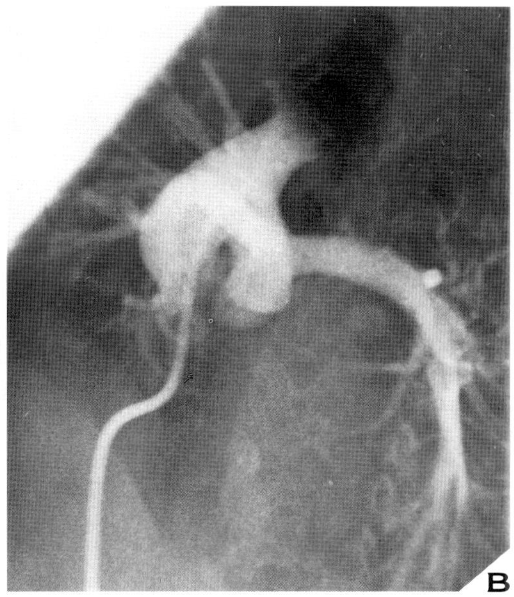

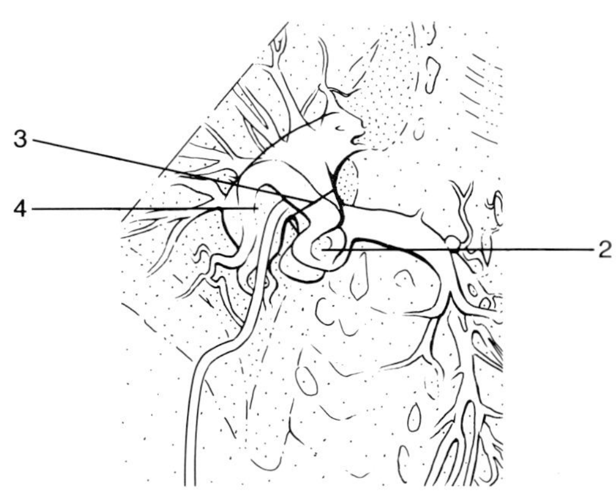

Fig. 14.1 Aortopulmonary window. (A) Left ventriculogram (frontal projection) and (B) thoracic aortogram (long axis projection) show a large aortopulmonary septal defect connecting the aorta and pulmonary trunk. The aortic and pulmonary valves are both well formed.

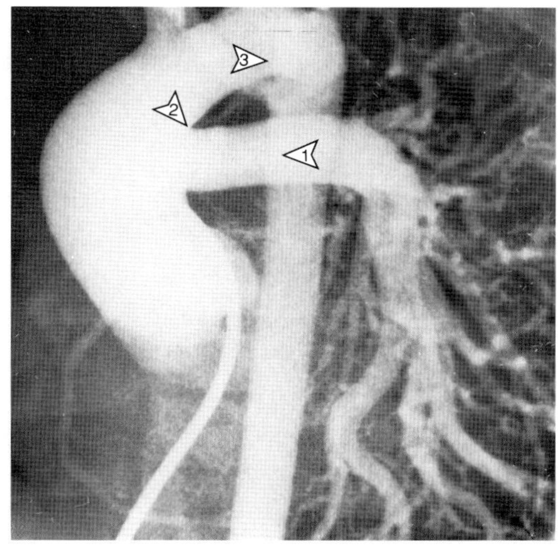

Fig. 14.2 Anomalous origin of left pulmonary artery from ascending aorta. Frontal projection of thoracic aortogram shows the left pulmonary artery (*arrow* 1) arising posteriorly from the ascending aorta (*arrow* 2). The distribution of pulmonary branches in the left lung is normal. Note left aortic arch with aberrant origin of the right subclavian artery (*arrow* 3).

MORPHOLOGY

The various anatomic arrangements are shown schematically in Figure 14.3. In patients with left aortic arch and a left-sided duct, the PDA connects the descending thoracic aorta and the left pulmonary artery. In patients with a right arch, the PDA connects the left subclavian or left innominate artery with the left pulmonary artery. In patients with a right aortic arch and a right-sided PDA, the connection is between the proximal descending thoracic aorta and the right pulmonary artery. In patients with left arch and a right-sided PDA, the connection is between the right innominate or right subclavian artery and the right pulmonary artery. Patients with bilateral PDAs may have either a right or a left aortic arch.

HEMODYNAMICS AND CLINICAL FEATURES

The clinical manifestations reflect the magnitude of the left to right shunt, which is determined by the size of the communication and the systemic and pulmonary vascular resistance, and by the age of the patient.

In the neonate with a large PDA, the magnitude of the left to right shunt increases as pulmonary resistance falls, usually culminating in severe congestive heart failure by about 1 month of age. Such infants typically present with a history of poor feeding, slow weight gain, and recurrent respiratory infections. Physical examination reveals a precordial systolic thrill, reflecting the cardiac enlargement. The pulses are jerky or collapsing, and there is a corresponding widening of the pulse pressure. Auscultation reveals a systolic murmur maximal at the pulmonic area, with late systolic accentuation and minimal spillover into diastole. Patients with a large left to right shunt may exhibit a progressive increase in pulmonary vascular resistance, becoming cyanotic when the pulmonary vascular resistance rises above systemic vascular resistance.

Patients with a small PDA are asymptomatic in infancy. Because the left to right shunt is relatively small, pulmonary resistance remains normal. The condition often remains undiagnosed until a continuous murmur (best heard with the patient sitting or standing) is detected on routine physical examination.

Small premature infants with idiopathic respiratory distress syndrome (hyaline membrane disease) and other respiratory disorders that cause significant hypoxemia commonly have left to right shunting through a PDA. This phenomenon, which results from the inhibitory effect of prostaglandins E_1 and E_2 on the musculature of the immature ductus, can sometimes be reversed by drugs that interfere with prostaglandin synthesis

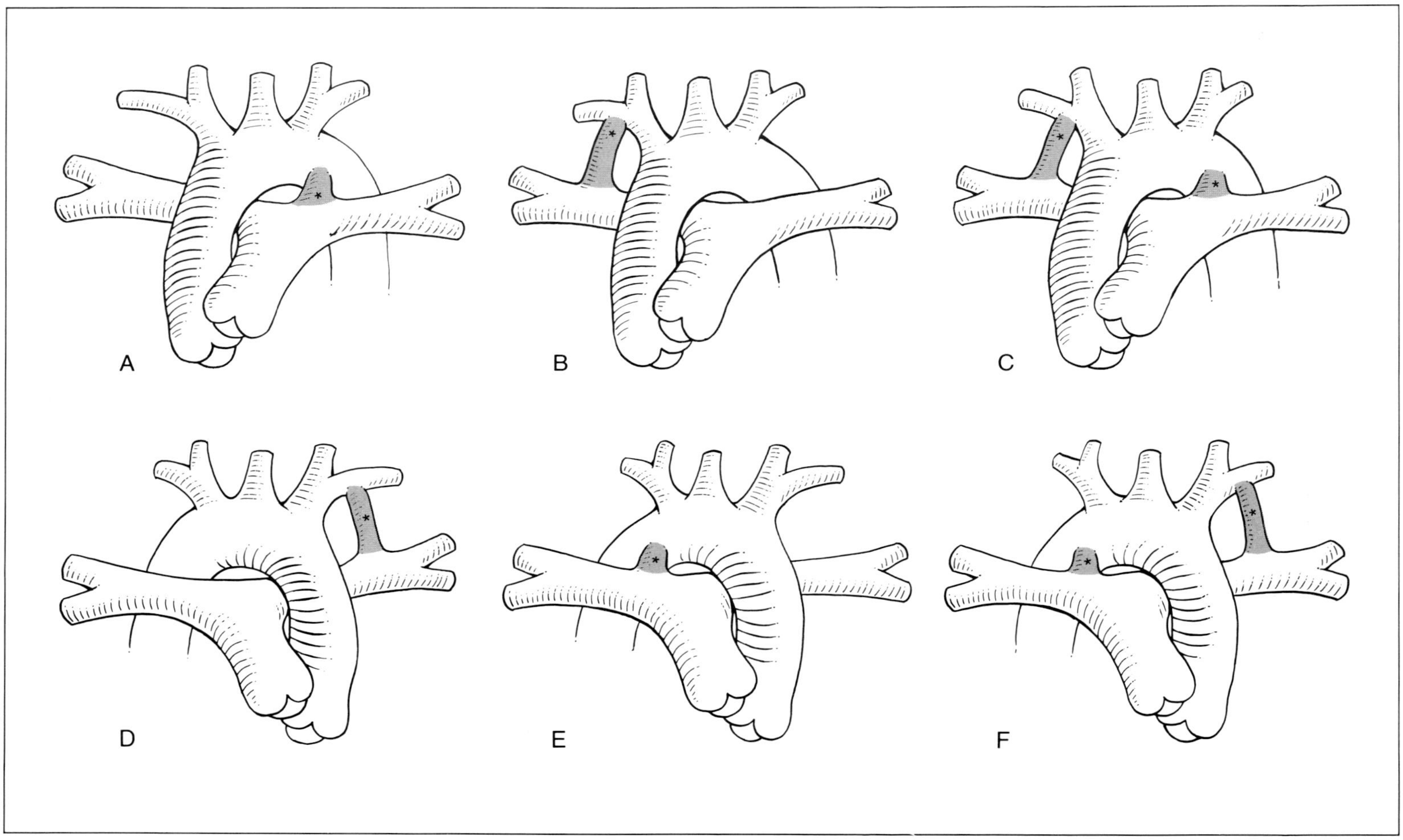

Fig. 14.3 Types of PDA. The position of the PDA is indicated by * (A–C) Associated with left aortic arch. (D–F) Associated with right aortic arch. The most common location is between the aortic arch and the left pulmonary artery (A). Less often, the PDA connects the right subclavian artery and right pulmonary artery (B). Bilateral PDAs are rare (C). In individuals with a right arch, the PDA usually connects the left subclavian artery and the left pulmonary artery (D); connections between the arch and the pulmonary artery (E) and bilateral PDAs are rare.

(eg, indomethacin). A large-volume shunt may cause congestive heart failure with flooding of the lungs, compounding the effects of the underlying lung disease. If drug therapy is ineffective, surgical closure of the ductus may be necessary.

IMAGING AND INVASIVE DIAGNOSIS

Plain Films

By far the most common arrangement is a left PDA connecting the upper descending thoracic aorta with the left pulmonary artery. Plain films show a normal-sized heart, prominence of the ascending aorta and aortic arch, and dilatation of the pulmonary trunk and the right and left pulmonary arteries (Fig. 14.4). Occasionally the dilated ductus can be identified as a local prominence of the left mediastinal border, between the aortic arch and the left pulmonary artery. Calcification of the aortic arch is not uncommon in older patients (Fig. 14.5).

Depending on the size of the left to right shunt, the plain film findings may remain stable or change over time. In patients with a small shunt the pulmonary resistance remains normal; in such individuals the radiographic appearance of the pulmonary vasculature will remain stable over a period of many years. On the other hand, when there is a large left to right shunt, pulmonary resistance tends to rise progressively, ultimately resulting in reversal of the shunt (Eisenmenger syndrome). Chest films at this stage typically show enlarged central pulmonary arteries with attenuation of the peripheral branches (see Fig. 9.4).

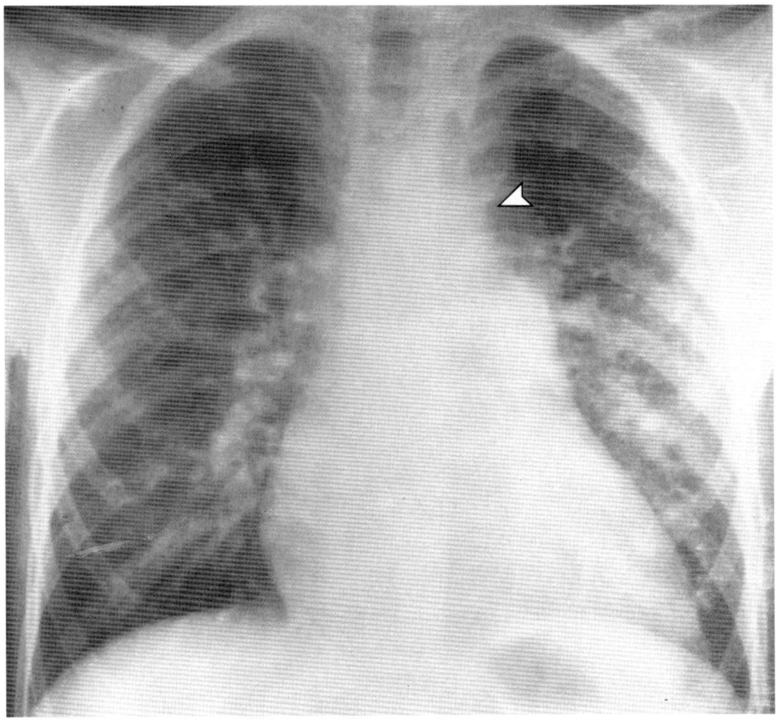

Fig. 14.4 PDA. In this 12-year-old patient a posteroanterior chest film shows an enlarged heart with a left ventricular configuration and moderate pulmonary plethora indicating the presence of a left to right shunt. The PDA appears as a linear density (*arrow*) along the left upper mediastinal border, between the aortic arch (above) and the dilated pulmonary trunk (below).

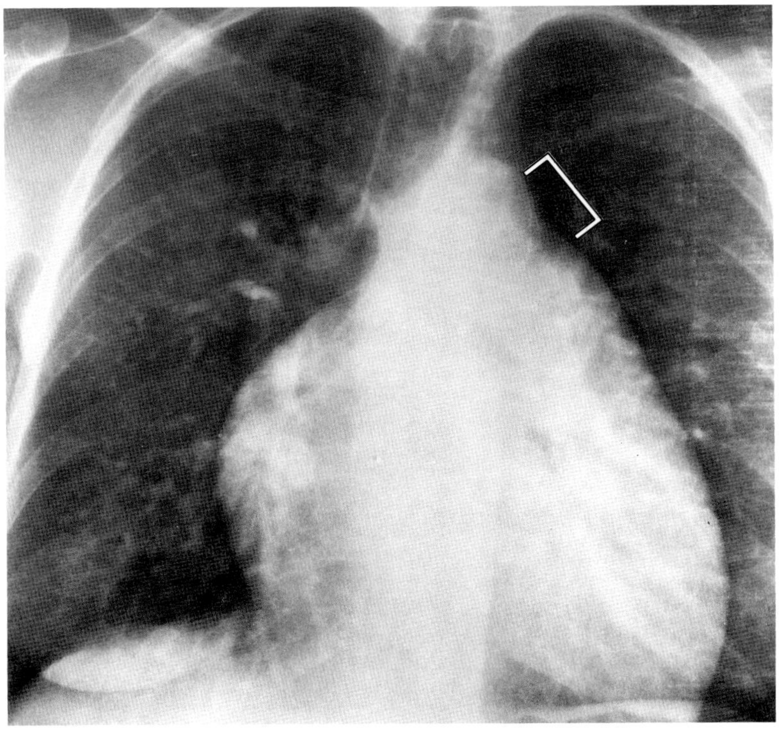

Fig. 14.5 Calification of aortic arch associated with PDA. Frontal chest film of an adult patient with a PDA shows dilation of the pulmonary trunk and aortic arch. Note the linear calcifications (*brace*) in the ductus arteriosus and aortic arch.

Chest films of a premature infant with a large PDA typically show cardiomegaly and pulmonary edema; in some instances, engorged pulmonary arteries and veins can be identified. The lung changes associated with the PDA may be obscured by parenchymal abnormalities resulting from hyaline membrane disease, bronchopulmonary dysplasia, or other lung pathology. Pharmacological closure of the ductus is often followed by rapid clinical and radiographic improvement (Fig. 14.6).

Echocardiography

Echocardiography plays an important role in the diagnosis of PDA. Short axial or long axial sections via an apical or parasternal window show the connection between the aortic arch and the left pulmonary artery (Fig. 14.7). Using color Doppler imaging, one can ascertain the direction of the shunt.

Cardiac Catheterization and Angiocardiography

Because of the sensitivity and specificity of echocardiography, cardiac catheterization and angiocardiography are seldom necessary in patients with typical clinical findings. However, both studies are indicated in patients with an atypical murmur or when increased pulmonary vascular resistance is suspected.

When pulmonary resistance is below systemic levels, an injection into the upper descending thoracic aorta will opacify the PDA (Fig. 14.8). Conversely, an injection into the pulmon-

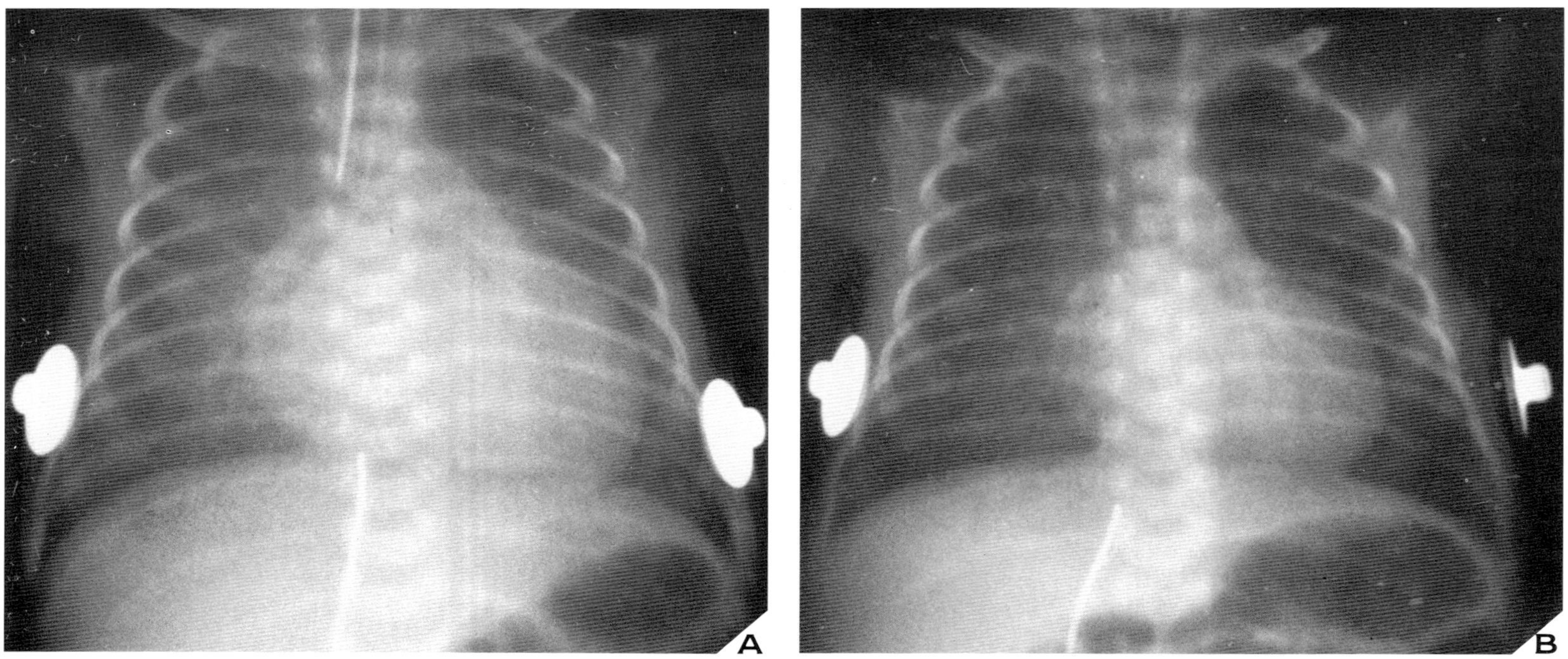

Fig. 14.6 Premature infant with PDA (response to indomethacin). (A) Frontal chest film shows cardiac enlargement with marked pulmonary plethora. (B) Follow-up chest film 3 days after indomethacin therapy shows marked improvement.

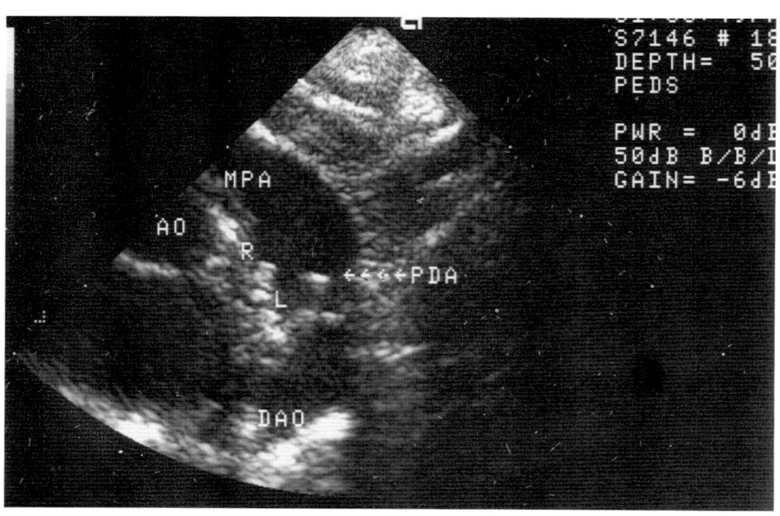

Fig. 14.7 PDA (echocardiographic findings). Parasternal short-axis view demonstrates a wide connection (PDA) between the left pulmonary artery L) and the descending thoracic aorta (DAO). [R = right pulmonary artery; AO = ascending aorta; MPA = main pulmonary artery (pulmonary trunk).

ary artery will opacify the PDA in a patient with reversal of the shunt secondary to increased pulmonary vascular resistance (Eisenmenger syndrome).

SYSTEMIC ARTERIOVENOUS SHUNTS AND FISTULAS (ARTERIOVENOUS MALFORMATIONS)

Extracardiac arteriovenous shunts and fistulas are an infrequent cause of increased flow and cardiac overload in neonates and young infants (rarely in older children and adults). The most common sites of hemodynamically significant vascular malformations are the brain, liver, extremities, lungs, and body wall. The most frequently encountered lesion of this type is the so-called "vein of Galen aneurysm." (This is a misnomer, because the lesion is actually an arteriovenous malformation involving the anterior, middle, and/or posterior cerebral arteries.) The anomalous vessels drain directly or indirectly into the vein of Galen, which in turn drains into the straight and lateral sinuses (all of these venous channels are markedly dilated secondary to the increased flow). Because the dilated vein of Galen lies above the roof of the third ventricle and the aqueduct of Sylvius, it may obstruct CSF flow, resulting in hydrocephalus.

HEMODYNAMIC AND CLINICAL FEATURES

Large extracardiac arteriovenous shunts and fistulas manifest hemodynamically with cardiac overload and high flow; most patients present with congestive heart failure of unknown

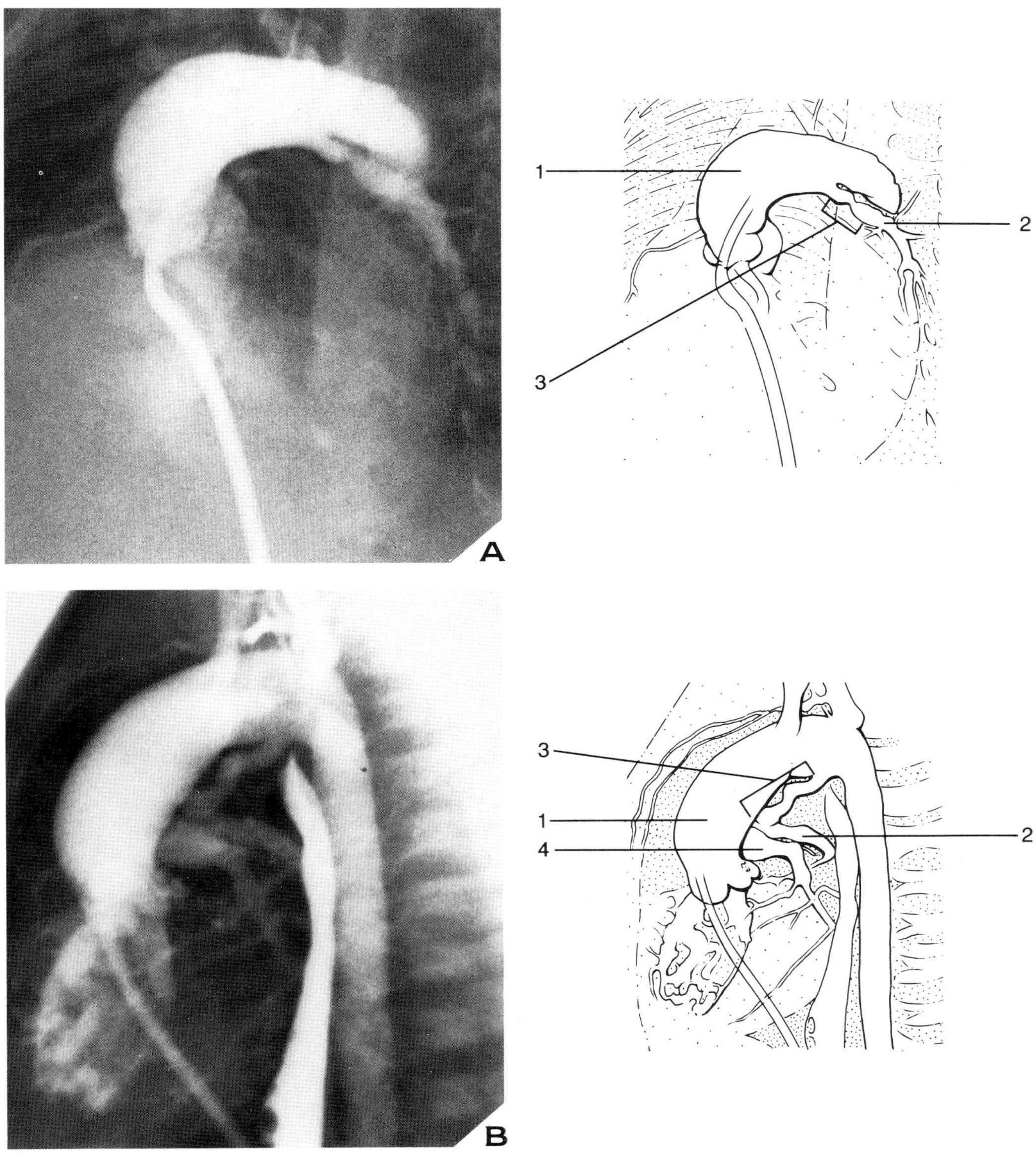

Fig. 14.8 PDA (angiographic features). (A) Thoracic aortogram (left anterior oblique projection) demonstrates a PDA originating on the inferior wall of the aortic arch and connecting distally with the left pulmonary artery. (B) Thoracic aortogram (lateral view) in a patient with a double aortic arch demonstrates a PDA connecting the left arch and the left pulmonary artery.

1	ascending aorta	3	PDA
2	left pulmonary artery	4	right pulmonary artery

cause. A thorough physical examination will usually point to the correct diagnosis. For example, a bruit in the head or neck (or a systolic murmur over the eye or neck) suggests the presence of an intracranial arteriovenous fistula; such patients may have other clinical manifestations of intracranial pathology (eg, hydrocephalus, seizures, headaches, hemorrhage). A bruit over the liver in a neonate or young infant is virtually pathognomonic of a hepatic hemangioendothelioma. Cutaneous hemangiomas are common in patients with vascular malformations of various types and provide an important diagnostic clue.

IMAGING AND INVASIVE DIAGNOSIS

Chest films typically show an enlarged heart and pulmonary plethora (Fig. 14.9). The definitive diagnosis is usually made by angiography, which demonstrates dilatation of the feeding artery or arteries, visualization of the AVM (which usually consists of a cluster of small channels), and early opacification of the draining veins (Fig. 14.10). Sonography, which can performed at the bedside, may be diagnostic in a neonate with an intracranial AVM (vein of Galen aneurysm) or a hemangioendothelioma of the liver.

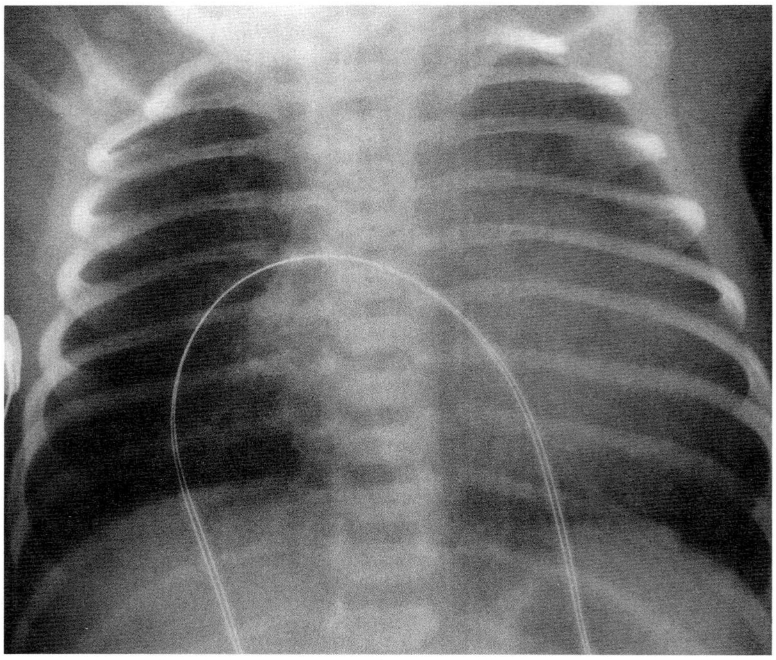

Fig. 14.9 Intracranial arteriovenous fistula ("vein of Galen aneurysm"). Frontal chest film of an infant with clinical signs of congestive heart failure shows moderate cardiomegaly with right atrial and right ventricular enlargement and pulmonary plethora. A bruit was audible over the head.

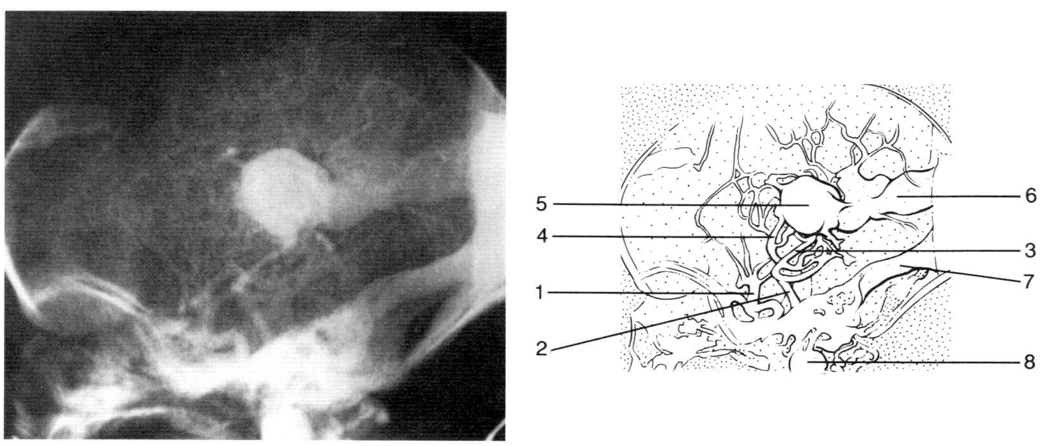

Fig. 14.10 Intracranial arteriovenous fistula ("vein of Galen" aneurysm"). Same patient as shown in Fig. 14.9. Lateral projection of skull obtained after left ventricular injection demonstrates significant enlargement of the middle and posterior cerebral arteries, which are supplying a large arteriovenous malformation. The vein of Galen, straight sinus, lateral venous sinuses, and jugular veins are all markedly dilated

1	carotid arteries	5	vein of Galen
2	vertebral artery	6	straight sinus
3	posterior cerebral artery	7	lateral sinus
4	arteriovenous malformation	8	jugular vein

CHAPTER 15

Anomalies of the Aortic Arch and Pulmonary Arteries

Anomalies of the aortic arch system and pulmonary arteries are found in about 3 percent of the population. Although certain malformations may compromise the upper aerodigestive tract, most are asymptomatic.

The most frequently encountered abnormalities of the arch system are left aortic arch with aberrant origin of the right subclavian artery, right aortic arch with aberrant origin of the left subclavian artery, and double aortic arch. Unusual malformations include cervical aortic arch and origin of the left pulmonary artery from the right pulmonary artery ("pulmonary artery sling").

Most aortic arch anomalies result from abnormal retention (or deletion) of portions of the fourth and sixth branchial arches (Figs. 15.1–15.6). (A cervical aortic arch is believed to result from abnormal retention of portions of the second or third branchial arch.) Fourth branchial arch anomalies result in vascular rings that encircle the trachea and esophagus. Vascular rings may be complete ("closed") or incomplete ("open"); the latter are much more common. The commonest type of *open ring* is left arch with aberrant right subclavian artery. In this anomaly, which occurs in about 0.5 percent of the general population, the ring is incomplete anteriorly (between the aorta and the pulmonary trunk). However, individuals with an unusually short left ligamentum arteriosum, or an unusually large Kommerell diverticulum, may be symptomatic. An analogous situation occurs in individuals with a right arch, aberrant left subclavian artery, and left ligamentum arteriosum. (Rarely, the ligamentum arteriosum is on the right; because the connection is between the right-sided descending thoracic aorta and the right pulmonary artery, this arrangement does not result in a vascular ring.) The commonest type of complete vascular ring is a double aortic arch. In this malformation, both arches are usually patent, although there may be an atretic segment.

Fewer than 20 percent of patients with aortic arch anomalies

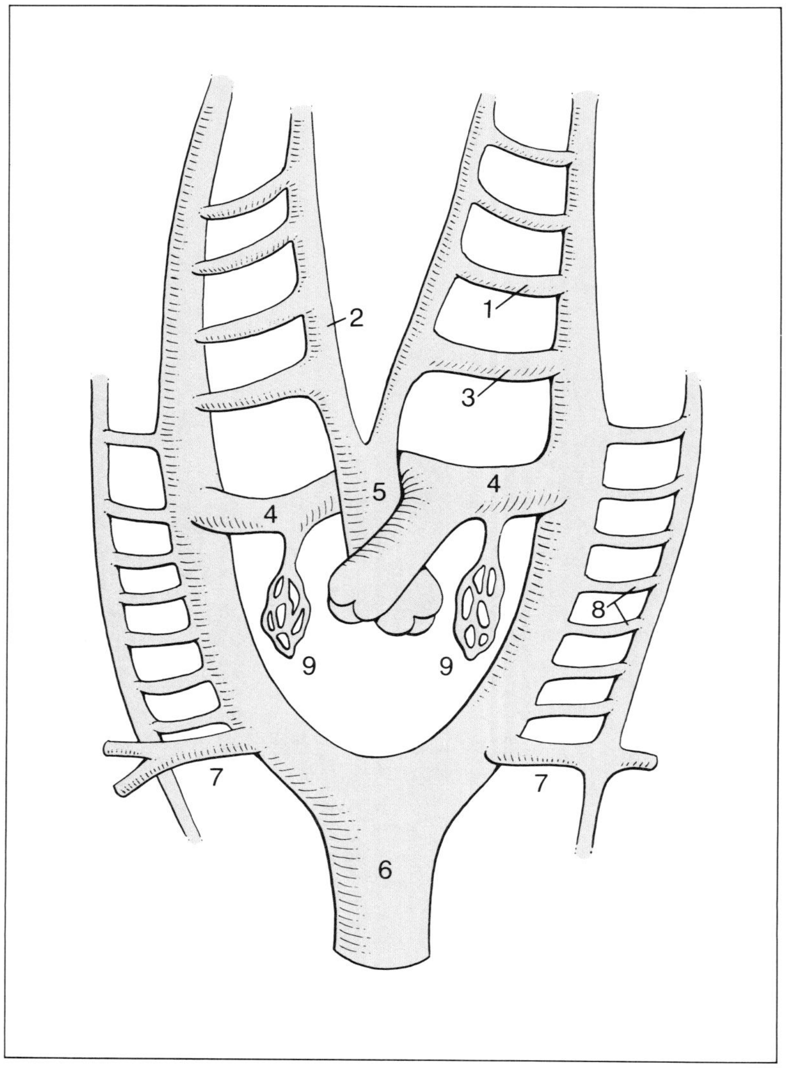

Fig. 15.1 Embryologic development of the aortic arch system. The ventral and dorsal aortic roots, the branchial arches and the connections to the longitudinal anastomoses are shown. (Adapted from Patten BM: The Cardiovascular System. In *Harris's Human Anatomy*, Section VI. 10th edition. Philadelphia: Blakiston, 1968)

1 third branchial arch
2 ventral aortic arch between branchial arches 3 and 4
3 fourth branchial arch
4 sixth branchial arch
5 ventral aortic root between branchial arches 4 and 6
6 dorsal aortic arch
7 seventh dorsal intersegmental artery
8 longitudinal anastomoses
9 lung buds

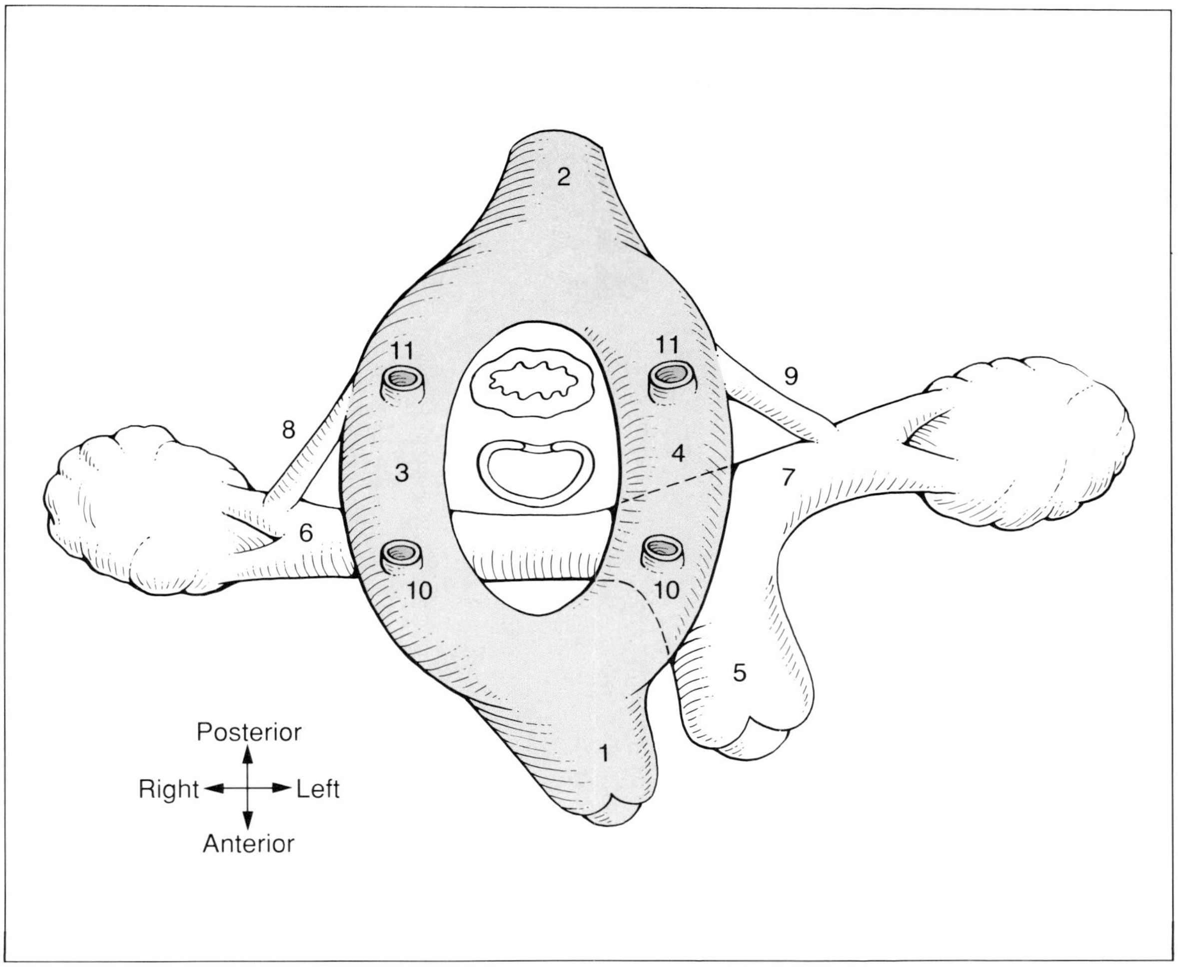

Fig. 15.2 Primitive vascular ring. Primitive double aortic arch and pulmonary arteries as seen from above. The right and left aortic arches originate from the aortic root and connect with the descending thoracic aorta, embracing the trachea (anterior) and esophagus (posterior). The pulmonary trunk and left pulmonary artery lie to the left of the aortic root. The right pulmonary artery passes behind the ascending aorta to reach the developing right lung. Each aortic arch communicates with the ipsilateral pulmonary artery via a ductus arteriosus. Four arteries originate from the primitive aortic arch: the paired common carotid arteries (closer to the aortic valve) and the paired subclavian arteries.

1 aortic root
2 descending thoracic aorta
3 right aortic arch
4 left aortic arch
5 pulmonary trunk
6 right pulmonary artery
7 left pulmonary artery
8 right ductus arteriosus
9 left ductus arteriosus
10 common carotid arteries
11 subclavian arteries

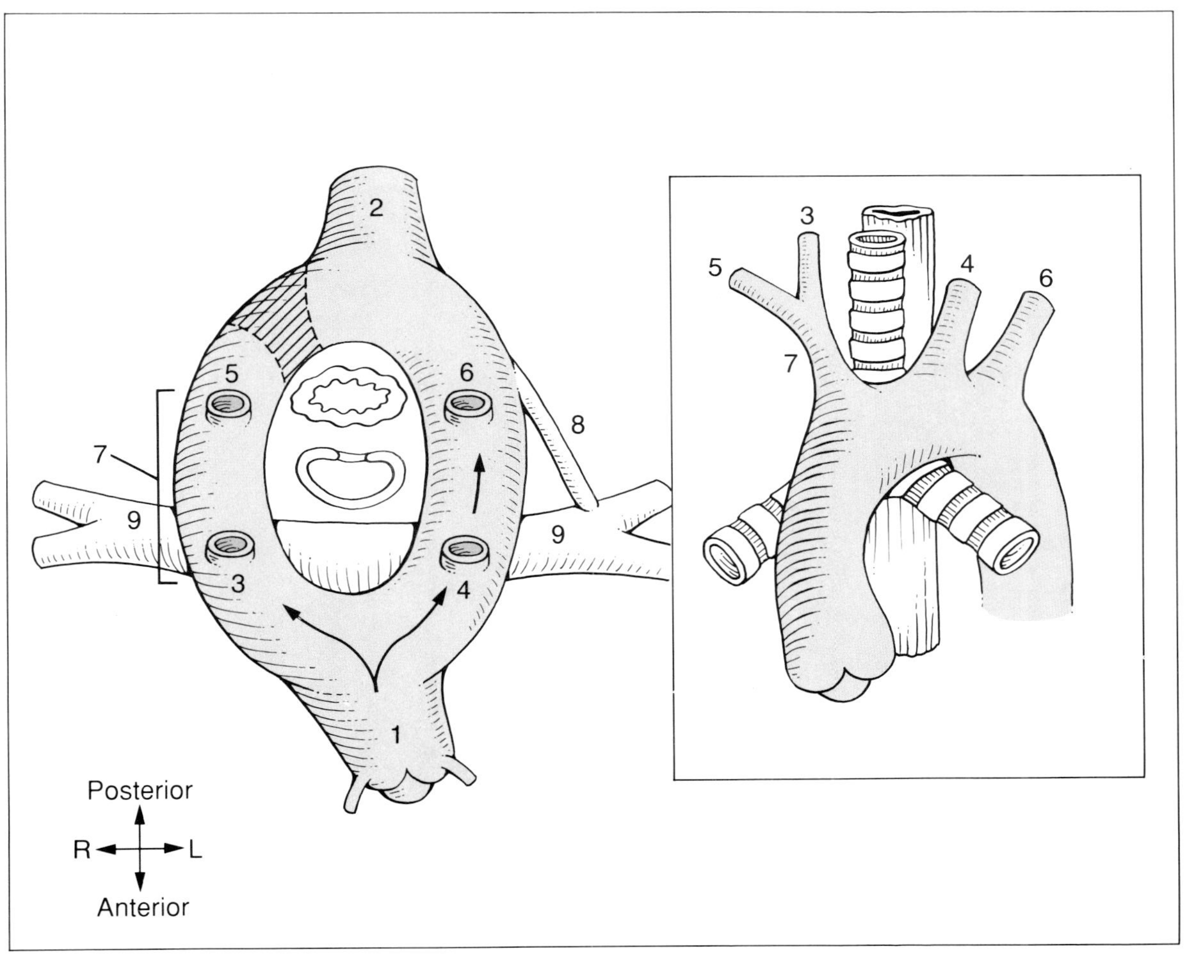

Fig. 15.3 Development of the normal left aortic arch. During normal development, the primitive vascular ring is disrupted distal to the origin of the right subclavian artery and proximal to the junction of the right arch and descending thoracic aorta. Thus, the first branch of the aortic arch is the right innominate artery, followed by the left carotid and left subclavian arteries. The left ductus arteriosus connects the upper descending aorta with the left pulmonary artery; the right ductus arteriosus, which connected the right subclavian and right pulmonary arteries, has disappeared.

1 aortic root
2 descending thoracic aorta
3 right carotid artery
4 left carotid artery
5 right subclavian artery
6 left subclavian artery
7 innominate artery
8 left ductus arteriosus
9 pulmonary arteries

hatched, site of disruption of primitive vascular ring (arrows indicate direction of blood flow)

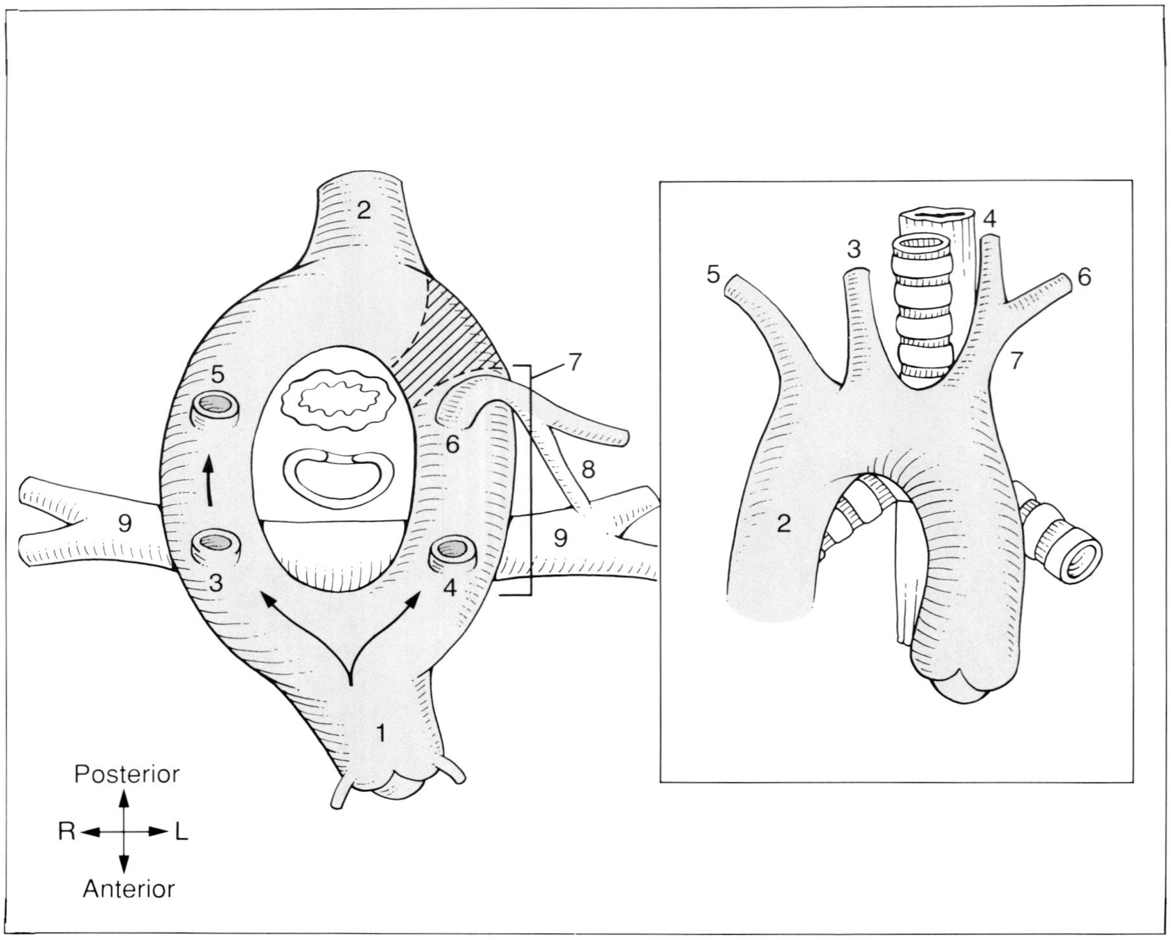

Fig. 15.4 Development of right aortic arch with mirror image branching. Interruption of the primitive vascular ring between the left subclavian artery and the junction of the left aortic arch with the descending thoracic aorta results in a mirror image of the normal left arch, ie, a right arch with mirror-image branching. The first branch is the left innominate artery, followed by the right common carotid and right subclavian. The descending thoracic aorta is usually to the right of the spine in the upper thorax and to the left of the spine in the lower thorax.

1 aortic root
2 descending thoracic aorta
3 right carotid artery
4 left carotid artery
5 right subclavian artery
6 left subclavian artery
7 innominate artery
8 left ductus arteriosus
9 pulmonary arteries

hatched, site of disruption of primitive vascular ring

(arrows indicate direction of blood flow)

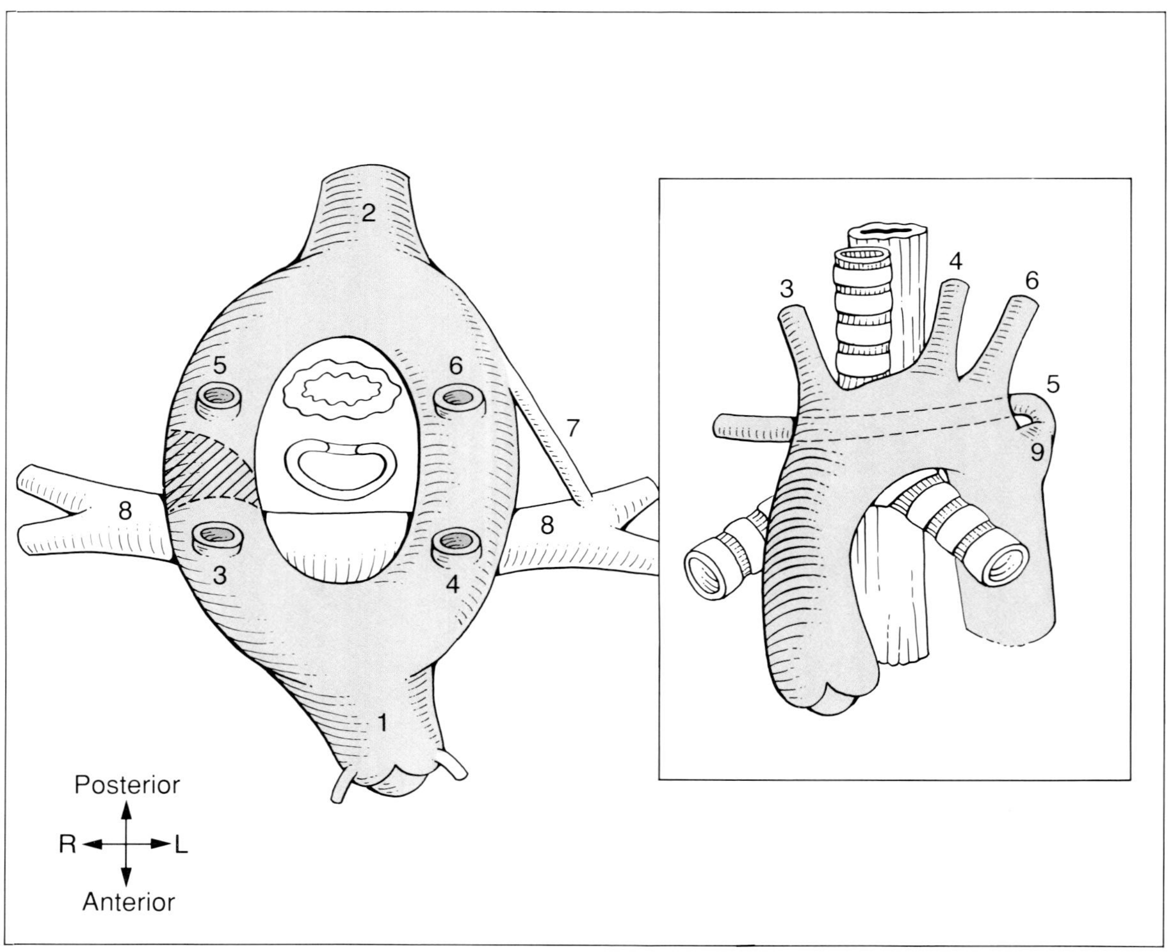

Fig. 15.5 Development of left aortic arch with anomalous (aberrant) right subclavian artery. If the right aortic arch is interrupted between the right carotid and right subclavian arteries, the first branch of the aortic arch will be the right carotid, followed by the left carotid, left subclavian, and right subclavian arteries. The right subclavian artery crosses behind the esophagus to reach the right arm. A Kommerell diverticulum (a localized widening at the origin of the right subclavian artery which represents the remnant of the distal right arch) is commonly present.

1 aortic root
2 descending thoracic aorta
3 right carotid artery
4 left carotid artery
5 right subclavian artery
6 left subclavian artery
7 left ductus arteriosus
8 pulmonary arteries
9 Kommerell diverticulum

hatched, site of disruption of primitive vascular ring

have congenital heart disease. However, certain cardiac defects are commonly associated with a right aortic arch, a finding that may be helpful in differential diagnosis (Fig. 15.7).

CLINICAL FEATURES

Presenting symptoms include stridor, cyanotic spells, recurrent respiratory infections, and dysphagia. Complete (closed) rings usually cause more distress than incomplete (open) ones and are usually symptomatic in infants and young children.

IMAGING

The role of imaging in the preoperative evaluation of patients with vascular rings remains controversial. Many authors believe that chest radiographs and barium esophagography are usually sufficient for this purpose. In their view, angiography can usually be omitted because there is no need to differentiate between a double aortic arch (the most common type of symptomatic vascular ring in infancy) and the right arch/short left ligamentum arteriosum complex: a left posterolateral thoracotomy is the standard surgical approach in either instance.

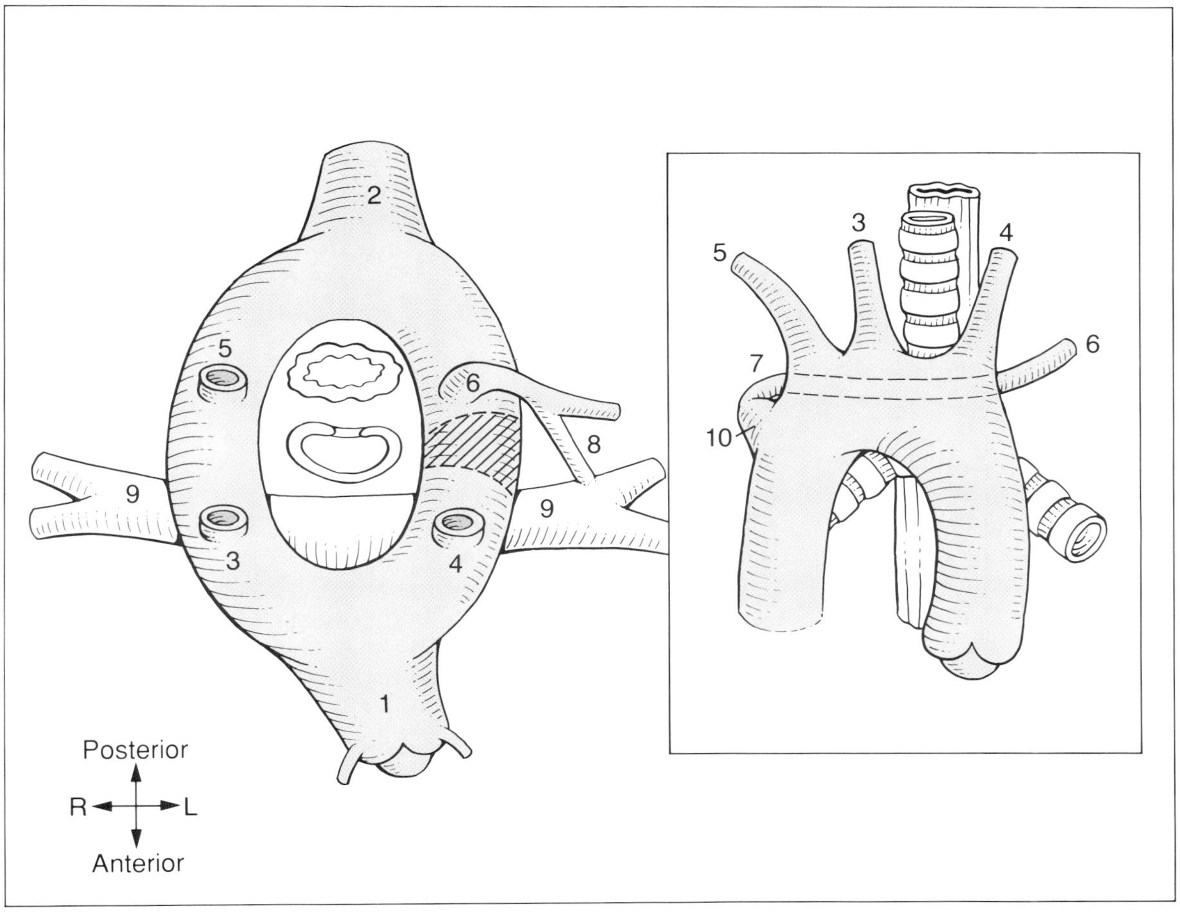

Fig. 15.6 Development of right aortic arch with anomalous (aberrant) left subclavian artery (schematic). Interruption of the left aortic arch between the left carotid and left subclavian arteries results in a right arch with an anomalous branching pattern. The first branch is the left carotid artery; the second is the right carotid; the third is the right subclavian; and the fourth is the left subclavian, which passes behind the esophagus to reach the left arm. A portion of the distal left arch persists as a localized widening at the origin of the anomalous left subclavian artery (Kommerell diverticulum). The descending thoracic aorta may be on the right or the left.

1 aortic root
2 descending thoracic aorta
3 right carotid artery
4 left carotid artery
5 right subclavian artery
6 left subclavian artery
7 innominate artery
8 left ductus arteriosus
9 pulmonary arteries
10 Kommerell diverticulum
hatched, site of disruption of primitive vascular ring

Fig. 15.7 ASSOCIATION OF RIGHT AORTIC ARCH WITH CONGENITAL HEART DISEASE.*

Malformation	Frequency of right aortic arch
Truncus arteriosus	40–50%
Tetralogy of Fallot	25–30%
Double outlet right ventricle	30%
Pulmonary atresia with VSD	20%
Tricuspid atresia	6–10%
Transposition of the great arteries	3–5%

Data derived from several autopsy and clinical series.

Fig. 15.6 Association of right aortic arch with congenital heart disease.

Proponents of angiography argue that anatomic variants are sufficiently common to warrant a more thorough preoperative evaluation, pointing out that 10 to 20 percent of vascular rings are best approached through a right thoracotomy and that other cardiovascular abnormalities are present in a small percentage of cases. In a patient with an unsuspected coarctation of the right arch, for example, dividing the left arch may result in a hemodynamically significant aortic coarctation.

Cineangiography in the anteroposterior, lateral, and axial four-chamber projection accurately depicts the abnormal vascular anatomy. (The latter projection is particularly useful in patients with complex or atypical malformations.) By instilling barium paste through a nasogastric tube, it is possible to combine angiography with esophagography in an anesthetized patient. Pulmonary angiography is performed when an aberrant left pulmonary artery ("pulmonary artery sling") is suspected.

Intravenous digital subtraction angiography (DSA), although it lacks the spatial resolution of film-screen angiography, is less invasive than conventional cineangiography and is highly accurate, even in small infants. Because intravenous DSA requires less contrast material than conventional cineangiography, a complete study with multiple projections, including four-chamber and axial views, can be obtained with a total dose that does not exceed safe limits (less than 3 to 5 mL/kg). Intravenous DSA is much less expensive than conventional angiocardiography and can be done on an outpatient basis.

Noninvasive imaging techniques (echocardiography, MRI, conventional and cine CT) offer attractive alternatives to angiography. MRI, which avoids ionizing radiation and allows multiplanar imaging, is particularly promising. In one recent pediatric series the only detail that could not be depicted by MRI was the exact site of the ligamentum arteriosum (Bisset et al, 1987). Similar accuracy has been claimed for cine CT, although this technique requires intravascular injection of contrast material and exposes the patient to ionizing radiation. Because of motion artifacts, which degrade images of the mediastinum, and the difficulty of maintaining optimal levels of contrast material over large portions of the chest (owing to limitations in the amount of contrast material that can be administered), conventional contrast-enhanced CT is less successful than cine CT in demonstrating aortic arch anomalies.

Like MRI, echocardiography avoids ionizing radiation and allows multiplanar imaging; it is also much less expensive. Although echocardiography accurately depicts aortic arch anomalies in infants and young children, it may not be possible to image the entire thoracic aorta in older children and adults.

ANOMALIES ASSOCIATED WITH LEFT AORTIC ARCH

INNOMINATE ARTERY COMPRESSION SYNDROME

An "anomalous" origin of the innominate (brachiocephalic) artery, ie, anterior or to the left of the trachea, is sometimes listed as a cause of symptomatic tracheal compression in infants and young children. Patients with the "innominate artery compression syndrome" typically present with cough, stridor, and apneic spells. Lateral films of the chest or neck show a prominent impression on the anterior tracheal wall at or just below the thoracic inlet; in some instances the tracheal lumen is markedly narrowed or even obliterated Fig. 15.8.

Recent observations have challenged the concept of an "anomalous" innominate artery. Imaging studies and bronchoscopy indicate that this vessel crosses the trachea in the great majority of infants and young children, both symptomatic and asymptomatic (Fig. 15.9). This relationship, which is clearly seen on both angiography and MRI (Fig. 15.10), presumably accounts for the slight indentation of the anterior tracheal wall that is commonly seen in asymptomatic children under 2 years of age.

There is little doubt that the crossing innominate artery can cause symptomatic airway compression in an infant with a "tight" or "crowded" mediastinum secondary to congenital heart disease or chronic esophageal distension (eg, following surgery for esophageal atresia). These patients usually benefit from surgical decompression (aortopexy or repositioning and reattachment of the innominate artery). It is not clear, however, that the crossing innominate artery is responsible for obstructive symptoms and apneic spells in other infants. Many authors have reported dramatic results following aortopexy, with cessation of

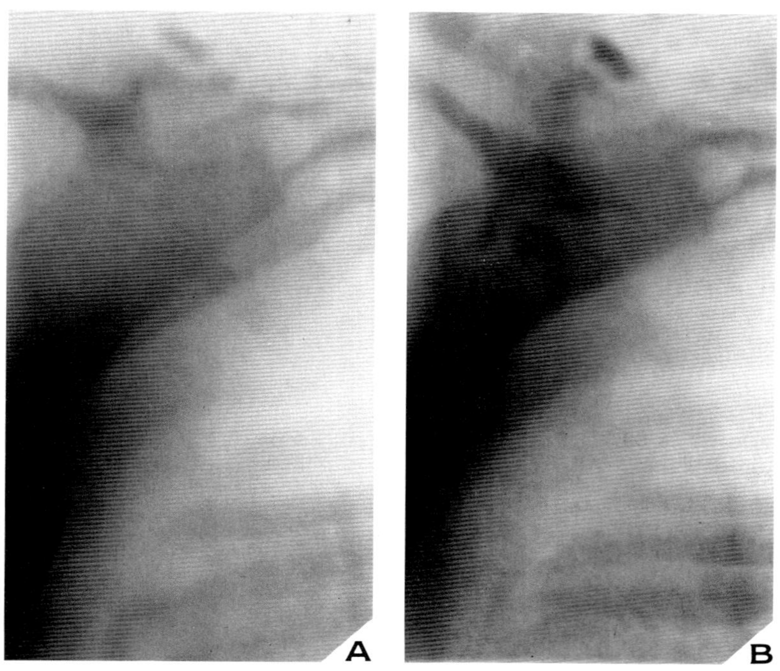

Fig. 15.8 Innominate artery compression syndrome. This 2.5-month-old infant was admitted in respiratory arrest, with a history of inspiratory stridor and feeding difficulty during the preceding month. Lateral spot films show partial (A) and complete (B) obliteration of tracheal lumen at the level of the thoracic inlet. Bronchoscopy revealed marked indentation of the anterior tracheal wall with prominent transmitted arterial pulsations, presumably produced by the innominate artery. The patient's symptoms abated after aortopexy.

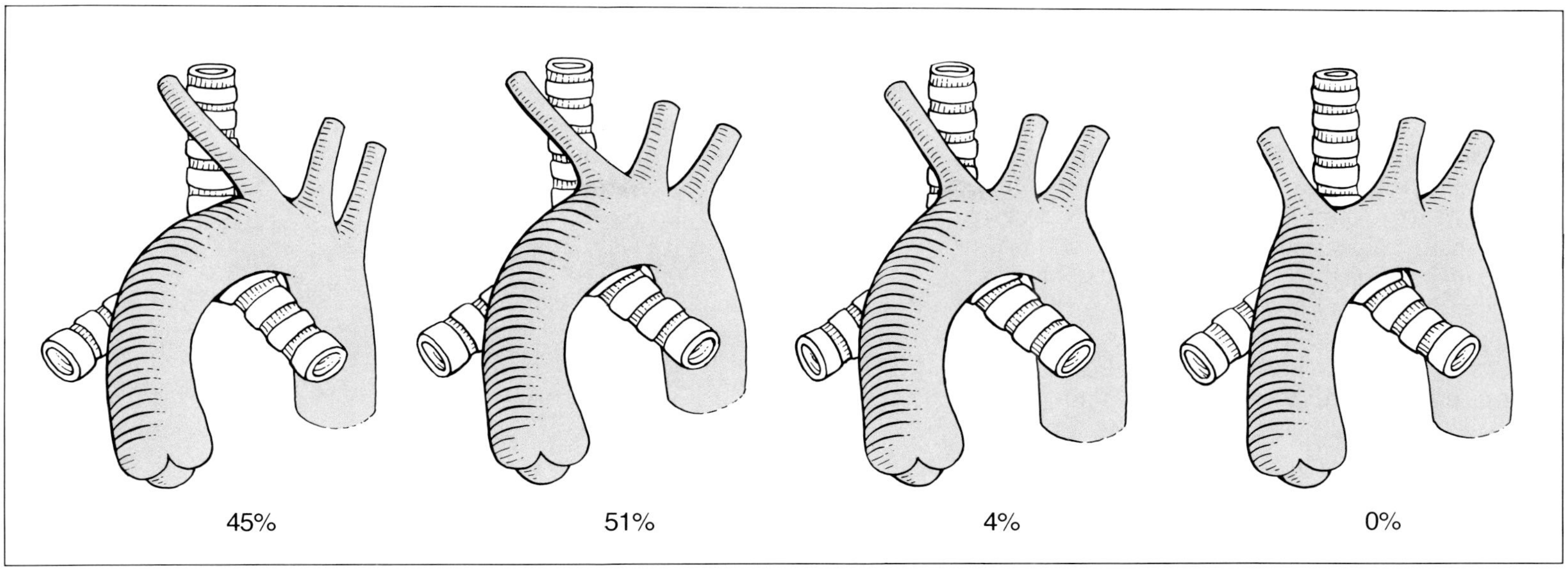

Fig. 15.9 Relationship of right innominate artery to trachea in children. Data based the anteroposterior projections of 172 aortograms and angiocardiograms in children and adolescents with congenital heart disease (excluding patients with transposition of the great arteries or tetralogy of Fallot). The innominate artery originated partially (51%) or completely (45%) to the left of the trachea. In 4% its origin was anterior to the trachea. The presumed "adult" relationship of the innominate artery and trachea (ie, both walls of the artery to the right of the trachea) was not observed in any of these patients. (Adapted with permission from Strife JL, et al: Tracheal compression by the innominate artery in infancy and childhood. *Radiology* 1981; 139:73)

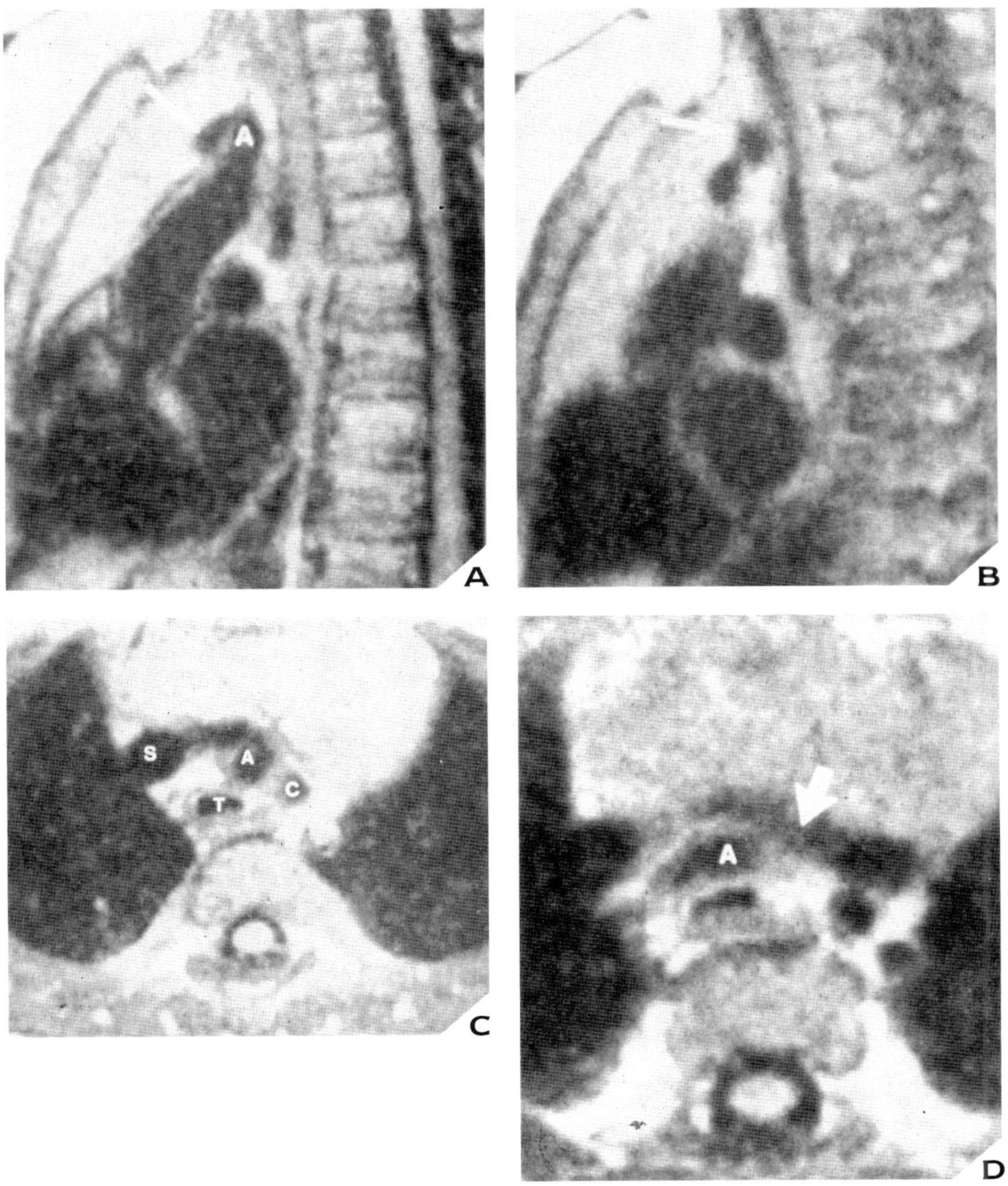

Fig. 15.10 Normal relations of innominate artery. Gated MR images of 8-month-old infant with clinically suspected airway obstruction. (A) Sagittal section through thorax at level of ascending aorta. The innominate artery is seen to arise from ascending aorta. The innominate vein is more anterior. (B) Sagittal section slightly to the right of A. The innominate artery is seen adjacent to the indented tracheal wall. (C) Axial section. Origin of innominate artery is anterior and slightly to the left of the compressed trachea. (D) Axial section slightly cephalad to C. The innominate artery is seen crossing anterior to the flattened trachea. The innominate vein is anterior to innominate artery. (Reproduced with permission from Fletcher BD, Cohn RC: Tracheal compression and the innominate artery in infants and children. *Radiology* 1989; 170:104)

A	innominate artery
S	superior vena cava
C	left common carotid artery
T	trachea
arrow	innominate vein

apneic spells and abatement of clinical airway obstruction. However, most infants who are treated conservatively improve spontaneously even though the relationship of the innominate artery and trachea is unchanged. Indeed, the innominate artery compression syndrome is rarely encountered after 18 months of age. These observations suggest that the underlying problem is an intrinsic abnormality of the tracheal cartilage ("tracheomalacia"), which may be aggravated during infancy by vascular compression resulting from a crowded upper mediastinum.

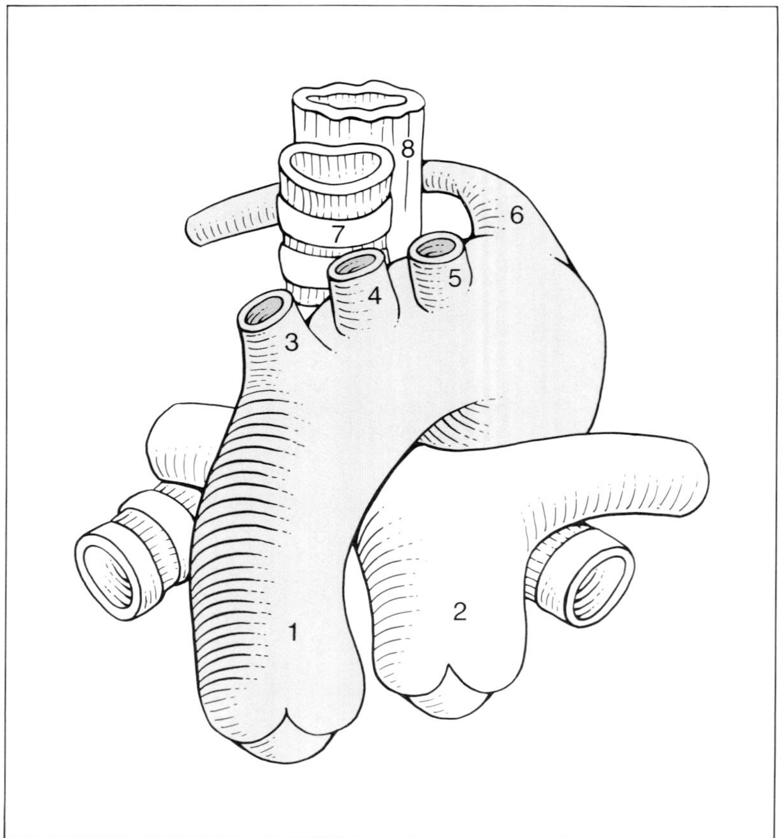

1	ascending aorta	5	left subclavian artery
2	pulmonary trunk	6	right subclavian artery
3	right common carotid artery	7	trachea
4	left common carotid artery	8	esophagus

Fig. 15.11 Left aortic arch with anomalous right subclavian artery. Viewed from above. The right common carotid artery arises as the first branch of the aortic arch, followed by the left common carotid and left subclavian arteries. The right subclavian artery is the last branch. It passes behind the trachea and esophagus to reach the right arm. A Kommerell diverticulum is generally present at the origin of the right subclavian artery.

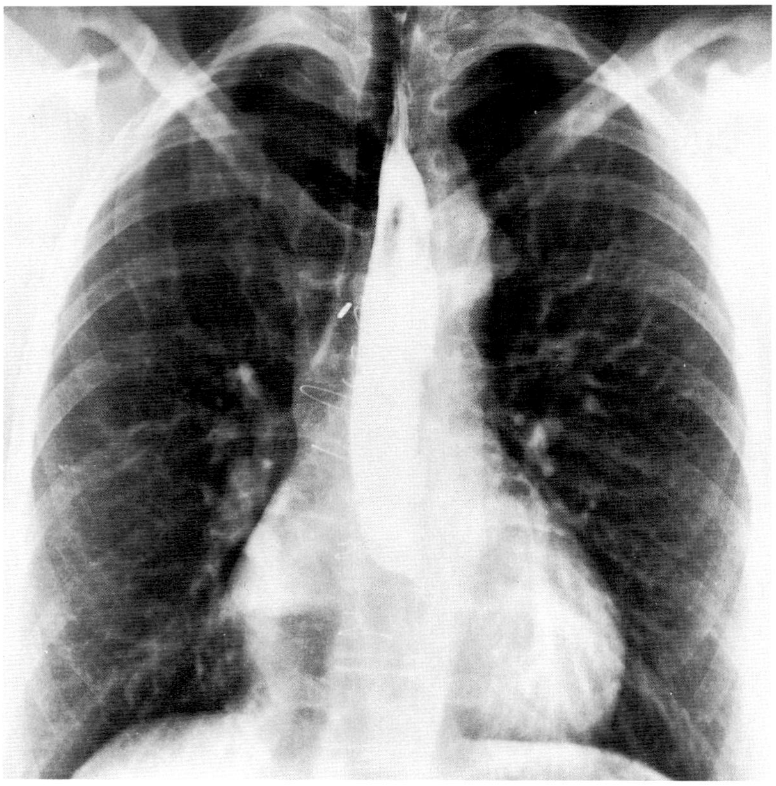

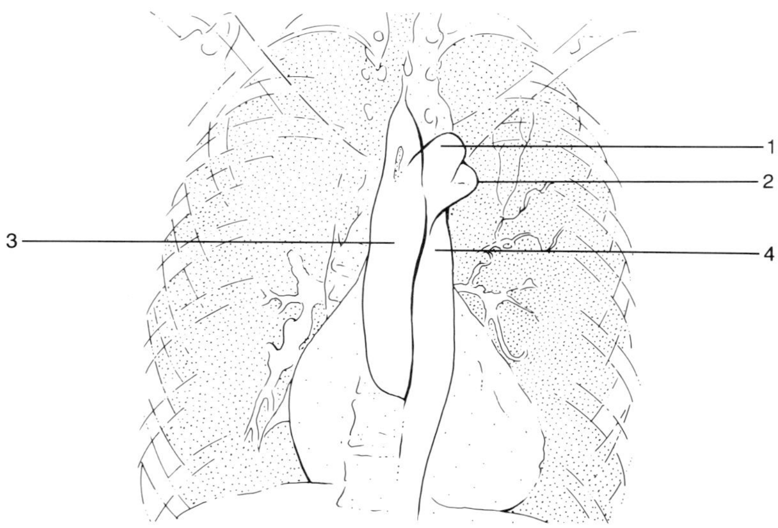

1	aortic arch	3	esophagus
2	right subclavian artery	4	descending thoracic aorta

Fig. 15.12 Left aortic arch with anomalous right subclavian artery. The aortic arch is well visualized on the frontal chest film. The anomalous right subclavian artery appears as a soft tissue density cephalad to the aortic arch.

LEFT AORTIC ARCH WITH ABERRANT ORIGIN OF THE RIGHT SUBCLAVIAN ARTERY

Normally, the right ventral fourth arch and the seventh intersegmental artery develop into the right subclavian artery. Resorption of the right ventral fourth arch, with persistence of the right dorsal aorta caudal to the third arch, results in an aberrant right subclavian artery. In this anomaly, which occurs in about 0.5 percent of the general population, the right subclavian artery arises as the last branch of the aortic arch and courses posterior to the esophagus to reach the right upper extremity (Fig. 15.11). Together with the left ligamentum arteriosum, the vascular structures form an incomplete ("open") vascular ring. Although most patients with this arrangement are asymptomatic, some infants and children have recurrent aspiration episodes secondary to esophageal compression. Dysphagia secondary to esophageal compression ("dysphagia lusoria") may also occur in the elderly.

IMAGING

The aberrant right subclavian artery can often be identified on frontal chest films as a convex density along the left upper mediastinal border. The aortic arch (which indents the left side of the trachea) and the descending thoracic aorta are both on the left. On the lateral projection, the anomalous right subclavian artery appears as a large, rounded superior mediastinal mass posterior to the trachea, which is displaced anteriorly.

The frontal esophagram shows an oblique filling defect beginning just above the aortic arch and ascending from left to right, which represents the aberrant right subclavian artery crossing behind the esophagus. The left side of the esophagus is indented by the left aortic arch (Fig. 15.12). A prominent impression on the posterior aspect of the esophagus, produced by the remnant of the right aortic arch (Kommerell diverticulum) and the aberrant right subclavian artery, is seen on the lateral projection (Fig. 15.13).

On the thoracic aortogram, the aberrant right subclavian artery is seen to arise as the most distal (ie, fourth) branch of the

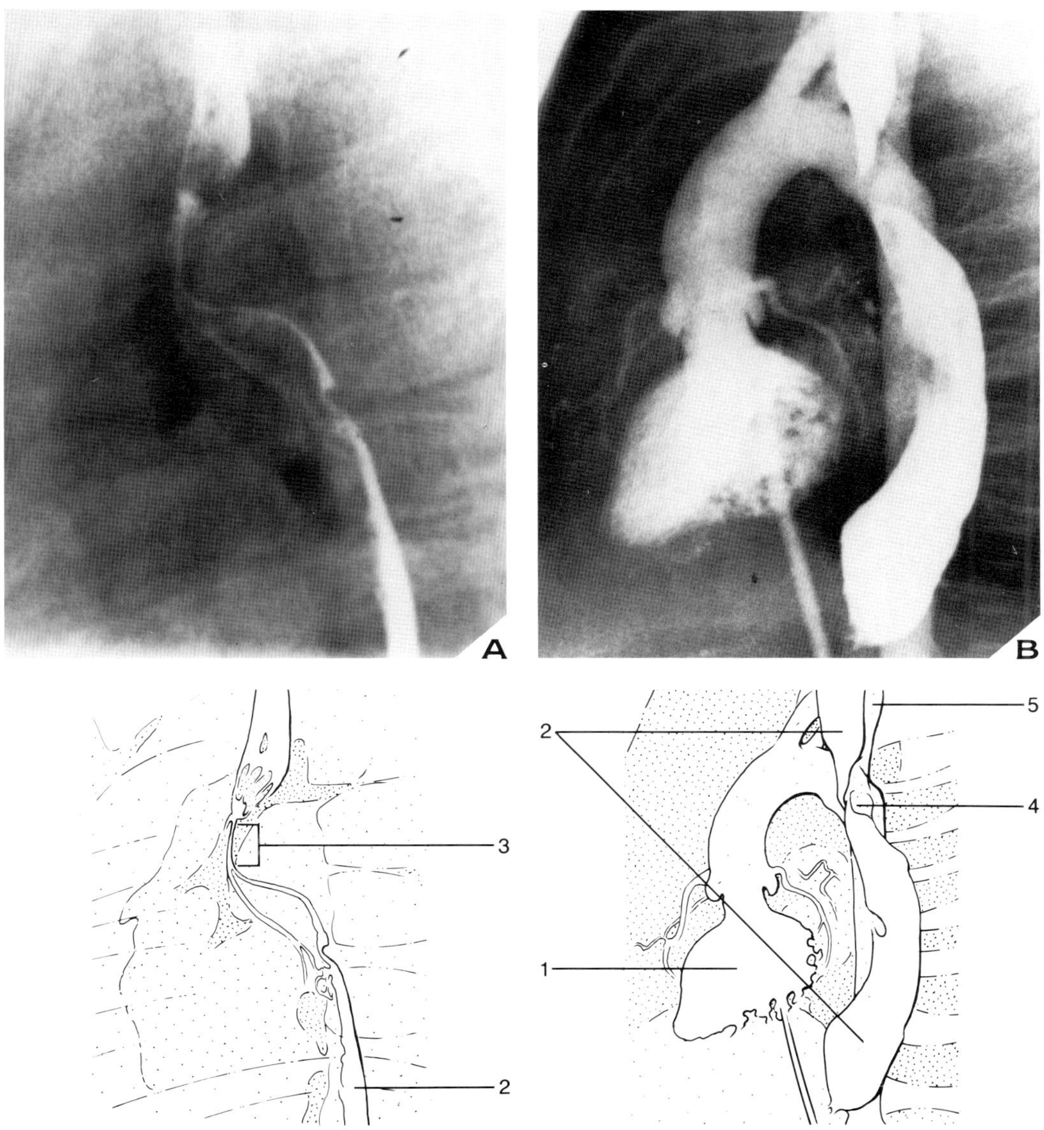

Fig. 15.13 Left aortic arch with aberrant right subclavian artery. Lateral views of barium esophagram (A) and thoracic aortogram (B) show posterior indentation of the esophagus by a Kommerell diverticulum and the anomalous right subclavian artery. The trachea is not compressed.

1 left ventricle
2 esophagus
3 indentation caused by Kommerell diverticulum
4 Kommerell diverticulum
5 right subclavian artery

aortic arch (Fig. 15.14). Noninvasive imaging techniques (echocardiography, MRI, or CT) can be used in lieu of angiography (Fig. 15.15). The left ligamentum arteriosum, which completes the vascular ring, cannot be demonstrated by imaging techniques.

RIGHT AORTIC ARCH

Resorption of the left ventral fourth arch results in a right aortic arch, which may be associated with an aberrant left subclavian artery or with mirror-image branching of the great arteries. The latter may be associated with a right or left descending thoracic aorta.

RIGHT AORTIC ARCH WITH MIRROR-IMAGE BRANCHING AND LEFT DESCENDING THORACIC AORTA

Right aortic arch with mirror-image branching and a right descending thoracic aorta is a normal anatomic variation. Rarely, the descending thoracic aorta crosses behind the esophagus and descends on the left (Fig. 15.16). The latter arrangement results in an incomplete vascular ring which is often symptomatic.

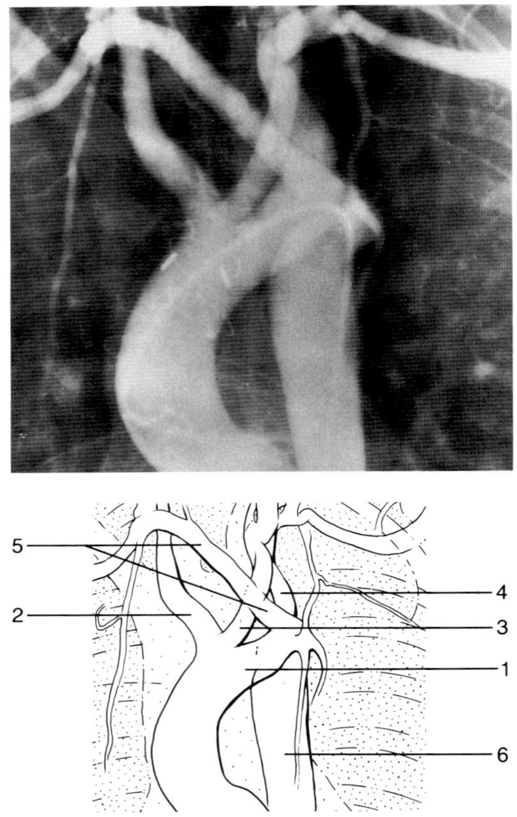

Fig. 15.14 Left aortic arch with aberrant right subclavian artery. Frontal projection of thoracic aortogram shows the right subclavian artery arising from the distal portion of the left aortic arch and coursing superiorly and to the right.

1 left aortic arch
2 right carotid artery
3 left carotid artery
4 left subclavian artery
5 anomalous right subclavian artery
6 descending thoracic aorta

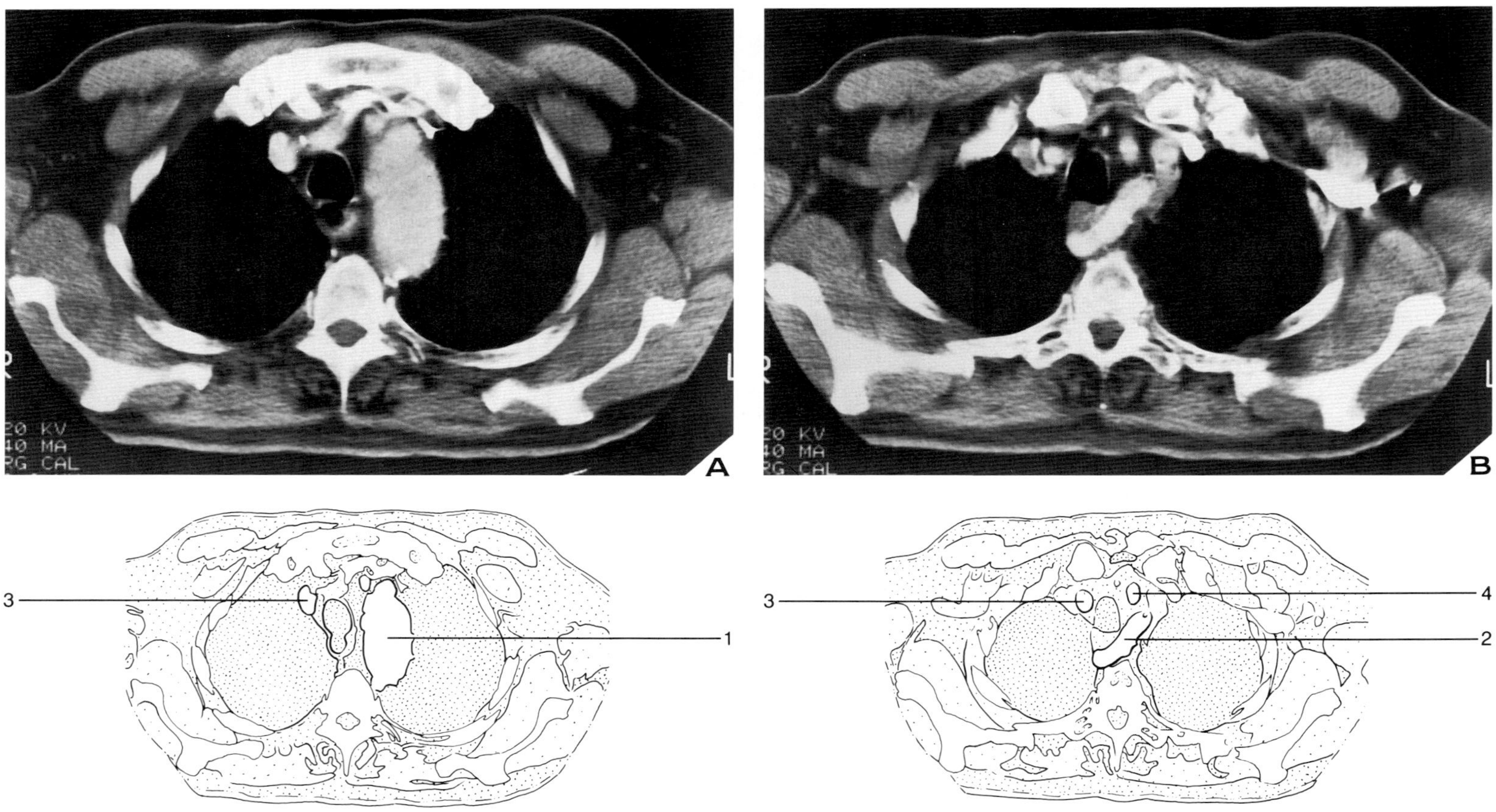

Fig. 15.15 Left aortic arch with anomalous right subclavian artery. (A) CT scan at level of aortic arch shows the aortic arch to the left of the trachea. (B) CT section above the aortic arch shows the right subclavian artery coursing behind the trachea. The right common carotid, left common carotid, and left subclavian arteries arise independently.

1 left aortic arch
2 anomalous right subclavian artery
3 right common carotid artery
4 left common carotid artery

IMAGING

On the frontal chest film the right aortic arch can often be identified as a right paratracheal density. In older children and adults, the supracarinal portion of the trachea is typically in the midline or displaced to the left; however, this is often not the case in infants and young children. When the descending thoracic aorta is on the right, it can be identified as a linear density just to the right of the spine; when it is on the left, it

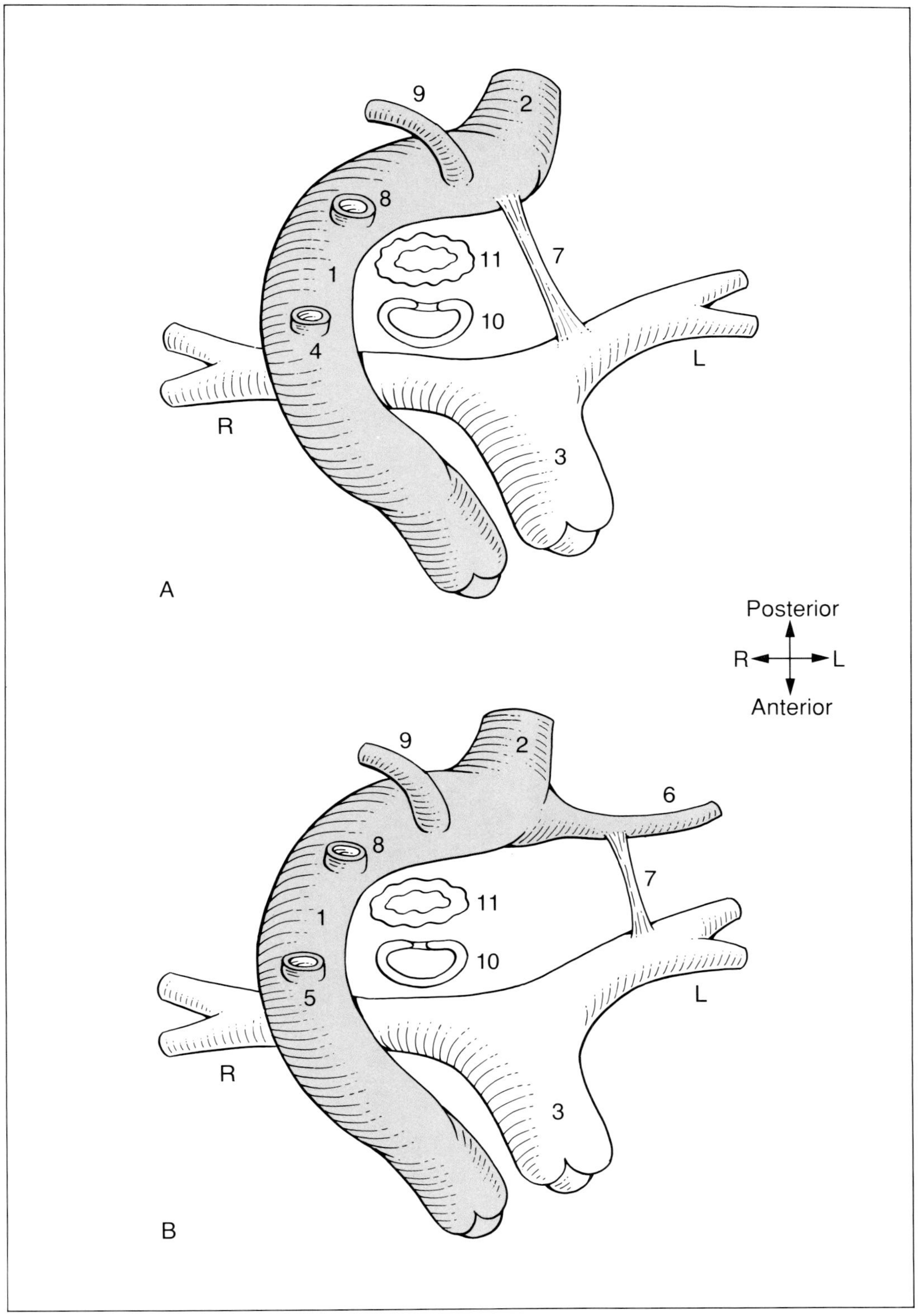

Fig. 15.16 Right aortic arch and left descending thoracic aorta. (A) The right aortic arch lies to the right of the trachea and courses behind it to join the descending thoracic aorta. The branches of the aortic arch arise in the usual way. The right subclavian artery courses from left to right, crossing the innominate and right subclavian arteries. This arrangement (the least common) creates an incomplete vascular ring consisting of the right aortic arch, the descending thoracic aorta (which crosses behind the esophagus), the left ductus or ligamentum arteriosus, and the left pulmonary artery. (B) In the most common form of the anomaly, there is an anomalous origin of the left subclavian artery, which arises as the last branch of the aortic arch. This creates an incomplete vascular ring consisting of the aortic (Kommerell) diverticulum, the left subclavian artery, and the left ligamentum arteriosum. The ring is usually lax and does not compress the trachea or esophagus.

1 right aortic arch
2 descending thoracic aorta
3 pulmonary trunk and left pulmonary artery
4 left innominate artery
5 left carotid artery
6 left subclavian artery
7 left ligamentum (or ductus) arteriosum
8 right common carotid artery
9 right subclavian artery
10 trachea
11 esophagus

appears as a linear retrocardiac density just to the left of the spine (Fig. 15.17). When the descending thoracic aorta is on the right, the lateral esophagram is unremarkable. When it is on the left, the aorta produces a prominent impression on the posterior aspect of the esophagus (Fig. 15.18). Anterior tracheal compression may be evident on the lateral chest film. On the thoracic aortogram, the aortic arch lies to the right of the trachea. The first branch of the arch is the left innominate artery, which gives rise to the left subclavian and left carotid arteries; the second branch is the right carotid artery; and the last branch is the right subclavian artery, which crosses the left subclavian and left carotid arteries to reach the right arm (Fig. 15.19). This anomaly can also be demonstrated by noninvasive techniques (echocardiography, MRI, or CT).

RIGHT AORTIC ARCH WITH ABERRANT LEFT SUBCLAVIAN ARTERY

This anomaly results when the left ventral fourth arch is resorbed and the left dorsal aorta persists, the latter fusing with the seventh left intersegmental artery to form the left subclavian artery. The aberrant left subclavian artery arises as the last branch of the aortic arch and courses behind the esophagus to reach the left upper extremity (Fig. 15.20). The thoracic aorta usually descends on the right (rarely, it is in the midline or on the left). The ductus remnant is usually on the right. In some instances a persistent left ductus or ligamentum arteriosum (which may be associated with a prominent Kommerell diverticulum) produces a symptomatic vascular ring.

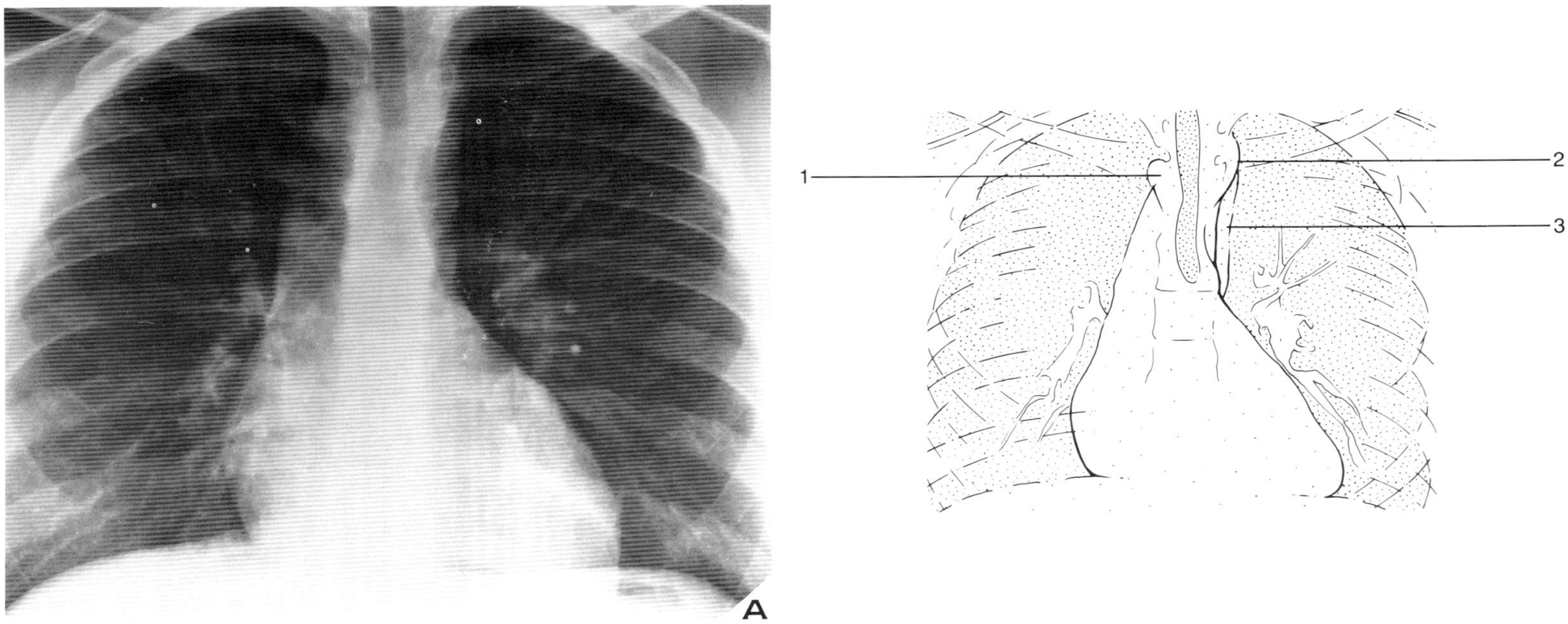

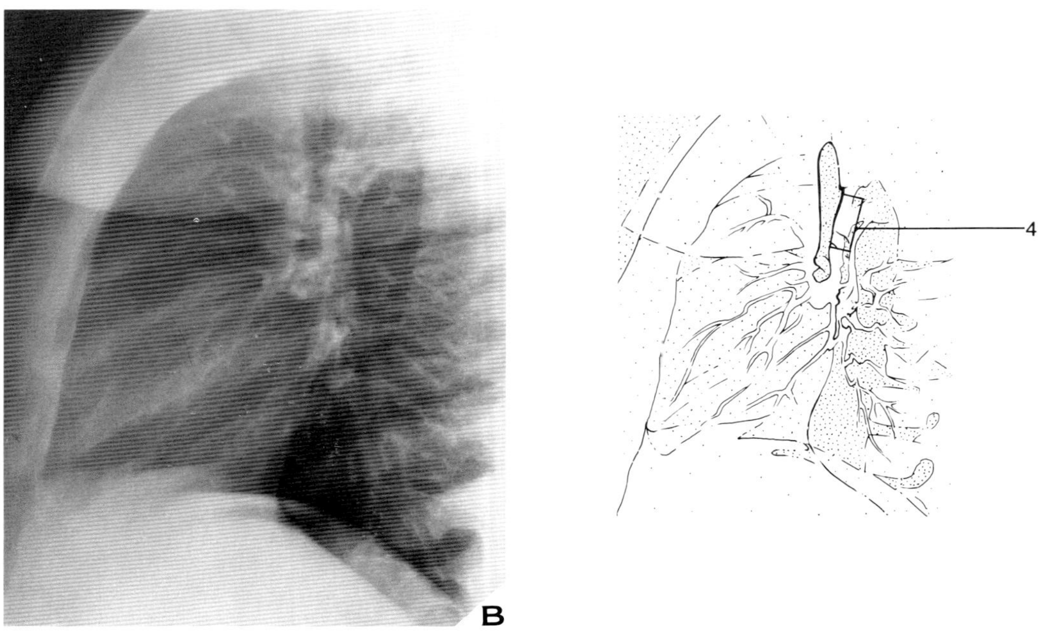

1	right aortic arch (to right of trachea)	3	descending thoracic aorta
2	upper part of descending thoracic aorta (to left of trachea)	4	displacement of trachea by descending thoracic aorta

Fig. 15.17 Right aortic arch and left descending thoracic aorta. (A) Frontal projection. The right aortic arch appears as a density to the right of the trachea and produces a shallow impression on the tracheal wall. The density to the left of the trachea represents the upper part of the descending thoracic aorta. The distal descending thoracic aorta appears as a linear density to the left of the spine. (B) Lateral projection. Note slight anterior displacement of trachea produced by the descending thoracic aorta, which crosses from right to left at this level.

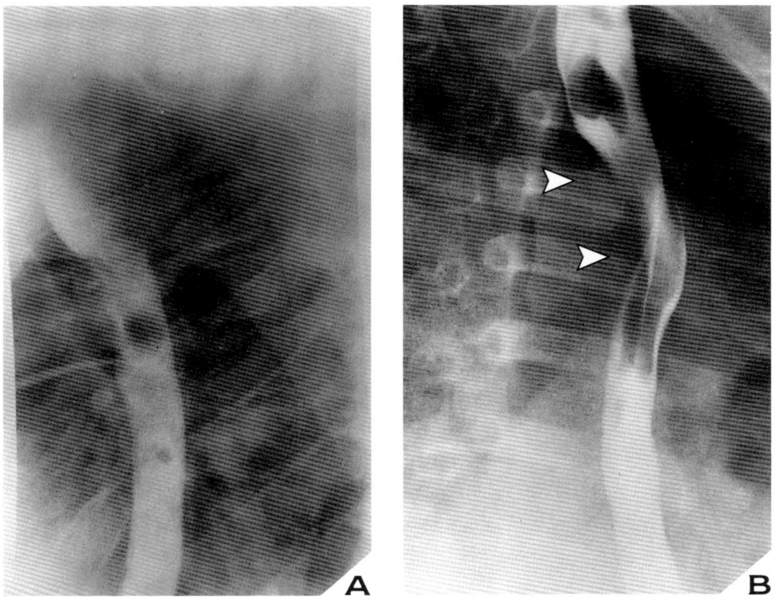

Fig. 15.18 Right aortic arch and left descending thoracic aorta. Lateral (A) and right anterior oblique (B) projections of esophagram show anterior displacement of the esophagus (*arrows*) at the level of the aortic arch, caused by the abnormally positioned upper descending thoracic aorta.

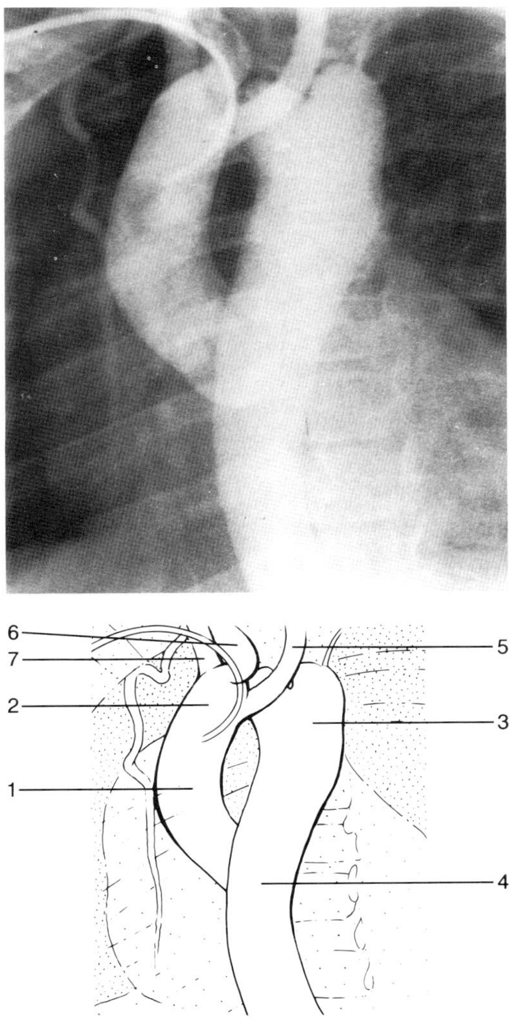

Fig. 15.19 Right aortic arch and left descending thoracic aorta. Frontal projection of thoracic aortogram. Both the ascending aorta and the aortic arch are on the right. The aortic arch is narrow. The upper descending thoracic aorta is on the left side of the mediastinum, descending on the left for several vertebral segments before crossing to the right.

1 ascending aorta
2 aortic arch
3 upper segment of descending thoracic aorta
4 middle segment of descending thoracic aorta
5 left innominate artery
6 right common carotid artery
7 right subclavian artery

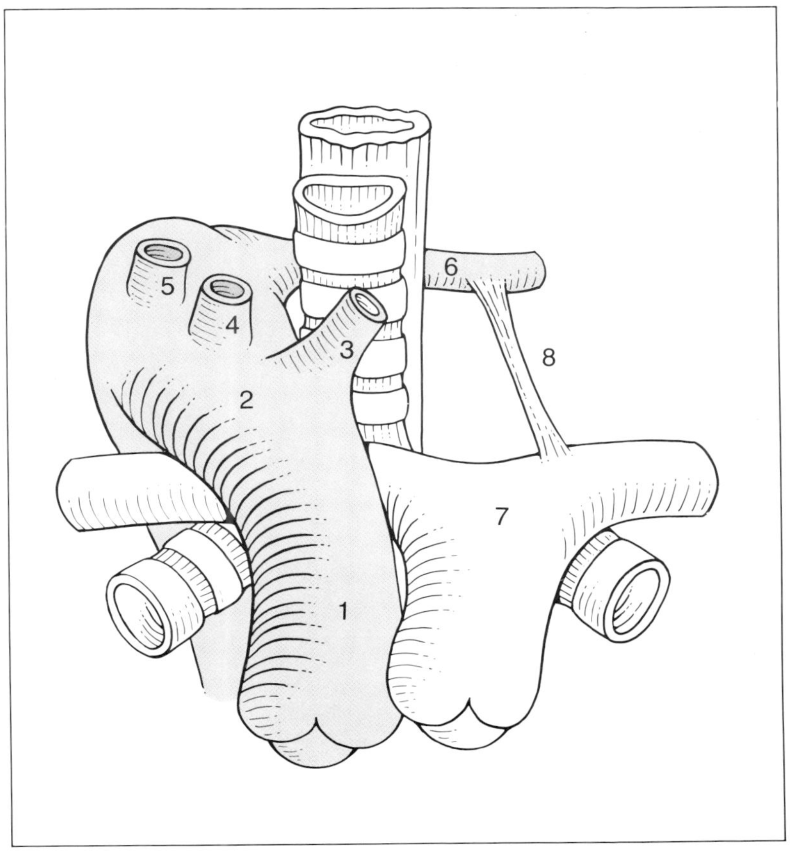

1 ascending aorta
2 right aortic arch
3 left common carotid artery
4 right common carotid artery
5 right subclavian artery
6 aberrant left subclavian artery
7 pulmonary trunk and left pulmonary artery
8 ligamentum arteriosum

Fig. 15.20 Right aortic arch with aberrant origin of left subclavian artery. The left subclavian artery arises as the last branch of the aortic arch and courses behind the trachea and esophagus to reach the left arm.

IMAGING

The frontal chest film typically reveals a right aortic arch, which appears as a right paratracheal density; an extra shadow to the left of the trachea represents the aberrant left subclavian artery (Fig. 15.21). The lateral esophagram shows a prominent indentation of the posterior wall of the esophagus at the level of the aortic arch. On the thoracic aortogram, the left subclavian artery arises as the last branch of the aortic arch and courses to the left (Fig. 15.22). Noninvasive imaging techniques (echocardiography, MRI, CT) are also diagnostic (Fig. 15.23).

DOUBLE AORTIC ARCH

Persistence of the right ventral fourth branchial arch results in a double aortic arch (see Figs. 15.1 and 15.2). The right arch is usually larger (ie, dominant); the left is often hypoplastic, although it is usually patent. The descending thoracic aorta is usually on the right, but occasionally lies to the left of the spine or in the midline. Together with the ascending aorta, these structures form a vascular ring, portions of which may be atretic (see Fig. 15.29).

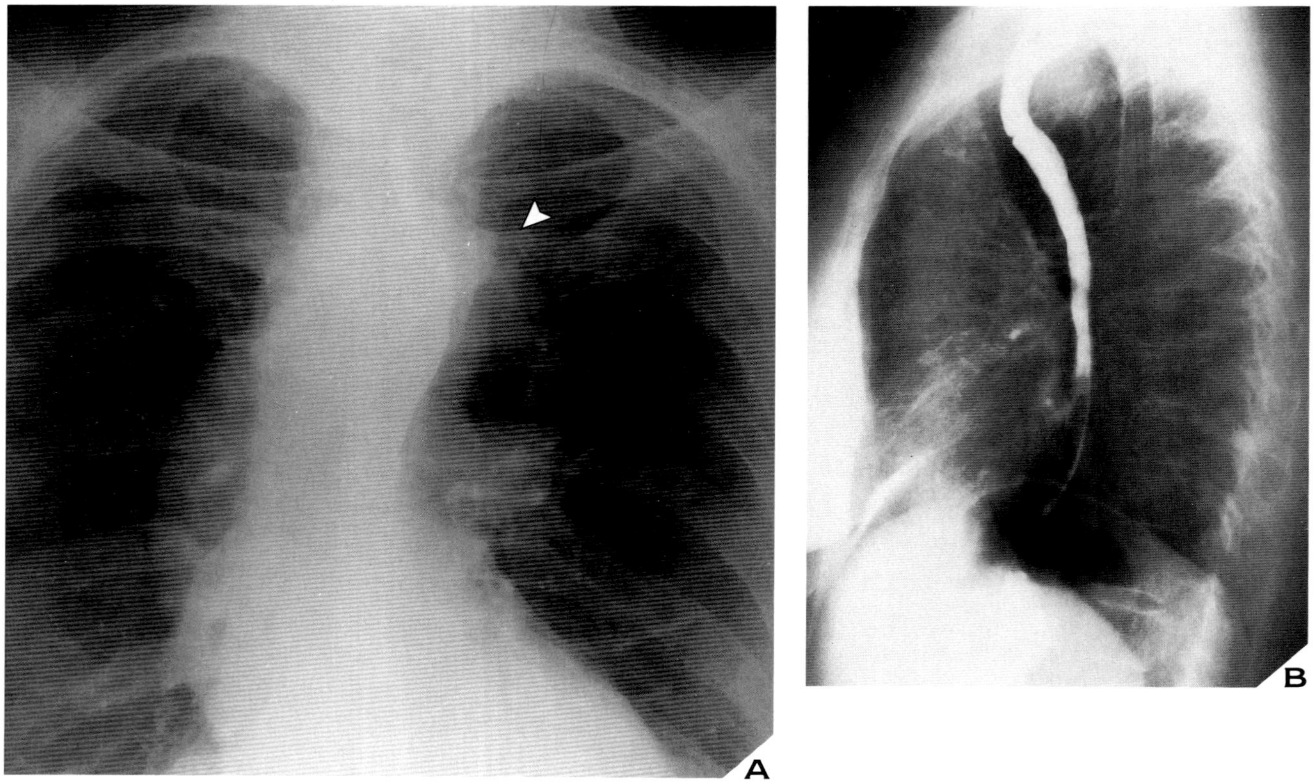

Fig. 15.21 Right aortic arch with aberrant (anomalous) left subclavian artery. (A) Frontal projection. The right aortic arch displaces the trachea to the left. The anomalous left subclavian artery can be seen as an extra shadow to the left of the trachea (*arrow*). (B) On the lateral view, the posterior aspect of the esophagus is indented by the anomalous subclavian artery. The trachea is also displaced anteriorly.

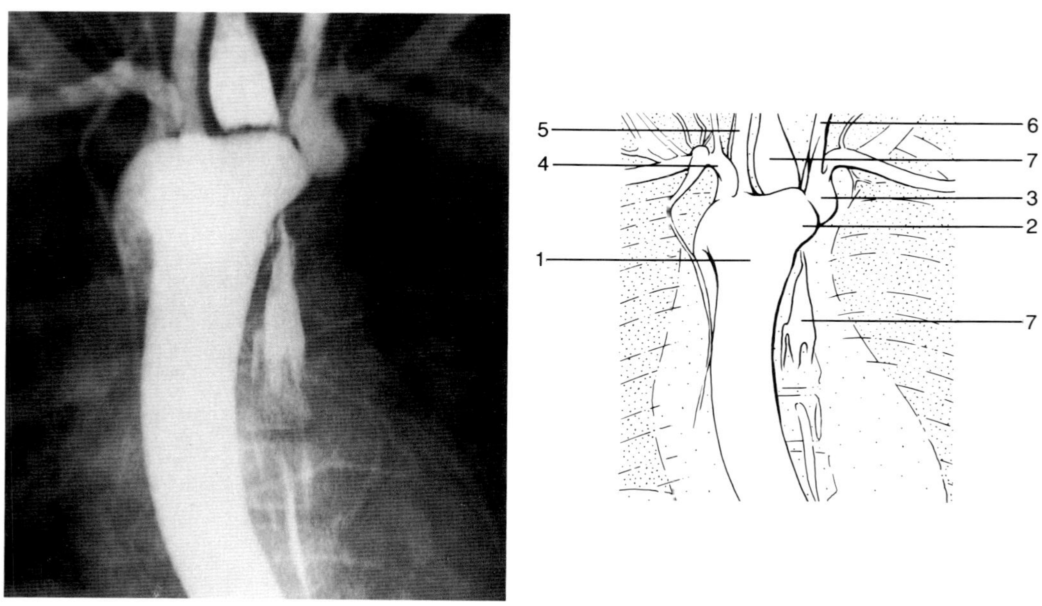

Fig. 15.22 Right aortic arch with anomalous left subclavian artery. Frontal projection of thoracic aortogram shows a right arch. The left subclavian artery arises as the fourth (and last) branch of the aortic arch. The widening of the origin of the left subclavian artery (Kommerell diverticulum) represents the remnant of the distal left aortic arch.

1 aortic arch
2 Kommerell diverticulum
3 anomalous left subclavian artery
4 right subclavian artery
5 right carotid artery
6 left carotid artery
7 esophagus

There are four brachiocephalic arteries. The right carotid and right subclavian arteries arise from the right aortic arch; the left carotid and left subclavian arteries arise from the left arch.

CLINICAL FEATURES

Symptoms and signs of tracheal and esophageal compression usually appear during the first year of life, often during the neonatal period. Breathing difficulties generally overshadow feeding problems. Stridor, often accompanied by cyanosis, is the typical presenting complaint. Dysphagia, vomiting, and recurrent episodes of aspiration pneumonia are less frequent. Older children and teenagers generally present with cough or dysphagia.

IMAGING

PLAIN FILMS AND ESOPHAGRAM

The abnormal position of the aortic arch is seldom appreciated on plain films in infants and young children. An "empty" tracheal segment may be apparent on the frontal projection; this finding, which indicates tracheal compression, is best appre-

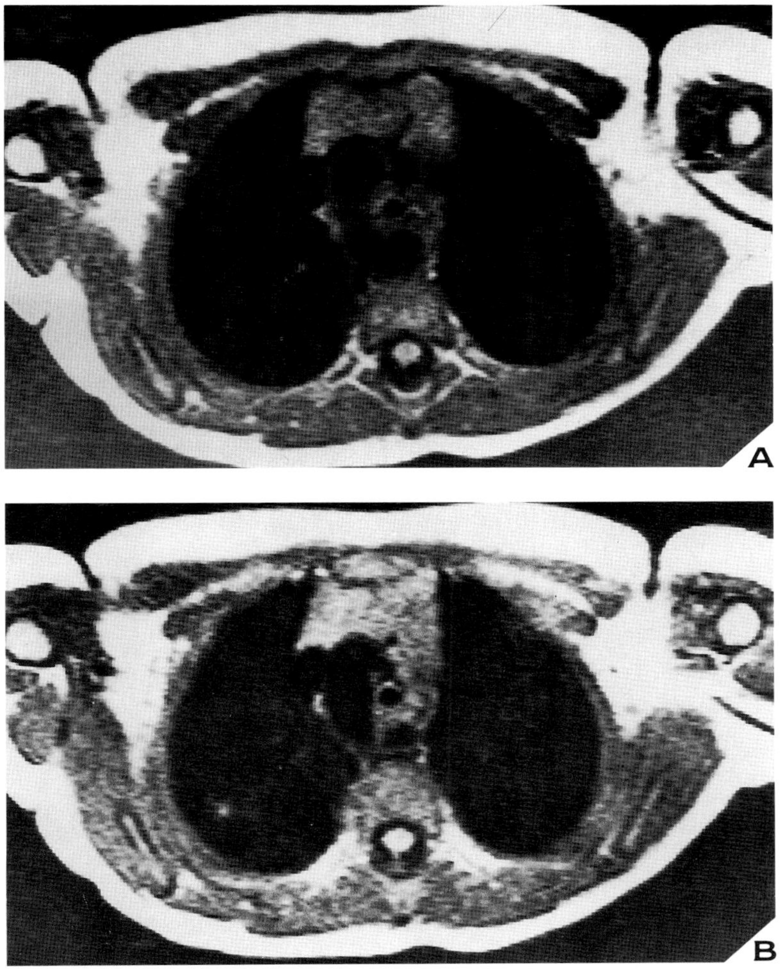

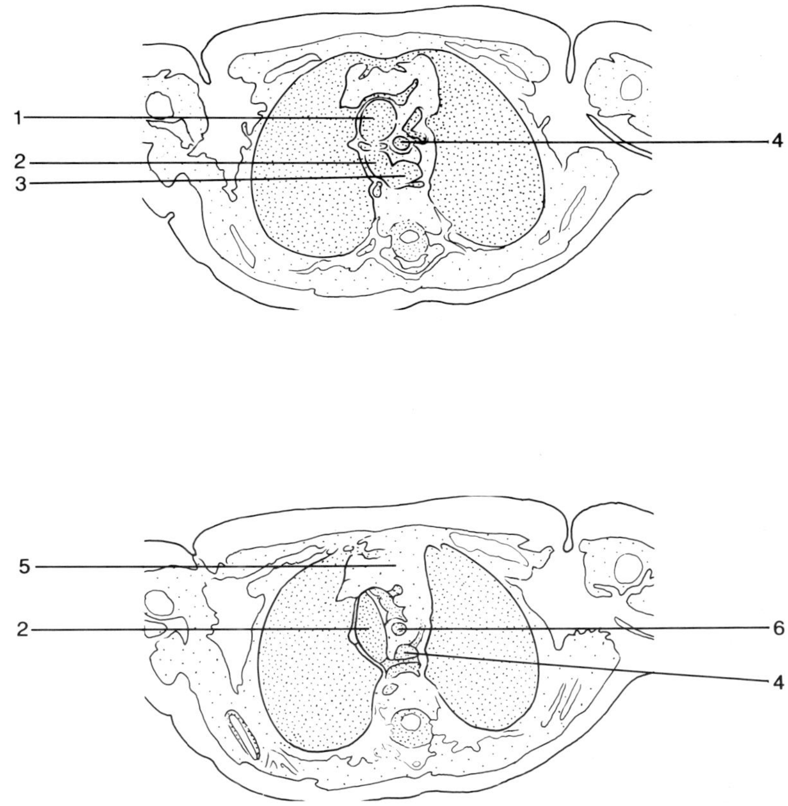

Fig. 15.23 Right aortic arch with anomalous left subclavian artery. Axial spin–echo MR images. (A) The ascending aorta and aortic arch are both on the right. The localized bulge along the left side of the distal aortic arch represents an aortic (Kommerell) diverticulum. (B) A slightly more cephalic cut demonstrates the left subclavian artery, which arises from the aortic diverticulum. (Courtesy of Ina Tonkin, MD, Memphis, Tennessee)

1 ascending aorta
2 right aortic arch
3 aortic (Kommerell) diverticulum
4 left subclavian artery
5 thymus
6 trachea

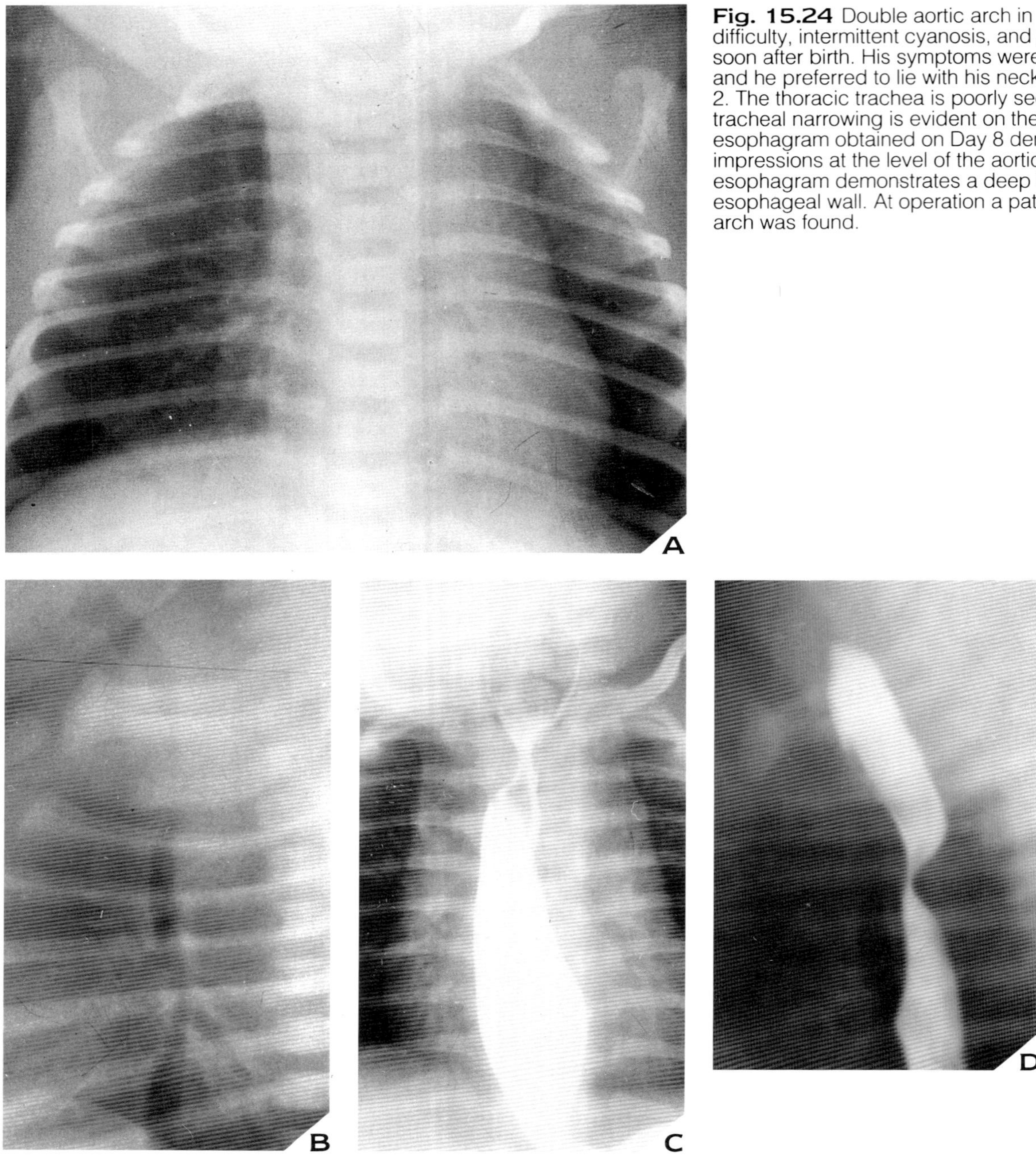

Fig. 15.24 Double aortic arch in infant. This neonate had respiratory difficulty, intermittent cyanosis, and persistent inspiratory stridor beginning soon after birth. His symptoms were exacerbated by crying and feeding, and he preferred to lie with his neck extended. (A, B) Chest films on Day 2. The thoracic trachea is poorly seen on the frontal view (A). Marked tracheal narrowing is evident on the lateral (B). (C) Frontal projection of esophagram obtained on Day 8 demonstrates prominent bilateral impressions at the level of the aortic arch. (D) Lateral projection of esophagram demonstrates a deep indentation of the posterior esophageal wall. At operation a patent double arch with a dominant left arch was found.

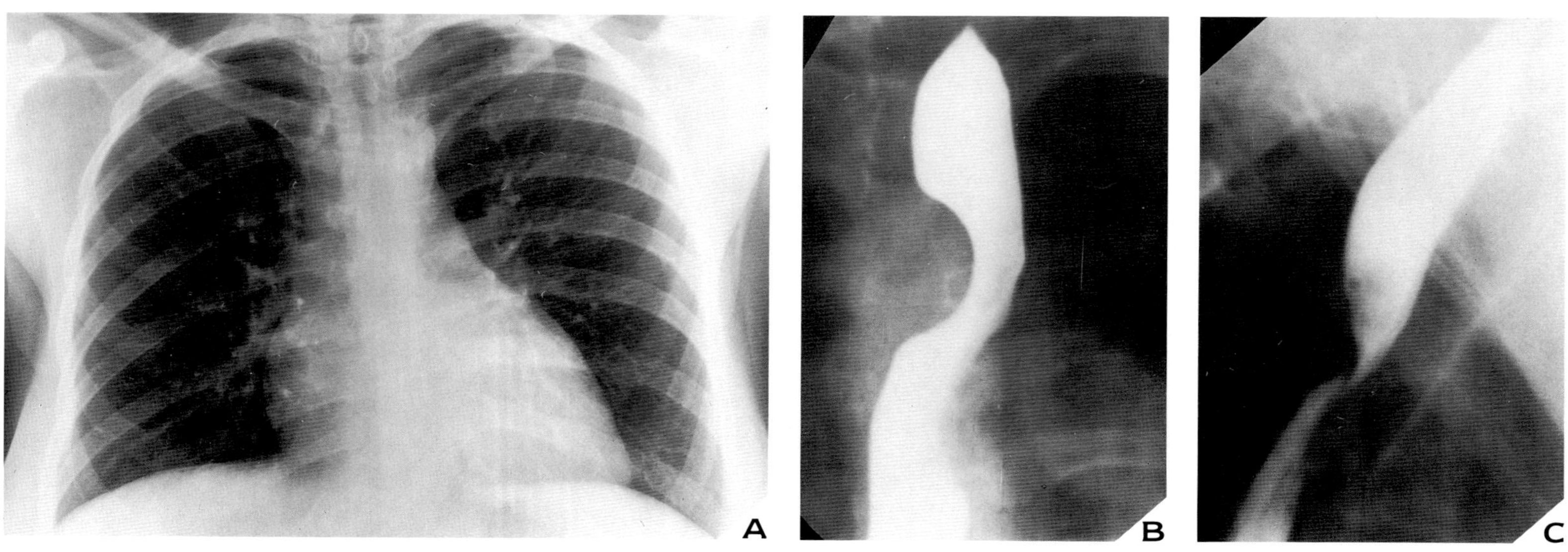

Fig. 15.25 Double aortic arch in adult. (A) Frontal chest film shows an inconspicuous left aortic arch and a small, convex density to the right of the trachea. Note the shallow indentation on the right side of the trachea. Frontal (B) and lateral (C) views of esophagram show mass effects typical of a double aortic arch. The left arch produces a shallow impression on the left side of the esophagus. The right arch indents the right side of the esophagus at a slightly higher level and crosses the posterior mediastinum, compressing the esophagus from behind.

ciated with the high-kilovoltage magnification technique (Fig. 15.24). In most instances, however, the only abnormality on the frontal projection is a right-sided or medially placed descending thoracic aorta. Anterior displacement of the trachea at the level of the aortic arch may be evident on the lateral projection; the trachea may be narrow as well (Fig. 15.24). The esophagram demonstrates a prominent posterior impression on the esophagus at the level of the aortic arch (Fig. 15.24D).

In older patients, the frontal chest film usually shows mediastinal widening, with bilateral paratracheal shadows representing the right and left aortic arches (Fig. 15.25). If the left arch is hypoplastic, only the right arch may be visible on the frontal projection. The presence of a right-sided or medially placed descending thoracic aorta strongly suggests a double aortic arch. Anterior displacement of the trachea is a constant finding on the lateral chest film.

Bilateral impressions on the barium-filled esophagus are seen on the frontal esophagram (Fig. 15.25B; see also Fig. 15.24C). An oblique defect caused by the retroesophageal right aortic arch can usually be appreciated also. In patients with a dominant right arch, the defect is directed upward and to the right (when the left arch is dominant, the defect is directed upward and to the left). The lateral projection reveals a deep impression on the posterior esophageal wall produced by the posterior component of the encircling vascular ring (Fig. 15.25C; see also Fig. 15.24D).

ANGIOGRAPHY

The aortic arch and its branches are best seen on oblique projections (Fig. 15.26). In patients in whom portions of the

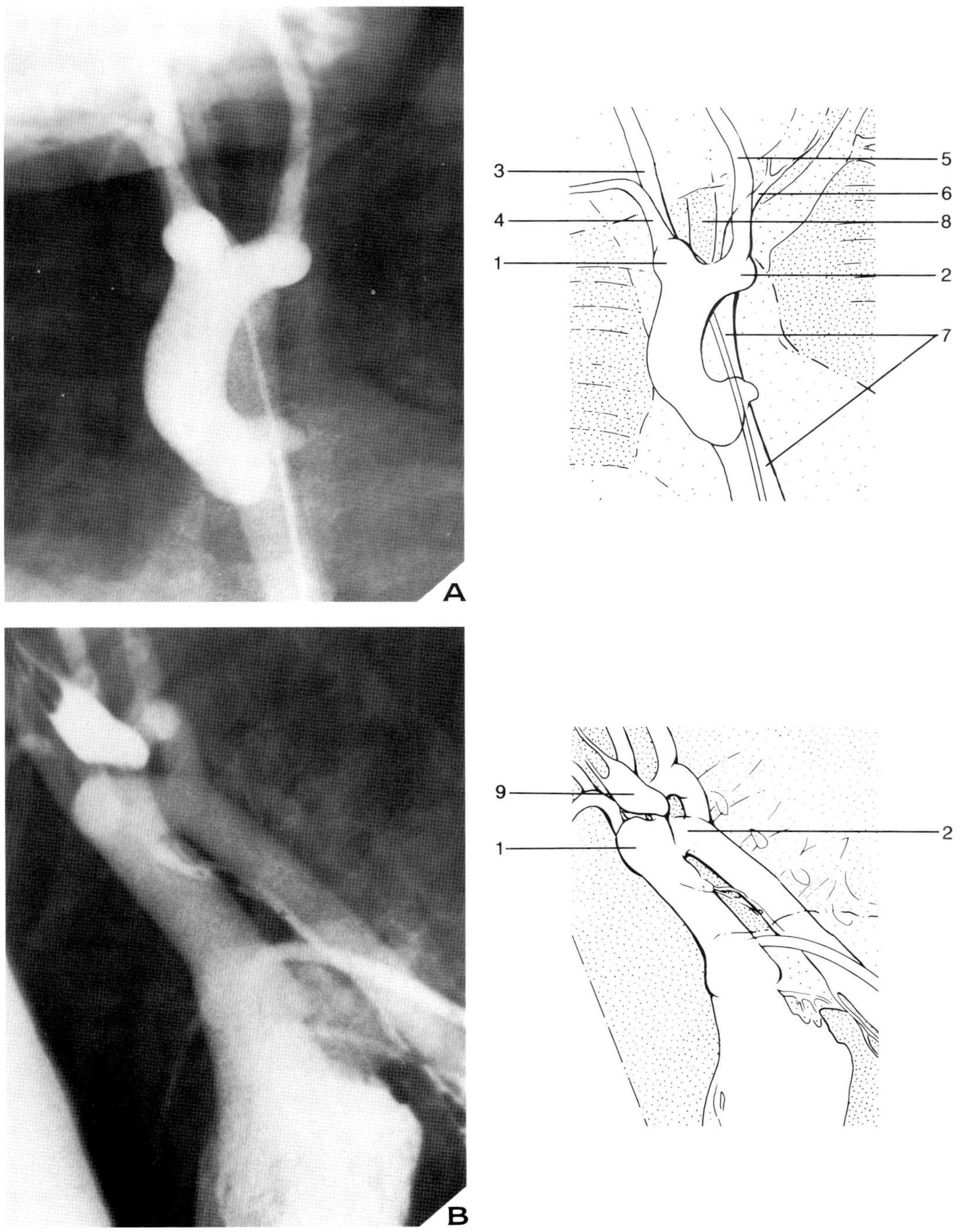

Fig. 15.26 Double aortic arch. (A) Frontal projection of thoracic aortogram shows right and left aortic arches of equal size; each arch gives rise to two brachiocephalic arteries. The descending thoracic aorta is in the midline. (B) Right anterior oblique view in another patient. The right aortic arch is larger than the left in this patient. The esophagus is partially compressed between the aortic arches.

1 right aortic arch
2 left aortic arch
3 right common carotid artery
4 right subclavian artery
5 left common carotid artery
6 left subclavian artery
7 descending thoracic aorta
8 trachea
9 esophagus

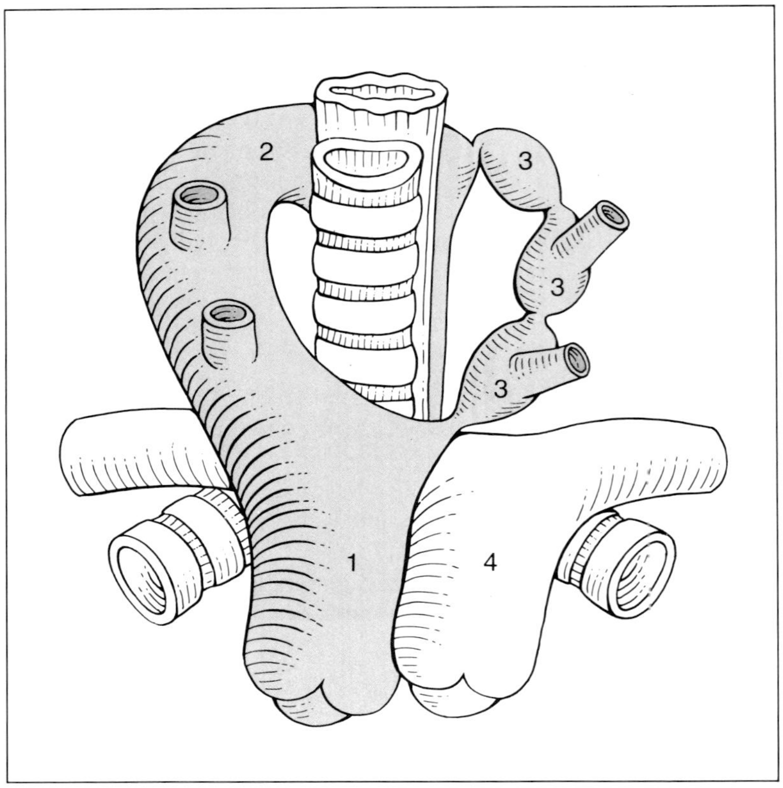

Fig. 15.27 Double aortic arch with multiple atretic segments. In this example, there are several interruptions of the left aortic arch.

1 ascending aorta 2 right aortic arch	3 left aortic arch with atretic segments	4 pulmonary trunk

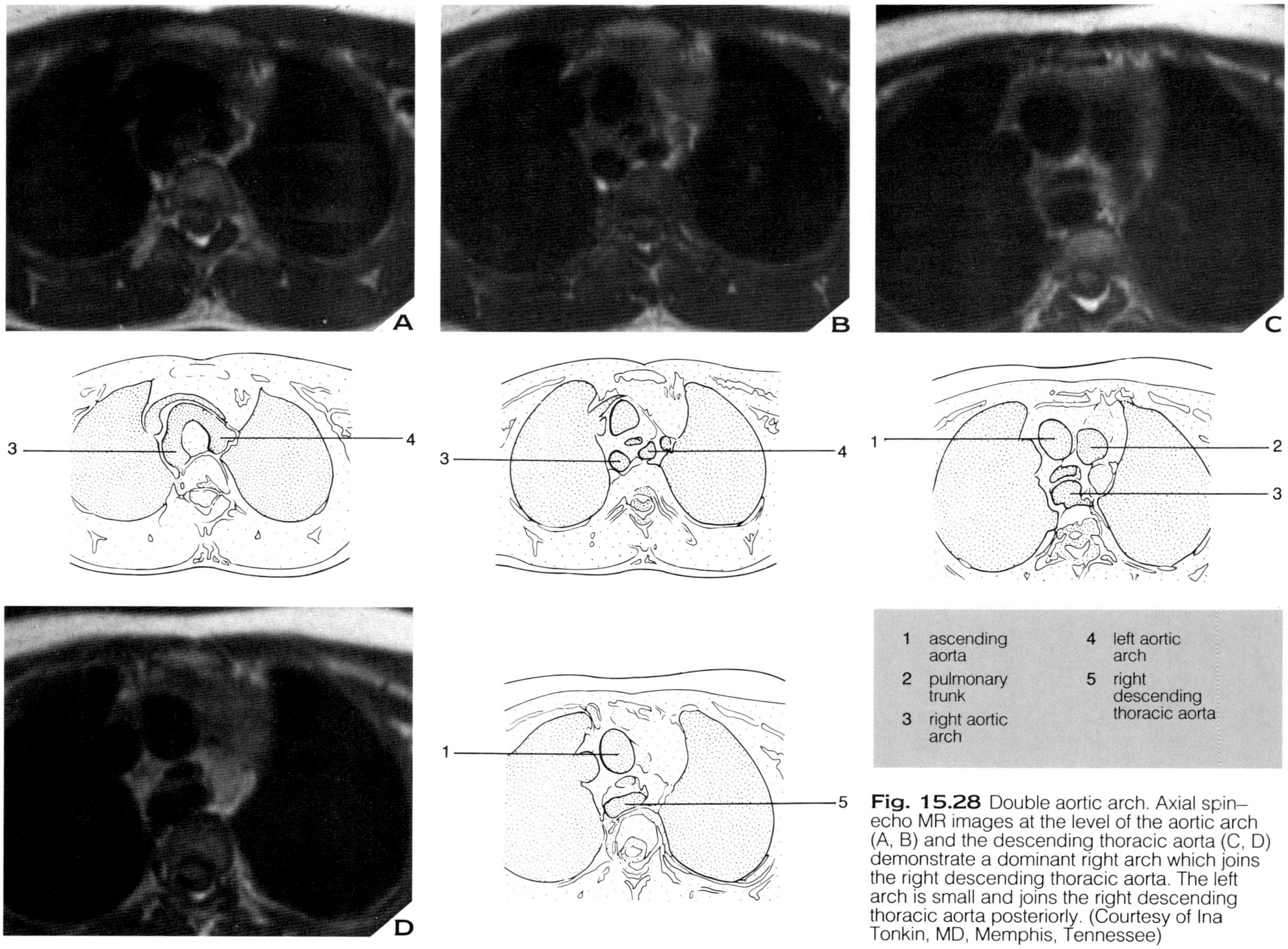

1 ascending aorta 2 pulmonary trunk 3 right aortic arch	4 left aortic arch 5 right descending thoracic aorta

Fig. 15.28 Double aortic arch. Axial spin–echo MR images at the level of the aortic arch (A, B) and the descending thoracic aorta (C, D) demonstrate a dominant right arch which joins the right descending thoracic aorta. The left arch is small and joins the right descending thoracic aorta posteriorly. (Courtesy of Ina Tonkin, MD, Memphis, Tennessee)

double arch are obliterated, the angiographic findings are determined by which segments are patent and whether there is a persistent ductus arteriosus or other associated anomaly (Fig. 15.27).

NONINVASIVE IMAGING TECHNIQUES

The pertinent features can be demonstrated by echocardiography, MRI, or CT (Fig. 15.28)

OTHER MALFORMATIONS OF THE AORTIC ARCH AND PULMONARY ARTERIES

CERVICAL AORTIC ARCH

This rare malformation of uncertain embryogenesis can occur on either side. Most investigators believe that a cervical arch is derived from the ipsilateral third or second branchial arch, in which case the ipsilateral second or first branchial arch persists as the proximal internal carotid artery (Fig. 15.29).

CLINICAL FEATURES

The patient typically presents with a pulsating neck mass which can be mistaken for a carotid artery aneurysm. Children with this anomaly are usually asymptomatic or have a relatively benign course. An occasional child, however, will present with stridor, recurrent upper or lower respiratory infection, or exertional dyspnea.

IMAGING

The frontal film demonstrates absence of the normal aortic knob and an apparent cut-off of the tracheal air column at the level of the superior mediastinum. The cervical arch can be identified as a mediastinal "mass" which displaces the trachea to the opposite side. The descending thoracic aorta may be on the same side or on the side opposite the cervical arch; the latter is usually the case when the cervical arch is on the right. The lateral projection shows en bloc anterior displacement of the

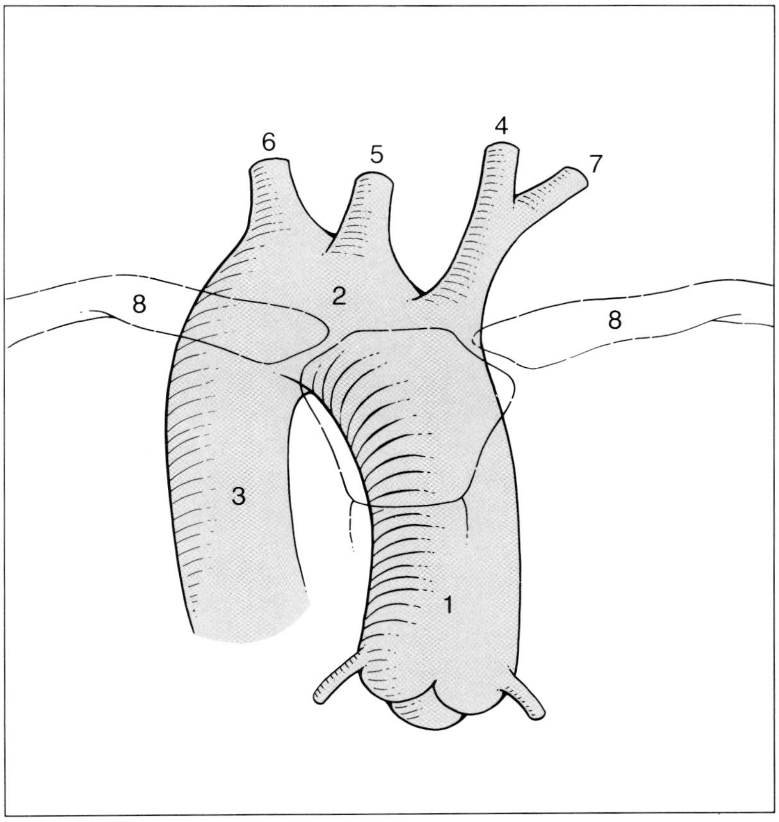

Fig. 15.29 Cervical aortic arch. In this hypothetical example the right aortic arch is above the level of the clavicles and gives rise to three arteries. The first branch is the left common carotid artery, followed by the right common carotid and the right subclavian. The left subclavian artery arises independently from the descending thoracic aorta.

1 ascending aorta
2 right aortic arch
3 descending thoracic aorta
4 left common carotid artery
5 right common carotid artery
6 right subclavian artery
7 left subclavian artery
8 clavicles

trachea and esophagus (Fig. 15.30). Angiography demonstrates a redundant aortic arch, which can be anywhere from slightly cephalad to its normal position to high in the neck (Fig. 15.31).

ANOMALOUS ORIGIN OF THE LEFT PULMONARY ARTERY FROM THE RIGHT PULMONARY ARTERY (PULMONARY ARTERY SLING)

In this rare anomaly the left pulmonary artery arises as a branch of the right pulmonary artery, at the level of the right hilus, and courses between the trachea and esophagus to reach the hilus of the left lung, where it bifurcates into upper and lower lobe branches (Fig. 15.32). In some patients most of the blood supply goes to the left lower lobe, in which event the arteries supplying the left upper lobe are smaller than normal. Some patients have coexistent long-segment tracheal stenosis caused by complete cartilage rings ("O ring," "napkin ring," "stovepipe trachea") (Fig. 15.33). Other anomalies of the tracheobronchial tree (eg, tracheal bronchus, an abnormally long right main bronchus) are not uncommon.

CLINICAL PICTURE

The clinical picture and prognosis are determined by the presence or absence of coexistent long-segment tracheal stenosis:

Patients without tracheal stenosis (Group I) may be asymptomatic, or they may have respiratory distress at birth with radiologic evidence of air trapping or obstructive atelectasis (almost always on the right). The obstructive symptoms are readily explained by "sling-like" compression of the right mainstem bronchus or bronchus intermedius by the crossing left pulmonary artery. Group I patients are generally cured by

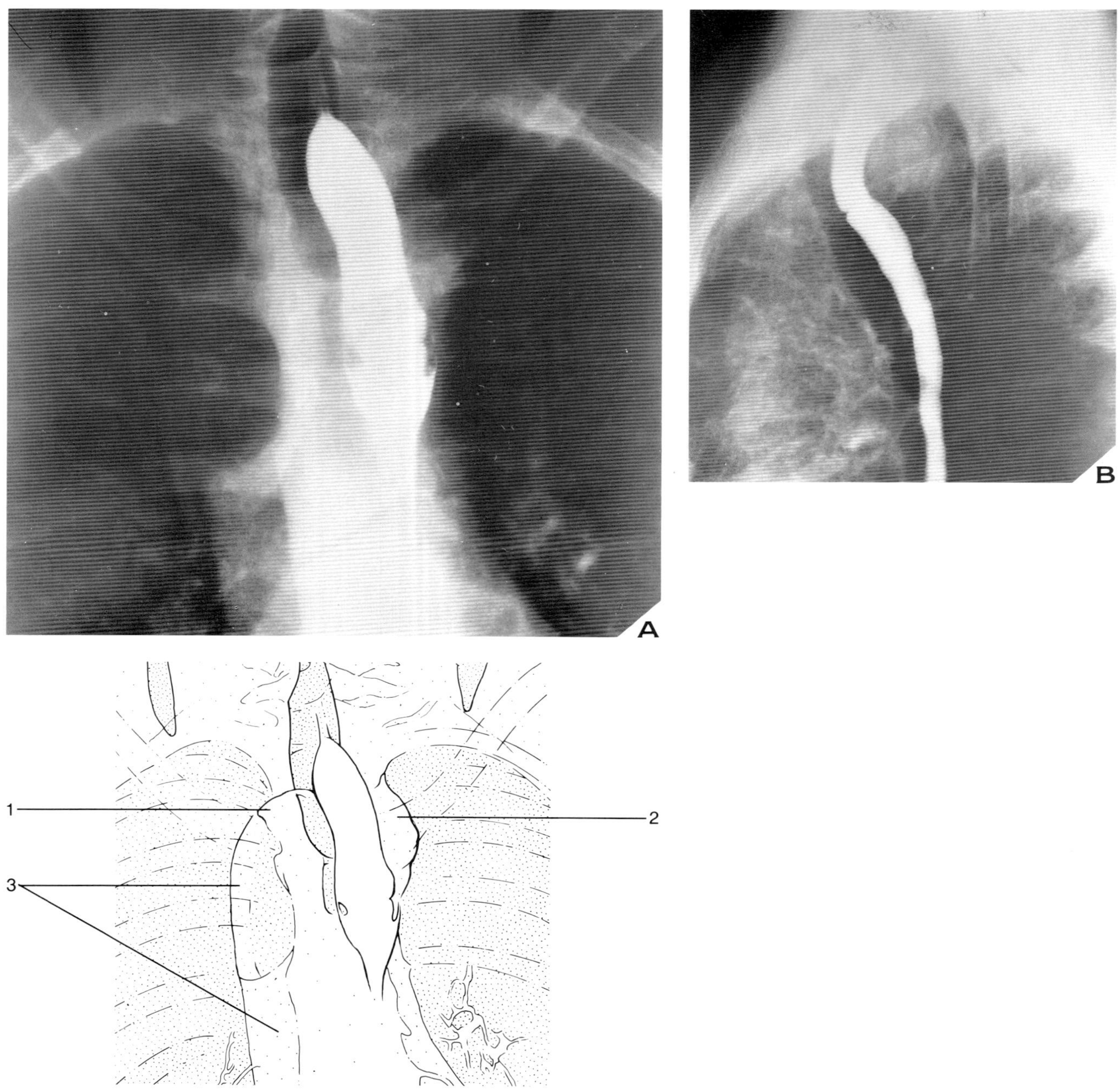

Fig. 15.30 Double cervical aortic arch. Frontal (A) and lateral (B) projections of cardiac series show a soft tissue density to the right of the esophagus at the level of the clavicles, which represents a right cervical aortic arch. A left cervical aortic arch is also present. The descending thoracic aorta is on the right. The esophagus is compressed from behind at the level of the aortic arches. The esophagus and trachea are both displaced forward.

1 right cervical aortic arch
2 left cervical aortic arch
3 descending thoracic aorta

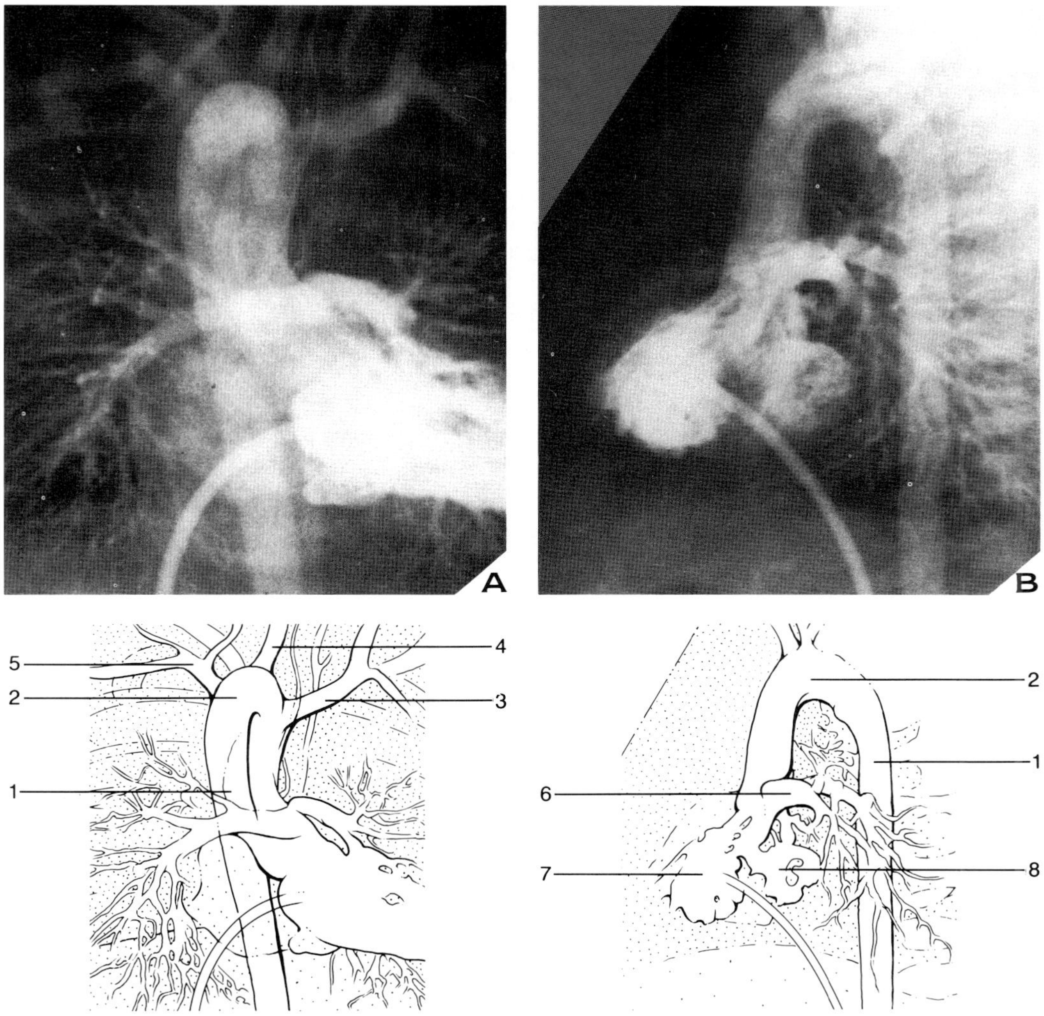

Fig. 15.31 Cervical aortic arch. Frontal (A) and lateral (B) projections of left ventriculogram in a patient with tetralogy of Fallot show a right-sided cervical aortic arch with a normal branching pattern. The ascending aorta and descending thoracic aorta are on the right.

1 descending thoracic aorta
2 right cervical aortic arch
3 left innominate artery
4 right common carotid artery
5 right subclavian artery
6 pulmonary trunk
7 right ventricle
8 left ventricle

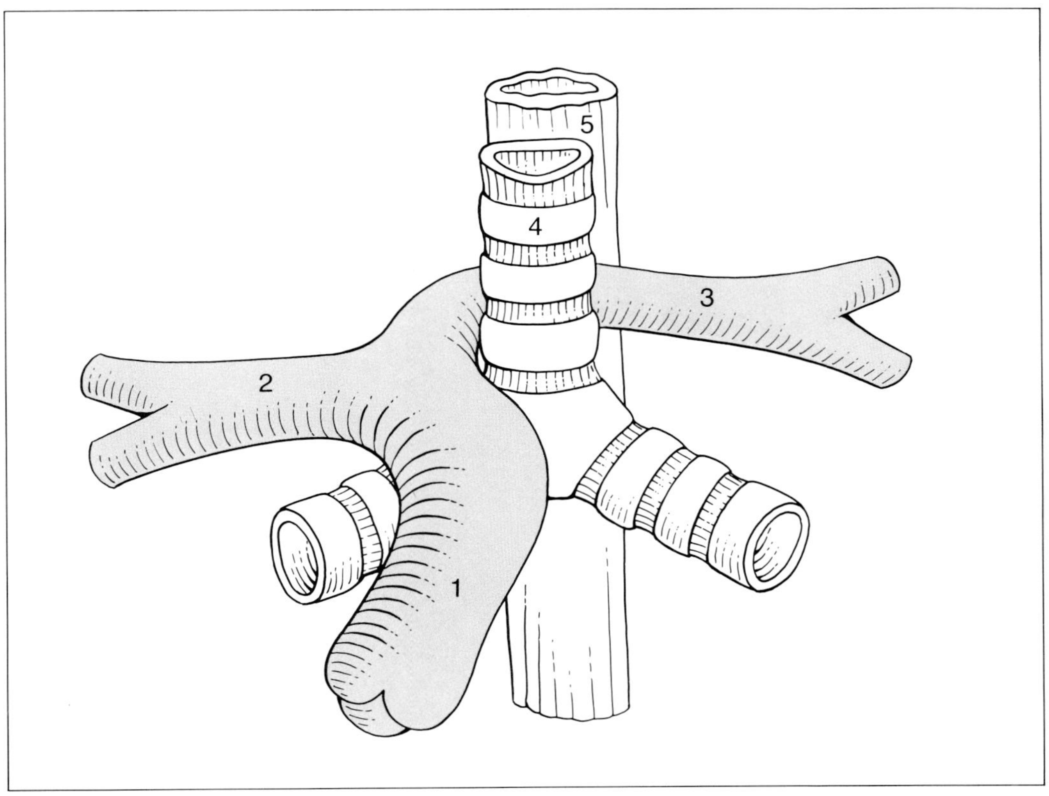

Fig. 15.32 Pulmonary artery sling. The pulmonary trunk continues as a right pulmonary artery. The left pulmonary artery arises from the right pulmonary artery to the right of the trachea and courses between the trachea and esophagus to reach the left lung.

1 pulmonary trunk
2 right pulmonary artery
3 left pulmonary artery
4 trachea
5 esophagus

surgery (division and reanastomosis of the left pulmonary artery with simultaneous division of the ligamentous ductal remnant).

Patients with associated tracheal stenosis (Group II)—the "ring-sling" complex—typically present in early infancy with repeated episodes of respiratory distress clinically thought to be bronchiolitis, and continue to have severe respiratory symptoms after surgical correction of the vascular anomaly. Group II patients die in infancy or have ongoing respiratory problems throughout childhood. The tracheal stenosis cannot be successfully dilated and is too long for surgical repair.

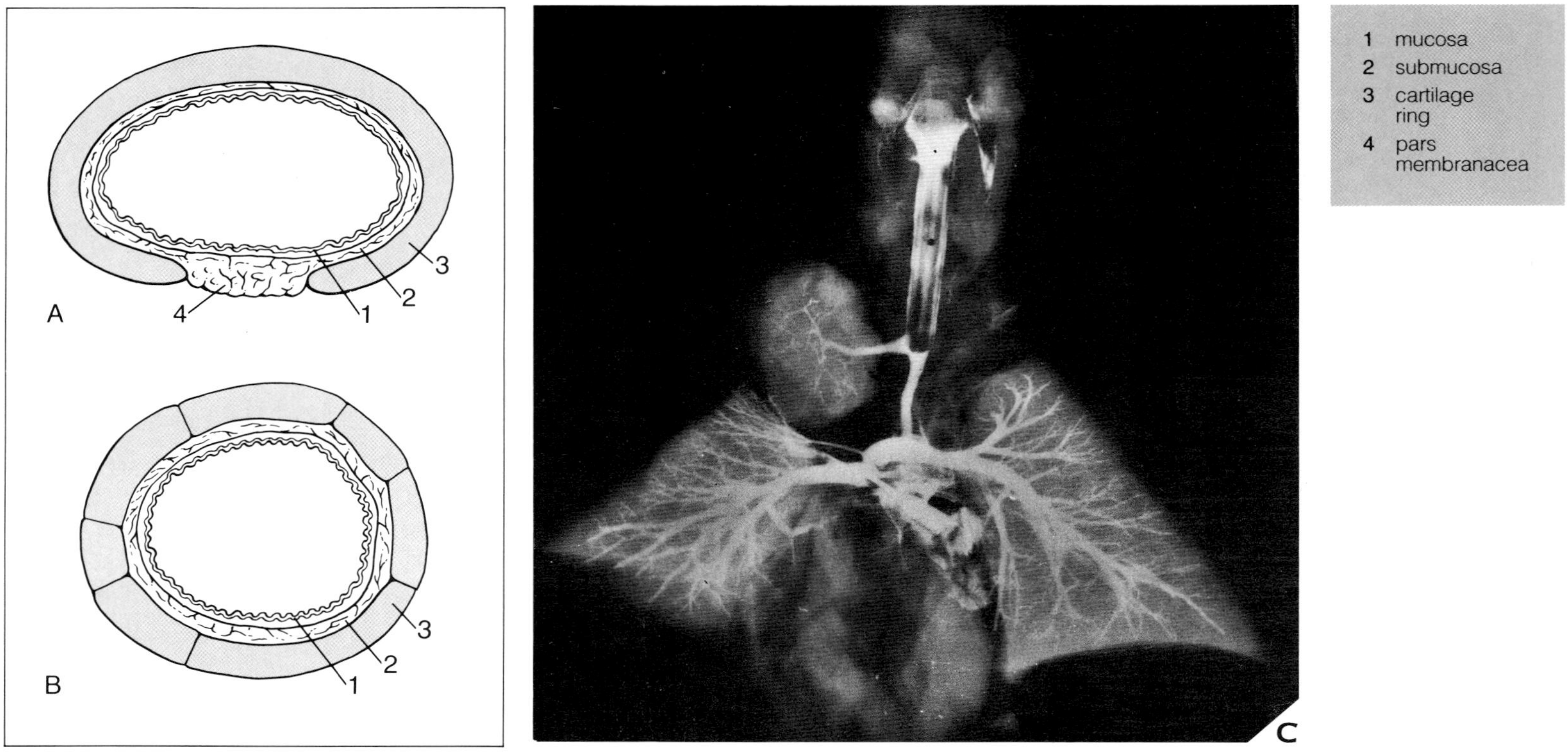

Fig. 15.33 Anomalous tracheal cartilages in pulmonary artery sling. (A) Cross-section of trachea cartilage from normal infant trachea shows oval shape with a large posterior pars membranacea. (B) Cross-section of tracheal cartilage from infant with "ring-sling" complex who died at 7 months of age. Note stenosis with absence of pars membranacea. Complete cartilage ring results in an "O" shape. (C) Postmortem bronchogram (with simultaneous opacification of anomalous left pulmonary artery) of patient shown in B demonstrates long segment tracheal stenosis. Note lack of correlation between length of tracheal stenosis and the site of the pulmonary sling. The right upper lobe is supplied by an anomalous tracheal bronchus. (A and B adapted and C reproduced from Berdon WE, et al: Complete cartilage-ring tracheal stenosis associated with anomalous left pulmonary artery: the ring-sling complex. *Radiology* 1984; 152:57

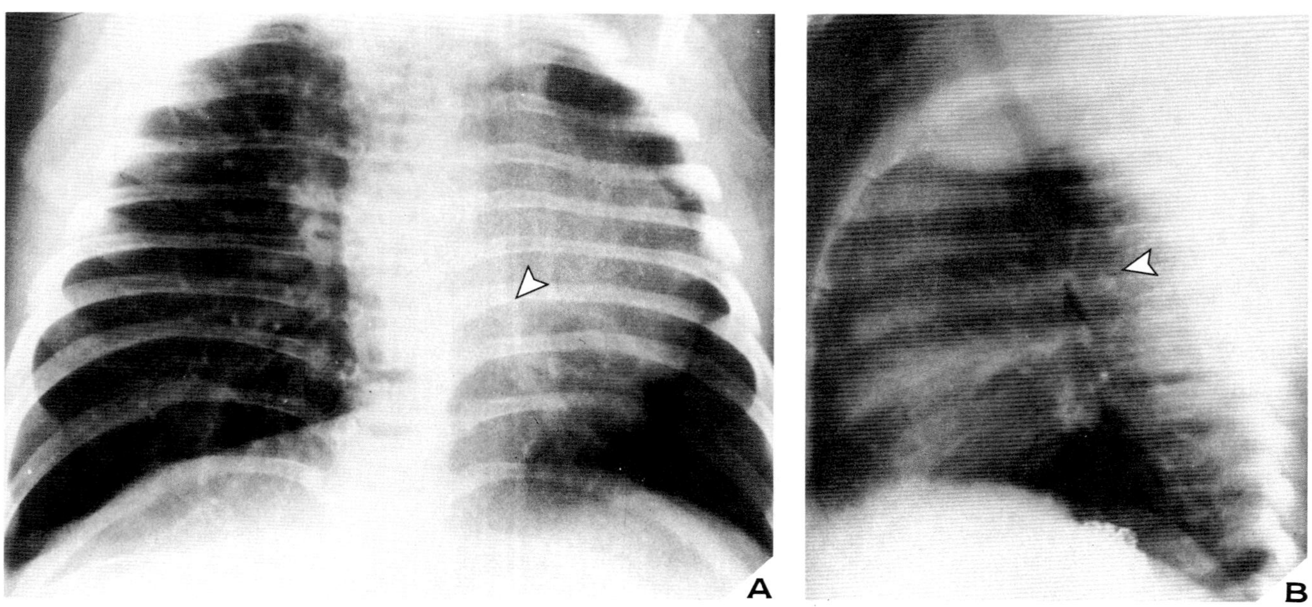

Fig. 15.34 Anomalous left pulmonary artery ("pulmonary artery sling") (Group 1). Newborn infant with respiratory distress. (A) Anteroposterior chest film shows marked hyperinflation of the right lung with a mediastinal shift to the left. The right pulmonary artery is prominent and its lobar and segmental branches are dilated, particularly in the upper zone. The left pulmonary artery (*arrow*) is small and in a lower position than normal. The asymmetry of the pulmonary vasculature reflects increased flow to the right lung secondary to hypoplasia of the left pulmonary artery, which is often present in this entity. (*B*) Lateral projection. The trachea is displaced anteriorly by a water density shadow (*arrow*), which represents the anomalous left pulmonary artery.

IMAGING

In symptomatic Group I patients, the frontal chest film typically shows emphysema or (less often) obstructive atelectasis of the right lung (Fig. 15.34). Neonates may have fetal fluid retention. The left pulmonary artery is smaller and in a lower position than normal. There may be a shallow indentation of the right side of the trachea just above the carina. The lateral esophagram reveals a soft tissue density interposed between the trachea and esophagus (Fig. 15.35). (This appearance is not pathognomonic, however, as it can also be seen in a patient with a bronchogenic cyst or other tumor between the trachea and esophagus, and in the "ductus arteriosus sling," a rare anomaly in which the PDA courses between the trachea and esophagus.)

In Group II patients, the lung fields are normal or symmetrically hyperinflated. The main bronchi typically have a horizontal course, resulting in an "inverted T" appearance; the left and right main bronchi are usually equal in length (Fig. 15.36). High-kV magnification films or bronchography (Fig. 15.37) demonstrate the extent of the tracheal or bronchial narrowing.

Pulmonary arteriography confirms the anomalous origin and

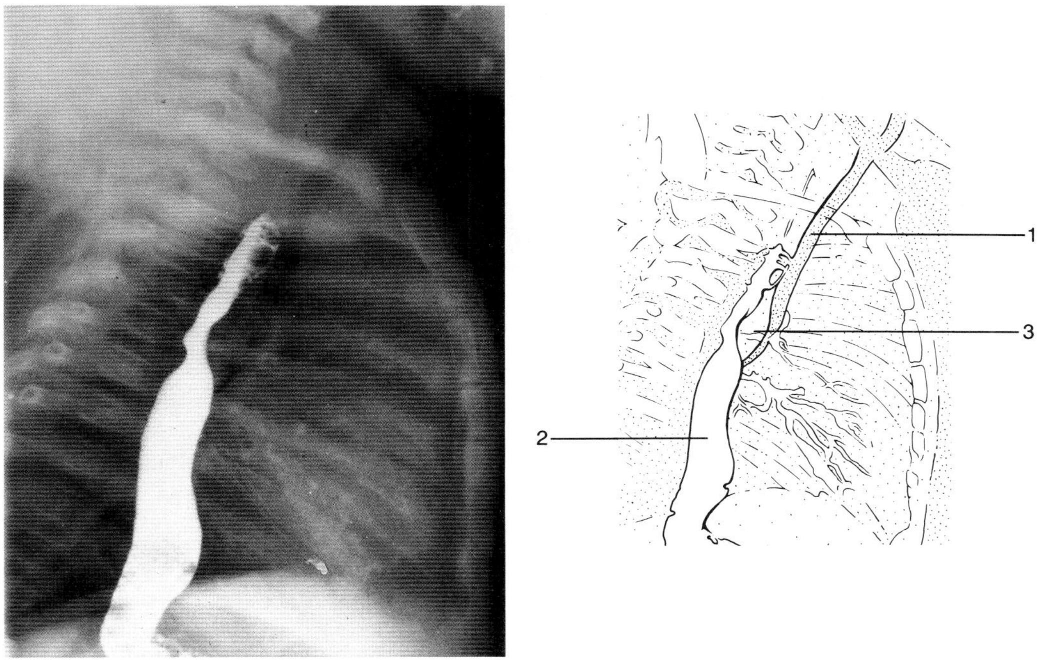

Fig. 15.35 Anomalous left pulmonary artery ("pulmonary artery sling") (Group I). Lateral chest with barium-filled esophagus shows trachea and esophagus separated by a small soft tissue mass which represents the anomalous left pulmonary artery.

1 trachea
2 esophagus
3 anomalous left pulmonary artery

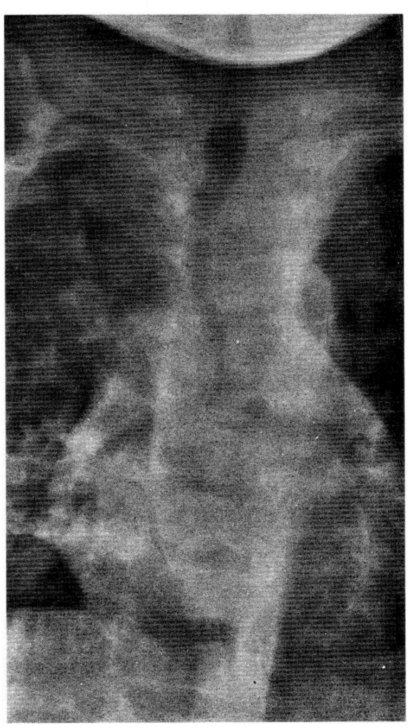

Fig. 15.36 Pulmonary artery sling with tracheal stenosis (Group II). After surgery for a pulmonary artery sling this infant continued to have attacks of respiratory distress characterized by stridor and wheezing. A high-kilovoltage magnification film shows a long-segment tracheal stenosis. Note the horizontal course of the right and left mainstem bronchi, which are of equal length. (Reproduced with permission from Berdon WE, et al: Complete cartilage-ring tracheal stenosis associated with anomalous left pulmonary artery: the ring–sling complex. *Radiology* 1984; 152:57)

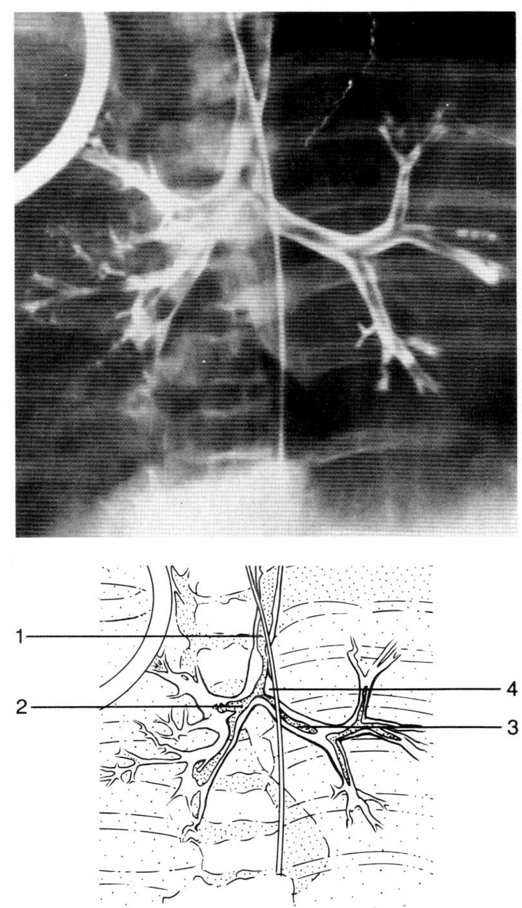

Fig. 15.37 Tracheal and bronchial stenosis associated with pulmonary artery sling. This infant continued to have respiratory symptoms after surgical treatment for a pulmonary artery sling. A bronchogram demonstrates focal narrowing at the origin of the left mainstem bronchus. The patient died of an unrelated cause; an anomalous "O" shaped bronchial cartilage was found at autopsy.

1 trachea
2 right mainstem bronchus
3 left mainstem bronchus
4 narrowing at origin of left mainstem bronchus

course of the left pulmonary artery (Fig. 15.38). MRI and CT accurately depict the vascular anatomy. Both of these noninvasive modalities can be used to define the extent and severity of the tracheal narrowing in Group II patients, thereby avoiding the hazards of bronchography.

CONGENITAL INTERRUPTION ("ABSENCE") OF A PULMONARY ARTERY

Congenital interruption ("absence") of the left or right pulmonary artery is almost always associated with hypoplasia of the ipsilateral lung. Only the proximal portion of the affected pulmonary artery is missing; the distal pulmonary artery, as well as the lobar and segmental branches, is normally developed. The anomaly typically occurs on the side opposite the aortic arch; therefore, interruption of the right pulmonary artery is far more common than absence of the left. Congenital interruption of the right pulmonary artery may occur as an isolated malformation or in association with congenital heart disease (patent ductus arteriosus, atrial septal defect, ventricular septal defect). Congenital interruption of the left pulmonary artery is usually associated with tetralogy of a Fallot.

The affected lung may be perfused by aortopulmonary collaterals arising from the descending thoracic aorta or from collaterals from the ipsilateral innominate or subclavian artery, or it may receive its blood supply from many small collateral vessels. The latter is nearly always the case in adults with isolated absence of the right pulmonary artery. Anomalous origin of the right pulmonary artery from the aorta is usually associated with congenital heart disease; only rarely is it encountered as an isolated anomaly in adults.

CLINICAL FEATURES AND HEMODYNAMIC FEATURES

Patients with interruption of the right pulmonary artery associated with congenital heart disease (eg, patent ductus arteriosus, atrial septal defect, ventricular septal defect) usually present early in life with congestive failure and respiratory distress. Because the entire cardiac output is directed to the normally perfused left lung, some of these infants develop pulmonary hypertension on the left. A minority of patients with isolated interruption of the right pulmonary artery present in infancy with pulmonary hypertension, presumably due to lack of regression of the fetal pulmonary vascular pattern. Patients with interruption of the right pulmonary artery who are symptomatic during infancy seldom survive beyond the age of 2 years. Those who are asymptomatic early in life go undetected or present as adults with an abnormal chest film. Most of the latter are asymptomatic, although hemoptysis has been reported in a small number of cases.

IMAGING

Plain Films

Chest films in adults with isolated interruption of the right pulmonary artery show volume loss of the affected hemithorax, with an ipsilateral tracheal and mediastinal shift, a small (or absent) hilar shadow, and abnormal vascular markings in the

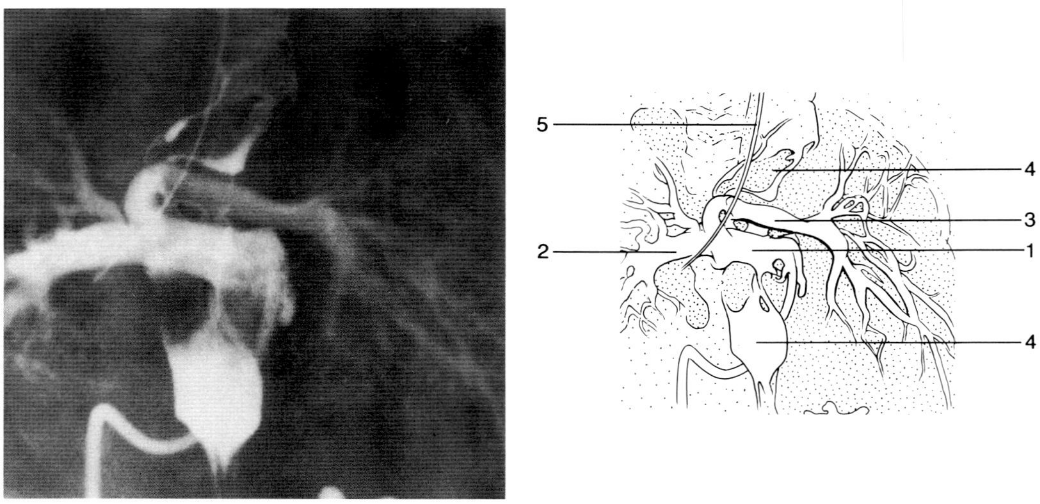

Fig. 15.38 Pulmonary artery sling. Right ventriculogram obtained with the patient semierect. The esophagus has been opacified with barium paste. The right pulmonary artery is the continuation of the pulmonary trunk. The left pulmonary artery arises as a branch of the right pulmonary artery, to the right of the trachea, and courses between the trachea and esophagus to supply the entire left lung.

1 pulmonary trunk
2 right pulmonary artery
3 left pulmonary artery
4 esophagus
5 endotracheal tube (tip in right mainstem bronchus)

affected lung (Fig. 15.39A). The latter is often hyperlucent, but expiratory films or fluoroscopy show no evidence of air trapping. Unilateral rib notching (Fig. 15.39B), caused by collaterals arising from the intercostal arteries, and vertebral abnormalities are common.

Nuclear Medicine

Lung scintigraphy demonstrates total absence of perfusion and homogeneous ventilation of the hypoplastic right lung (Figs. 15.39C and 15.39D). (Although there are fewer counts on the right, ventilation per unit of lung volume is almost the same in

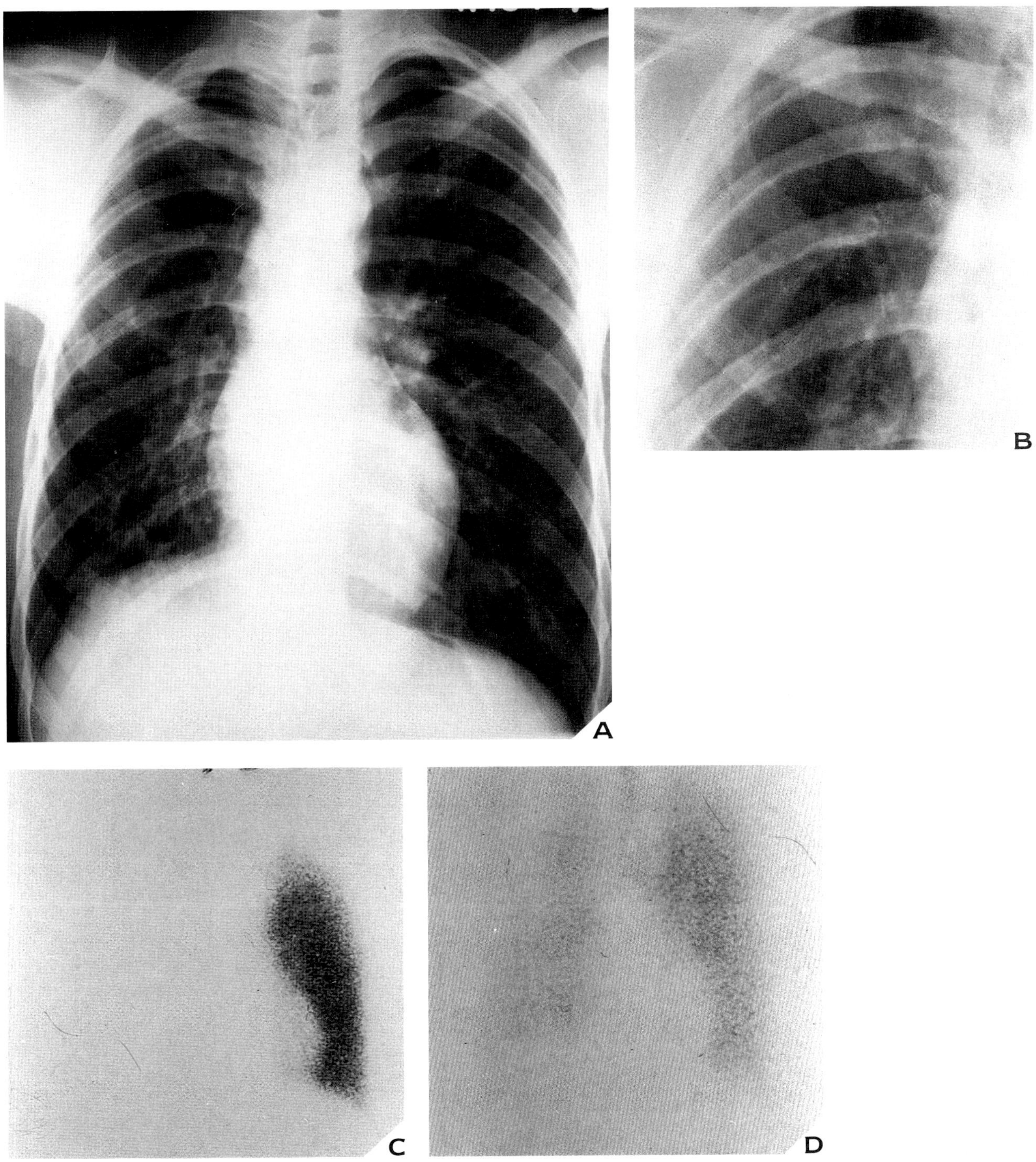

Fig. 15.39 Isolated absence of the right pulmonary artery. This 27-year-old man had recurrent hemoptysis and mild exercise intolerance. The posteroanterior chest film (A) shows slight decrease in the size of the right hemithorax (note the subtle mediastinal and tracheal shift and elevation of the right hemidiaphragm). The right hilum is very small, and abnormal vascular markings are seen throughout the right lung. Notching of the right 3rd-6th ribs can be appreciated on the detail view (B). A ^{131}I-macroaggregated albumen (MAA) perfusion lung scan (C) shows no perfusion of the right lung; the ^{81m}Kr ventilation scan (D) shows diminished but homogeneous perfusion of the right lung. (A, B courtesy of Eyal Barzel, MD, Brooklyn, NY. C, D courtesy of Arnold Strashun, MD, Brooklyn, NY)

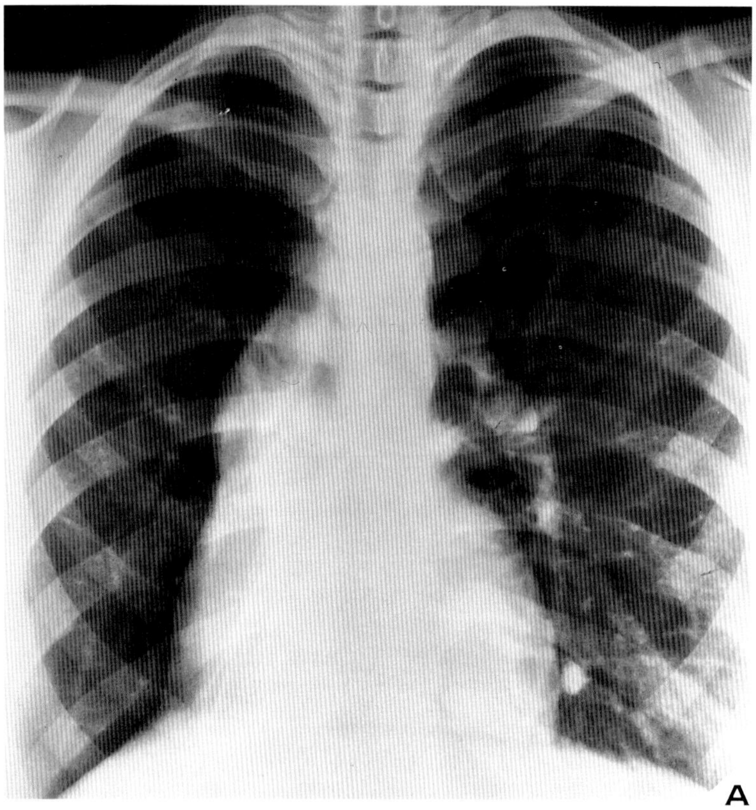

A

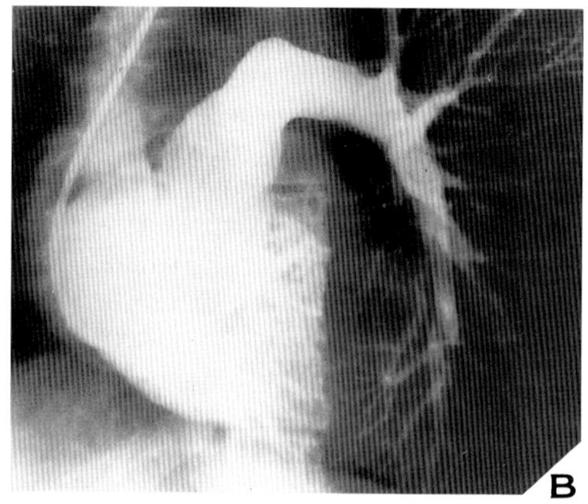

B

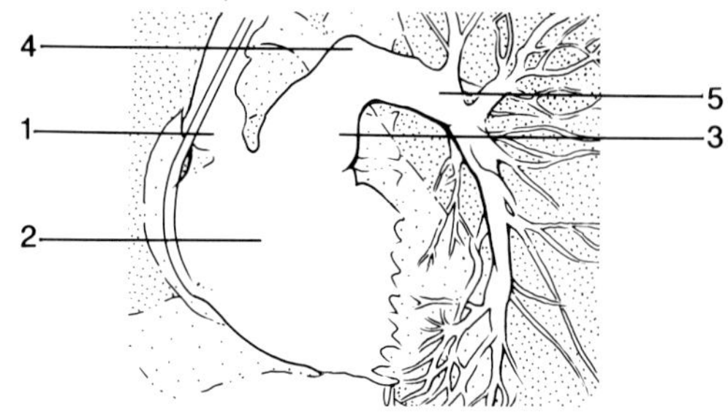

1 right atrium
2 right ventricle
3 pulmonary trunk
4 expected takeoff of missing right pulmonary artery
5 left pulmonary artery

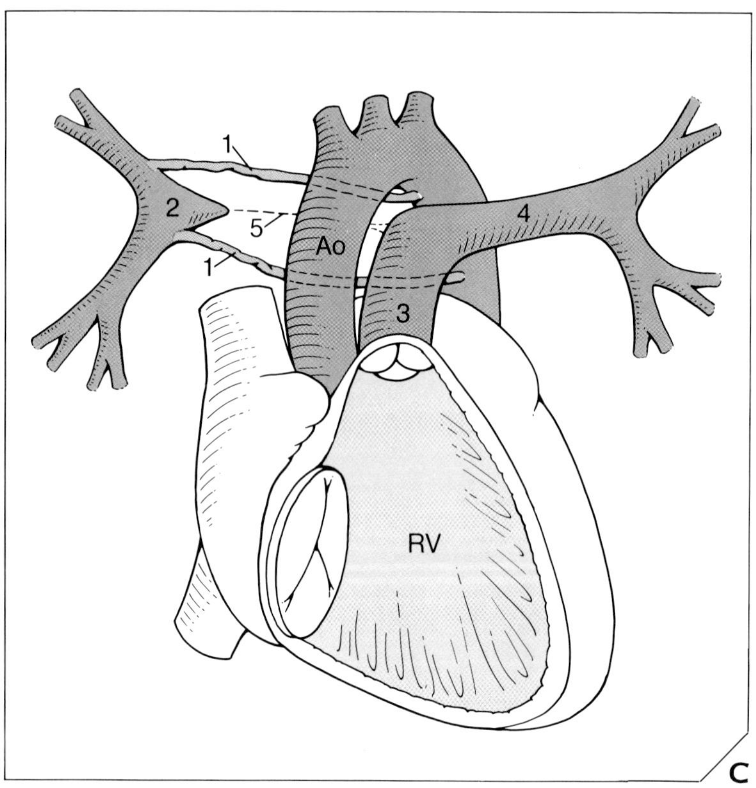

C

Fig. 15.40 Congenital interruption of the right pulmonary artery. (A) Posteroanterior chest film demonstrates displacement of the heart and mediastinum to the right. The cardiac axis is directed to the left and the aortic arch is left-sided. The right pulmonary artery cannot be identified. Vascular markings are sparsely distributed throughout the right lung. The left pulmonary artery is well developed and its peripheral branches are normally distributed. (B) Frontal projection of right ventriculogram. The right ventricle is displaced to the right and its outflow tract is left-sided. The pulmonary trunk and left pulmonary artery are normally developed. The proximal segment of the right pulmonary artery is absent. (C) The portion of the right pulmonary artery between the pulmonary trunk and the hilus is atretic. The lobar, segmental, and intraparenchymal branches of the right lung are well developed.

1 aortopulmonary collaterals
2 lobar and intraparenchymal branches of right pulmonary artery
3 pulmonary trunk
4 left pulmonary artery
5 atretic right pulmonary artery

both lungs, suggesting that the apparent hypoventilation is due primarily to the decreased volume of the hypoplastic lung.) A similar scintigraphic pattern (absent perfusion and homogeneous ventilation) is seen in patients with severe unilateral proximal pulmonary branch stenosis and in those with chronic thrombotic occlusion of the right pulmonary artery. However, the former usually have a characteristic murmur, whereas the latter almost always have a history of an acute episode compatible with an acute pulmonary artery occlusion. In patients with branch stenosis or chronic thrombotic occlusion, the affected lung is usually of normal size (ie, there is no mediastinal or tracheal shift or elevation of the diaphragm). In patients with acquired lung disease (eg, severe unilateral parenchymal disease, Swyer–James–McLeod syndrome), ventilation scans usually demonstrate patchy defects; perfusion is seldom entirely absent.

Angiography

Pulmonary arteriography confirms the absence of the proximal right pulmonary artery (Fig. 15.40). Aortography demonstrates the collateral blood supply to the right lung. Angiography is usually unnecessary, however, since the anomaly is clearly depicted by noninvasive techniques (CT, MRI, or intravenous digital subtraction angiography).

CHAPTER 15A

Imaging the Fetal Heart

EDWARD C. COLVIN, M.D.
W. ROBERT MORROW, M.D.

INTRODUCTION

The ability to observe the human fetus in utero with transabdominal ultrasound has revolutionized obstetric diagnosis and created new opportunities to diagnose and treat fetal disease. The application of echocardiography to fetal diagnosis has paralleled the development of echocardiographic technology, permitting the early diagnosis of structural and functional abnormalities. The initial application of M-mode cardiac ultrasound in the human fetus was reported by Garrett and Robinson in 1970. Egeblad, in 1975, identified the atrioventricular septum in the fetus using M-mode echocardiography. M-mode

CHAPTER LABELING KEY			
RA	right atrium	LV	left ventricle
LA	left atrium	Ao	aorta
RV	right ventricle	AZ	azygos vein

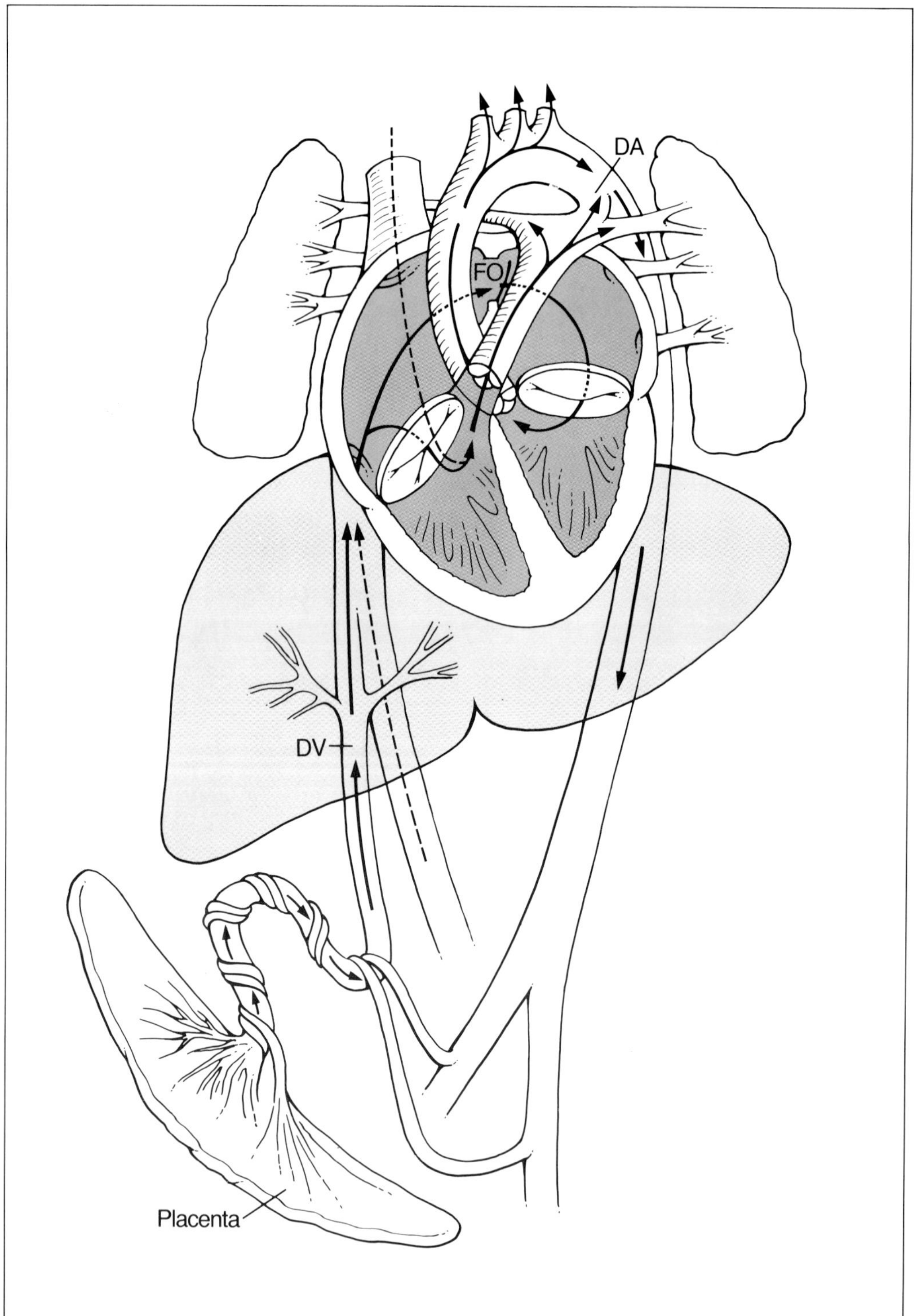

Fig. 15A.1 Fetal circulation. Unique features of the fetal circulation include the presence of the ductus arteriosus (DA), ductus venosus (DV), foramen ovale (FO), and placenta. (See text for details.)

parameters of ventricular size and function have subsequently been developed. The use of two-dimensional echocardiography in the diagnosis of structural malformations was pioneered by Allan (1980) and Kleinman (1980), and has subsequently been refined by many investigators. Advances in M-mode, pulsed Doppler, and color M-mode echocardiography now permit the accurate diagnosis and effective treatment of fetal arrhythmias. Thus, the full range of fetal cardiac disease can now be investigated noninvasively, allowing appropriate and timely treatment of the affected fetus.

FETAL CIRCULATION

Accurate diagnosis of fetal heart disease requires an appreciation of the basic differences between the circulation of the fetus and that of the neonate adapted to extrauterine life. In the fetus, the placenta is the organ of gas exchange, nutrient supply, and waste elimination; therefore, it receives a major portion of the cardiac output. The fetal lungs and bowel do not contribute directly to gas exchange or nutrient supply. Three cardiovascular shunts—the ductus arteriosus, the ductus venosus, and the foramen ovale—exist in the fetus to distribute oxygen and nutrients to the fetus and conduct carbon dioxide and other products of metabolism to the placenta. Consequently, the fetal circulation functions in parallel, rather than in series (as in the adult). Fetal cardiac output can therefore be described only in terms of combined ventricular output.

The fetal circulation is shown schematically in Fig. 15A.1. Total umbilical venous flow represents placental blood returning to the fetus. The oxygen-rich umbilical venous return ultimately reaches the left ventricle, whence it is distributed to the fetal head and upper body. In the fetus, the left ventricular output represents approximately 30 percent of the combined ventricular output and has an oxygen saturation of approximately 65 percent.

Systemic venous blood returning to the heart via the inferior vena cava (IVC) is directed mainly to the foramen ovale and left atrium by the eustachian valve; however, a small amount is directed to the tricuspid valve. The inferior vena caval return consists mostly of umbilical venous blood, which is directed to the IVC by the ductus venosus, and is augmented by portal and hepatic venous flow. The superior vena caval return, which represents venous flow from the fetal head and upper body, is directed mainly through the tricuspid valve to the right ventricle. The superior vena caval return and a portion of the inferior vena caval return is ejected from the right ventricle.

Approximately 60 percent of the combined ventricular output enters the ductus arteriosus and supplies the descending aorta. In the fetal lamb, approximately 10 percent of the ascending aortic flow enters the descending aorta via the aortic isthmus. The paired umbilical arteries arise from the descending aorta; umbilical arterial flow, which represents the arterial supply to the placenta from the fetus, accounts for approximately 40 to 50 percent of combined ventricular output. In the human fetus, as well as the fetal lamb, the right ventricle accounts for most of the blood supply to the descending aorta. Therefore, fetal heart failure is often initially manifested by right ventricular enlargement and ultimately by signs of right ventricular failure (eg, ascites, edema, pleural and pericardial effusions).

The proportion of blood flow distributed to various fetal organs varies with gestational age, the metabolic activity of the organ, organ growth, and species. The proportion of blood flow to the fetal head and lungs increases with increasing gestational age, whereas the proportion of the blood flow to the fetal heart remains approximately the same throughout gestation. In the human fetus the proportion of the combined ventricular output ejected by the left ventricle is greater than in the fetal lamb, a phenomenon that has been attributed to the greater mass of cerebral tissue in the human fetus.

FETAL ECHOCARDIOGRAPHY

INDICATIONS

The uses of fetal echocardiography include the diagnosis of structural malformations, evaluation of fetal arrhythmias, and assessment of ventricular function. In general, any screening sonographic examination of the fetus should include a four-chamber view of the heart, which will detect most major cardiac malformations. A detailed examination is warranted when there is reason to suspect a fetal cardiac abnormality. For example, when a parent has a congenital defect, the risk of a cardiac malformation in the offspring is 8 to 14 percent. When a couple has had a previous child with a heart defect the risk in subsequent pregnancies is 3 to 4 percent; if they have had two previous children with heart defects the risk in subsequent pregnancies is 15 percent. Other indications include poorly controlled maternal diabetes, maternal rubella infection, fetal exposure to teratogens (eg, lithium, anticonvulsants, ethanol) and known chromosomal abnormalities.

Certain chromosomal abnormalities are associated with a high incidence of cardiac malformations. More than 90 percent of fetuses with trisomy 13 or 18 have congenital cardiac defects; 50 percent of fetuses with trisomy 21 have detectable cardiac malformations (usually ventricular septal defect, atrioventricular canal, or tetralogy of Fallot). Cardiac malformations are also common in Turner's syndrome (XO and other karyotypes). Chromosomal abnormalities occur in about 5 percent of fetuses with congenital heart malformations. Therefore, when a fetal heart defect is identified, a careful fetal morphological assessment is necessary. All of the trisomies, as well as a number of other syndromes associated with congenital cardiac malformations, have characteristic morphologic features that can be detected by careful fetal sonographic examination in the second trimester (Fig. 15A.2). Cytogenetic studies may be needed in some instances.

The indications for a detailed fetal echocardiographic evaluation are summarized in Fig. 15A.3.

INSTRUMENTATION

There is no system ideally suited to every application of fetal echocardiography. Conventional linear array instruments routinely used for obstetric imaging offer the advantages of excellent depth penetration, excellent resolution, and a rectangular format that allows visualization of the entire fetus. A major disadvantage of linear array scanners is the large, cumbersome transducer (scanhead), which is difficult to rotate about an axis while keeping the fetal heart at the center of rotation. In addition, standard linear array scanners do not incorporate duplex Doppler imaging, a feature necessary for detailed fetal cardiac evaluation. Although some newer instruments provide an independent offset crystal for Doppler imaging, Doppler sampling is more cumbersome than with dedicated cardiac imaging systems that provide a steerable cursor.

Combined two-dimensional and M-mode imaging, both of which are essential for obtaining accurate chamber dimensions and diagnosing fetal arrhythmias by M-mode echocardiography, are standard features of modern dedicated cardiac imaging systems. The latest designs incorporate in-line M-mode and duplex Doppler. Dedicated cardiac imaging systems utilize mechanical or electronic (phased array) transducers for *sector* scanning. Although both types of transducer provide good image resolution, significant constraints are imposed by the need to examine the fetus in utero. To achieve adequate penetration it is necessary to use a relatively low carrier frequency (in the range of 3 to 5 mHz). Therefore, image quality can never approach that which is possible with the high-frequency (7.5 to 10 mHz) transducers used postnatally. Dynamically focused annular array transducers appear to provide better image resolution than other types of mechanical transducer. With any sector scanner, far-field images are inferior owing to the decrease in line density as distance from the transducer increases. The restricted expansion (RES) function available on some machines allows improved sector imaging at greater depths.

Pulsed and continuous wave Doppler and color flow mapping can be performed with linear array, phased array, or mechanical systems, using carrier frequencies ranging from 2 to 7 mHz. Lower carrier frequencies allow greater depth of penetration with fewer aliasing artifacts. When continuous wave Doppler interrogation of the fetus is necessary, two-dimensional guidance of the continuous wave beam is essential.

To sum up, linear array and sector scanners each offer advantages to the fetal echocardiographer, and both should be used in complementary fashion to maximize diagnostic accuracy.

Fig. 15A.2 FETAL SONOGRAPHIC FINDINGS IN CHROMOSOMAL AND GENETIC DISORDERS ASSOCIATED WITH CONGENITAL HEART DISEASE.

Syndrome	Extracardiac Sonographic Findings*	Commonly Associated Cardiac Malformations**
Trisomy 13	Holoprosencephaly (absent falx, monoventricle, fused thalami), abnormal midfacial development (midline cleft, hypotelorism, cyclopia), postaxial polydactyly, horseshoe kidneys, polycystic kidneys, omphalocele, posterior encephalocele	VSD, double outlet right ventricle
Trisomy 18	Severe growth retardation, polyhydramnios, clubfoot or rockerbottom feet, clenched fist with overlapping index finger, shortened radial ray, diaphragmatic hernia, omphalocele	VSD, complete atrioventricular canal, double outlet right ventricle
Trisomy 21	Thickened nuchal folds, slightly shortened femurs, hypoplastic middle phalanx of fifth finger (incurved fifth finger), duodenal atresia (after 22nd week)	Complete atrioventricular canal, VSD, tetralogy of Fallot
Turner (XO)	Bilateral cervical cystic hygroma (web neck), horseshoe kidneys	Aortic coarctation, aortic stenosis
Holt–Oram	Radial hypoplasia, radial aplasia	ASD, VSD
Ellis–van Crevald	Postaxial polydactyly, small thoracic cage, mild dwarfing (third trimester)	ASD, single atrium

**Detectable before 20th fetal week except where noted.*
***Minor cardiac defects (VSD, ASD) are difficult to detect in the second trimester*

Fig. 15A.2 Sonographic features of malformation syndromes associated with congenital heart disease.

THE TWO-DIMENSIONAL FETAL ECHOCARDIOGRAM

INITIAL OBSTETRIC SONOGRAPHIC EVALUATION

A complete obstetric ultrasound examination should be performed in conjunction with the fetal echocardiographic evaluation. An accurate assessment of gestational age and fetal growth (utilizing biparietal diameter, abdominal circumference, femur length, and other parameters as appropriate) should be available at the time of the fetal echocardiographic study, since some fetuses with cardiac disorders are growth-retarded or large for gestational age. The obstetric sonographic examination may also reveal body wall edema, ascites, and pleural and/or pericardial fluid in a hydropic fetus with congestive heart failure secondary to a structural malformation or a fetal arrhythmia (Fig. 15A.4). In monitoring the response to therapy, it is important to assess the severity of the hydrops on serial examinations. It is also important to identify fetal anomalies or malformations of other organ systems, as these may be associated with congenital cardiac defects (see Fig. 15A.2). A four-chamber projection of the heart will detect most cardiac malformations, and should be obtained as part of the routine obstetric sonographic assessment.

MORPHOLOGIC ASSESSMENT

After a thorough obstetric examination has been performed and an accurate assessment of gestational age has been obtained, attention is directed to the fetal heart. After a careful echocardiographic examination, it is usually possible to exclude serious congenital heart disease in the great majority of fetuses of more than 18 weeks' gestation. In some instances the fetal echocardiographic examination may be limited by fetal mobility, particularly early in gestation, and fetal position. As the fetus matures, ossification of the ribs and vertebral bodies adds to the difficulty of obtaining adequate images. The combination of an occiput anterior position and an anterior placenta is especially troublesome, since this places the fetal spine and the placenta between the transducer and the fetal heart. Other factors that may limit the study include maternal obesity, extreme fetal edema, oligohydramnios, and polyhydramnios. Owing to the paucity of adipose tissue in the midline, using the

Fig. 15A.3 INDICATIONS FOR A DETAILED EXAMINATION OF THE FETAL HEART

Familial

Parent or sibling with congenital heart disease
History of syndrome with cardiac involvement

Maternal

Drug exposure
- Alcohol
- Hydantion
- Thalidomide
- Trimethadione
- Lithium
- Isotretinoin
- Progestins
- Amphetamines

Illness
- Diabetes
- Lupus erythematosis
- Phenylketonuria
- Rubella

Fetal

Noncardiac structural abnormality
Suspected cardiac abnormality on screening scan
Chromosomal abnormality
Nonimmune hydrops
Polyhydramnios
Arrhythmia

Fig. 15A.3 Indications for detailed echocardiographic evaluation of the fetal heart.

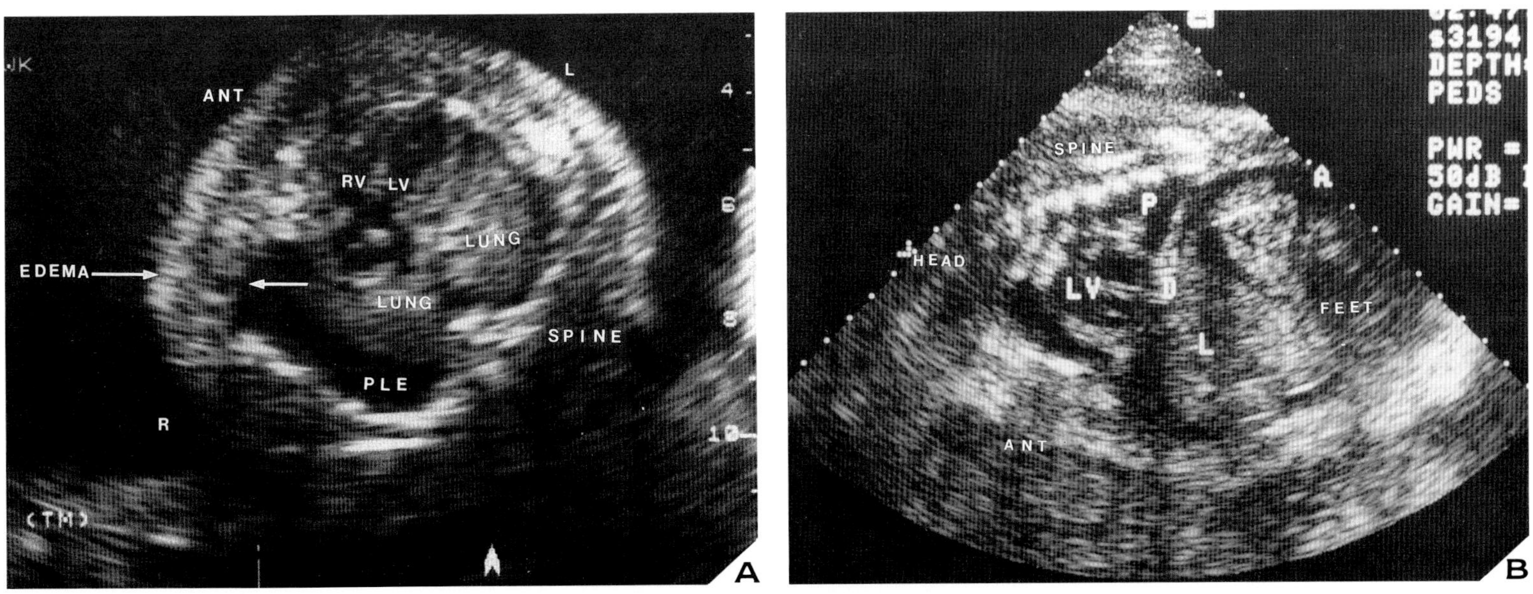

Fig. 15A.4 Fetal hydrops secondary to congestive heart failure. (A) Transverse section of the fetal thorax demonstrates skin edema (*arrows*) and pleural effusion (PLE). (B) Sagittal section of the fetal torso demonstrates pleural effusion (P) and ascites (A).

maternal umbilicus as a "window" or positioning the transducer just above the pubic symphysis may be helpful in a problem case.

A traditional "view-oriented" approach (see Chapter 2) is unsuitable for fetal echocardiography, since the examiner's inability to control fetal position results in an unconventional orientation of the cardiac images. In our experience, it is more practical to employ a segmental approach that emphasizes the visualization of venous, atrial, ventricular, and arterial connections. However, an attempt should be made to obtain images in at least three conventional imaging planes: the short-axis, four-chamber, and long-axis planes. In addition, images comparable to the suprasternal notch views obtained postnatally can often be obtained in the fetus.

FETAL POSITION

The initial requirement is to establish the position of the fetus with respect to the maternal abdomen. In the standard cross-sectional display of the maternal abdomen, the mother's left side is displayed on the right-hand side of the video screen; on sagittal images, the mother's head is on the right and the symphysis pubis is on the left. In this way, maternal landmarks can be used to orient the examiner to the fetal position (Fig. 15A.5). Once the orientation of the fetus to the mother is established, the fetus is examined to ascertain the position of the fetal head and spine, thus establishing its anterior/posterior and left/right orientation. Unfortunately, the fetus is likely to change its position with respect to the maternal abdomen, so

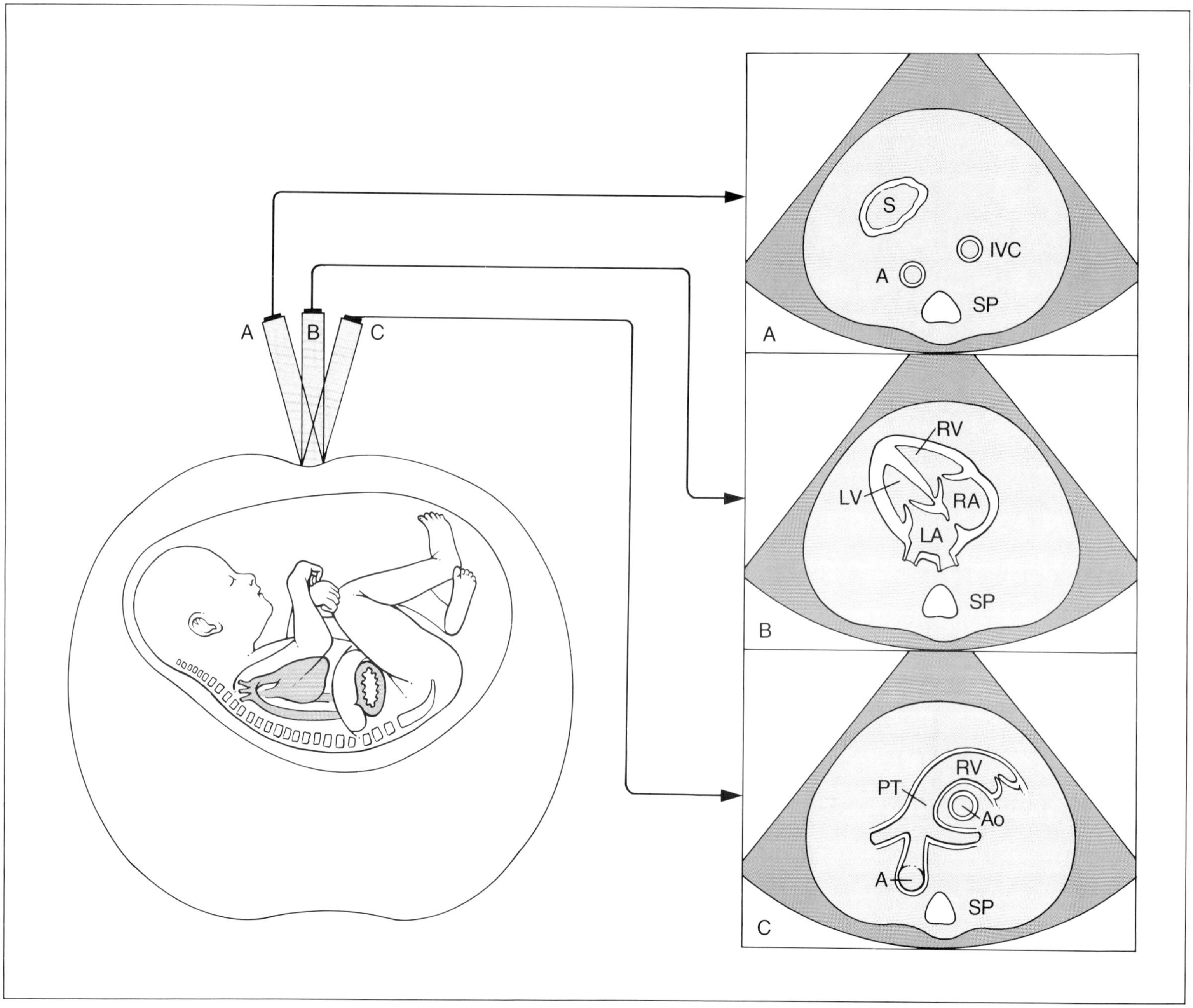

Fig. 15A.5 Method of determining fetal laterality. The transducer placed on the maternal abdomen can be tipped from a transverse plane which demonstrates the fetal abdomen, spine, and stomach bubble (a) to a more cephalic cross-section which demonstrates a four-chamber view of the fetal heart in the midportion of the fetal thorax (b), and finally to a transverse section through the upper portion of the fetal thorax in which the great vessels can be identified (c). The operator can thus establish the cephalocaudad orientation of the fetus; by imagining himself in the same cephalocaudad orientation, he can be confident of the left/right orientation of the fetus. Note that the location of the fetal stomach bubble is not an adequate indicator of laterality, since abnormal visceral situs (heterotaxy) is not uncommon in patients with congenital heart disease. (S = stomach; A = descending aorta; SP = spine; IVC = inferior vena cava; Pa = pulmonary trunk; Ao = aortic root)

that it is necessary to continually reestablish these relationships as the examination proceeds. The examiner must avoid the temptation to obtain conventionally oriented cardiac images or to reverse the orientation of the video image when fetal position changes, as this could result in confusing the left/right orientation of the fetus, leading to incorrect assessment of the cardiac or visceral situs or the ventriculoarterial connections.

CARDIAC POSITION

After establishing fetal position, the examiner's attention is directed to the fetal thorax and abdomen. By scanning in a cephalocaudad direction in the transverse plane (ie, by obtaining successive axial images of the fetal trunk), it is possible to establish the orientation of the heart within the chest and the position of the abdominal aorta and inferior vena cava at the level of the diaphragm. Because the fetal lungs are filled with fluid and the fetal liver is relatively large, the usual orientation of the heart is to the left and horizontal, with the apex clearly directed to the left. Thus, scanning in a sagittal plane parallel to the fetal spine produces short-axis images (Fig. 15A.6). A diagnosis of dextrocardia is warranted when the bulk of the cardiac mass is in the right chest (usually with the cardiac apex directed to the right). However, when dextrocardia is produced by displacement of the heart from the left hemithorax, as in a congenital diaphragmatic hernia, the apex may be in the midline or directed to the left. In such cases, the presence of abdominal contents in the left hemithorax confirms the diagnosis of a congenital diaphragmatic hernia (Fig. 15A.7)

ATRIAL AND VISCERAL SITUS

In assessing atrial and visceral situs, it is essential to determine the position of the inferior vena cava (IVC) and abdominal aorta. In atrial situs solitus the IVC courses to the right and anterior to the fetal spine and abdominal aorta; the abdominal aorta is to the left and anterior to the fetal vertebral bodies. In abdominal situs inversus this relationship is reversed: the IVC is to the left and anterior to the fetal spine and the abdominal aorta is on the right.

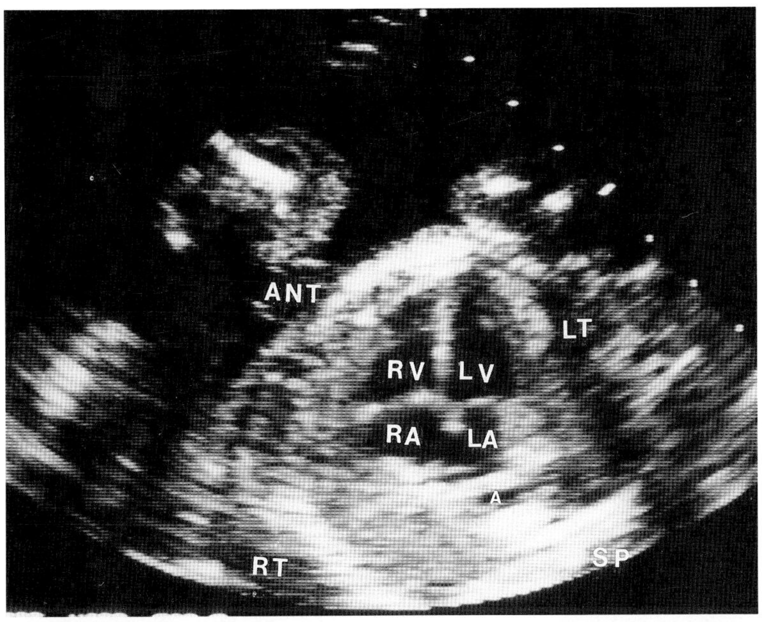

Fig. 15A.6 Normal fetal heart. (A) Four-chamber view of a normal fetal heart as seen in a transverse scan of the fetal chest. The apex is directed to the left. The right ventricle and left ventricle are of approximately equal size. The left atrium is immediately anterior to the fetal spine (SP). (ANT = anterior; RT = right; LT = left).

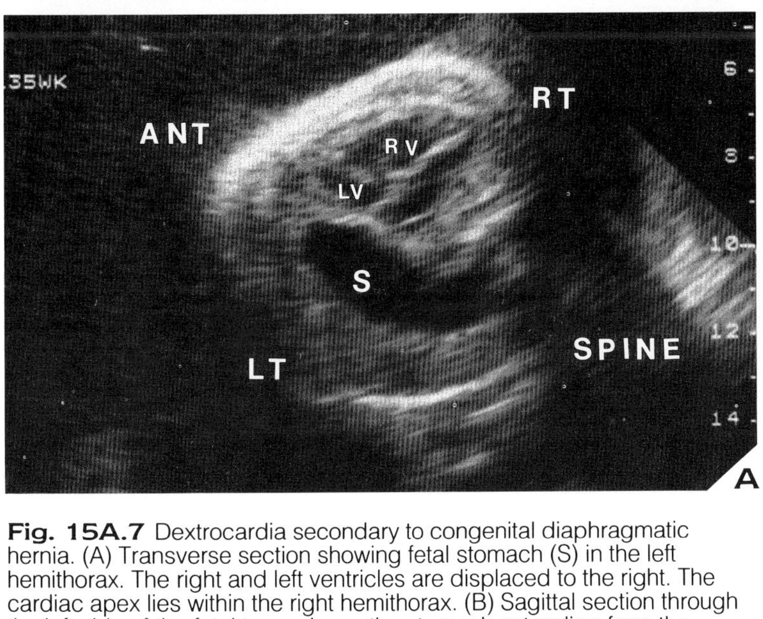

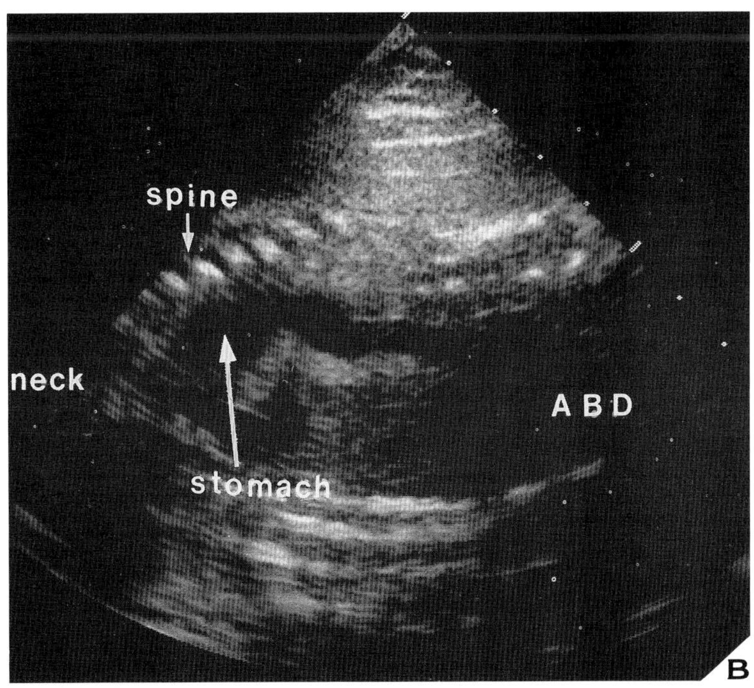

Fig. 15A.7 Dextrocardia secondary to congenital diaphragmatic hernia. (A) Transverse section showing fetal stomach (S) in the left hemithorax. The right and left ventricles are displaced to the right. The cardiac apex lies within the right hemithorax. (B) Sagittal section through the left side of the fetal torso shows the stomach extending from the abdomen (ABD) into the left hemithorax.

In the normal heart, the IVC and superior vena cava (SVC) enter the morphologic right atrium, and the morphologic left atrium has no systemic venous connection. (The atrium that receives the systemic veins can usually be accepted as the morphologic right atrium. However, a left SVC may enter the left atrium in fetuses with an unroofed coronary sinus. Rarely, the hepatic veins may enter the morphologic left atrium.) In right atrial isomerism the abdominal aorta and IVC are usually on the same side of the fetal spine, with the IVC anterior to the aorta; the systemic venous connections to the right atrium are usually (but not always) normal. In left atrial isomerism the aorta is usually midline; typically, there is absence of the suprarenal segment of the IVC with azygos continuation (Fig. 15A.8). The azygos vein is almost always posterior to the abdominal aorta; however, it may be either to the right or the left of the fetal spine. Left atrial isomerism is usually associated

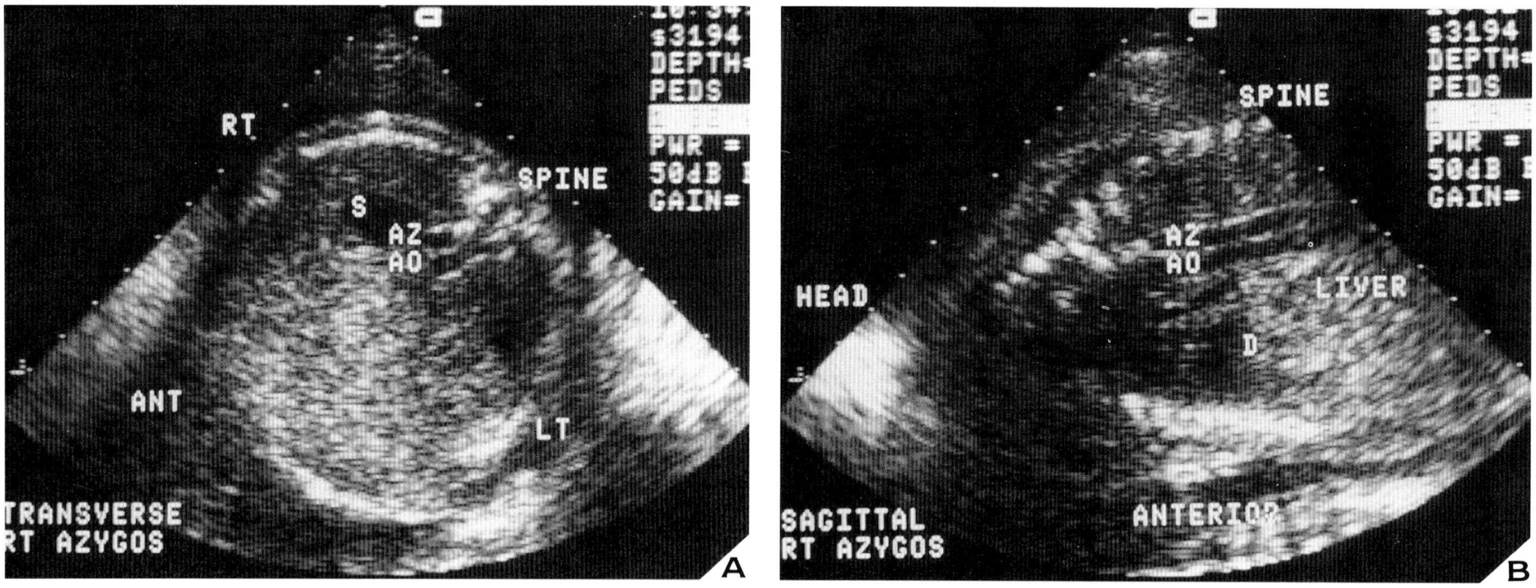

Fig. 15A.8 Absence of the suprarenal inferior vena cava with azygos continuation. (A) Transverse and (B) sagittal two-dimensional echocardiograms of the fetal abdomen. The azygos vein is posterior to the aorta; the suprarenal segment of the inferior vena cava cannot be identified. In atrial situs solitus with normal systemic venous return, the aorta is anterior to the fetal spine and the inferior vena cava is to the right of and anterior to the aorta. Therefore, the findings in this fetus are compatible with left atrial isomerism. (RT = right; LT = left; ANT = anterior; S = stomach; D = diaphragm)

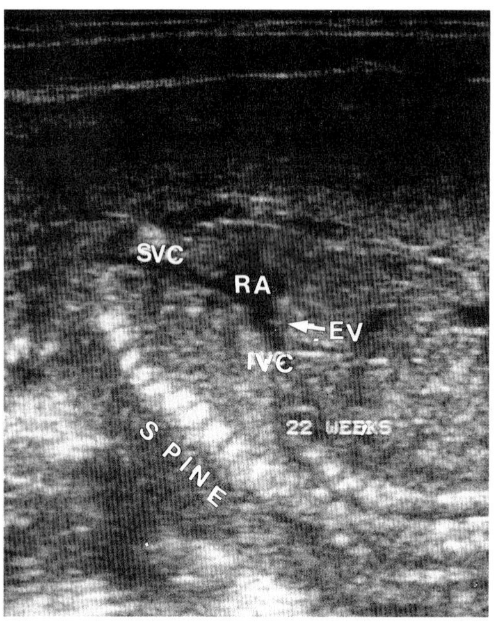

Fig. 15A.9 Eustachian valve. Sagittal section shows the eustachian valve (EV) at the junction of the inferior vena cava (IVC) and right atrium. The function of the eustachian valve is to direct inferior vena caval flow posteriorly, towards the foramen ovale. (SVC = superior vena cava)

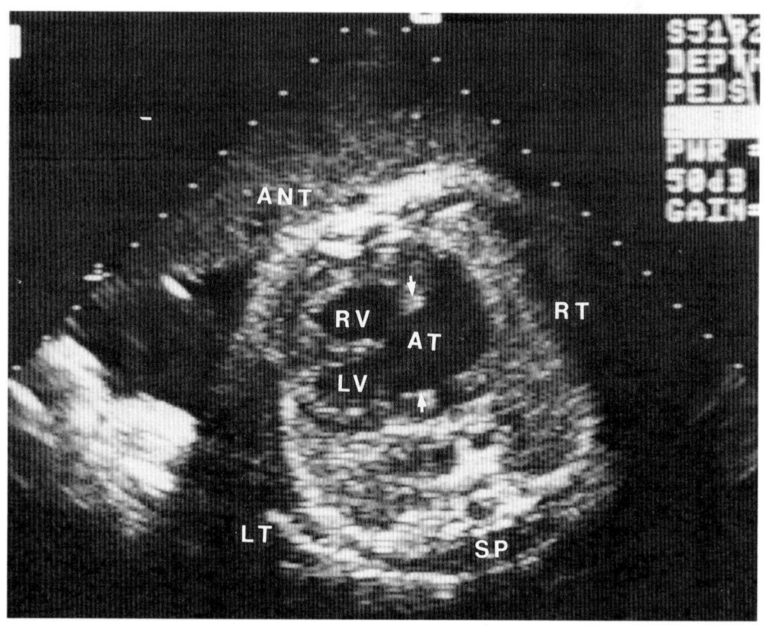

Fig. 15A.10 Atrioventricular septal defect (atrioventricular canal). Four-chamber view demonstrates a common atrium (AT) and a common atrioventricular orifice (*arrow*). (RT = right; LT = left; ANT = anterior; SP = spine)

with anomalous hepatic venous connection, with the hepatic veins connecting directly to the atria. Atrial situs can also be ascertained by identifying the characteristic morphologic features of the atrial appendages (see below; see also Chapter 8).

ATRIAL MORPHOLOGY

After assessing the systemic venous connections to the heart, the next step is to evaluate atrial morphology. In the normal heart, the eustachian valve can often be identified in the right atrium (Fig. 15A.9). (The eustachian valve directs the inferior vena caval return towards the foramen ovale.) Because the foramen ovale is patent during fetal life, the presence of a secundum atrial septal defect (ASD) cannot be excluded in utero. However, a common atrium and the atrial component of a complete or partial atrioventricular canal are readily identified on images obtained in the four-chamber plane (Fig. 15A.10).

The morphology of the atrioventricular valves can also be assessed in the four-chamber plane. Normal valve motion can be appreciated on both two-dimensional and M-mode echocardiography. The relative size of the tricuspid and mitral valves should be noted; both orifices are approximately the same size in a normal fetus.

ATRIOVENTRICULAR CONNECTIONS

To establish the atrioventricular connections it is necessary to demonstrate the characteristic morphologic features of each ventricle. In a normal heart, the tricuspid valve is closer to the cardiac apex than the mitral valve. (In a fetus with Ebstein's malformation, which results in "atrialization" of the right ventricle, there may be extreme apical displacement of the tricuspid valve.) Other morphologic features of the normal right ventricle include lack of atrioventricular–semilunar valve continuity, the presence of a muscular conus, the presence of an infundibular or "outflow" segment, the presence of a moderator band, and poorly defined papillary muscles (Fig. 15A.11).

Several morphologic features characteristic of a normal left ventricle can usually be identified echocardiographically. These include fibrous continuity of the atrioventricular and semilunar valves, well-defined papillary muscles, and absence of a muscular conus. In the fetus, the most easily identified feature is atrioventricular–semilunar valve continuity, which is seen to best advantage in the long-axis plane (Fig. 15A.12).

VENTRICLES

Next, the relative size of the ventricles is evaluated in the four-chamber plane. The right and left ventricles should be approximately equal in size in this projection. Although the dimensions of both ventricles may be comparable, analysis of right ventricular geometry reveals a pattern of right ventricular dominance. Thus, the fetal left ventricle has an elliptical shape instead of the circular configuration seen in infants and children.

Right ventricular enlargement is seen in a number of conditions, including some forms of pulmonary atresia with right

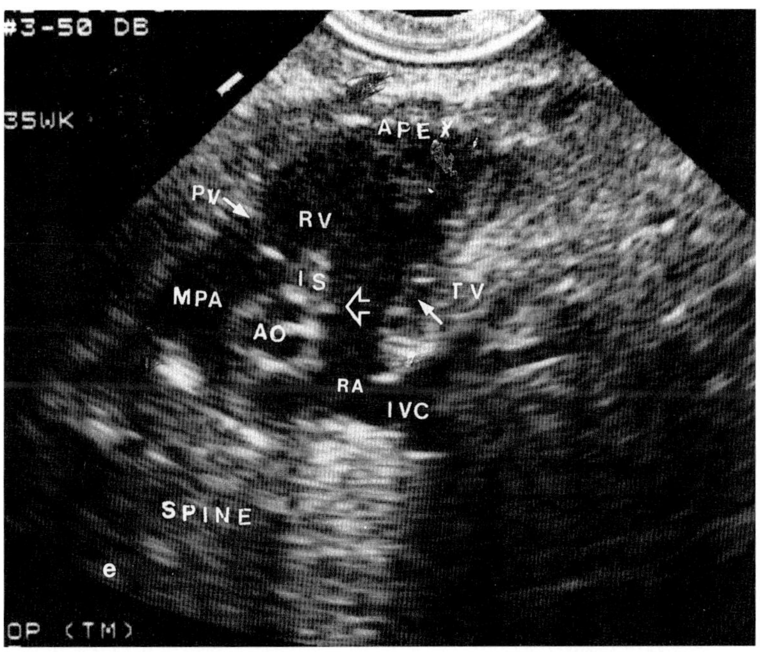

Fig. 15A.11 Normal right ventricular morphology. This oblique section through the right ventricle demonstrates the lack of fibrous continuity between the pulmonic valve (PV) and the septal leaflet (*open arrow*) of the tricuspid valve (TV). The infundibular septum (IS) separates these two structures. [MPA = main pulmonary artery (pulmonary trunk); IVC = inferior vena cava]

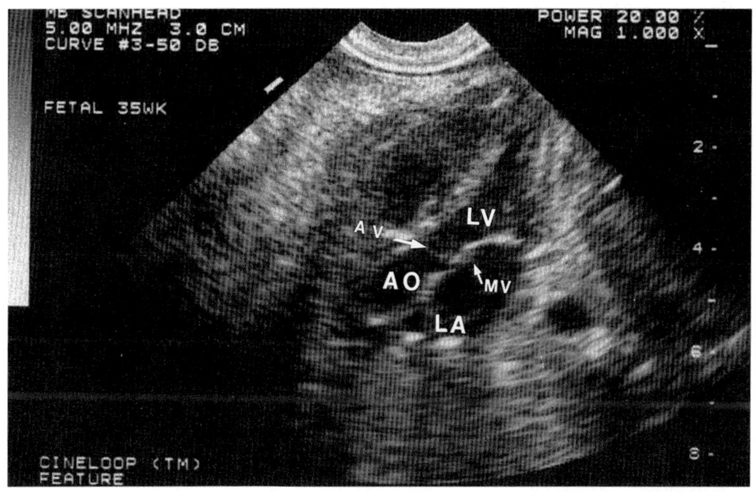

Fig. 15A.12 Normal left ventricular morphology. Apical long-axis scan shows that the mitral valve (MV) is in fibrous continuity with the aortic valve. The demonstration of atrioventricular valve/semilunar valve fibrous continuity is the most useful morphologic feature for identifying the anatomic left ventricle.

ventricular dilatation, right ventricular dominant atrioventricular canal, hypoplastic left heart syndrome (Fig. 15A.13), coarctation of the aorta, and congestive heart failure with nonimmune hydrops.

Left ventricular enlargement (usually accompanied by right ventricular enlargement) is seen in critical aortic stenosis (Fig. 15A.14, Appendix), endocardial fibroelastosis, cardiomyopathy, and congestive heart failure of undetermined cause.

The inlet portion of the ventricular septum is best assessed in the four-chamber plane. The inlet VSD and malformations of the atrioventricular valves associated with a complete atrioventricular canal ("endocardial cushion defect") are clearly depicted in this imaging plane (Fig. 15A.15). Septal hypertrophy and reduced cardiac function are commonly seen in fetuses of poorly controlled diabetic mothers. Absence of the ventricular septum or extreme dominance of one ventricle is usually obvious in hearts with a univentricular atrioventricular connection; the type and mode of atrioventricular connection are best appreciated in the four-chamber plane (Fig. 15A.16). Although VSDs of moderate size are accurately diagnosed in utero (Fig. 15A.17), both false-positive and false-negative diagnoses are common in fetuses with small VSDs. Spontaneous closure of a VSD in utero has been documented echocardiographically.

VENTRICULOARTERIAL CONNECTION

After establishing the atrioventricular connections and evaluating left ventricular morphology and the ventricular septum, the next step is to establish the ventriculoarterial connections. This is accomplished by imaging in both the long-axis and short-axis planes. The first step in establishing the existence of normal ventriculoarterial connections is to demonstrate that the morphologic right ventricle connects with the pulmonary trunk and ductus arteriosus (Fig. 15A.18). (Owing to the normal continuity of the large fetal ductus arteriosus and the descending thoracic aorta, it is easy to mistake the pulmonary trunk and ductus arteriosus for the ascending aorta and aortic arch. This pitfall can be avoided by demonstrating the origin of the brachiocephalic arteries, which are usually easily identified, from the aortic arch. Additional echocardiographic features that are helpful in differentiating the ductus arteriosus from the aortic arch are the more cephalic course and smaller size of the latter, and the continuity of the arch with the descending thoracic aorta. In the human fetus the aortic isthmus is relatively small with respect to the ductus arteriosus, which is nearly the same size as the descending thoracic aorta.)

This phase of the examination is completed by establishing that the ventriculoarterial connection on the left side of the

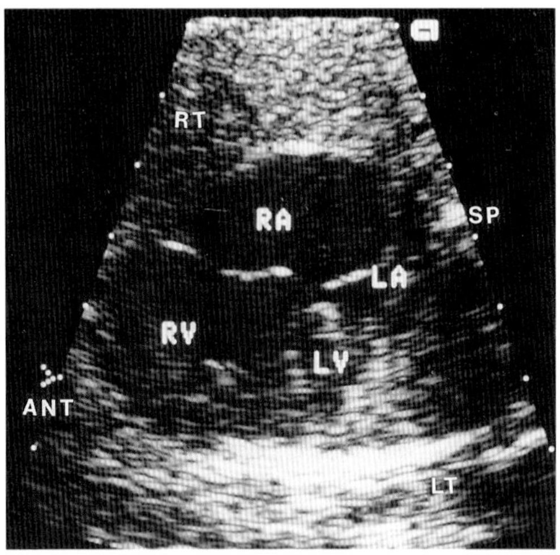

Fig. 15A.13 Right ventricular enlargement. Four-chamber view demonstrates right ventricular enlargement in a fetus with mitral atresia. (RT = right; LT = left; ANT = anterior; SP = spine)

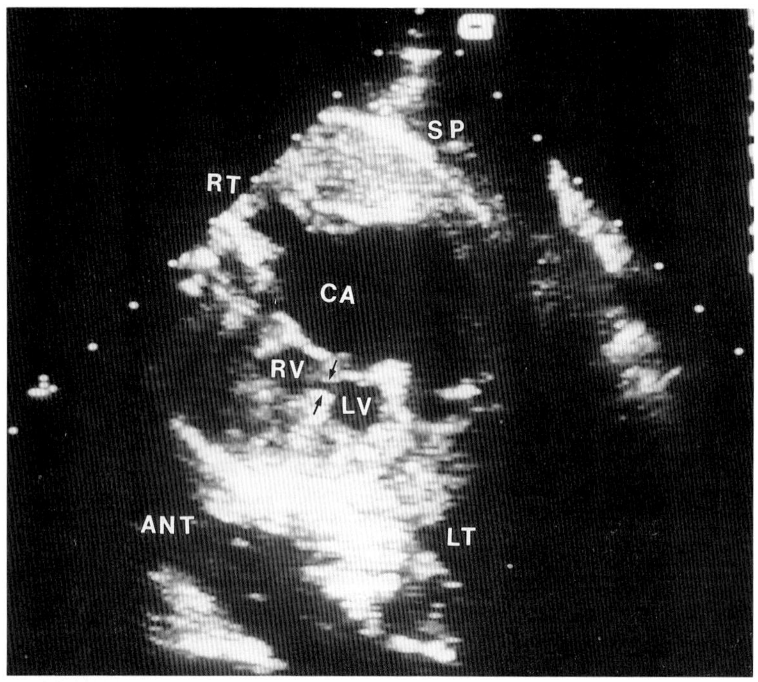

Fig. 15A.15 Complete atrioventricular canal. Transverse scan of the fetal chest (four-chamber view) demonstrates a common atrium (CA), a common atrioventricular valve orifice, and an inlet ventricular septal defect (*arrows*). (RT = right; LT = left; ANT = anterior; SP = spine)

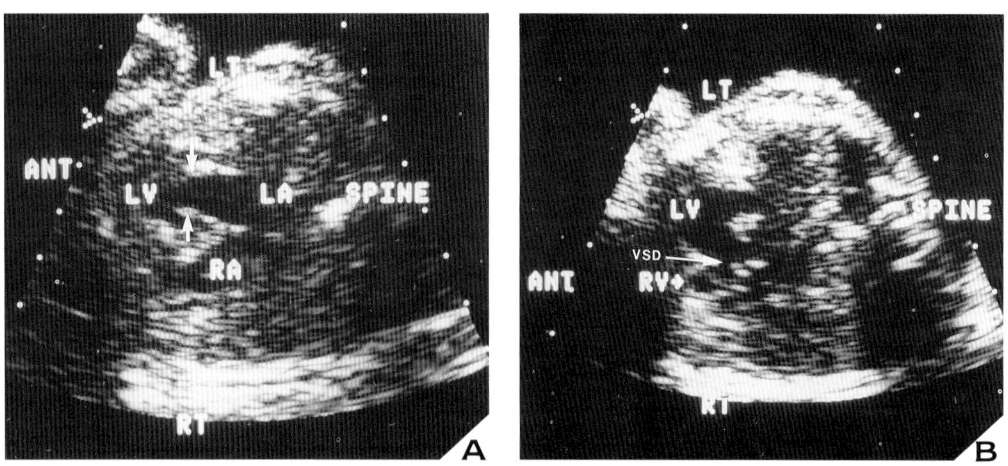

Fig. 15A.16 Tricuspid atresia. (A) Four-chamber view demonstrates absence of the right atrioventricular connection. A single atrioventricular valve (*arrows*) opens from the left atrium into the large left ventricle. (B) By angling the transducer superiorly, a small, anterior right ventricular outlet chamber (RV) and ventricular septal defect (VSD) are visualized. (RT = right; LT = left; ANT = anterior; SP = spine)

heart is normal, ie, that there is a normal connection between the morphological left ventricle and the aorta, with fibrous continuity of the atrioventricular (mitral) and semilunar (aortic) valves.

ARTERIAL (SEMILUNAR) VALVES

The normal morphology and function of the semilunar valves can be demonstrated by both two-dimensional and M-mode echocardiography. Demonstration of a normal-sized, normally functioning pulmonic valve is helpful in excluding pulmonary atresia. In fetuses with pulmonary atresia it is usually possible to demonstrate abnormal anatomy and function of the pulmonic valve, hypoplasia of the pulmonary trunk and ductus arteriosus, and relative enlargement of the ascending aorta; abnormalities of right ventricular size (dilated or hypoplastic) and function are commonly present as well. Echocardiograms in fetuses with tetralogy of Fallot demonstrate various degrees of hypoplasia of the right ventricular outflow tract and pulmonary trunk, as well as a large VSD with an overriding aorta. Aortic atresia is characterized echocardiographically by extreme hypoplasia of

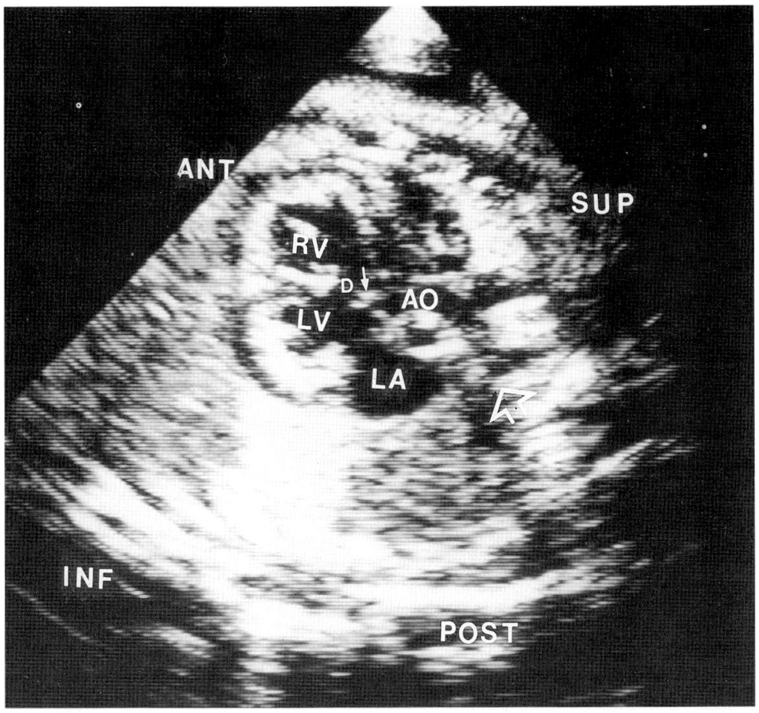

Fig. 15A.17 Ventricular septal defect. Long-axis view of the left ventricular outflow tract demonstrates a moderate-sized muscular ventricular septal defect (D). Subaortic stenosis (*small arrow*) and coarctation (*large arrow*) of the aorta are also present. (SUP = superior; INF = inferior; ANT = anterior)

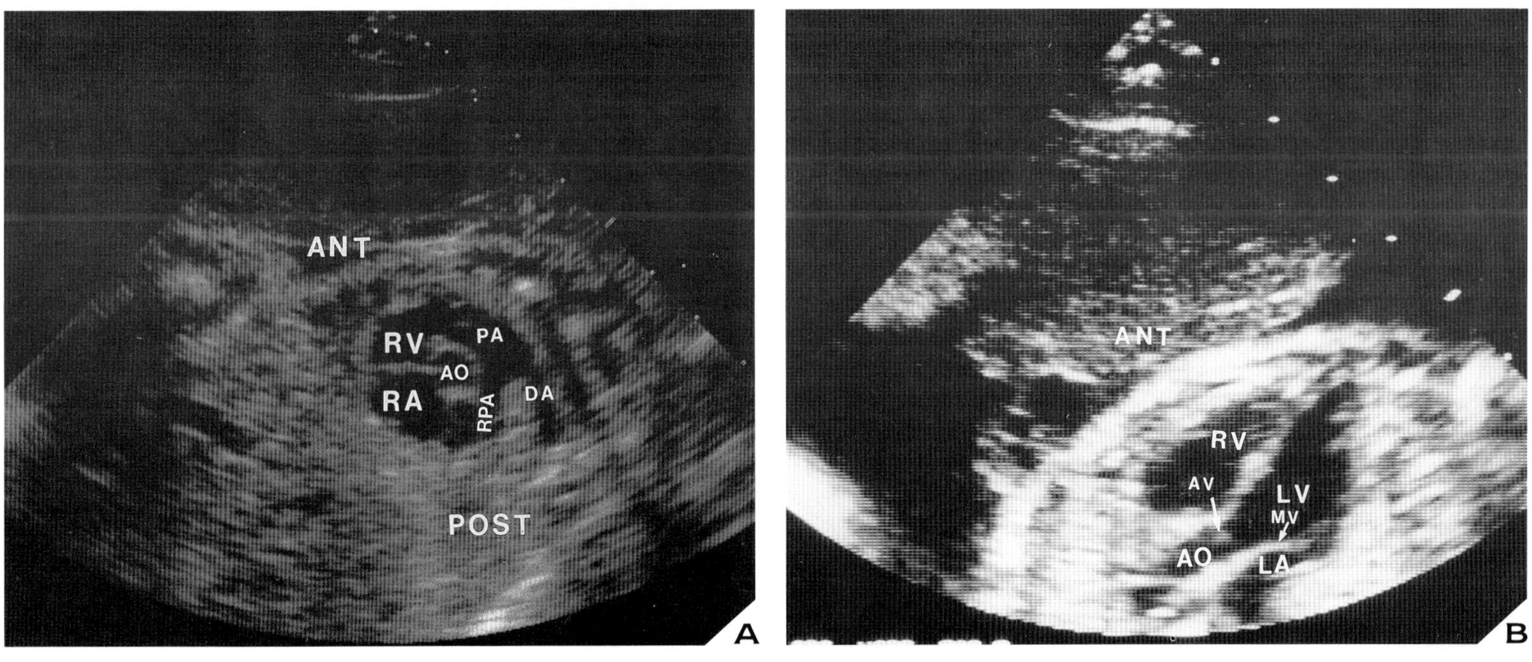

Fig. 15A.18 Normal ventriculoarterial connection. The normal connection between the ventricles and the great arteries is established by demonstrating that the pulmonary trunk connects with the morphologic right ventricle and the aorta connects with the morphologic left ventricle. The pulmonary trunk can be identified as the great artery which gives rise to the right and left pulmonary arteries and communicates posteriorly with the ductus arteriosus; the aorta can be identified as the great artery which gives rise to the subclavian and carotid arteries. (A) Short-axis view of the right ventricular outflow tract demonstrates the pulmonary trunk, which rise to the right pulmonary artery (RPA) and ductus arteriosus (DA). (B) Long-axis view of left ventricular outflow tract demonstrates normal connection of left ventricle and aorta. Note fibrous continuity of mitral (MV) and aortic (AV) valves. (ANT = ant; POST = post)

the ascending aorta and aortic arch, gross right ventricular enlargement, and enlargement of the pulmonary trunk and ductus arteriosus (Fig. 15A.19).

A lesion causing aortic arch obstruction (eg, coarctation of the aorta, interrupted aortic arch) should be suspected in any fetus with right ventricular enlargement that is not associated with obstruction at the level of the aortic valve or left ventricular outflow tract. Echocardiographic demonstration of coarctation or arch interruption is difficult owing to the small size of the aortic isthmus in the normal fetus. For this reason, aortic coarctation is one of the most difficult diagnoses to make on fetal echocardiography. However, hypoplasia of the transverse arch and enlargement of the pulmonary trunk, which are characteristically seen on echocardiograms of infants with isolated aortic coarctation, can also be appreciated in the fetus, and should suggest the presence of this anomaly. Critical aortic stenosis is manifested echocardiographically by a small aortic annulus, poststenotic dilatation of the ascending aorta, and (frequently) the presence of endocardial fibroelastosis (Fig. 15A.20). The latter is manifested by bright endocardial echoes in the left ventricle, with poor left ventricular function.

RESULTS OF MORPHOLOGIC ASSESSMENT

The spectrum of cardiac malformations that can be detected in utero differs considerably from that encountered in postnatal life. The indications that lead to referral for fetal echocardiography will result in the identification of a disproportionate number of fetuses with severe malformations causing congestive heart failure and fetal hydrops, fetal arrhythmias, and gross abnormalities of the ventricles and atrioventricular valves detected on routine obstetric sonography. Many of the malformations commonly encountered in postnatal life are diagnosed with difficulty in the fetus (eg, aortic coarctation), or are recognized only in their most severe forms (eg, aortic stenosis, pulmonic stenosis). Augmenting the two-dimensional echocardiographic examination with conventional and/or color Doppler may improve diagnostic accuracy in fetuses with milder degrees of semilunar valve stenosis, as well as in those with complex malformations.

EVALUATION OF FETAL HEART RATE AND RHYTHM

As the use of antepartum fetal heart rate monitoring increases, an increasing number of pregnant women are being referred for echocardiographic evaluation of abnormalities of fetal heart rate and rhythm, which occur in a small percentage of pregnancies. Southall et al (1980) documented transient fetal bradycardia in 1.1 to 1.3 percent and transient fetal tachycardia in less than 1 percent of otherwise normal pregnancies. Premature contractions are detected in fetuses at a rate only slightly higher than that observed in normal neonates (1.7 percent).

Although fetal bradycardia, tachycardia, or arrhythmia is infrequently observed in normal pregnancies, the detection of an abnormal heart rate or rhythm on routine antenatal heart rate monitoring raises the question of a fetal cardiac abnormality. Unfortunately, owing to the normal absence of P-waves, the extraneous electrical noise, and the difficulty in identifying abnormal QRS morphology, fetal ECGs are difficult to interpret. The most important role of fetal echocardiography has been in the diagnosis of fetal rhythm disturbances.

Echocardiographic assessment of fetal heart rate and rhythm assumes that the electrical activation sequence in the atria and ventricles can be inferred from mechanical events that are depicted echocardiographically. Although a normal activation sequence may be appreciated on two-dimensional echocardiography, accurate analysis of arrhythmias and other rhythm disturbances requires either two-dimensionally directed M-mode echocardiography or duplex pulsed Doppler echocardiography. Detailed analysis of fetal rhythm should be preceded by a careful two-dimensional echocardiographic evaluation to document the presence or absence of congestive heart failure (manifested by cardiac enlargement and hydrops) or congenital

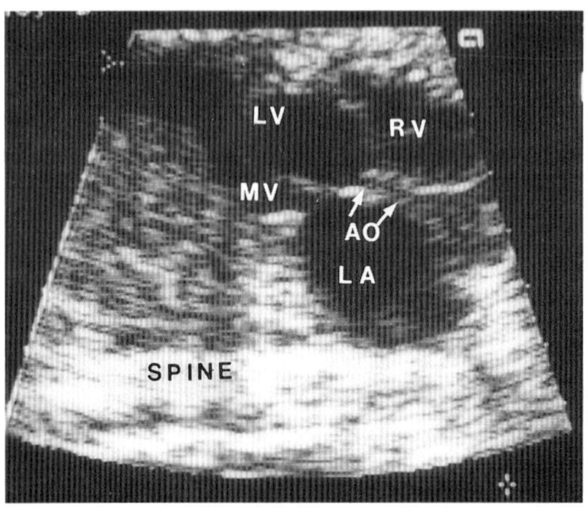

Fig. 15A.19 Aortic valve atresia and hypoplastic aorta. Long axis view demonstrates a hypoplastic ascending aorta and dilatation of the left ventricle and left atrium. An associated premature closure of the foramen ovale was responsible for the enlargement of the left-sided chambers in this fetus. (MV = mitral valve)

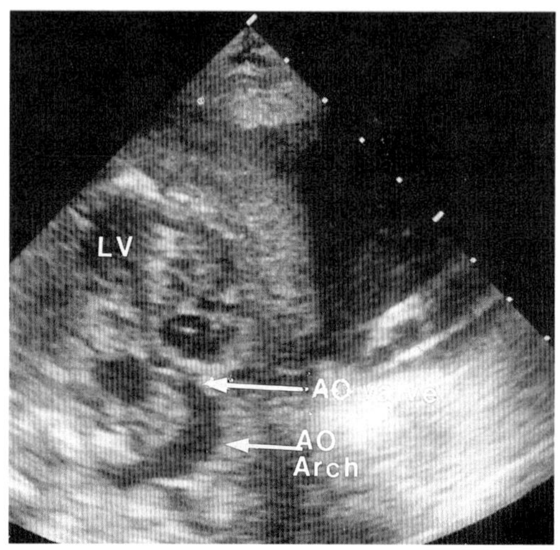

Fig. 15A.20 Subvalvar and valvar aortic stenosis. Long axis view of left ventricular outflow segment (LV) demonstrates poststenotic dilatation of the ascending aorta (AO arch). (AO valve = aortic valve)

heart disease. The precise nature of the rhythm disturbance can then be established by either M-mode or Doppler echocardiography.

M-MODE ECHOCARDIOGRAPHY

In this technique, the line of M-mode interrogation is directed by two-dimensional imaging of various cardiovascular structures, including the right atrial and right ventricular walls, the tricuspid or mitral valve, the aortic root, and the left atrium. Atrial contraction is manifested by atrial wall motion or an A-wave of the atrioventricular valve. Ventricular contraction is manifested by ventricular wall motion, atrioventricular valve closure, and/or opening of the semilunar valves. Superimposing the color Doppler image on the M-mode tracing, which relates blood flow to the mechanical events of contraction, may facilitate recognition of the activation sequence.

Premature Contractions

An irregular fetal rhythm detected on routine obstetric evaluation is the usual reason for referral for echocardiographic evaluation of a "fetal arrhythmia." In such cases the irregular rhythm is almost always caused by a premature contraction, which is followed by a compensatory pause. Premature contractions that are preceded by atrial wall motion or an early A-wave represent premature atrial contractions (Fig. 15A.21). Ventricular premature contractions are characterized by early ventricular wall motion or atrioventricular valve closure without evidence of a preceding atrial contraction (Fig. 15A.22, Appendix). Mixed atrial and ventricular premature contractions may occur in the same patient.

Bradycardia

Fetal bradycardia, defined as a sustained heart rate of less than 100 beats per minute, is usually a sinus bradycardia, with an atrial contraction preceding each ventricular contraction. (Sinus bradycardia associated with intrapartum fetal distress will not be considered here.) Transient sinus bradycardia is occasionally observed during echocardiography, and is believed by some investigators to be caused by pressure of the transducer on the maternal abdomen or by movements of the fetus. Sustained fetal bradycardia may be due to blocked premature atrial contractions, blocked atrial bigeminy, complete heart block, or second degree heart block with fixed or variable rates of atrioventricular conduction. In fetuses with blocked premature atrial contractions, M-mode tracings demonstrate early atrial wall motion or A-waves without an ensuing ventricular contraction, after which there is a compensatory pause. In fetuses with blocked atrial bigeminy, M-mode tracings reveal an irregular atrial rate, with a ventricular contraction following every other atrial contraction (Fig. 15A.23). In complete heart block, atrial contraction is unrelated to ventricular contraction, resulting in a ventricular bradycardia with a rate of 60 to 80 beats per minute. M-mode echocardiography reveals A-waves "marching through" regular atrioventricular valve closure or

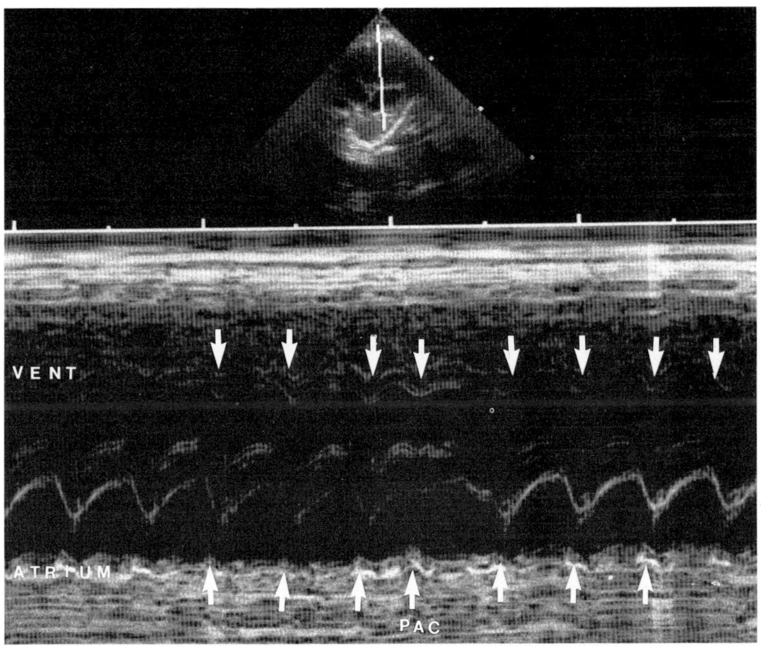

Fig. 15A.21 Sinus rhythm with a premature atrial contraction. In this M-mode tracing the lower arrow marks the onset of atrial contraction. The upper arrow marks the onset of ventricular contraction. The early beat (PAC) demonstrates first atrial, then ventricular contraction.

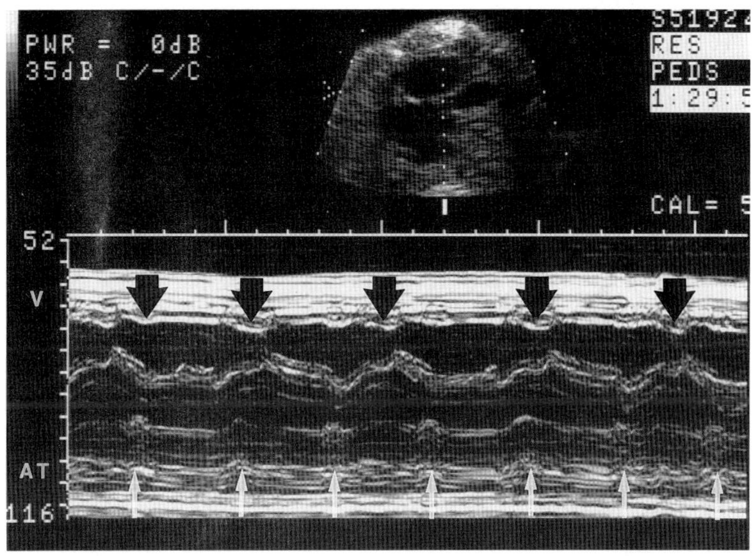

Fig. 15A.23 Complete heart block. M-mode echocardiogram. The large arrows mark ventricular contraction and the small arrows mark atrial contraction. The atrial rate is greater than the ventricular rate (atrioventricular dissociation).

atrial wall motion that is unrelated to ventricular wall motion (Fig. 15A.23). Second-degree heart block with fixed or variable rates of atrioventricular conduction can also be detected by M-mode echocardiography.

It is important to establish the mechanism of fetal bradycardia before therapy is instituted. Failure to recognize that fetal bradycardia is due to complete heart block or blocked premature atrial contractions can lead to unnecessary cesarian delivery for presumed fetal distress.

Tachycardia

Supraventricular tachycardia is characterized by atrial rates above 180 beats per minute, with an atrial contraction or A-wave preceding each ventricular contraction (Fig. 15A.24, Appendix). Supraventricular tachycardia cannot be distinguished echocardiographically from ventricular tachycardia with 1:1 retrograde conduction to the atrium. However, many fetuses with a presumptive diagnosis of supraventricular arrhythmia who were diagnosed and treated in utero have had recurrence of this arrhythmia in the neonatal period, providing retrospective confirmation of the antenatal echocardiographic diagnosis. Another cause of fetal tachycardia is atrial flutter, which is characterized on M-mode echocardiography by very high atrial contraction rates, usually above 400 beats per minute. Atrial flutter is associated with variable ratios of atrioventricular block. In a typical case the atrial contractions are followed by ventricular contractions in a ratio of 2:1 to 4:1 (Fig. 15A.25).

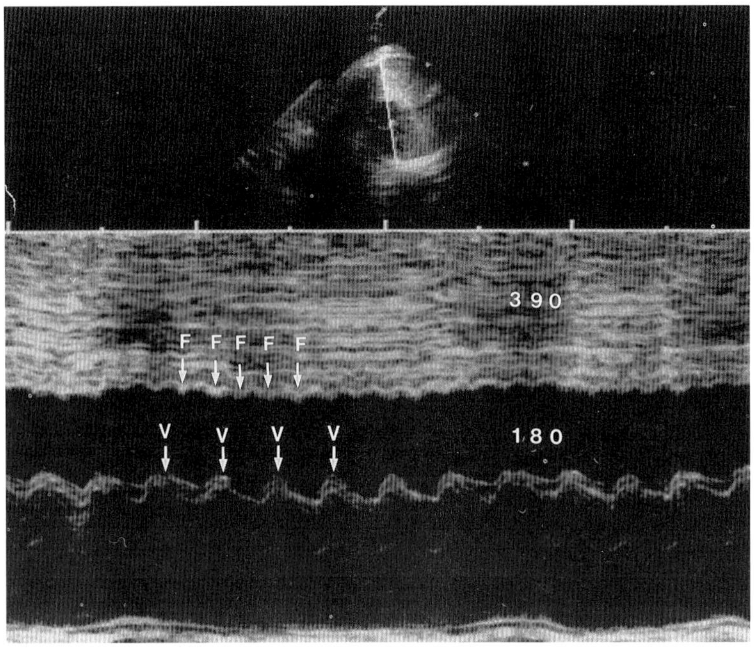

Fig. 15A.25 Atrial flutter. M-mode tracing demonstrates atrial flutter with a 2:1 atrioventricular block. The atrial rate is approximately 390 beats per minute and the ventricular rate is approximately 180 beats per minute. (F = movement of the fluttering atrium; V = movement with ventricular contraction)

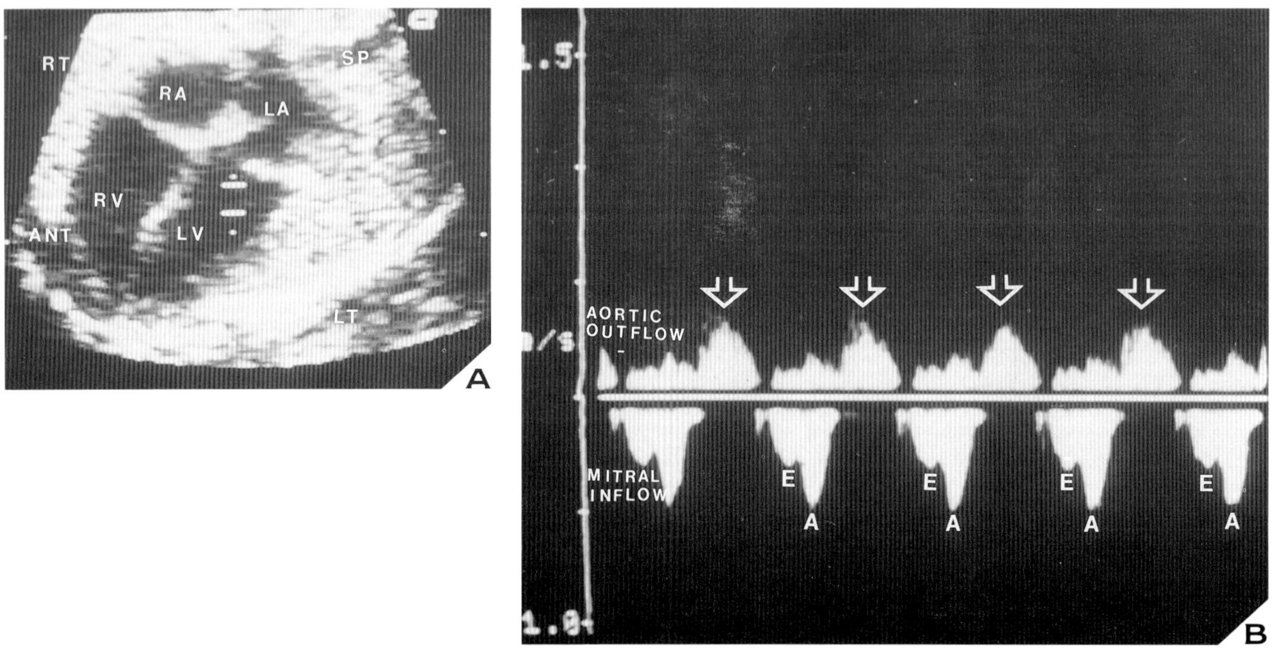

Fig. 15A.26 Left ventricular flow velocities: Doppler analysis. (A) Four-chamber view. The Doppler sample volume is in the left ventricular (LV) inlet. By analyzing the Doppler signal in this region it is possible to evaluate both diastolic (mitral) inflow and systolic (aortic) outflow. (RT = right; LT = left; ANT = anterior; SP = spine) (B) Doppler wave form. The diastolic inflow velocity is shown below the zero line and the systolic outflow is shown above the line. Note that the peak caused by active atrial contraction (A) is more prominent than the peak caused by passive ventricular filling (E). This pattern is typical of diastolic inflow in the fetus. The mitral inflow velocity (shown below the zero line) goes to 0 during systole, when the mitral valve closes. In this tracing the aortic outflow velocity (*open arrows*) peaks at less than 0.5/m/sec.

DOPPLER ECHOCARDIOGRAPHY

The sensitivity and specificity of Doppler echocardiography in the diagnosis of fetal arrhythmias are comparable to those of M-mode echocardiography. The principle of the Doppler technique is that the electrical activation sequence can be deduced from the sequence of flow detected by range-gated pulsed Doppler. Thus, by sampling the flow across an atrioventricular valve or the foramen ovale, it is possible to describe the pattern of atrial contraction. Similarly, by sampling flow in the left ventricular outflow tract or a great artery, it is possible to describe the pattern of ventricular contraction. Doppler interrogation of the left ventricular inlet permits simultaneous analysis of flows across the atrioventricular valve and left ventricular outflow tract; thus, by sampling in one location, it is possible to describe the activation sequence (Fig. 15A.26).

Sinus Rhythms

In normal sinus rhythm and sinus bradycardia, an atrial A-wave precedes each systolic velocity profile. Premature atrial contractions are characterized by early occurrence of the A-wave, accentuation of peak atrioventricular valve velocity, or early accentuation of peak velocity through the foramen ovale (Fig. 15A.27). The early atrial flow is followed by ventricular flow at a velocity less than that of the preceding sinus beat. Prolonged passive ventricular filling and accentuation of ventricular flow velocities (post-extrasystolic potentiation) occurs after a compensatory atrial pause. In the presence of atrioventricular block, early atrial flow may not be followed by ventricular flow.

Premature Ventricular Contractions

Premature ventricular contractions (PVCs) result in early ventricular systole; consequently, atrioventricular valve flow is abbreviated. Therefore, early ventricular flow is of lower velocity than that of the preceding normal beat. PVCs may be associated with systolic insufficiency of the atrioventricular valve. The Doppler image demonstrates a compensatory pause with prolonged passive ventricular filling and accentuated ventricular velocity on the beat following the PVC.

Bradycardia and Complete Heart Block

Complete heart block is characterized by an atrial A-wave that is dissociated from ventricular or arterial flow. In some fetuses with complete heart block, Doppler images may demonstrate diastolic atrioventricular valve insufficiency, which results from failure of atrioventricular valve closure after atrial systole. As with M-mode echocardiography, atrial bigeminy can be distinguished from complete heart block by the presence of early atrial flow without subsequent ventricular flow, alternating with a 1:1 ratio of atrial and ventricular flow.

Tachyarrhythmias

In fetuses with supraventricular tachycardia and atrial flutter, rapid atrial contraction produces low amplitude A-waves which merge with passive atrial filling and are followed by low amplitude ventricular flow. Rapid atrial contraction can also be demonstrated by pulsed Doppler sampling within the foramen ovale. Careful analysis of the Doppler images usually (but not always) enables the echocardiographer to differentiate atrial flutter with 1:1 conduction from supraventricular tachycardia. Atrial flutter is characterized by atrial rates of 400 beats per minute and is usually associated with atrioventricular block, whereas supraventricular tachycardia is characterized by rates of 200 to 300 beats per minute with 1:1 atrioventricular conduction.

CLINICAL SIGNIFICANCE

The echocardiographic methods described above have greatly enhanced our understanding of the spectrum and outcome of fetal arrhythmias. It is now clear that isolated premature contractions (usually of atrial origin) account for the great majority of fetal rhythm disturbances. Although an occasional fetus with isolated premature atrial contractions may develop supraventricular tachycardia, the tachycardia nearly always resolves in utero or soon after birth. Premature ventricular contractions, although uncommon, appear to have a similarly benign prognosis. Transient bradycardia, with rates dropping below 100 beats per minute for short intervals, is not uncommon and is of no clinical significance. Although the mechanism is unclear, most investigators believe that it is due to fetal movement or to transducer pressure on the maternal abdomen. The causes of sustained bradycardia (heart rate persistently below 100 beats per minute) include sinus bradycardia secondary to fetal distress, blocked atrial bigeminy, and complete heart block. Maternal lupus erythematosus is frequently associated with fetal heart block. When an arrhythmia is associated with congenital heart disease, the malformation is usually complex. Abnormalities of the atrial septum and inflow portion of the ventricular septum (eg, right or left atrial isomerism with a common atrium, common atrioventricular valve, and abnormal systemic venous return) are typically present in such cases.

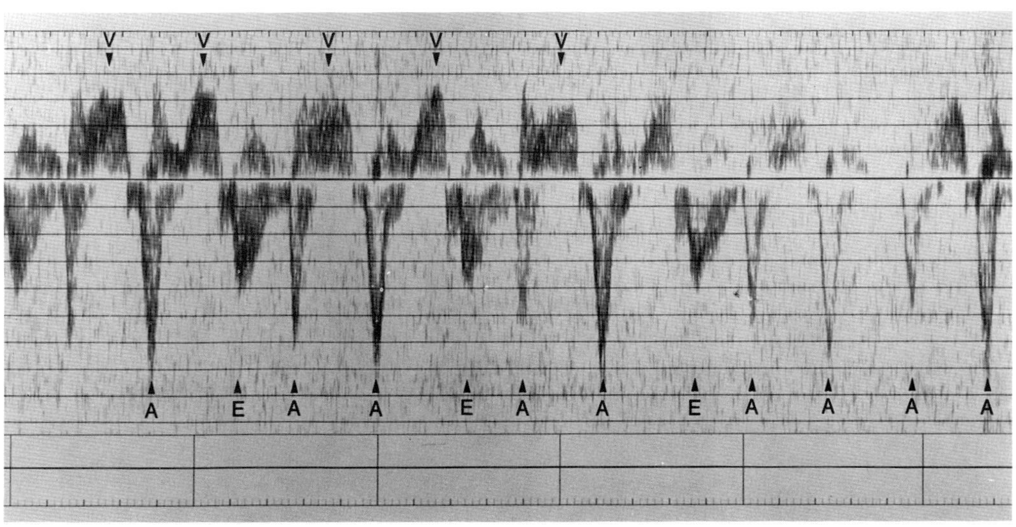

Fig. 15A.27 Premature atrial contractions (bigeminy pattern). Doppler tracing shows that during each sinus beat there is a normal E peak followed by an A peak. During the subsequent premature atrial contraction there is no E peak, since the atrium contracts during early diastolic filling; however, this results in a greater than normal A peak. The subsequent beat shows a normal filling pattern, with an E wave and an A wave. The pattern repeats (bigeminy).

EVALUATION OF FETAL CIRCULATORY FUNCTION

CLINICAL MANIFESTATIONS OF CARDIAC DYSFUNCTION

Fetal cardiac dysfunction may result from a variety of causes, most of which are not primarily cardiac in origin. Nonimmune hydrops fetalis (NIHF) is often the first sign of fetal cardiac failure observed by the obstetrician. It may be the initial manifestation of fetal heart failure in such diverse conditions as maternal anemia, preeclampsia, fetal arteriovenous malformations, and sacrococcygeal teratoma. Cardiac enlargement is often noted in hydropic fetuses, irrespective of the cause of the hydrops. Other indices of reduced cardiac function (eg, decreased shortening and ejection fractions) may be present as well. Because it provides most of the fetal blood flow that ultimately reaches the placenta, the right ventricle is disproportionately affected in NIHF. Extracardiac malformations are commonly present in fetuses with NIHF; however, NIHF is most likely to be present when the anomalies include a major cardiac malformation. NIHF is a frequent sequela of unsuccessfully treated fetal arrhythmias.

After excluding an arrhythmia or major cardiac malformation, a careful echocardiographic assessment of heart size and function by means of two-dimensional, M-mode, and Doppler echocardiography is the next step in evaluating a fetus with NIHF.

TWO-DIMENSIONAL AND M-MODE ECHOCARDIOGRAPHY

Ventricular Size

Disparities in chamber size often provide strong evidence of congenital heart disease in the fetus. When the right and left ventricles are compared, one or the other may appear larger. However, unless one knows the size and relationships of the ventricles in the normal fetus, it is difficult to decide whether one is abnormally large or abnormally small or whether both are abnormal. On two-dimensional echocardiography, the right and left ventricles appear approximately equal in size on both four-chamber and short-axis projections (see Fig. 15A.6), a relationship that remains constant throughout gestation.

Normal standards for ventricular size in the human fetus (related to standard parameters of fetal growth such as biparietal diameter, abdominal circumference, and femur length) have been established by both two-dimensional and M-mode echocardiography. Owing to differences in methodology, the normal range varies from author to author. Nevertheless, these quantitative data are useful in detecting abnormal ventricular size and/or dysfunction.

Measurements of ventricular size in the fetus are subject to a number of important limitations. For example, because it is not possible to synchronize the M-mode tracing with the ECG, standard measurement techniques cannot be used to determine diastolic ventricular size. Owing to the presence of flat or paradoxical septal motion in the normal fetus, as well as differ-

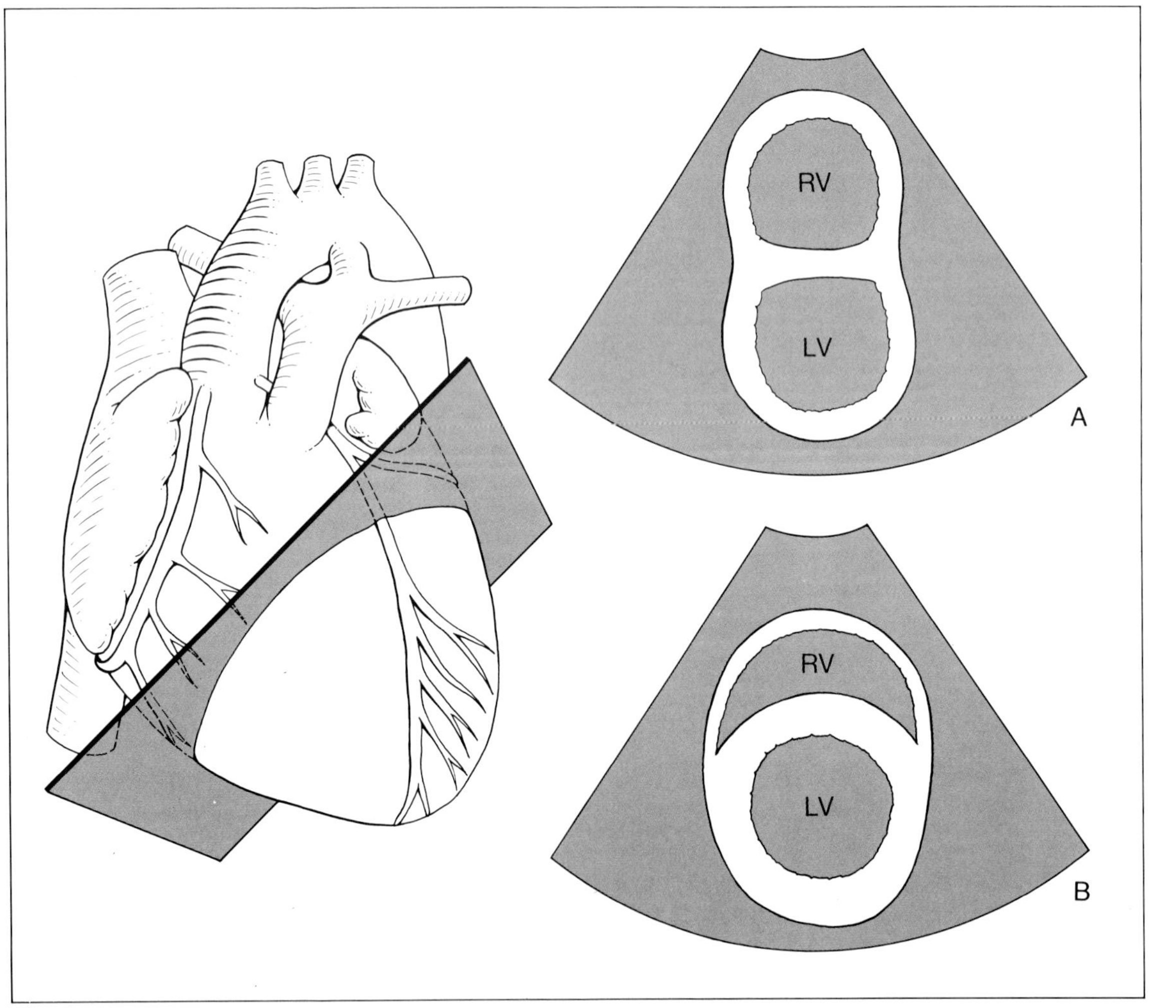

Fig. 15A.28 Changing configuration of ventricles and ventricular septum from prenatal to postnatal life. (A, B) Diagrammatic cross-section through the mid-portions of the right and left ventricles. In the fetus (A) both ventricles have a relatively circular shape when viewed in cross-section. The ventricular septum is relatively flat and encroaches on each ventricle to approximately the same degree. After birth (B) the ventricular septum bulges into the right ventricle. The left ventricular cavity becomes much more circular than it was during fetal life. The right ventricular cavity becomes flattened as it wraps around the concentric mass of the left ventricle.

ences in ventricular geometry in the fetus and newborn (which presumably reflect the relatively greater right ventricular volume load in the former), comparisons of ventricular size and shortening fraction before and after birth are meaningless.

Various studies have shown that the diameters of the right and left ventricles are approximately equal throughout gestation. However, this does not imply that ventricular volume and/or stroke volume are equal. Indeed, it has been shown that because of substantial differences in ventricular geometry the end diastolic and end systolic volumes are greater in the right ventricle. As a result, ventricular stroke volume is considerably greater on the right than on the left. Anzacot (1983) has described a characteristic developmental pattern for the fetal left ventricle. On short-axis images, a cross-section of the left ventricle resembles a flattened ellipse in the fetus and a circle in older infants (neonates exhibit a transitional configuration) (Fig. 15A.28). Thus, the left ventricular configuration in a normal fetus resembles that of an older infant with a congenital cardiac defect causing right ventricular pressure or volume overload. Stated another way, three-dimensional analysis of ventricular geometry clearly indicates right ventricular dominance even though the transverse diameters of the ventricles (as seen in the four-chamber projection) are equal (Fig. 15A.29).

Ventricular Function

Echocardiographic parameters of ventricular functions are load dependent and are therefore of limited use for assessing the contractile state. The parameters employed in postnatal life are primarily ejection phase indices (eg, pre-ejection/ejection period ratio, shortening fraction, mean velocity of shortening, ejection fraction). Although the systolic time interval can be measured on transabdominal fetal echocardiograms in the human fetus, such measurements are affected by changing afterload and are technically difficult to obtain. Kleinman and

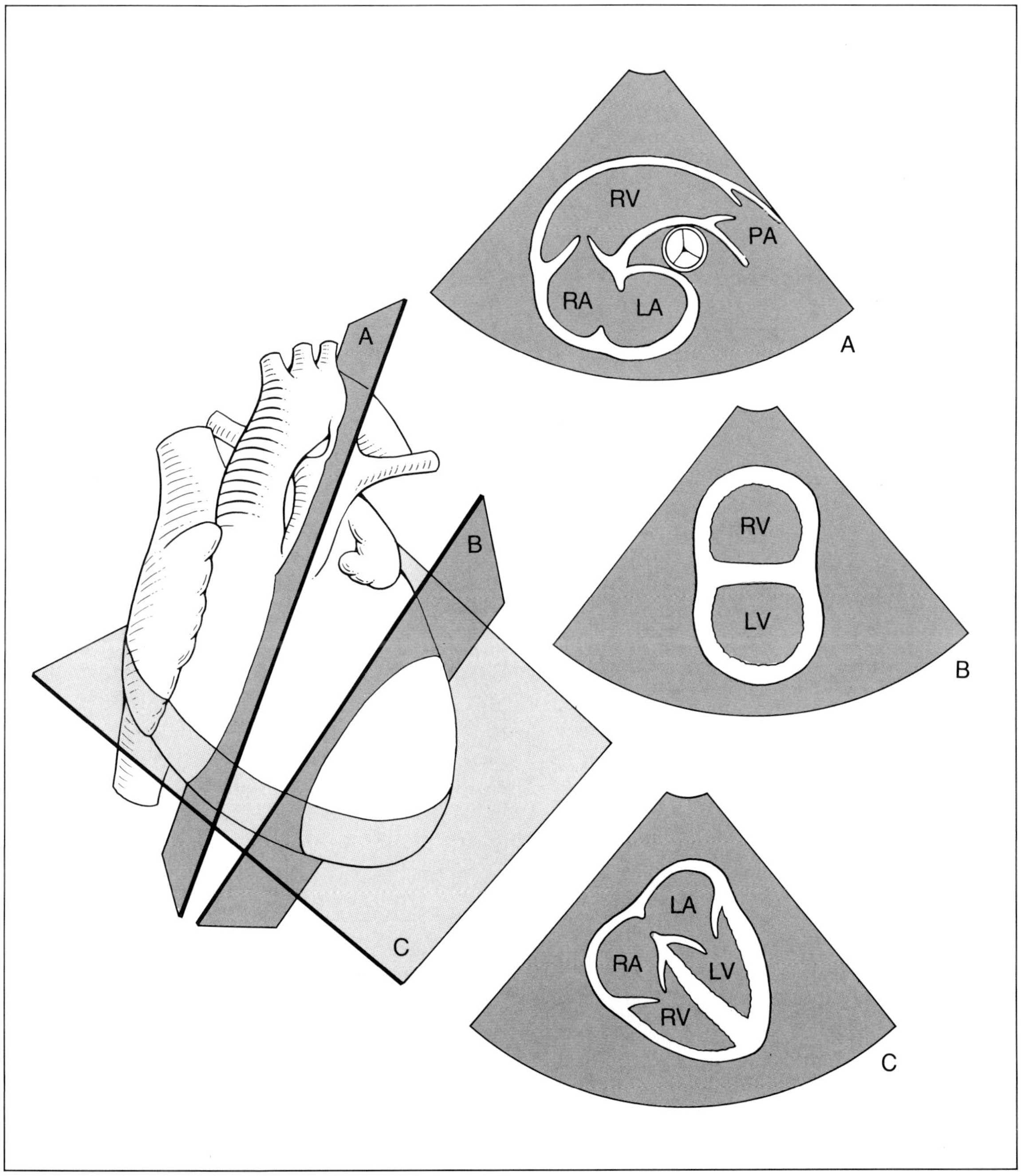

Fig. 15A.29 Normal prominence of right ventricular outflow tract. The right and left ventricles appear to be of equal size on a cross-sectional view of the midportion of the ventricular cavities (B) and a section corresponding to the four-chamber view (C). However, a section including the inlet and outlet portions of the right ventricle (A) demonstrates that the outlet portion of the right ventricle differs from that of the left, enabling the right ventricle to have a greater stroke volume during systole.

Donnerstein (1985) have demonstrated that the pre-ejection/ejection period ratio increases with gestational age.

Post-extrasystolic potentiation has been demonstrated in the human fetus by assessing shortening fraction and peak systolic wall velocity on M-mode recordings. The presence of post-extrasystolic potentiation presumably reflects increased preload, thus confirming the existence of a Starling response in the normal human fetus. Fractional shortening appears to be similar in both ventricles (approximately 32 percent), with the value decreasing slightly from 20 weeks to term.

Because of the inability to assess changes in fetal loading conditions, it is not possible to infer the contractile state of the fetal myocardium in a given clinical setting. Moreover, because of the changes in ventricular geometry that occur after birth it is not possible to compare the left ventricular shortening fraction in the fetus, neonate, and older infant. Ultimately, conventional obstetric sonography will reveal evidence of congestive heart failure (eg, right ventricular enlargement, pleural and pericardial effusions, scalp edema) in various disease states; however, these are late changes.

PULSED AND CONTINUOUS WAVE DOPPLER

As described above, pulsed Doppler is useful in the diagnosis of fetal arrhythmias; it can also be used to estimate fetal blood flow, detect valvular insufficiency, demonstrate turbulent flow in the great arteries, and detect constriction of the fetal ductus arteriosus. However, a number of technical factors limit the application of Doppler imaging techniques in the human fetus (Fig. 15A.30). Despite these limitations, the pulsed Doppler examination is a useful adjunct to cardiac imaging in the fetus.

Pulsed and continuous wave Doppler expose the fetus to higher energy ultrasound energy than two-dimensional or M-mode imaging. Although adverse effects have not been demonstrated in the human fetus, the Doppler examination should not be considered a routine part of the fetal echocardiographic study. Indications for pulsed Doppler include demonstration of abnormal flow in fetuses with suspected congenital heart disease; evaluation of fetal arrhythmias; and assessment of cardiac function in fetuses at risk for congestive heart failure. The risk can be minimized by using the lowest possible energy output and the smallest possible sample volume size.

COLOR DOPPLER FLOW IMAGING

Color Doppler flow imaging ("color Doppler") can enhance the fetal echocardiographic examination in a number of ways. Because of the lower pulse repetition time of color Doppler systems, the energy intensity is less in any given tissue volume, so that the risk to the fetus is less than with conventional pulsed or continuous wave Doppler imaging. The addition of color Doppler may allow differentiation of structures that are not clearly depicted by two-dimensional echocardiography alone, particularly in the presence of maternal obesity, polyhydramnios, or advanced fetal gestational age. The use of color Doppler may shorten the examination by enabling the echocardiographer to quickly recognize normal or abnormal flow. The presence of a regurgitant jet caused by mitral or tricuspid insufficiency (see Fig. 15A.14B, Appendix) or a turbulent jet caused by semilumnar valve stenosis will alert the examiner to interrogate the region of interest with conventional pulsed Doppler. Finally, the use of color Doppler enables the examiner to quickly identify the direction of flow and to select the optimal angle to measure flow velocity.

Technical Considerations

A number of important technical considerations are associated with the use of color Doppler in the human fetus. The low pulse repetition frequency, as well as the need for sampling at a relatively great depth, leads to frequency aliasing at low flow velocities. Sampling at greater depths, coupled with the small volume flows encountered in the fetus, may lead to low signal amplitude owing to reduced intensity of the backscattered ultrasonic pulses. Currently available color Doppler systems have relatively poor resolution because of the relatively low carrier frequencies employed, and relatively poor temporal resolution owing to the slow frame rates required for color Doppler signal processing. Because Doppler signal amplitude is greatest along the axis of flow, the optimal imaging plane for color Doppler sampling is often at right angles to the optimal imaging plane for two-dimensional echocardiography.

Clinical Application

Because standard image orientation is often not possible in the fetus, the usual color patterns of intracardiac flow cannot be seen in a high percentage of cases. The color of the Doppler flow signal depends on the orientation of the heart with respect to the scanhead (transducer). For example, when recorded from an apical position in the four-chamber plane in a normal fetus, atrioventricular valve flow appears as a red jet in diastole. However, it is depicted in blue if the four-chamber view is recorded from base to apex (Fig. 15A.31, Appendix). The blue jet of semilunar valvular regurgitation can be identified in the apical four-chamber plane or in a modified long-axis image recorded from the apex. The enhanced recognition of atrioventricular valvular insufficiency may aid in the early diagnosis of congestive heart failure in the fetus. Increasing severity of fetal tricuspid insufficiency correlates with increasing severity of fetal congestive heart failure progressing to hydrops (Fig. 15A.32, Appendix).

In the modified long-axis projection, flow in the great arteries

Fig. 15A.30 FACTORS LIMITING DOPPLER ECHOCARDIOGRAPHIC EXAMINATION

Depth of structures
- Requires higher energy to penetrate
- Results in poor signal-to-noise ratio and frequency aliasing
- Decreased accuracy of diameter measurement for flow calculation

Fetal position and movement
- Limit alignment with flow
- May not allow interrogation of all valves

Fig. 15A.30 Technical factors limiting Doppler echocardiographic examination of the fetus.

appears as a region of contrasting colors, with flow in the pulmonary trunk and ductus arteriosus encoded in blue (ie, away from the transducer) and flow in the ascending aorta encoded in red (ie, towards the transducer). The ductal sample may exhibit aliasing owing to the relatively high velocity of ductal flow in the fetus.

Right to left flow across the foramen ovale is usually easily demonstrated in the normal fetus (Fig. 15A.33, Appendix). Left to right flow implies a severe degree of inflow obstruction at the level of the mitral valve secondary to mitral atresia (hypoplastic left heart syndrome) or mitral stenosis. Streaming of inferior vena caval flow to the left atrium and of superior vena cava flow to the right atrium can be demonstrated in some normal fetuses. The characteristic spiral course of the umbilical vessels with alternating red and blue color is beautifully depicted by color Doppler.

With further refinements in technology, it can be anticipated that color Doppler will play an increasing role in fetal cardiac diagnosis.

RISKS AND BENEFITS OF FETAL ECHOCARDIOGRAPHY

RISK FACTORS

Although fetal echocardiography is associated with a theoretical hazard of fetal injury, the magnitude of the risk has not been established. It can be assumed that any adverse effects on fetal tissues are related to the amount of ultrasonic energy absorbed by the target tissue. Very many factors affect the amount of ultrasonic energy delivered to and absorbed by fetal tissues (Fig. 15A.34). Of these, the major potential determinant of adverse fetal effects is the relatively high frequency [2 to 10 cycles per second (mHz)] used for fetal echocardiography. The duration and pattern of exposure (eg, pulsed versus continuous) has a major impact on the total amount of ultrasonic energy delivered to fetal tissues. With pulsed ultrasound, the duration of the exposure varies with the pulse repetition frequency (repetition rate) and the duration of the exposure. Thus, the tissue effects at a given carrier frequency are greatest with continuous ultrasound exposure and least with pulsed exposures of short duration at a low repetition rate. Because adverse tissue effects are proportional to the amount of ultrasonic energy absorbed, they decrease with increasing distance from the transducer. The amount of transmitted ultrasonic energy is also affected by the characteristics of the maternal and fetal tissues interposed between the transducer and the target tissue. Finally, various biologic events induced by the ultrasonic exposure modify the tissue effects in the fetus.

PATHOGENESIS OF TISSUE INJURY

Ultrasonic exposure may damage fetal tissue in a number of ways. When ultrasonic energy is absorbed by tissue, heat is generated, the amount of which is inversely related to the distance from the transducer (ie, depth of the target tissue). The degree of local heating is related to the rate of heat removal in the target tissue, which in turn is a function of blood flow and the interval between ultrasonic pulses (or, in the case of continuous Doppler, exposure periods); the extent of tissue injury depends on the temperature threshold for cell damage. Another mechanism of tissue injury is the formation of gas bubbles (cavitation). The extent to which cavitation occurs is largely determined by the frequency (greater at higher frequencies) and duration of the exposure. Both local heating and cavitation can lead to cell death.

RECOMMENDATIONS

Assessing the risk to the fetus is no simple task, since the potential hazards vary with both technical factors (eg, type of instrumentation, operating mode, type of examination performed, duration of exposure) and biologic factors (eg, fetal and maternal size, presence of fetal edema, amount of amniotic fluid). However, threshold intensity levels have been established at which there is no measurable risk to the fetus even with continuous exposure. In general, higher threshold intensities are tolerated with pulsed ultrasound. There appears to be little risk to the fetus at the carrier frequencies and repetition rates used for two-dimensional and M-mode echocardiography. However, evaluation of the fetal heart by Doppler echocardiography entails a higher fetal energy exposure than conventional imaging because of the higher repetition rates utilized by Doppler imaging. Therefore, fetal exposure during Doppler echocardiography may exceed current federal guidelines, which state that the spatial peak temporal average may not exceed 100 mW/cm^2.

Although it is difficult to estimate fetal exposure, the risk can be minimized by keeping the duration of the echocardiographic examination as short as possible and using the lowest possible energy output [decibels (Db)]. Doppler should be employed

Fig. 15A.34 FACTORS DETERMINING MAGNITUDE OF FETAL TISSUE EFFECTS IN OBSTETRIC ULTRASONOGRAPHY AND FETAL ECHOCARDIOGRAPHY.

Technical Factors	Biologic Factors
Energy level (decibels)	Maternal and fetal tissue characteristics
Ultrasonic frequency (2 to 10 mHz)	Maternal size
Duration and pattern of exposure (continuous versus pulsed)	Maternal obesity
With pulsed ultrasound:	Fetal size
Pulse repetition frequency	Fetal edema
Duration of exposure	Amount of amniotic fluid
Distance of target tissue from transducer	Biologic effects induced by ultrasonic energy

Fig. 15A.34 Factors determining magnitude of fetal tissue effects in obstetric ultrasonography and fetal echocardiography.

only when there is a clear clinical indication—never as a screening method. Continuous wave Doppler should never be employed when pulsed Doppler will yield equivalent information. When repeated echocardiographic examinations are required, Doppler should only be used to evaluate a potentially life-threatening abnormality. Direct Doppler sampling should be confined to the heart, great arteries, and umbilical vessels, strictly avoiding the central nervous system, eyes, and gonads.

Judiciously utilized and carefully performed, the benefits of fetal echocardiography far outweigh the risks. It is difficult to quantitate the positive psychological (and perhaps physical) benefit of excluding a serious fetal cardiac defect when there is a history of congenital heart disease in a sibling or parent. If a significant structural defect or arrhythmia is detected, the obstetrician should discuss the natural history of the condition (both before and after birth) with the parents, and present the available options for medical and surgical treatment. Unfortunately, because the natural history of some defects detected in utero is not clear, the ultimate severity may be over- or underestimated. This is particularly likely when more than one malformation is present (eg, tetralogy of Fallot associated with atrioventricular canal).

The medical and surgical management of many types of congenital heart disease is continuously evolving. An exciting prospect on the imminent horizon is that it may soon be possible to treat certain potentially lethal defects (eg, hypoplastic left heart syndrome, pulmonary atresia with intact ventricular septum) in utero. An important benefit of antenatal diagnosis is that arrangements can be made to deliver a baby at a medical center equipped to care for critically ill infants with congenital heart disease. For example, administration of prostaglandin E_1 before ductal closure may be lifesaving in a neonate with severe right or left ventricular outflow obstruction. Prenatal fetal assessment may sometimes reveal a lethal cardiac malformation, or it may detect a potentially treatable cardiac malformation in a fetus with a malformation complex or a genetic disorder likely to lead to early postnatal death (trisomy 13, trisomy 18) or survival with severe disabilities (trisomy 21, VACTERL syndrome). The decision to terminate pregnancy is ultimately an ethical and moral one: it calls for an assessment of life expectancy and quality of life if the fetus should survive, and should be considered only after all of the options have been thoroughly explored with the parents.

CHAPTER 16

Treatment of Congenital Heart Disease by Surgery and Catheter Techniques

INTRODUCTION

The era of surgical treatment of congenital heart disease began in 1938, when Gross ligated a patent ductus arteriosus. He later performed the first successful operation for coarctation of the aorta, in 1944. Extracardiac palliative procedures were introduced soon thereafter: pulmonary artery to subclavian artery shunt (Blalock and Taussig) in 1945, and pulmonary artery banding in 1952. The first intracardiac operation, pulmonary valvotomy, was performed by Brock in 1949 under inflow occlusion. The intensive surgical attack on congenital heart disease began in 1954 with the introduction of extracorporeal circulation (cardiopulmonary bypass) by Lillehei and his colleagues. The 1970s saw the introduction of conduits. During the same decade, the techniques of intracardiac surgery were refined and used in younger patients; the concept of primary repair of a variety of defects evolved concomitantly. By the early 1980s, cardiac surgeons had devised theoretically feasible operations for all but a handful of congenital malformations. The 1980s also saw the introduction of transcutaneous interventional techniques for treatment of pulmonic stenosis, aortic stenosis, coarctation of the aorta, and patent ductus arteriosus.

Early statistics indicate that approximately half of all patients with congenital heart disease died before reaching adulthood, with most deaths occurring in infancy. Until quite recently, almost all cardiac surgery was performed in the select few who survived infancy. In recent years, the thrust of invasive cardiology and cardiac surgery has clearly shifted towards definitive treatment of neonates and infants. The first such operations were done during the 1970s; by the early 1980s, more than 6000 infants and young children per year were surviving definitive repairs in North America alone. Today, more than 70 percent of infants with symptomatic congenital heart disease survive beyond their first birthday—a remarkable advance in only a few years. The great majority are enjoying a normal childhood and adolescence and can look forward to a productive life.

PALLIATIVE SURGERY

Three main types of palliative procedures are available: procedures that increase blood flow through the pulmonary circulation (eg, by connecting a systemic artery to the pulmonary artery or by connecting systemic veins with the pulmonary artery); procedures that permit intracardiac mixing of blood (eg, atrial septostomy, enlargement of a ventricular septal defect); and procedures that decrease pulmonary blood flow (ie, pulmonary artery banding).

SYSTEMIC TO PULMONARY SHUNTS

SUBCLAVIAN TO PULMONARY ARTERY (BLALOCK–TAUSSIG) ANASTOMOSIS

The first palliative shunt was the Blalock–Taussig subclavian artery–pulmonary artery anastomosis, introduced in 1945. This procedure was used to provide increased pulmonary blood flow in patients with pulmonary atresia, severe pulmonic stenosis, and tetralogy of Fallot. In the classical operation, the thoracotomy is performed on the side opposite the aortic arch. The right or left subclavian artery is sectioned, and the proximal segment is turned down and anastomosed to the ipsilateral pulmonary artery in the end to side fashion (Fig. 16.1). Postoperatively, the upper extremity is supplied by branches of the external carotid, intercostal, and mediastinal arteries (which connect with the distal segment of the subclavian artery). Shortening of the ipsilateral arm is a potential complication if the operation is performed at an early age. In a modification of the classical operation, introduced in 1980, the subclavian artery is not sacrificed; instead, a prosthetic (Goretex) tube is interposed between the subclavian and pulmonary arteries (Fig. 16.1). The modified Blalock–Taussig anastomosis is usually performed on the same side as the aortic arch.

The immediate hemodynamic effects of a functioning Blalock–Taussig shunt are increased heart rate and pulmonary blood

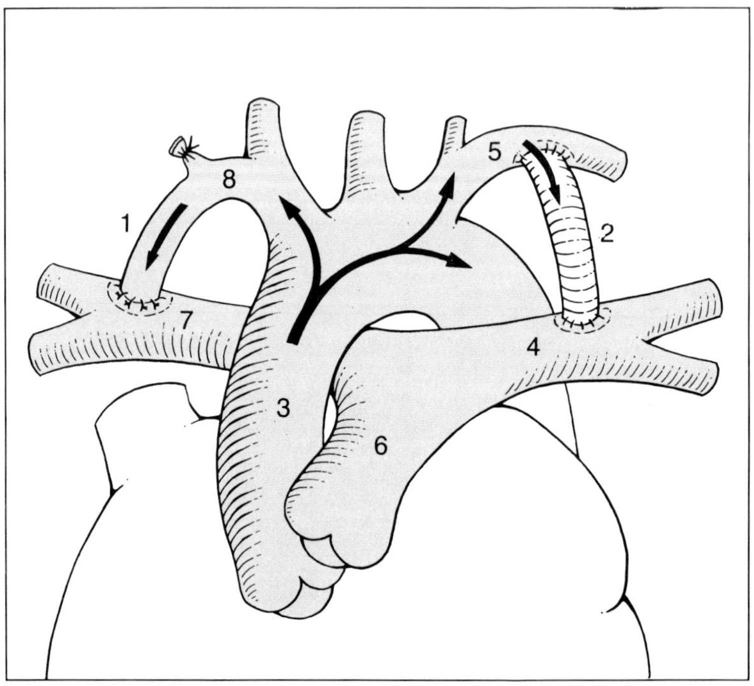

Fig. 16.1 Blalock–Taussig anastomosis. In the classical Blalock–Taussig anastomosis, shown on patient's right, the subclavian and pulmonary arteries are directly connected. The distal subclavian artery is severed from the aortic arch. In the widely used modification shown on patient's left, the left subclavian and left pulmonary arteries are connected via a prosthetic (Goretex) conduit. The distal subclavian artery remains in continuity with the aortic arch.

1 conventional Blalock–Taussig anastomosis
2 modified Blalock–Taussig anastomosis (prosthetic conduit)
3 aorta
4 left pulmonary artery
5 left subclavian artery
6 pulmonary trunk
7 right pulmonary artery
8 right subclavian artery

flow; the latter is evident on chest films obtained immediately after surgery. After the classical operation there may be systemic hypotension and ischemia of the ipsilateral upper extremity owing to the surgically created fistula between the systemic and pulmonary circulations. Late sequelae include dilatation of the recipient pulmonary artery, which may reach enormous size, and left atrial enlargement. Occlusion or stenosis of the anastomosis (caused by kinking of the subclavian artery proximal to the anastomosis or narrowing of the anastomosis itself) renders the shunt useless. Another potential complication is thrombosis of the artery to the ipsilateral upper lobe. Shunt obstruction can be seen by angiography (Fig. 16.2) or MRI (Fig. 16.3).

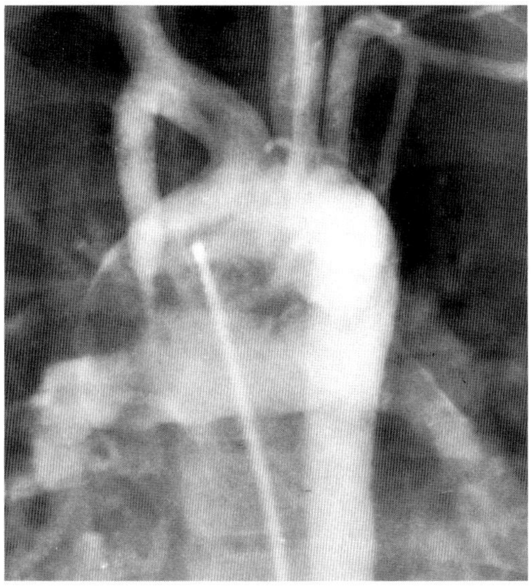

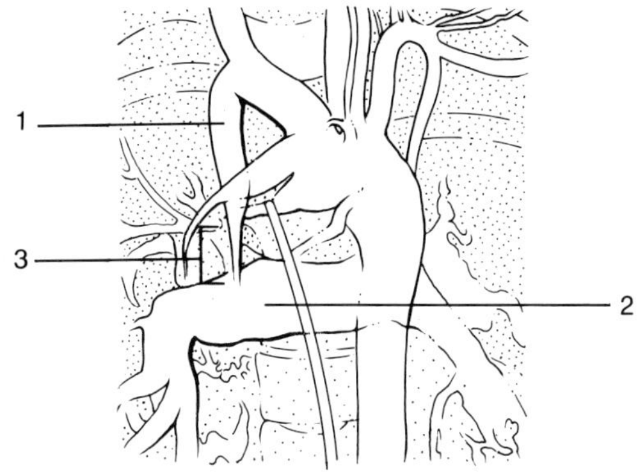

1	right subclavian artery	3	stenotic segment
2	right pulmonary artery		

Fig. 16.2 Stenosis of Blalock–Taussig anastomosis. Frontal projection of thoracic aortogram shows a long stenotic segment just proximal to the anastomosis between the right subclavian and right pulmonary arteries.

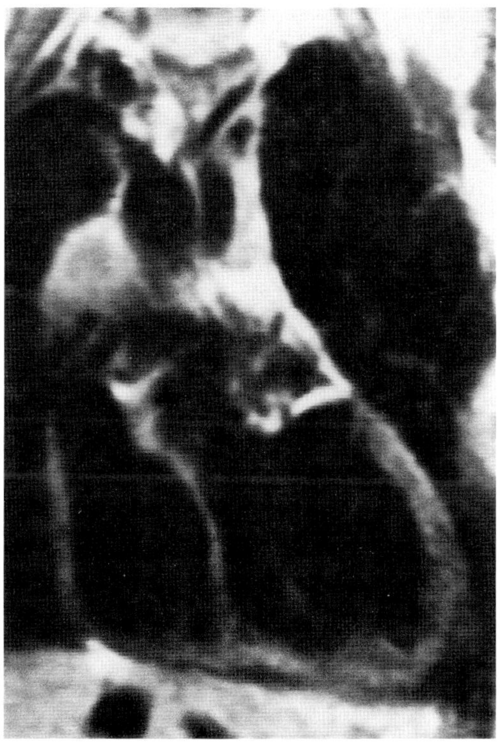

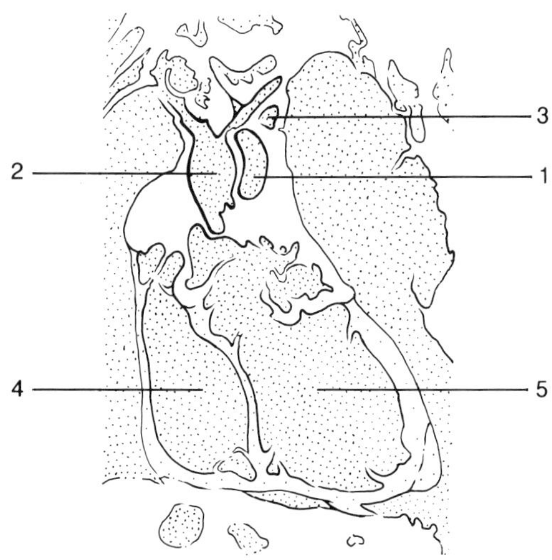

1	Prosthetic conduit between left pulmonary and left subclavian arteries	2	aorta
		3	left subclavian artery
		4	right atrium
		5	left ventricle

Fig. 16.3 Demonstration of Blalock–Taussig anastomosis by MRI. Coronal spin–echo image patient with tetralogy of Fallot shows a channel which represents the prosthetic conduit, to the left of the aorta. The conduit is anastomosed superiorly to the left subclavian artery and inferiorly to the left pulmonary artery. (The latter connection was shown to be patent on other images.)

DESCENDING AORTA TO PULMONARY ARTERY (POTT'S) ANASTOMOSIS

In this operation, used to increase pulmonary blood flow in malformations associated with decreased pulmonary perfusion, a window is made between the descending thoracic aorta and the left pulmonary artery (Figs. 16.4 and 16.5). Because it is difficult to regulate the volume of the resultant left to right shunt, marked flooding of the lungs may occur, culminating in increased pulmonary resistance. Chest films and angiograms of patients with this complication reveal marked enlargement of the left pulmonary artery (Fig. 16.6). Because of the problems associated with the Pott's anastomosis, this procedure is now only rarely employed.

ASCENDING AORTA TO PULMONARY ARTERY (WATERSTON) SHUNT

In this operation, which is also employed in patients with poor pulmonary perfusion, a window is made between the posterior aspect of the ascending aorta and the ipsilateral (usually the right) pulmonary artery (Figs. 16.7 and 16.8). As with the Pott's anastomosis, the volume of flow through the shunt is difficult to regulate, which may result in marked pulmonary overcirculation and dilatation of the ipsilateral pulmonary artery, eventually leading to increased pulmonary resistance (see Fig. 16.6). Hemorrhagic pulmonary edema of the ipsilateral lung (sometimes limited to the upper lobe) is not uncommon in the early postoperative period. This complication, believed to result

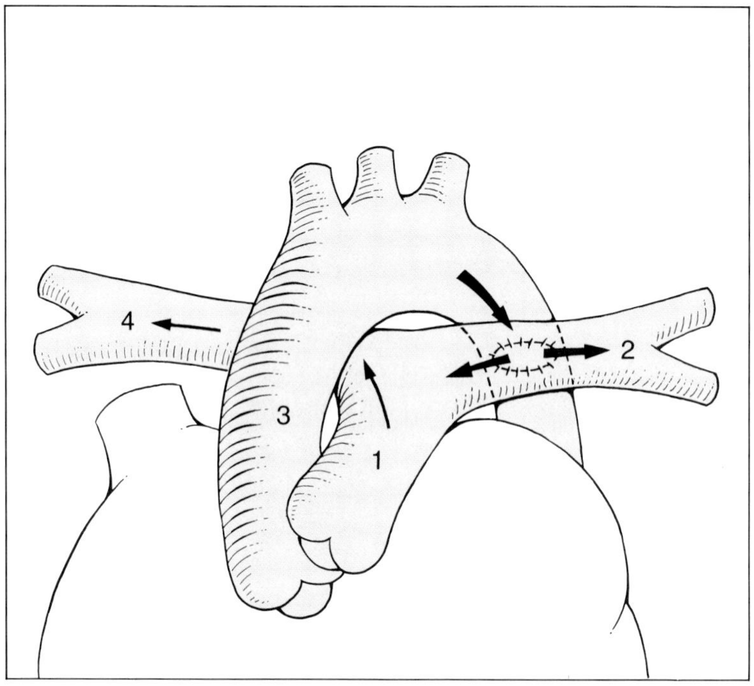

Fig. 16.4 Pott's anastomosis. The left pulmonary artery is connected to the descending thoracic aorta.

1	pulmonary trunk	3	aorta
2	left pulmonary artery	4	right pulmonary artery

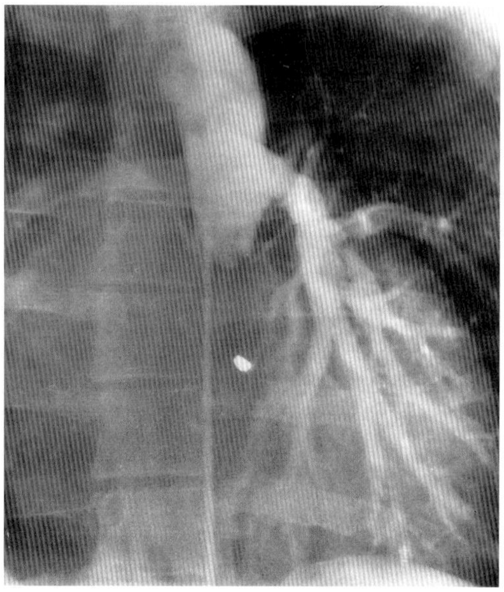

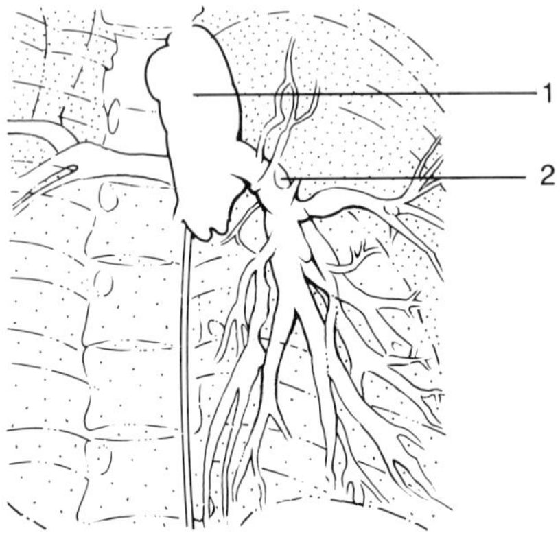

Fig. 16.5 Pott's anastomosis. Frontal projection of thoracic aortogram demonstrates a large-volume shunt through a wide anastomosis between the descending thoracic aorta and the left pulmonary artery.

1	descending thoracic aorta	2	left pulmonary artery

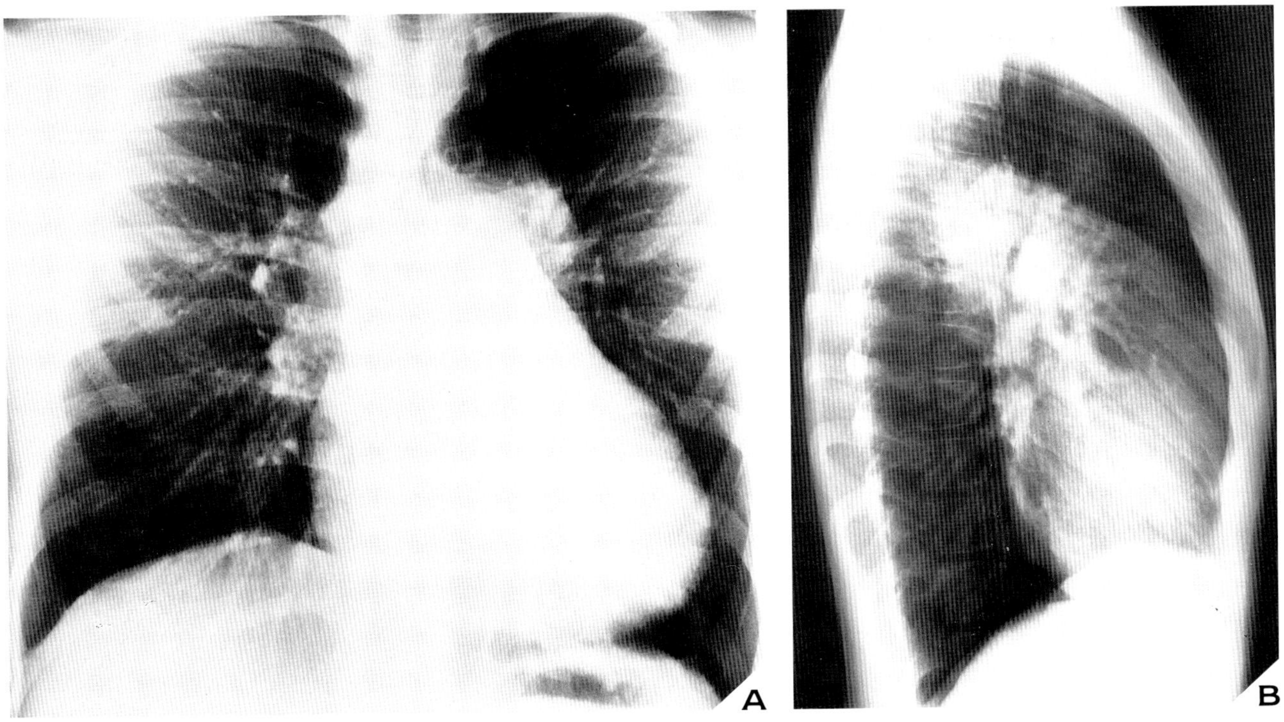

Fig. 16.6 Pulmonary arterial hypertension after a Pott's anastomosis. (A) Frontal and (B) lateral chest films show cardiomegaly with right ventricular enlargement. The main pulmonary arteries are markedly enlarged, the left more so than the right. The peripheral lung fields are poorly perfused.

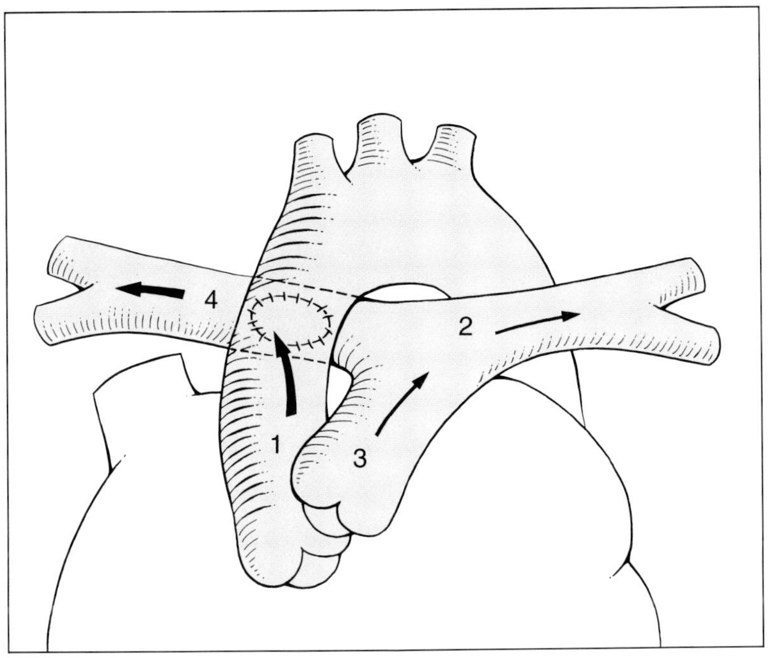

Fig. 16.7 Waterston anastomosis. The right pulmonary artery is connected to the ascending aorta.

1	ascending aorta	3	pulmonary trunk
2	left pulmonary artery	4	right pulmonary artery

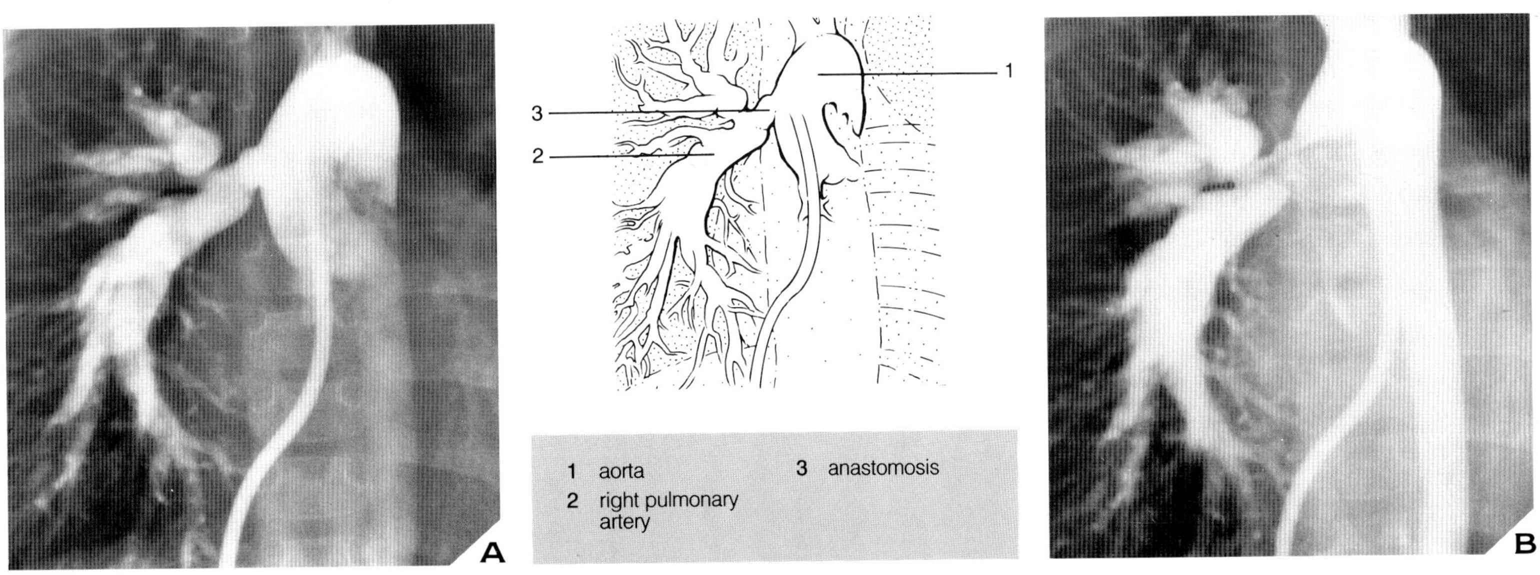

1	aorta	3	anastomosis
2	right pulmonary artery		

Fig. 16.8 Waterston anastomosis. (A, B) Sequential frames of thoracic aortogram (frontal projection) show the anastomosis between the right pulmonary artery and the ascending aorta.

from the sudden increase of blood flow in the abnormal pulmonary vascular bed, is accompanied by hypoxia and clinical deterioration. Immediate surgery is usually necessary to decrease the size of the anastomosis (this can sometimes be accomplished by transcutaneous catheter techniques). Because of the frequent late sequelae of the Waterston shunt, it is seldom employed nowadays.

CENTRAL SYSTEMIC TO PULMONARY ARTERY (REDO–AKER) ANASTOMOSIS

Introduced by Redo and Aker in 1963, this procedure connects the aorta and pulmonary trunk by means of a prosthetic (Gore-tex) conduit (Fig. 16.9). This anastomosis makes it possible to regulate the magnitude of the left to right shunt more precisely than with the Pott's and Waterston anastomoses, which connect aorta and pulmonary arteries directly.

SUPERIOR VENA CAVA TO PULMONARY ARTERY (GLENN) ANASTOMOSIS

In this operation, introduced by Glenn in 1954, a surgical connection is made between the superior vena cava (SVC) and the right pulmonary artery. The right pulmonary artery is divided centrally and its distal portion is anastomosed to the right posterior aspect of the SVC, close to the orifice of the azygos vein. The SVC is then ligated and divided close to the right atrium, directing the caval blood flow into the right pulmonary artery (Fig. 16.10). Unlike systemic artery to pulmonary artery anastomoses, the flow through a Glenn anastomosis is nonpulsatile. Postoperatively, the pulmonary blood flow is mainly distributed to the lower zones, with relatively poor perfusion of the mid and upper zones (Fig. 16.11). The Glenn anastomosis is used mainly in patients with tricuspid atresia, and occasionally in other malformations associated with poor pulmonary perfu-

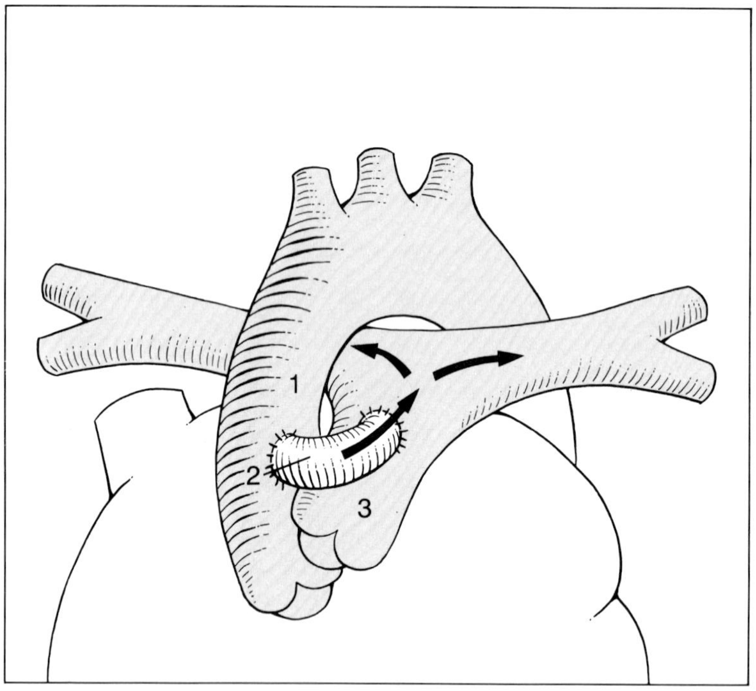

1 aorta
2 prosthetic tube
3 pulmonary trunk

Fig. 16.9 Central systemic to pulmonary artery (Redo–Aker) anastomosis. The ascending aorta is connected to the pulmonary trunk via a prosthetic tube.

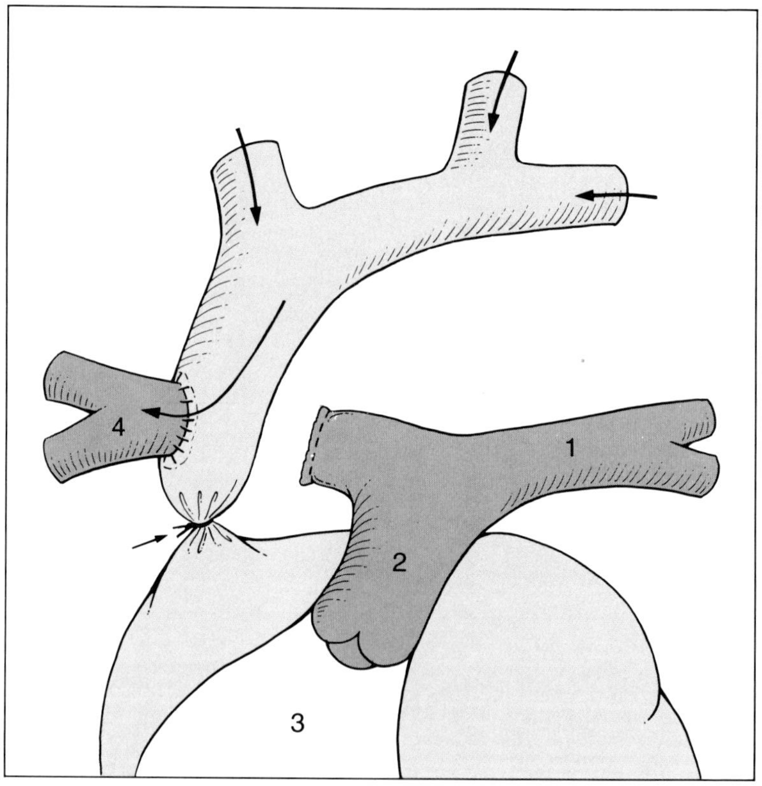

1 left pulmonary artery
2 pulmonary trunk
3 right atrium
4 right pulmonary artery

Fig. 16.10 Cavo–pulmonary (Glenn) anastomosis. The right pulmonary artery has been disconnected from the pulmonary trunk and anastomosed to the right side of the superior vena cava. The connection between the superior vena cava and the right atrium has been tied off (*arrow*). Therefore, blood returning from the upper part of the body flows into the right pulmonary artery.

sion (eg, univentricular atrioventricular connection with pulmonic stenosis).

PALLIATIVE INTRACARDIAC PROCEDURES

ATRIAL SEPTOSTOMY

The surgical creation of an atrial septal defect (ASD) was introduced by Blalock and Hanson in 1948 as a palliative treatment for transposition of the great arteries (TGA). This procedure, in which a portion of the atrial septum is resected, results in bidirectional blood flow at the atrial level, thereby increasing peripheral saturation. It has been life-saving in patients with TGA with an intact ventricular septum, tricuspid atresia with a restricted ASD, and other complex malformations. At present, palliative atrial septostomy is usually performed in the cardiac catheterization suite by means of a balloon catheter (Rashkind procedure). In this technique, introduced in 1964, the catheter is passed into the right atrium and advanced across the foramen ovale into the left atrium. The balloon is then inflated and the catheter pulled back into the right atrium, creating an ASD (Fig. 16.12). The Rashkind technique can also be used to enlarge a restricted ASD, although it is likely to be unsuccessful in patients with a thick atrial septum. More recently, transcutaneous knife

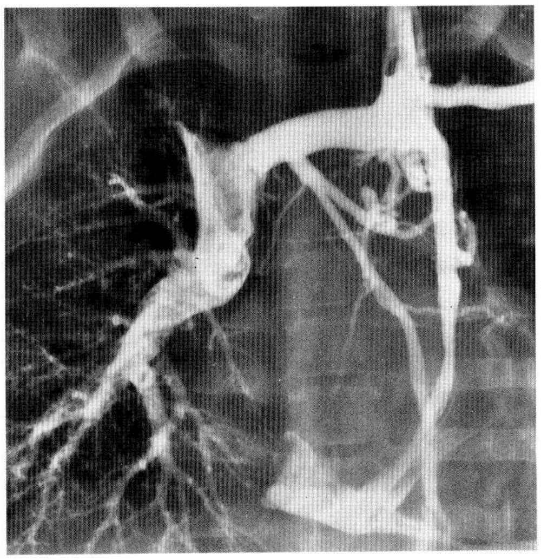

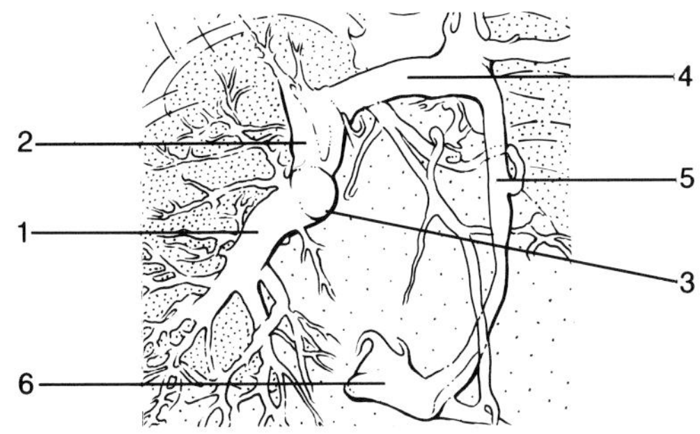

1	right pulmonary artery	4	left innominate vein
2	superior vena cava	5	collaterals
3	anastomosis	6	coronary sinus

Fig. 16.11 Glenn anastomosis. There is a wide anastomosis between the superior vena cava and the right pulmonary artery. The veins originating from the left innominate vein and draining into the coronary sinus represent collaterals.

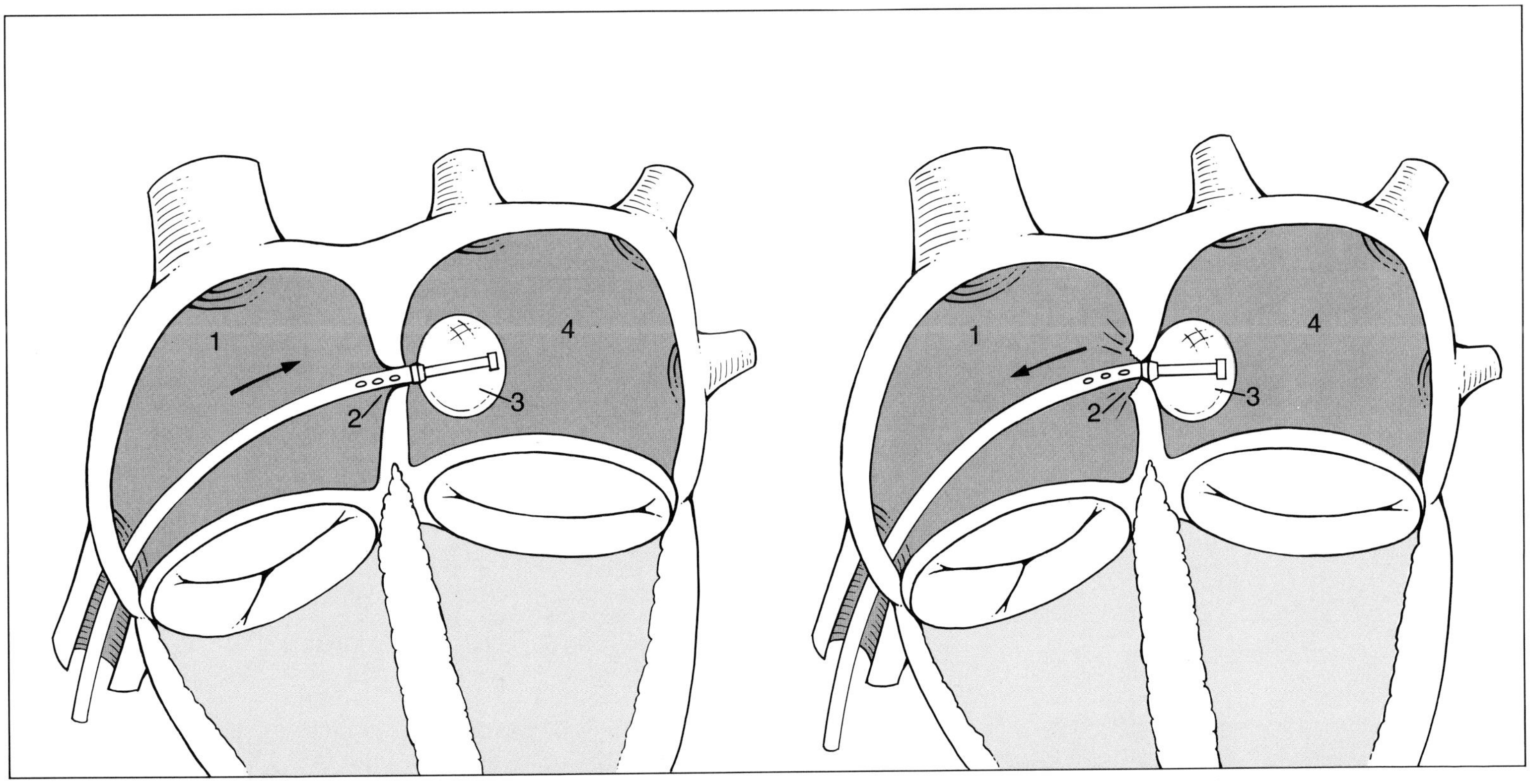

Fig. 16.12 Balloon atrial septostomy (Rashkind procedure). A balloon catheter has been introduced via the inferior vena cava into the right atrium and passed through the patent foramen ovale into the left atrium. The balloon is then inflated and traction is applied to the catheter, rupturing the atrial septum. The iatrogenic atrial septal defect enables blood in the atrial chambers to mix.

1	right atrium	3	balloon catheter
2	foramen ovale	4	left atrium

septostomy has been employed in selected cases. In this technique, first performed by Park and colleagues in 1978, a special blade-tipped catheter, introduced via a peripheral vein, is used to resect a portion of the atrial septum.

PALLIATIVE PROCEDURES TO REDUCE PULMONARY BLOOD FLOW

PULMONARY ARTERY BANDING

When the pulmonary arterial system is flooded with an excessive volume of blood, small pulmonary arteries and arterioles may become progressively narrowed or obliterated, leading to a fixed increase in pulmonary resistance. This is most likely to occur in patients with a large, high-pressure left to right shunt (eg, a large VSD). Pulmonary artery banding was introduced in 1952 as a palliative procedure to prevent this complication, which precludes corrective surgery. In this technique, umbilical tape or other material is placed around the pulmonary trunk and tightened until the distal pulmonary artery pressure has been reduced to one third or one half the systemic pressure. The band is then sutured in place (Figs. 16.13 and 16.14), to be removed later at the time of the definitive repair.

Serious complications (eg, cardiac failure, migration of the band, left ventricular outflow obstruction, shunt reversal with cyanosis) occur in as many as 50 percent of patients with pulmonary artery bands. It is now recognized that the cumulative mortality of two-stage repairs usually exceeds that of primary repair. For this reason, pulmonary artery banding is now largely restricted to infants with complex congenital defects and large left to right shunts in whom the risks associated with total correction are too great. Most infants with atrioventricular canal, once a common indication for banding, now undergo primary repair. Pulmonary artery banding is now only rarely employed for treatment of VSD. The indications are limited to patients with multiple ventricular septal defects (''Swiss cheese'' septum) and congestive heart failure, and patients with VSD and coarctation of the aorta with congestive heart failure.

CORRECTIVE SURGERY

The object of corrective surgery is to create a heart that is anatomically and physiologically normal. Even when these goals cannot be achieved, the resultant functional improvement leads to increased survival and an enhanced quality of life, both of which amply justify the effort.

CORRECTION OF TOTAL ANOMALOUS VENOUS CONNECTION

To correct total anomalous pulmonary venous connection (TAPVC), it is necessary to reattach the anomalous pulmonary veins to the left atrium (Fig. 16.15). The method varies according to the nature of the anomaly. In patients with TAPVC to the left vertical vein, the anomalous common pulmonary venous chamber is reattached to the top of the left atrium, enabling the pulmonary veins to empty into the morphologic left atrium (Fig. 16.16). This operation may be technically difficult in patients with TAPVC of the subdiaphragmatic type, in whom the left atrium may be quite distant from the common chamber; in

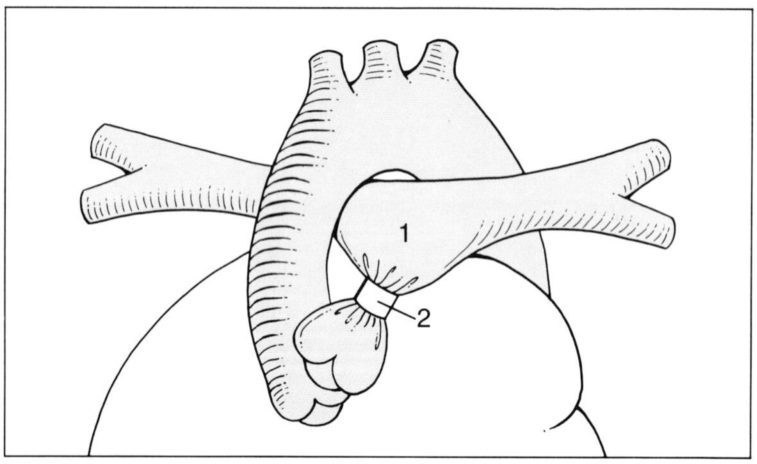

Fig. 16.13 Pulmonary artery banding. A band is placed around the pulmonary trunk, constricting the lumen and decreasing blood flow and pressure in the pulmonary arteries.

1 pulmonary trunk
2 extrinsic band

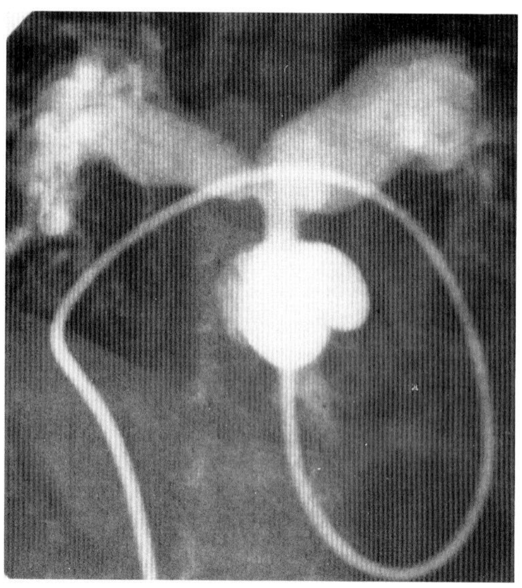

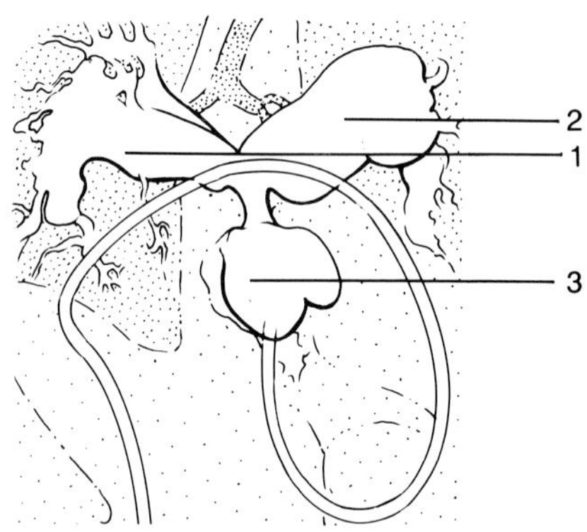

1 right pulmonary artery
2 left pulmonary artery
3 pulmonary trunk

Fig. 16.14 Pulmonary artery banding. Frontal projection of pulmonary arteriogram with cranial angulation demonstrates marked narrowing of the pulmonary trunk just above the sinuses of Valsalva. Note mild stenosis of the origin of the right pulmonary artery. The pulmonary arteries are markedly dilated.

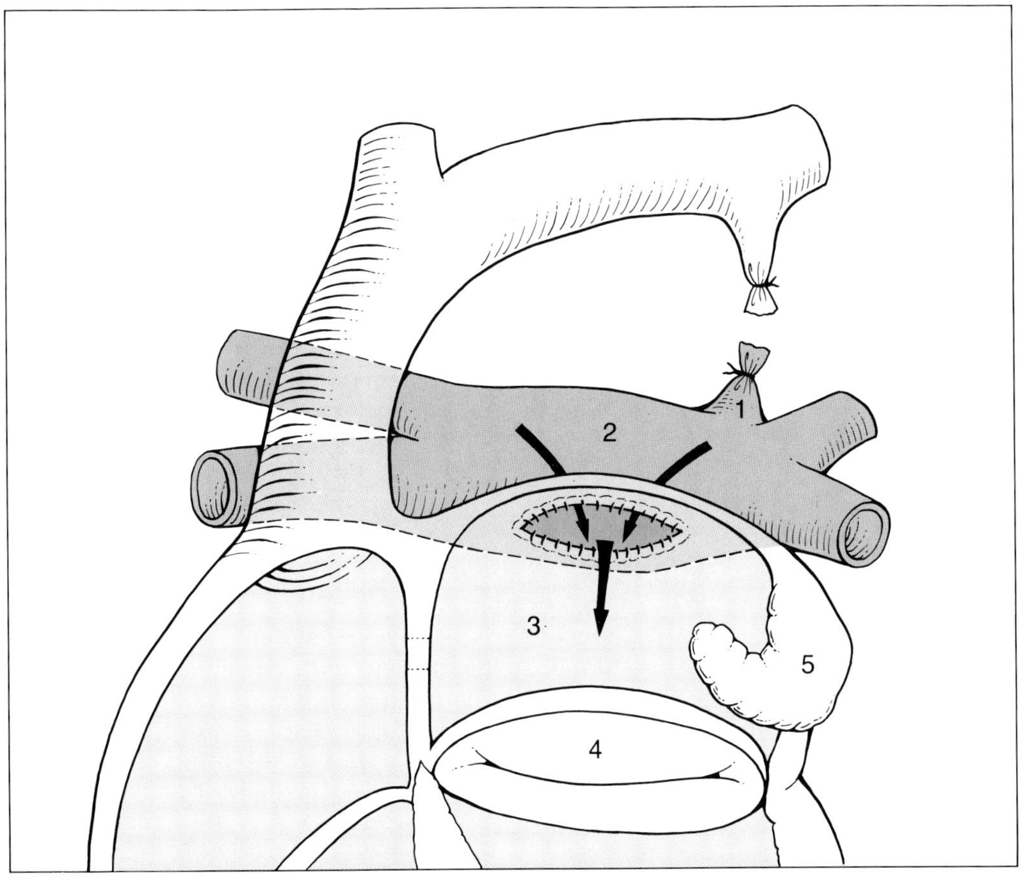

Fig. 16.15 Surgical correction of supracardiac type of total anomalous pulmonary venous connection. A wide communication has been created between the inferior wall of the common pulmonary venous chamber (which receives all the pulmonary venous return) and the superior aspect of the left atrium. The left vertical vein has been ligated.

1	left vertical vein	4	mitral valve
2	common pulmonary venous chamber	5	left atrial appendage
3	left atrium		

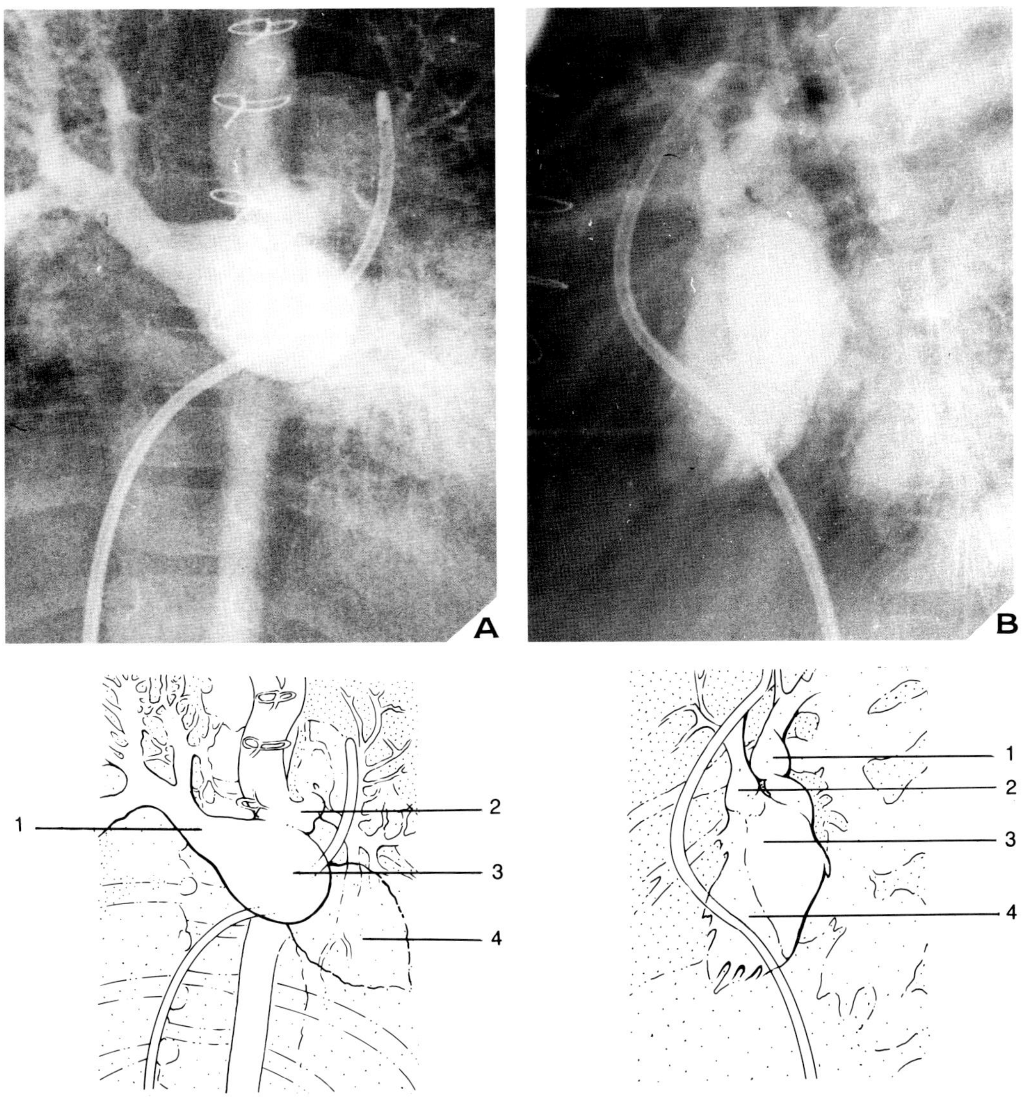

Fig. 16.16 Surgical correction of total anomalous pulmonary venous connection (supracardiac type). (A) Frontal and (B) lateral projections of levophase of pulmonary arteriogram shows that the pulmonary veins are now connected properly to the left atrium. The opacified pulmonary venous blood passes into the left ventricle and aorta in normal fashion.

1	right upper pulmonary vein	3	left atrium
2	left upper pulmonary vein	4	left ventricle

these patients the connection is made between the pulmonary veins and the left atrium (sometimes to the left atrial appendage). In patients with TAPVC to the right atrium, the anomalous pulmonary veins are reattached to the left atrium, either directly or indirectly (ie, by tunneling through the right atrium). To correct TAPVC via the coronary sinus, a large opening is made in the roof of the coronary sinus, after which the opening of the coronary sinus into the right atrium is sealed (Fig. 16.17).

To repair total anomalous systemic venous connection, the surgeon reattaches the abnormally draining systemic vein to the right atrium.

CORRECTION OF SEPTAL DEFECTS

Depending on the nature of the defect, ASD and VSD can be repaired either by suturing the defect or by insertion of a patch. The latter may be constructed of prosthetic material (eg, teflon) or pericardium.

ATRIAL SEPTAL DEFECT REPAIR

Patients with ASD typically present in adolescence or adulthood with congestive heart failure; fewer than 5% present with pulmonary arterial hypertension (Eisenmenger syndrome). Early repair of the defect avoids progression to pulmonary arterial hypertension. Surgery is usually performed as soon as the diagnosis is made.

Although repair of ostium secundum ASD is usually uncomplicated, other types of ASD occasionally present problems for the surgeon. In repairing a sinus venosus ASD, the patch is placed very close to the sinoatrial (SA) node, which may result in a "sick sinus" syndrome. Repair of a coronary sinus ASD (which actually represents a defect in the roof of the coronary sinus) can be done in either of two ways. When the coronary sinus is not connected to the left superior vena cava, the repair consists of closing the natural connection between the coronary sinus and the right atrium (some surgeons use pericardium or a patch for this purpose). In patients with a persistent left superior vena cava without a bridging vein, it is necessary to reconstruct the coronary sinus. In this technique, performed via a right or left atriotomy, the surgeon applies a patch over the roof of the coronary sinus. Ligating the left superior vena cava, which leaves an insignificant left to right shunt, is sufficient in cases with a patent bridging vein.

Because the sutures can interrupt the conducting system, arrhythmias are a potential complication of ASD repair. The atrioventricular node is at risk in patients with ostium primum ASD, owing to its location along the margin of the septal defect.

VENTRICULAR SEPTAL DEFECT REPAIR

Complications of VSD closure include arrhythmias (atrioventricular block and right bundle branch block) caused by damage to the conducting system, which runs close to the margins of the defect, and a residual shunt resulting from incomplete closure of the defect or breakdown of the repair. The latter can be demonstrated by echocardiography or angiocardiography (Fig. 16.18). Rarely, the surgeon may inadvertently suture a papillary muscle or tricuspid leaflet to the patch, resulting in tricuspid regurgitation. The most significant complication related to the patch itself is hemolysis, which is usually caused by patch failure. Complications of right ventriculotomy include aneurysm formation at the venticulotomy site and damage to the ventricular branches of the coronary arteries. (Cardiac aneurysms are readily diagnosed by echocardiography.) To avoid the risks associated with right ventriculotomy, many surgeons prefer to repair the VSD via a right atriotomy.

Multiple muscular VSDs ("Swiss cheese septum") are approached via a right ventriculotomy or right atriotomy. (In the past such defects were frequently repaired through a left ventri-

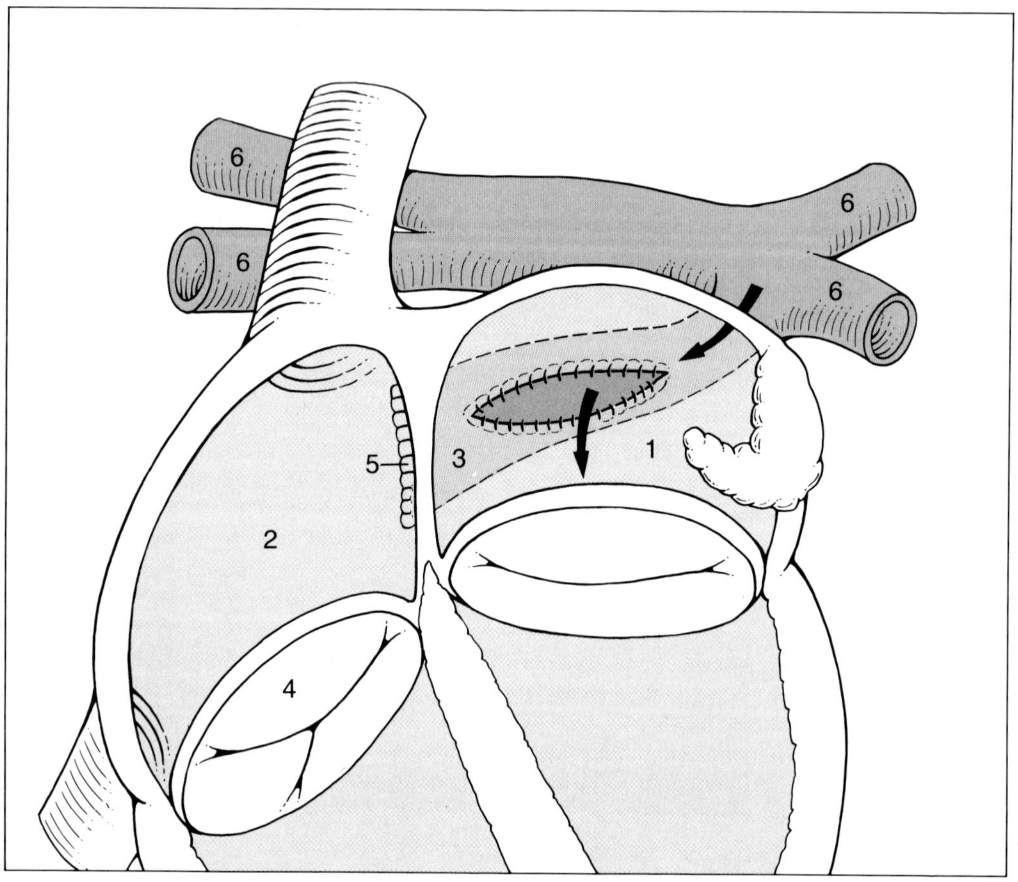

Fig. 16.17 Surgical repair of total anomalous pulmonary venous connection to coronary sinus and right atrium. The enlarged coronary sinus is connected to the left atrium by its atrial wall, after which the natural connection between the coronary sinus and the right atrium is sealed off. All the pulmonary venous return now flows into the left atrium and thence into the systemic circulation.

1	left atrium	5	closed-off entrance of coronary sinus into the right atrium
2	right atrium	6	pulmonary veins
3	coronary sinus		
4	tricuspid valve		

culotomy; however, because of the frequency of severe postoperative myocardial dysfunction, this approach is no longer employed.)

The problems present before VSD closure may remain after a technically successful repair in patients who have a fixed, increased pulmonary vascular resistance (the incidence of which depends on the age at which the operation is performed). Patients with a large VSD and pulmonary arterial hypertension who have normal pulmonary vascular resistance at the time of surgery may develop a fixed, elevated pulmonary resistance later in life. Patients with increased pulmonary vascular resistance (higher than 10 units/m^2 of body surface) at the time of surgery usually die within 5 years after closure of the defect. In general, the younger the child at the time of VSD, the better the chance of long-term survival and of having normal pulmonary artery pressure and normal pulmonary resistance 5 years after surgery.

REPAIR OF ATRIOVENTRICULAR SEPTAL DEFECT ("AV CANAL")

Complete correction of a complete atrioventricular septal defect (AVSD) entails closure of the interatrial and interventricular connections and repair of the malformed atrioventricular valves (Fig. 16.19). The interatrial and interventricular communications are repaired by patching. (The surgeon must take particular care not to suture into the bundle of His, which runs along the posterior border of the defect.) Repair of the left atrioventricular (mitral) valve is indicated only when it is incompetent. Although the valve is always malformed, it has three leaflets and is usually competent; if not, it must be repaired or replaced. The right atrioventricular (tricuspid) valve is usually competent; severely malformed valves are generally incompetent and must be repaired or replaced.

As with other left to right shunts, AVSD must be corrected before the patient develops a fixed, elevated pulmonary vascular resistance. It should be emphasized that patients with AVSD do not always present as infants with cardiac failure; children or teenagers often present with increased pulmonary vascular resistance at the time of diagnosis. In such cases it may be difficult to determine preoperatively if the increase is fixed, in which event there is no satisfactory surgical treatment.

REPAIR OF EBSTEIN'S MALFORMATION

Ebstein's malformation is characterized by a markedly enlarged and incompetent tricuspid valve whose leaflets are adherent to the wall of the right ventricle. The goal of surgery is to correct the tricuspid insufficiency, making the right ventricle a

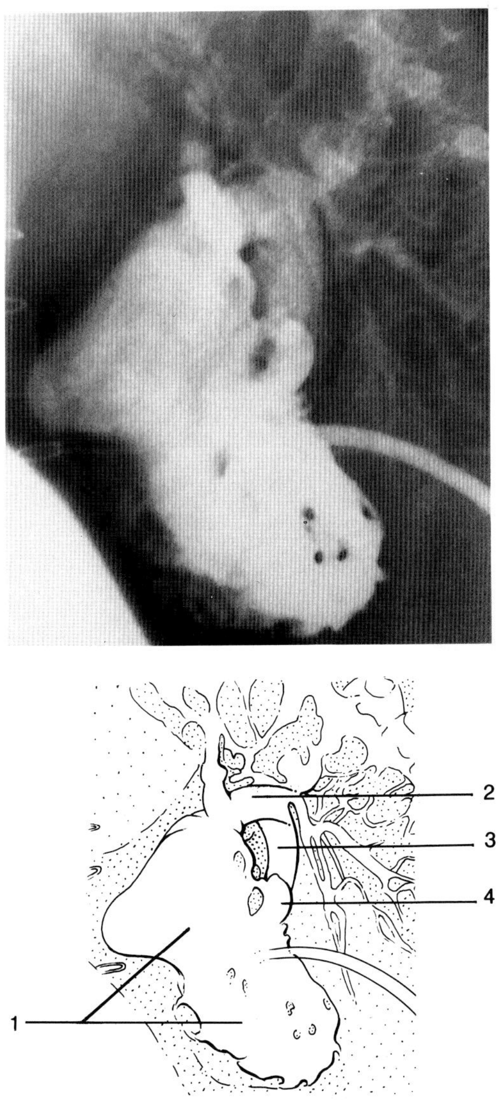

Fig. 16.18 Residual shunt after VSD repair. Lateral projection of right ventriculogram shows contrast material passing into the left ventricular outflow tract via a small ventricular septal defect.

1 right ventricle
2 pulmonary trunk
3 ascending aorta
4 residual ventricular septal defect

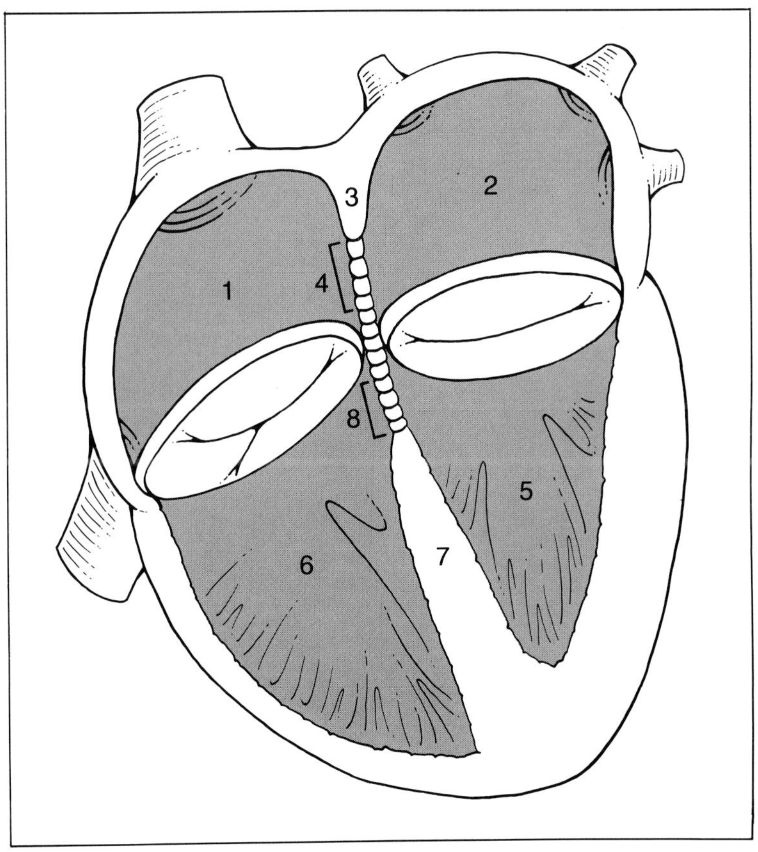

1 atrial septum
2 left atrium
3 atrial septum
4 patch closing ASD
5 left ventricle
6 right ventricle
7 ventricular septum
8 patch closing VSD

Fig. 16.19 Repair of complete form of atrioventricular septal defect ("AV canal"). A patch is applied to close the ASD, which is located just cephalad to the atrioventricular valve. Another patch is used to close the VSD, which is just caudal to the atrioventricular valves. The right and/or left atrioventricular valves are repaired if they are malfunctioning.

functional chamber. Surgical techniques include valve replacement, plication of the atrialized portion of the right ventricle, or a combination of the two. None of these surgical procedures is feasible if the right ventricular wall is severely malformed.

REPAIR OF HEARTS WITH ABSENCE OF ONE ATRIOVENTRICULAR CONNECTION OR WITH UNIVENTRICULAR ATRIOVENTRICULAR CONNECTION

In this group of malformations, the entire pumping function is provided by a single ventricle. The other ventricle is hypoplastic and has significant function only in exceptional cases. In the great majority of these patients the dominant ventricle is responsible for both the pulmonary and the systemic circulation. The most common surgical solution to this problem is to establish a connection between the systemic veins or the right atrium and the pulmonary artery, thereby relieving the overload on the dominant ventricle.

RIGHT TRICUSPID ATRESIA

In patients with right tricuspid atresia, systemic venous blood enters the right atrium, crosses the ASD, and passes into the left atrium. The Fontan procedure (1971), mainly used for treatment of this problem, involves anastomosis of the right atrial appendage to the pulmonary trunk or to the left or right pulmonary artery, anterior to the right ventricular outflow tract. In a variation of this procedure the rudimentary right ventricle is interposed between the right atrium and the pulmonary trunk. After the classical Fontan operation, systemic venous blood bypasses the rudimentary right ventricle (Fig. 16.20); pulmonary blood flow is nonpulsatile and slow, going mainly to the lower zones, and the upper zones are poorly perfused.

Many modifications of the Fontan procedure have been introduced. In Kreutzer's modification (1980), which has gained wide acceptance, the posterosuperior aspect of the right atrium is connected to the right pulmonary artery or to the bifurcation of the pulmonary trunk (Fig. 16.21). This arrangement avoids compression of the anastomosis by the anterior chest wall, a potential complication of the classical Fontan operation. Other possible complications of the Fontan operation and its variations include stenosis of the surgically created connection, occlusion of the pulmonary arteries, and pulmonary thromboembolism (Fig. 16.22).

LEFT TRICUSPID ATRESIA

When the atretic valve is on the left, the pulmonary venous return passes across the ASD from the left atrium to the right atrium, where it mixes with the systemic venous return. The mixed venous blood then passes through the right atrioventricular valve into the right-sided dominant ventricle (which may be a morphologic right or left ventricle). The pulmonary circulatory pattern depends on the nature of the ventricularterial connection. In most instances the pulmonary artery arises from the dominant ventricle, so that the lungs are perfused at systemic pressure; therefore, pulmonary vascularity is markedly increased. (Pulmonary perfusion may be normal or decreased in patients with severe pulmonic valvular or subvalvular stenosis.)

To decrease the pulmonary overcirculation, it is necessary to partition the right atrium such that the pulmonary venous return passes from the left atrium across the right atrioventricular valve into the dominant right ventricle. This is accomplished by creating a tunnel between the left atrium and the right atrioventricular valve. Outside this tunnel, the right portion of the right

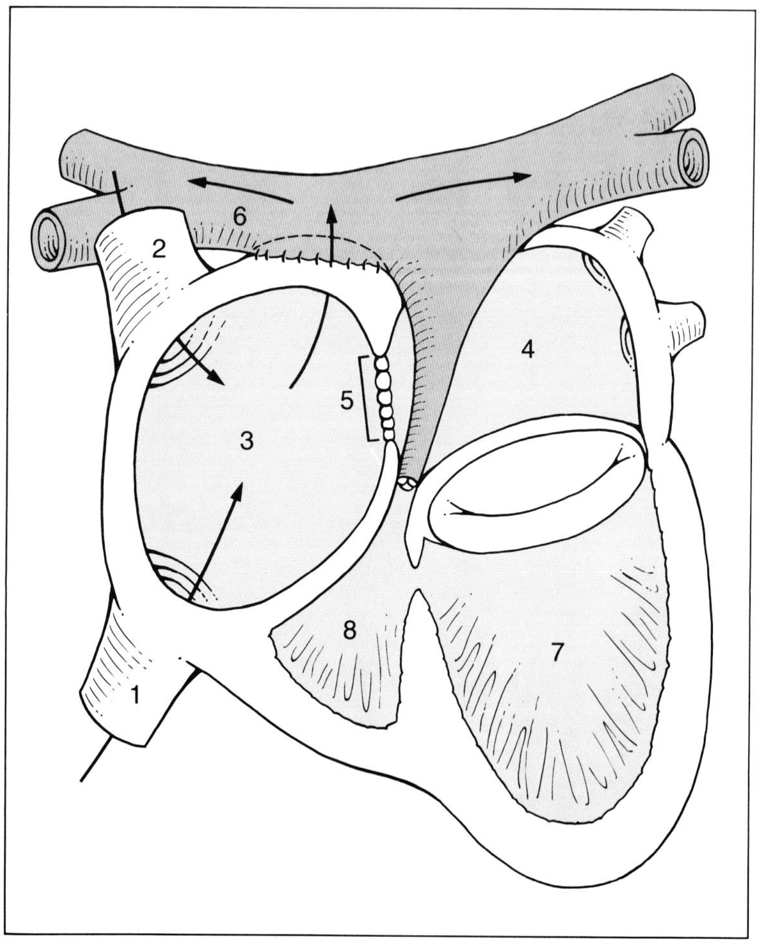

Fig. 16.20 Fontan anastomosis for tricuspid atresia. The right atrium has been anastomosed to the right pulmonary artery and the ASD has been closed. (The connection is made to the pulmonary trunk if an anastomosis with the right pulmonary artery is not feasible.) Systemic venous blood from the right atrium now flows into the pulmonary circulation, decreasing the left ventricular overload and increasing peripheral saturation.

1	inferior vena cava	5	patch closing ASD
2	superior vena cava	6	right pulmonary artery
3	right atrium	7	left ventricle
4	left atrium	8	hypoplastic right ventricle

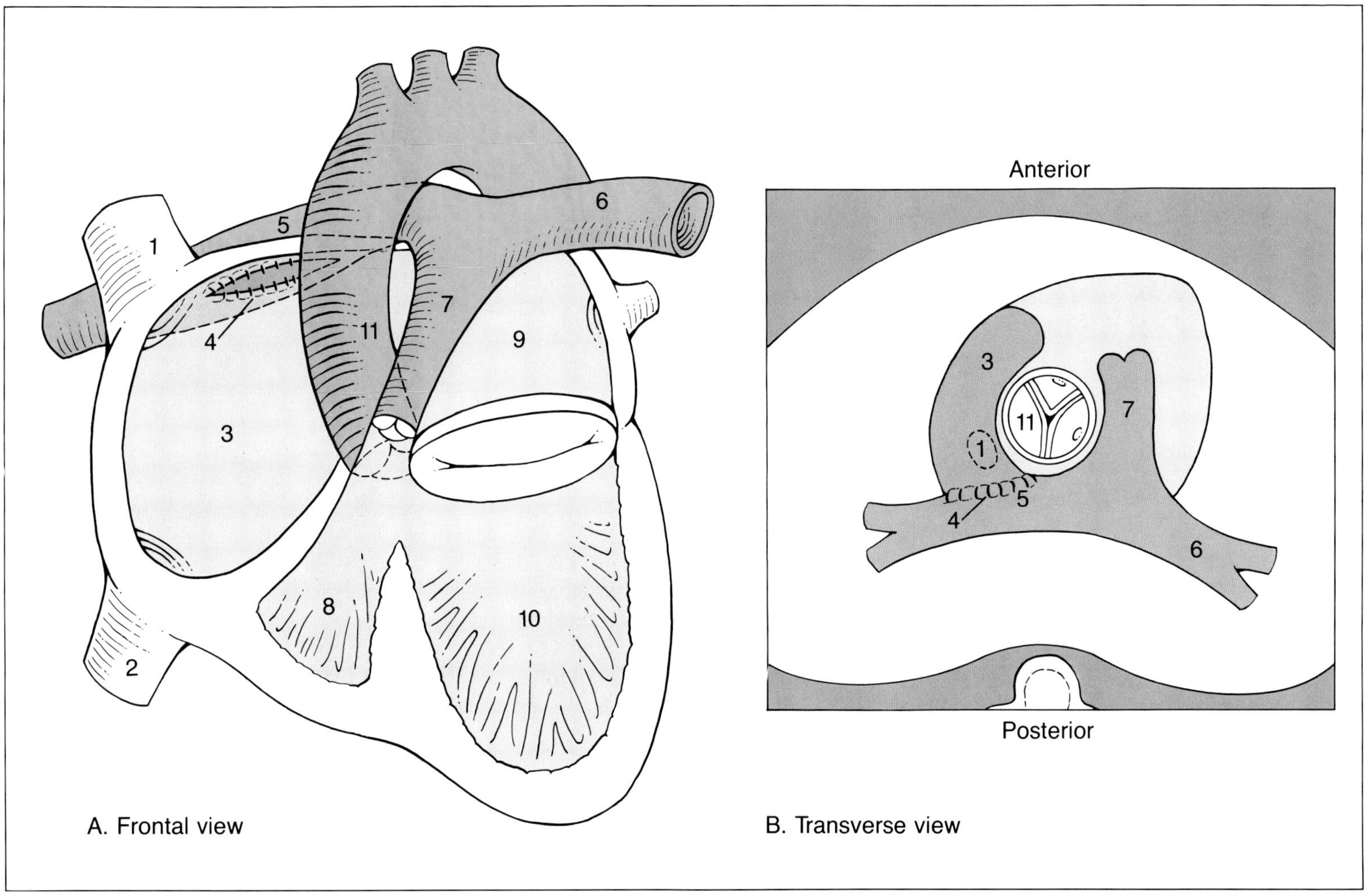

1 superior vena cava	4 Fontan anastomosis	7 pulmonary trunk	10 left ventricle
2 inferior vena cava	5 right pulmonary artery	8 right ventricle	11 aorta
3 right atrium	6 left pulmonary artery	9 left atrium	

Fig. 16.21 Kreutzer modification of Fontan operation. The anastomosis is made between the posterosuperior aspect of the right atrium and the right pulmonary artery or pulmonary trunk. Because the anastomosis is posterior to the ascending aorta, it cannot be compressed by the anterior chest wall, a theoretical limitation of the standard Fontan operation in infants and young children.

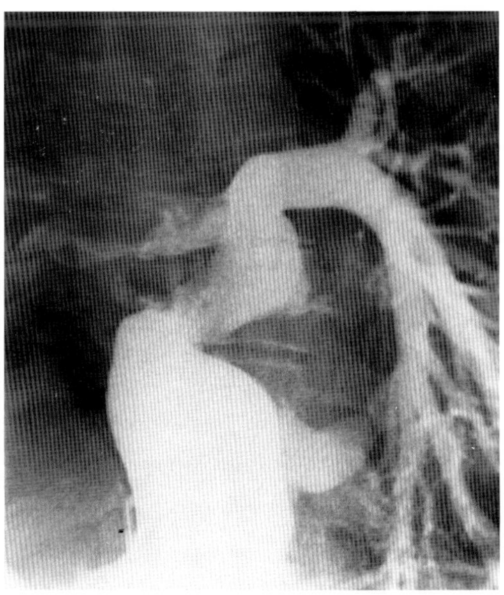

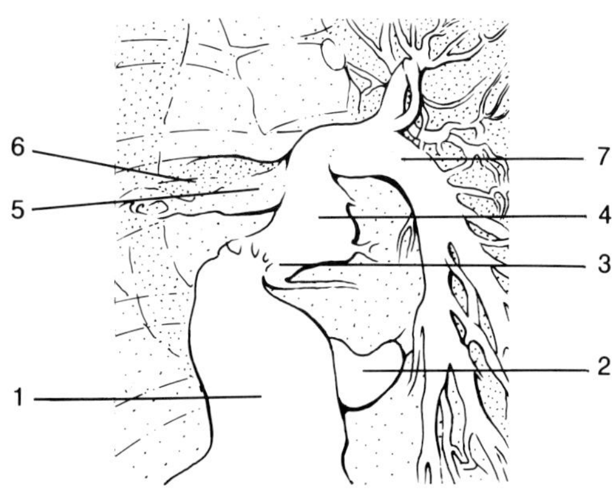

Fig. 16.22 Complication of Fontan anastomosis. Frontal projection of right atriogram shows opacification of the right atrium, coronary sinus, and pulmonary arteries. There is a surgically created connection between the right atrium and the pulmonary trunk. Contrast material opacifies the entire left pulmonary artery. Only the proximal portion of the right pulmonary artery is opacified, indicating the presence of thromboembolus in the distal portion.

1 right atrium	5 right pulmonary artery
2 coronary sinus	6 thromboembolus
3 surgically created connection	7 left pulmonary artery
4 pulmonary trunk	

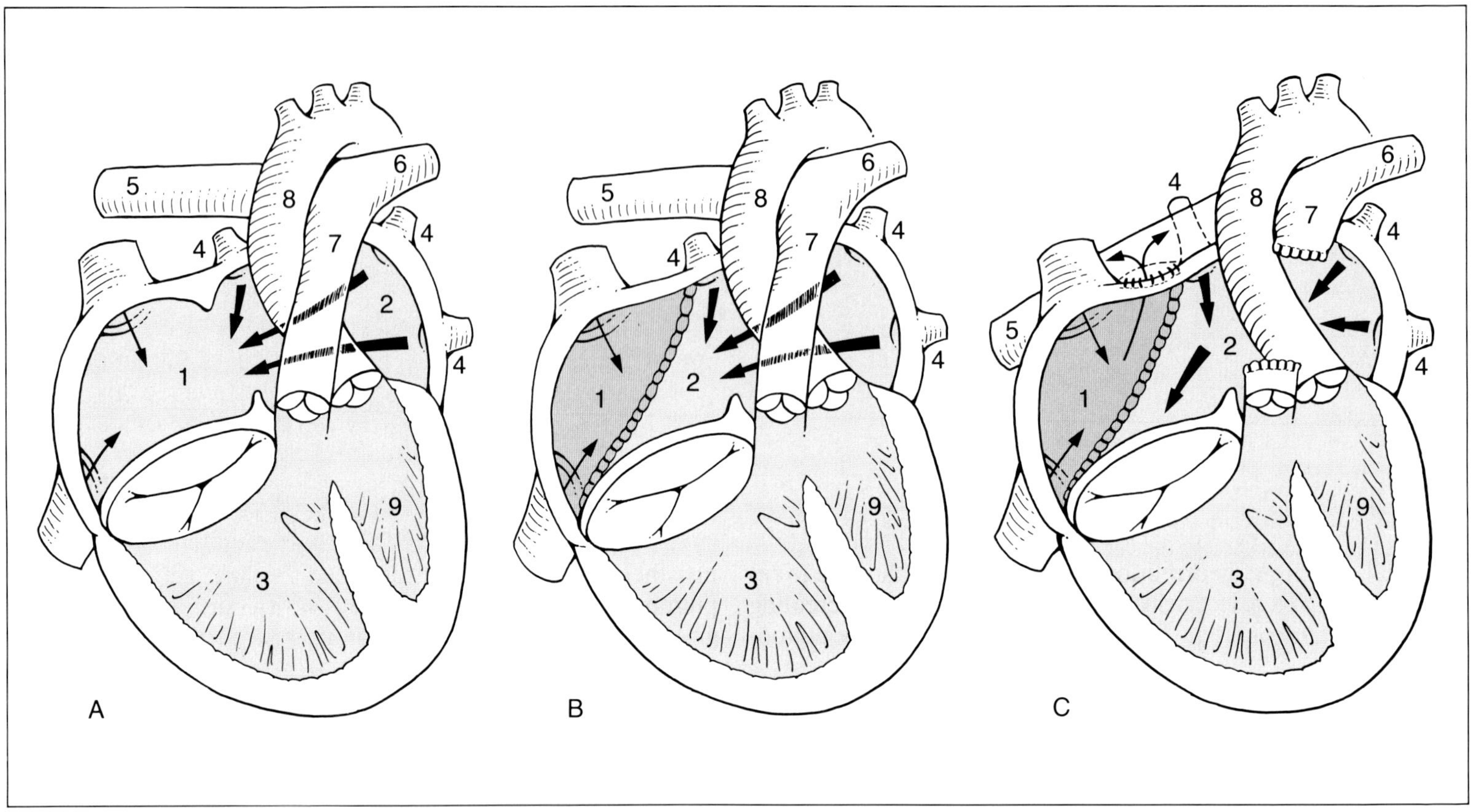

1	right atrium	4	pulmonary veins	6	left pulmonary artery	8	aorta
2	left atrium	5	right pulmonary artery	7	pulmonary trunk	9	left ventricle
3	right ventricle						

Fig. 16.23 Reverse Fontan operation. (A) Preoperative. In the absence of an atrioventricular valve related to the left atrium, the right atrium serves as a mixing chamber for the systemic and pulmonary venous return. (B, C) Reverse Fontan operation. A tunnel has been constructed in such a way that the entire venous return is directed to the right atrioventricular valve. (B) The operation is completed by anastomosing the right atrium to the right pulmonary artery and disconnecting the pulmonary trunk from its ventricular connection (C).

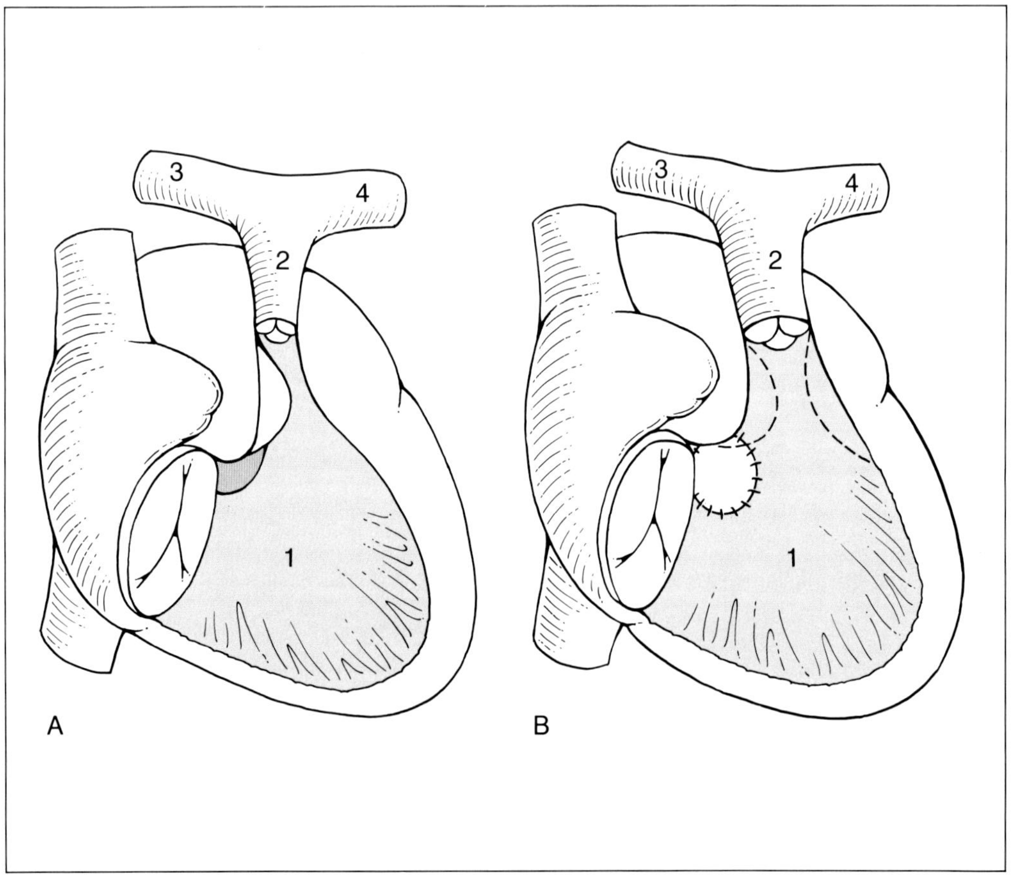

Fig. 16.24 Complete repair of tetralogy of Fallot with moderate stenosis of right ventricular outflow tract. The interior of the right ventricle is viewed from its anterior aspect. (A) Preoperative. Displacement of the infundibular septum causes a narrowing of the right ventricular outflow tract. Hypertrophy of the free wall of the right ventricle exacerbates the outflow stenosis. (B) Resection of the infundibulum and part of the free wall of the right ventricle reestablishes an unobstructed connection between the right ventricle and the pulmonary trunk. A teflon patch is then sutured over the VSD, completing the repair (not illustrated).

1	right ventricle	3	right pulmonary artery
2	pulmonary trunk	4	left pulmonary artery

atrium receives blood from the caval veins. The right atrium is then surgically connected to the right pulmonary artery or the pulmonary trunk. This operation, known as the *reverse Fontan procedure,* is completed by disconnecting the pulmonary trunk from its native ventricular connection (the aortic connection to the ventricle is maintained). The functional result is that the systemic veins are connected to the right-sided right atrium. Unsaturated venous blood passes across the surgically created right atrium–pulmonary artery connection into the pulmonary circulation. The oxygenated pulmonary venous return empties into the left atrium and passes through the surgically created tunnel into the right-sided atrioventricular valve. The oxygenated blood then passes into the left ventricle and out the aorta (Fig. 16.23).

COMPLETE CORRECTION OF TETRALOGY OF FALLOT

The goals of surgical correction of tetralogy of Fallot are to relieve the stenosis of the right ventricular outflow tract, creating an unobstructed pathway from the right ventricle to the pulmonary circulation, and to close the VSD in such a way that the overriding aorta is entirely connected to the left ventricle. Ideally, there will be no stenosis of the connection between the right ventricle and the pulmonary trunk; right ventricular pressure will not exceed 40 mm Hg; there will be no residual VSD; and there will be a normal sinus rhythm. (Although normal right ventricular pressure is ≤20 mg Hg, patients with pressure ≤40 mm Hg after total correction can expect to lead a normal life with unrestricted activity, and to have a normal life expectancy.)

The right ventricular outflow obstruction can be relieved in one of three ways: by resecting a portion of the infundibular septum and the other structures contributing to the obstruction (Fig. 16.24); by enlarging the pulmonary outflow by means of a transannular patch (constructed from pericardium or prosthetic material) applied to the anterior aspect of the right ventricle–pulmonary trunk connection (Figs. 16.25 and 16.26); or by inserting an external conduit, which usually incorporates a prosthetic pulmonic valve, between the right ventricle and the pulmonary trunk [a dacron conduit with a porcine valve heterograft (Hancock prosthesis) is commonly used for this purpose]

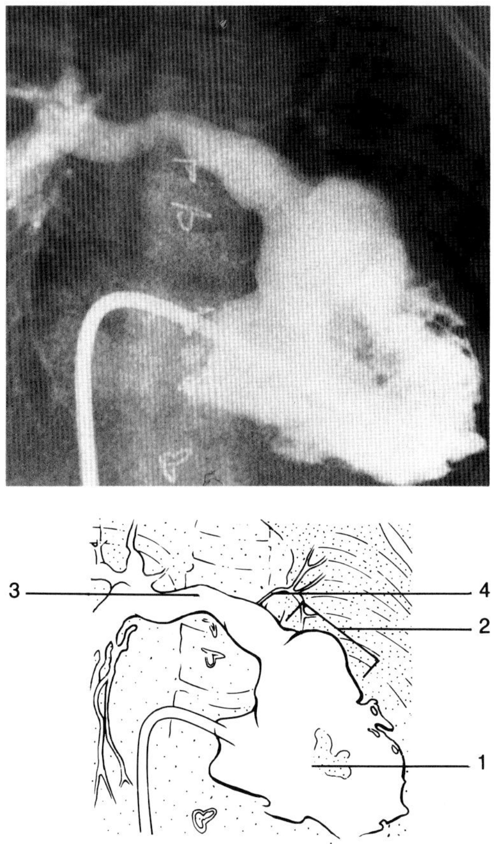

Fig. 16.26 Surgical correction of tetralogy of Fallot using transannular patch. Frontal projection of right ventriculogram shows dilatation of right ventricular outflow tract and pulmonary trunk and widening of pulmonic valve annulus after insertion of a transannular patch. Note severe stenosis of left pulmonary artery.

1 right ventricle
2 transannular patch
3 right pulmonary artery
4 left pulmonary artery

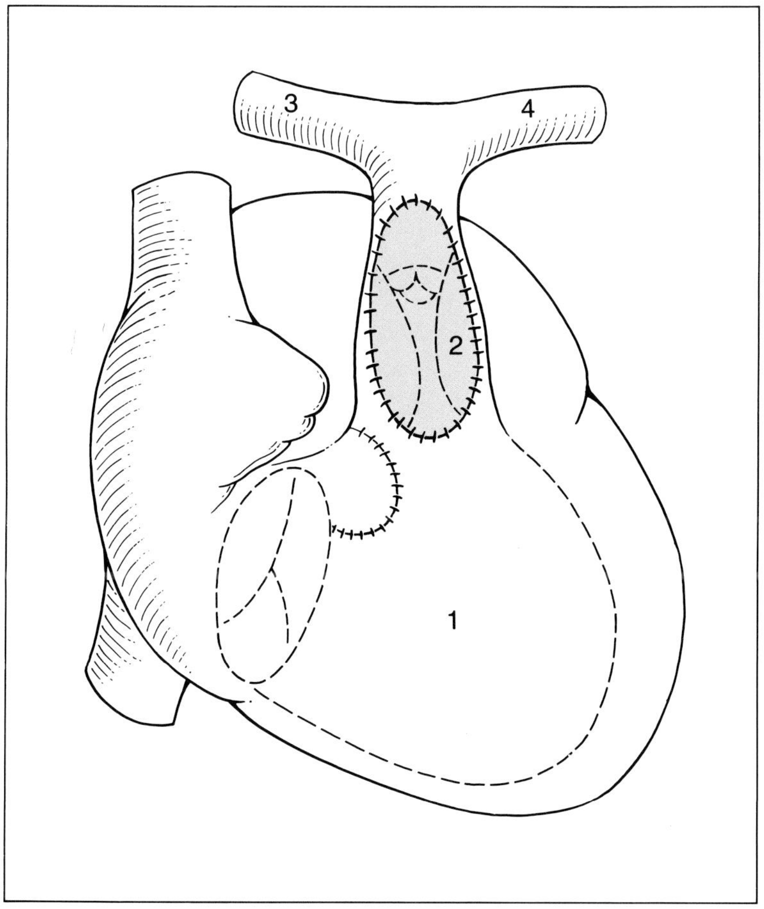

1 right ventricle
2 transannular patch
3 right pulmonary artery
4 left pulmonary artery

Fig. 16.25 Complete repair of tetralogy of Fallot with severe stenosis of right ventricular outflow tract. The interior of the right ventricle is viewed from its anterior aspect. A transannular patch (made from pericardium or a synthetic material, eg, dacron) is applied to the anterior wall of the infundibulum, annulus of the pulmonic valve, and the proximal part of the pulmonary trunk to enlarge the connection between the right ventricle and the pulmonary trunk. The VSD is closed with a teflon patch (not illustrated).

(Figs. 16.27 and 16.28). In each instance, the VSD is closed with a patch of prosthetic material applied in such a way that the overriding aortic valve is exclusively committed to the left ventricular outflow tract.

Before undertaking complete repair of tetralogy of Fallot, it is important to map the coronary arteries, because certain variations present serious hazards for the surgeon and potentially life-threatening complications for the patient. For example, the anterior descending artery may originate from the right coronary artery and course across the usual infundibulotomy site; if this variant is not recognized, the artery can be inadvertently transected, resulting in myocardial ischemia and probable myocardial infarction.

Pulmonic valvular insufficiency is not uncommon in patients in whom a transannular patch or unvalved external conduit has been used to correct the right ventricular outflow stenosis. Although mild to moderate pulmonic insufficiency is well tolerated, severe pulmonic insufficiency leads to right ventricular enlargement and eventually to tricuspid insufficiency (Fig. 16.29; see Appendix).

Progressive dilatation of the right ventricular outflow tract may occur when the obstruction has not been completely relieved, or when an excessive amount of myocardium has been resected; most often, however, it is caused by stretching of the prosthetic material used to construct the transannular patch. True aneurysms often stabilize, but false aneurysms are prone to rupture. A frequent late complication of external conduits is restenosis caused by proliferation of fibrous tissue within the conduit or the prosthetic valve. Calcification of the conduit or valve leaflets is rare within the first 5 years, but is quite common in conduits that have been in place for 10 years or more. A small percentage of patients with prosthetic valves have serious complications such as endocarditis, hemolysis, or thromboemboli.

In one large series, about 15 percent of patients who underwent complete repair had a residual VSD. Although small residual VSDs are usually well tolerated, large residual defects, usually due to dehiscence of the sutures, lead to right ventricular overload. Any patient with clinical or radiologic evidence of heart failure after a complete repair should have echocardiography or undergo recatheterization, as there is almost always an underlying cause, usually a residual VSD (Fig. 16.30; see Appendix).

SURGICAL CORRECTION OF TRANSPOSITION OF THE GREAT ARTERIES

The goal of corrective surgery in patients with transposition of the great arteries (TGA) is to convert two functionally separate (ie, parallel) circuits into a single circuit in which the pulmonary and systemic circulations connect in normal (ie, series) fashion. This can be accomplished by switching the arterial and venous circulation at the atrial level, at the ventricular level, or at the level of the great arteries. Because pulmonary vascular obstruc-

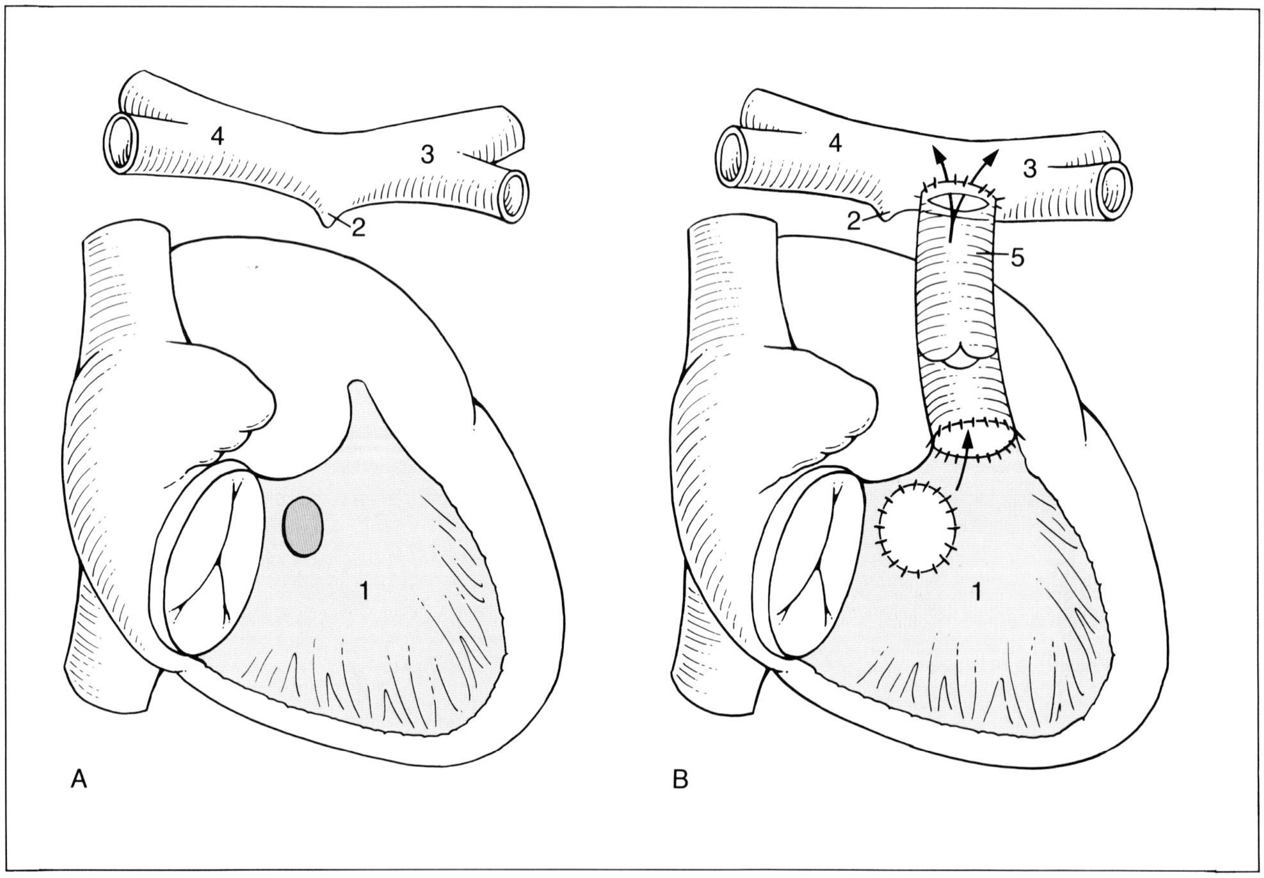

Fig. 16.27 Complete repair of tetralogy of Fallot with pulmonary atresia. The interior of the right ventricle is viewed from its anterior aspect. (A) Preoperative. The pulmonary trunk is atretic and there is no connection between the right ventricle and the pulmonary arteries. (B) An external conduit containing a porcine heterograft valve (Hancock valve) connects the right ventricle and the pulmonary arteries just proximal to the bifurcation, restoring normal blood flow. As in milder forms of tetralogy of Fallot, the VSD is closed with a teflon patch.

1 right ventricle
2 atretic pulmonary trunk
3 left pulmonary artery
4 right pulmonary artery
5 valved external conduit

tive disease may appear as early as 6 months of age when TGA is associated with a VSD, and as early as 1 year of age when the septum is intact, early correction is strongly recommended.

ATRIAL (INFLOW) SWITCH OPERATIONS

The goal of atrial (inflow) switch operations is to reroute desaturated systemic venous blood across the left atrioventricular (mitral) valve into the left ventricle, which supports the pulmonary trunk, and to reroute the oxygenated pulmonary venous return across the right atrioventricular (tricuspid) valve into the right ventricle, which supports the aorta. To accomplish this, a double channel, or baffle, is fashioned from the walls of the morphologic left and right atria (Fig. 16.31). In the *Mustard procedure,* introduced in 1964, synthetic material (eg, dacron or teflon) or pericardium is used to construct the baffle. The *Senning procedure* (1958) employs the patient's own atrial tissue for this purpose. When the "switch" is completed, desaturated systemic venous blood returning to the right atrium via the superior and inferior caval veins is directed across the left atrioventricular (mitral) valve into the left ventricle and thence to the

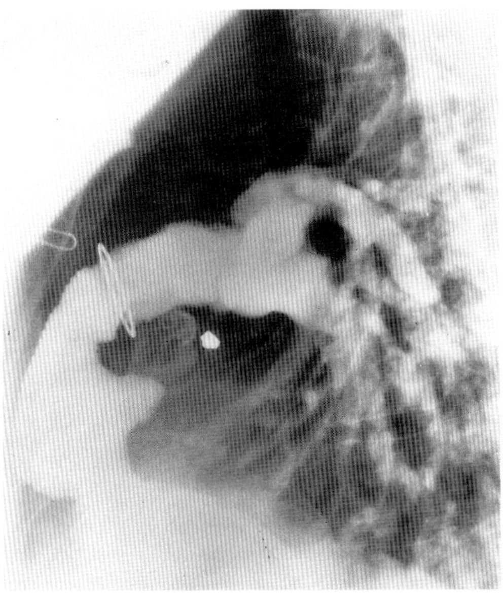

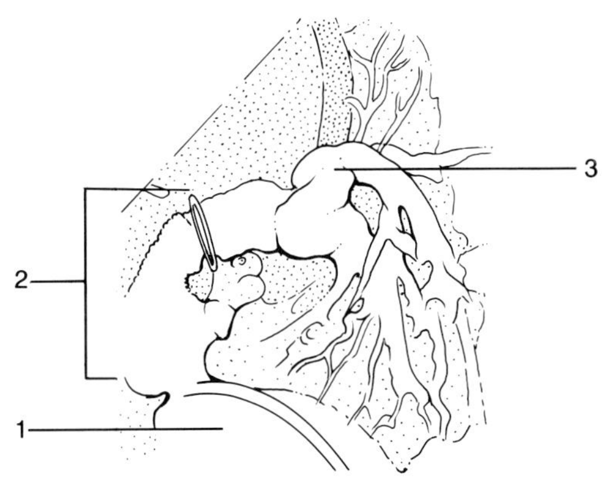

1	right ventricle	3	left and right pulmonary arteries
2	external conduit		

Fig. 16.28 Surgical correction of tetralogy of Fallot using a valved external conduit. Lateral projection of right ventriculogram shows an external conduit interposed between the right ventricle and the pulmonary trunk. The metallic ring marks the site of the prosthetic valve (porcine heterograft).

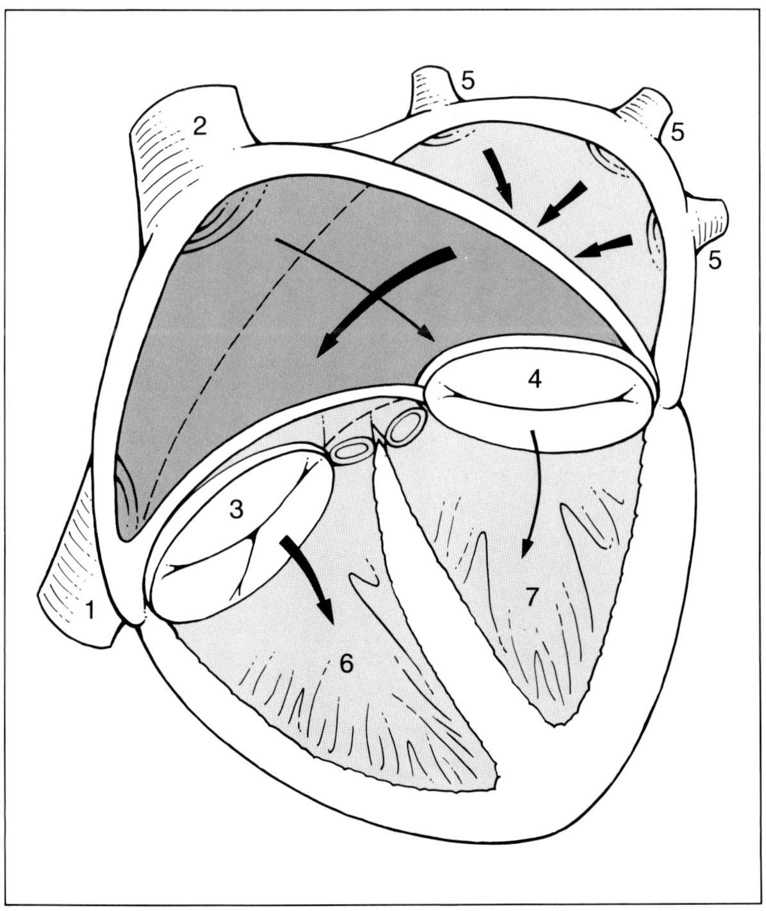

Fig. 16.31 Surgical correction of complete transposition of great arteries: atrial switch. In the various atrial switch operations, desaturated systemic venous blood is directed through a surgically created channel ("baffle") into the mitral valve. The desaturated blood passes into the left ventricle and is pumped into the pulmonary circulation. Oxygenated pulmonary venous blood is directed across the tricuspid valve into the right ventricle, whence it is distributed to the systemic circulation. In the Mustard procedure, synthetic material (dacron) or pericardium is used to construct the baffle. In the Senning procedure the patient's own atrial tissue is employed for this purpose.

1	inferior vena cava	5	pulmonary vein
2	superior vena cava	6	right ventricle
3	tricuspid valve	7	left ventricle
4	mitral valve		

lungs (Fig. 16.32). Oxygenated pulmonary venous blood returning to the left atrium passes across the right atrioventricular (tricuspid) valve into the right ventricle and is pumped into the systemic circulation.

Complications include arrhythmias, superior or inferior vena caval obstruction, baffle leaks (which may cause a significant left to right shunt), and pulmonary venous obstruction. Various imaging techniques, including angiography, echocardiography, and MRI, can be used to demonstrate these complications (Figs. 16.33 and 16.34). Because the right ventricle must continue to function as the systemic ventricle for the rest of the patient's life, right ventricular failure is a theoretical complication, although it appears to be quite rare. (Patients with corrected transposition of the great arteries typically develop right ventricular failure in the fifth or sixth decade of life; patients with TGA treated with an atrial switch operation probably do not survive long enough for this complication to appear.)

INTRAVENTRICULAR SWITCH OPERATIONS

The intraventricular rerouting technique, introduced by Rastelli in 1969, has been widely used in patients with TGA associated with a VSD; this is the operation of choice in patients in whom TGA is associated with VSD and subpulmonic stenosis. The goal of the operation is to direct oxygenated left ventricular blood across the VSD into the right ventricular outflow tract, which supports the aorta (Fig. 16.35). Using pericardium or synthetic material (eg, dacron), the surgeon constructs a chan-

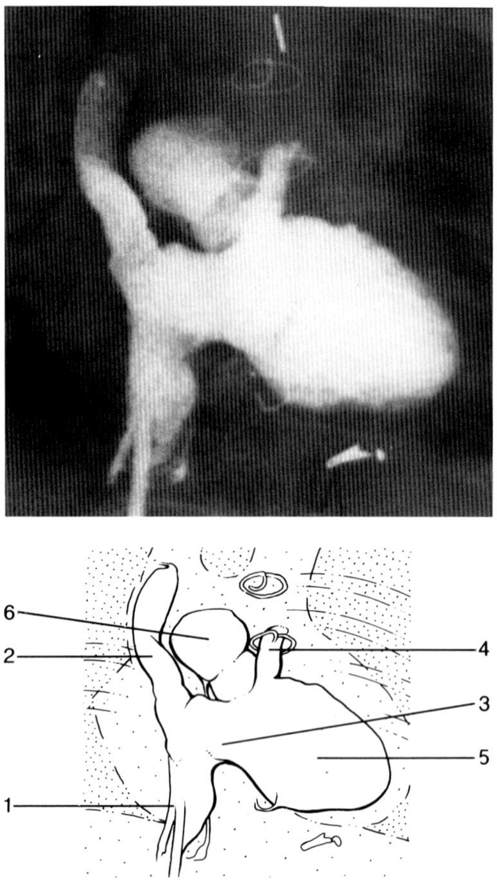

1	inferior vena cava	4	left atrial appendage
2	superior vena cava	5	left ventricle
3	surgically created channel ("baffle")	6	pulmonary trunk

Fig. 16.32 Atrial switch operation for TGA. Frontal projection of right atriogram shows opacified blood passing across the surgically created channel ("baffle") into the left atrium, opacifying the left atrial appendage, left ventricle, and pulmonary trunk.

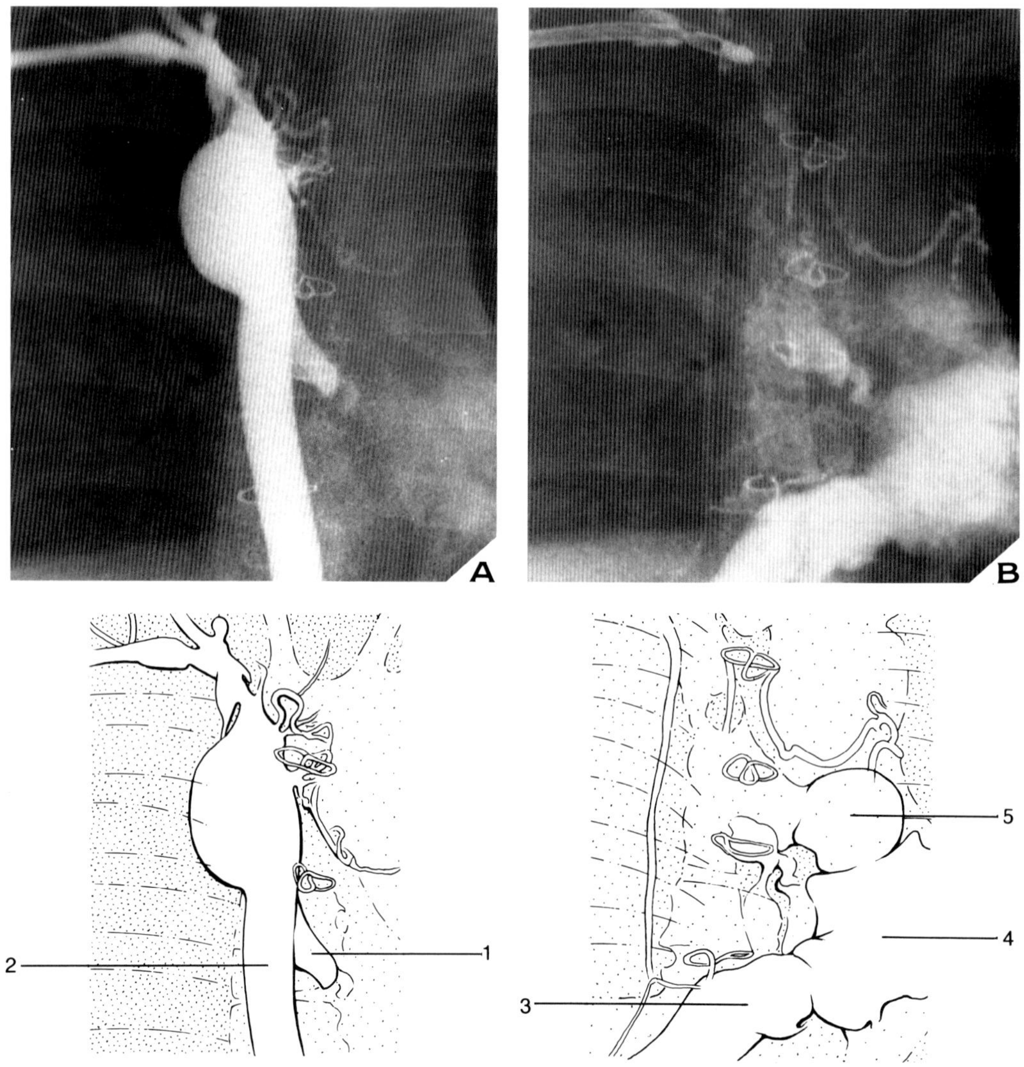

1	superior vena cava	3	inferior vena cava	5	pulmonary trunk
2	right azygos vein	4	left atrium		

Fig. 16.33 Obstruction of superior vena cava after atrial switch operation for TGA. Early (A) and late (B) phases of venogram obtained after injection of contrast material into the right subclavian vein demonstrates obstruction of the superior vena cava at its entrance into the right atrium (A). Opacified blood flows into the abdomen via the azygos system and returns to the heart via the inferior vena cava, whence it is distributed to the lungs (note opacification of pulmonary trunk). The connection between the inferior vena cava and the left atrium is widely patent.

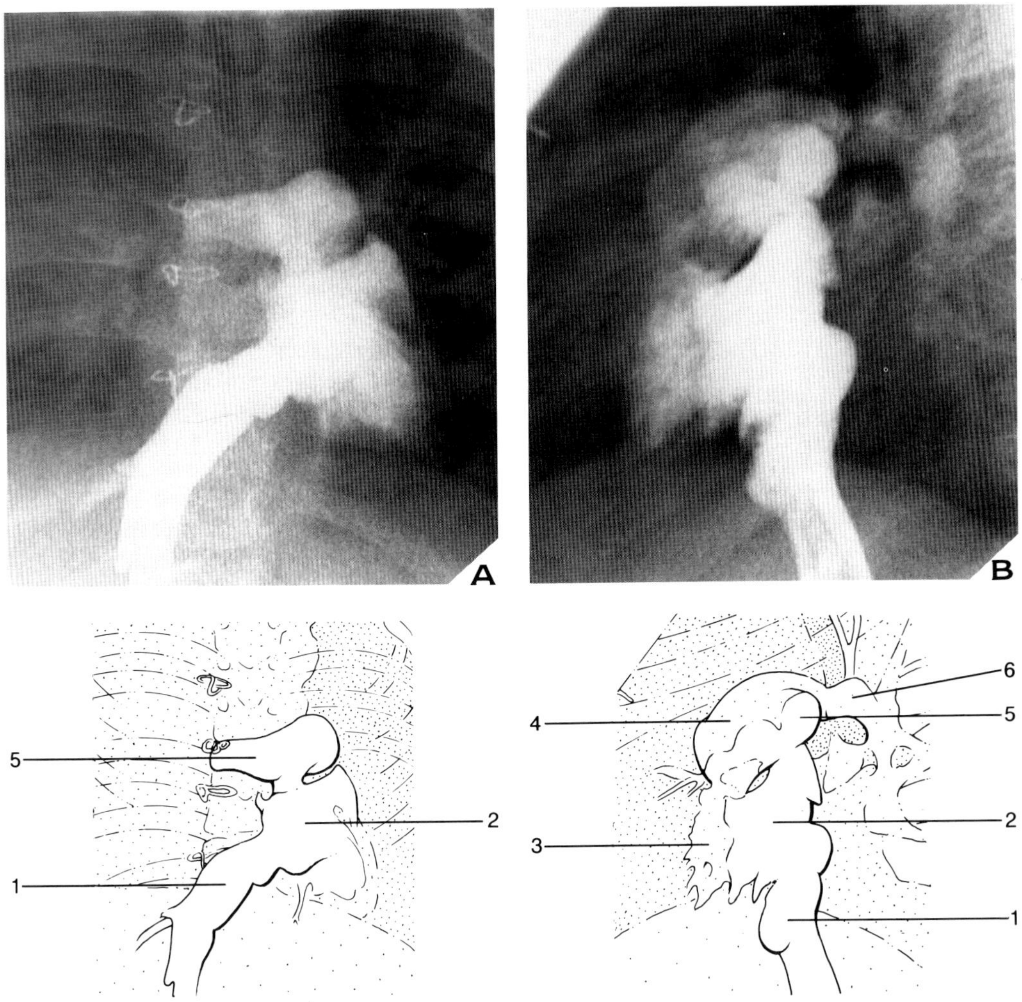

Fig. 16.34 Thrombosis of right pulmonary artery after atrial switch operation for TGA. Inferior vena cavogram in frontal (A) and lateral (B) projections demonstrates the connection of the inferior vena cava with the left atrium, which empties into a normal left ventricle. The pulmonary trunk and left pulmonary artery are normal. However, the proximal segment of the right pulmonary artery is occluded.

1 inferior vena cava
2 left atrium
3 left ventricle
4 pulmonary trunk
5 right pulmonary artery
6 left pulmonary artery

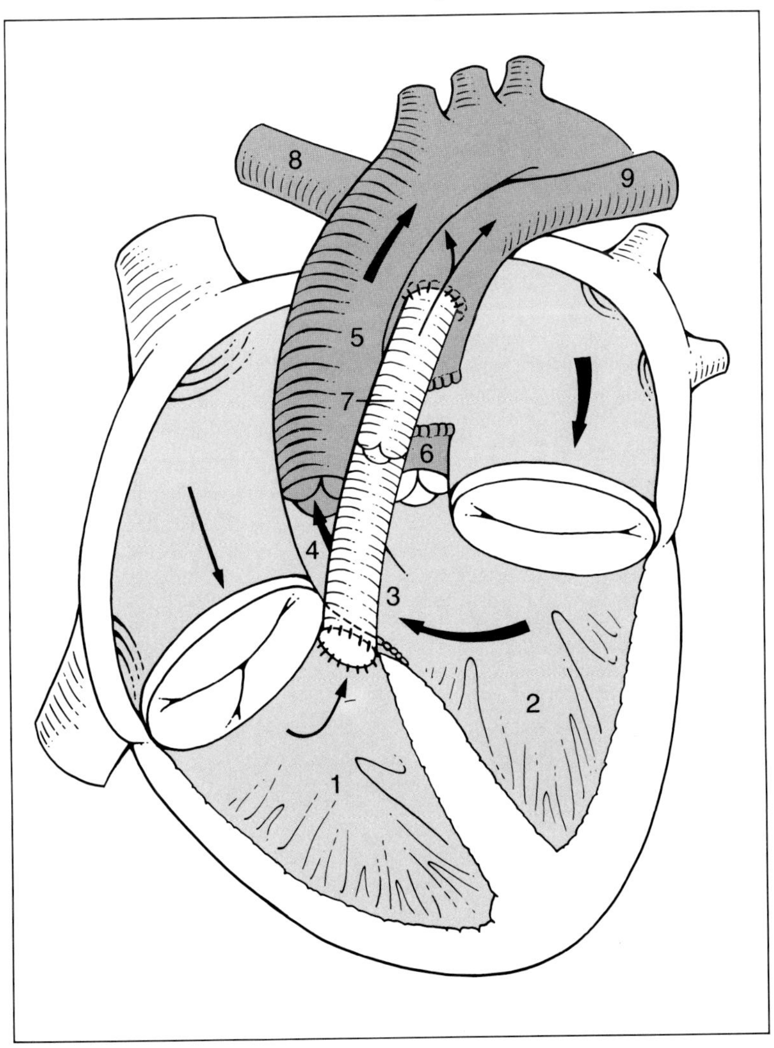

Fig. 16.35 Surgical correction of complete transposition of great arteries: intraventricular switch (Rastelli operation). Pericardium or synthetic material (eg, dacron) is used to construct an interventricular channel across the VSD. The surgically created channel directs oxygenated left ventricular blood into the right ventricular outflow tract, which supports the aorta. The pulmonic trunk has been divided and the pulmonic valve has been sutured shut. An external conduit containing a porcine heterograft valve (Hancock valve) connects the right ventricle with the pulmonary arteries.

1 right ventricle
2 left ventricle
3 surgically created channel across VSD
4 right ventricular outflow tract
5 aorta
6 pulmonary trunk (divided and sutured shut)
7 external conduit (with heterograft valve)
8 right pulmonary artery
9 left pulmonary artery

nel connecting the left ventricle and aorta via the VSD. (In some instances it is necessary to enlarge the VSD to provide adequate left ventricular outflow.) The pulmonary trunk is divided, and the pulmonic valve is sutured shut. An external conduit incorporating a porcine xenograft (Hancock valve) is inserted between the right ventricle and pulmonary trunk to conduct unsaturated blood to the lungs.

Complications of the intraventricular switch include atrioventricular block, residual VSD, subaortic stenosis, calcification of the conduit with valve dysfunction, and false aneurysms at the point where the conduit is sutured to the right ventricle (Fig. 16.36). Compression of the conduit against the sternum may lead to obstruction; because of problems related to the patient's size, conduits are seldom employed in children under 2 years of age.

Although the Rastelli operation restores normal ventriculoarterial connections, and the relative infrequency of postoperative arrthymias gives it an important theoretical advantage

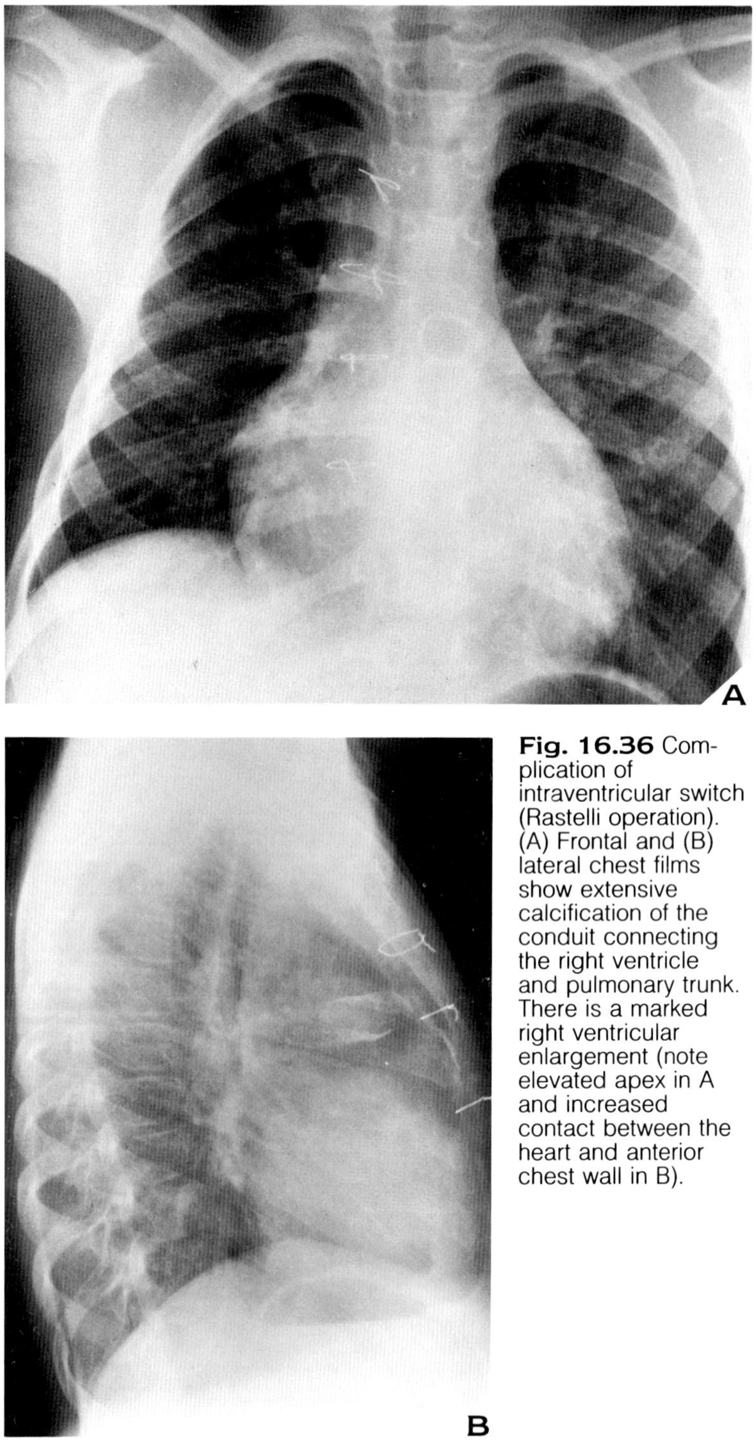

Fig. 16.36 Complication of intraventricular switch (Rastelli operation). (A) Frontal and (B) lateral chest films show extensive calcification of the conduit connecting the right ventricle and pulmonary trunk. There is a marked right ventricular enlargement (note elevated apex in A and increased contact between the heart and anterior chest wall in B).

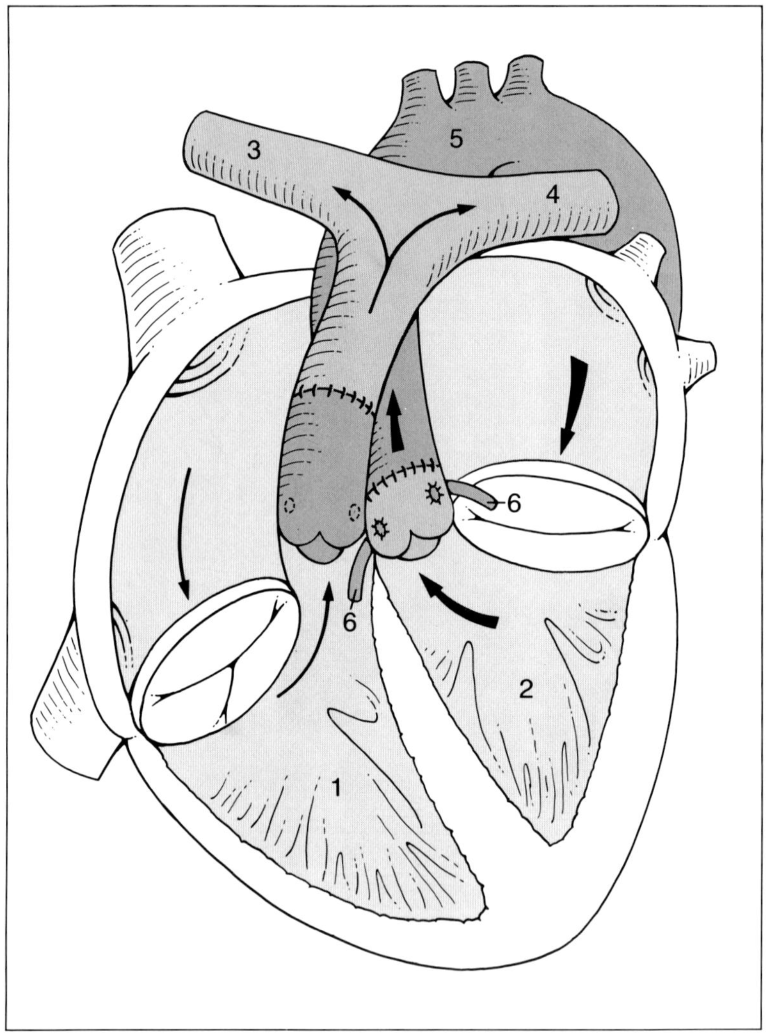

1	right ventricle	4	left pulmonary artery
2	left ventricle	5	aorta
3	right pulmonary artery	6	reattached cornary arteries

Fig. 16.37 Surgical correction of complete TGA by arterial switch (Jatene) operation. The aorta is sectioned above the sinuses of Valsalva and the pulmonary trunk is sectioned above the pulmonic valve. The distal aorta is connected to the native pulmonary trunk and the distal pulmonary trunk to the aortic root, completing the outflow switch. The coronary arteries are then reattached to the proximal pulmonary trunk, which now supports the systemic circulation.

over the Mustard and Senning repairs, the operative mortality of this procedure may be as high as 25 percent. Its most obvious limitation is that a prosthetic conduit cannot grow as the child grows, and must therefore be changed several times as body size increases.

ARTERIAL (OUTFLOW) SWITCH OPERATIONS

In the "outflow switch" operation, introduced by Jatene in 1975, the pulmonary trunk and aorta are sectioned above the sinuses of Valsalva. The distal connections of the great arteries are switched so that the distal aorta connects with the proximal pulmonary trunk and the distal pulmonary trunk connects with the proximal aorta. When the switch is completed, the morphologic left ventricle supports the aorta and the morphologic right ventricle supports the pulmonary trunk; thus the normal circulatory pattern is restored (Figs. 16.37 and 16.38).

To supply the myocardium with oxygenated blood, the coronary arteries must be reattached to the proximal pulmonary trunk, which presents formidable technical problems for the surgeon. The mortality of the Jatene operation was initially very high; in recent series, however, the mortality has been as low as 4.2 percent, making the outflow switch a reasonable choice for many patients with TGA.

Late complications include coronary artery obstruction (leading to myocardial ischemia), left ventricular dysfunction, and stenosis of the arterial anastomoses.

SURGICAL CORRECTION OF TRUNCUS ARTERIOSUS

To correct this malformation the surgeon must disconnect the pulmonary artery from the truncus, reestablish the connection between the right ventricle and the pulmonary arteries (usually

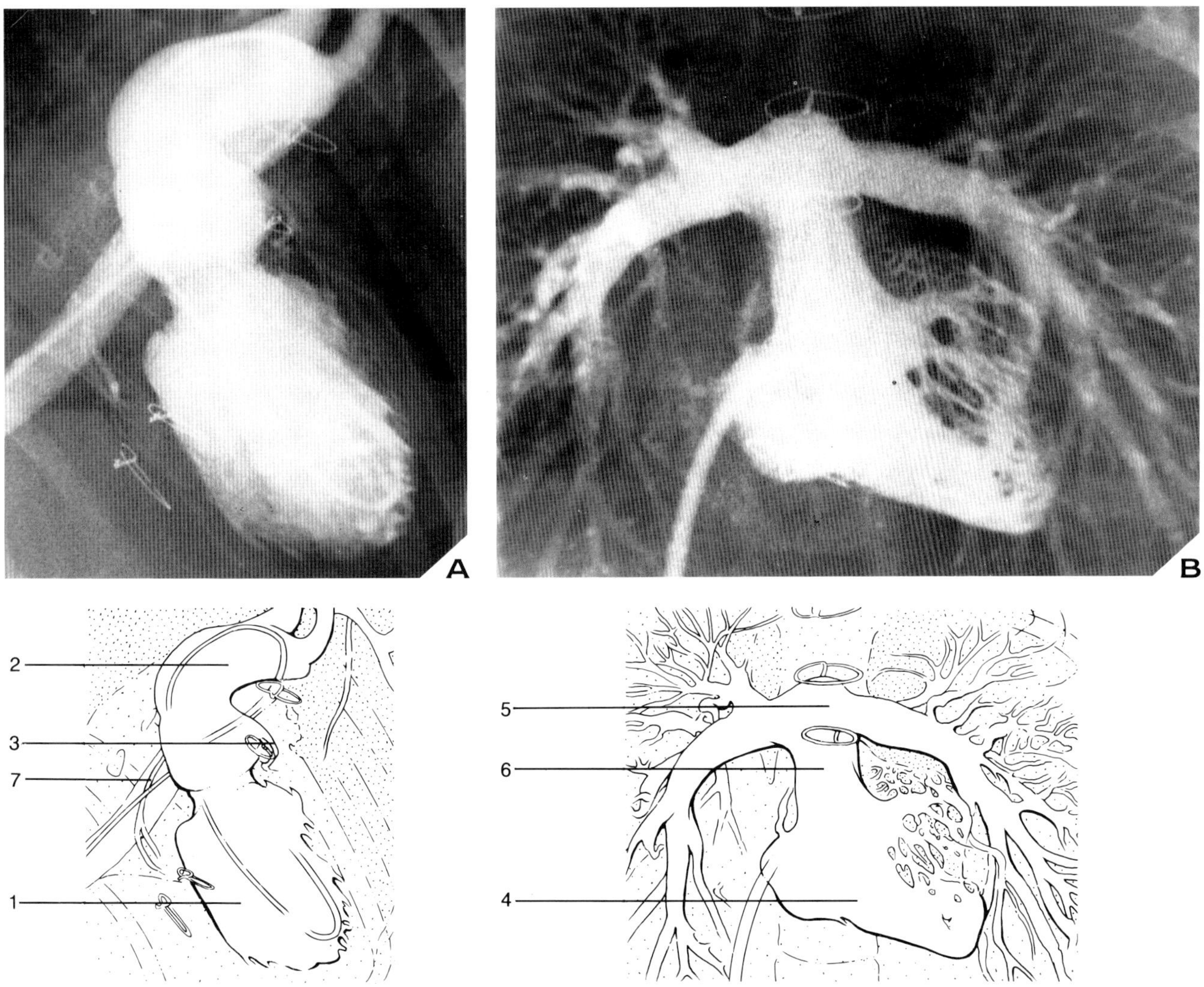

Fig. 16.38 Surgical repair of complete TGA by arterial switch (Jatene) operation. Right anterior oblique projection of left ventriculogram (A) and frontal projection of right ventriculogram (B) show the left ventricle emptying into the aorta. The reattached right and left coronary arteries are patent. The right ventricle and aorta are connected via the native aortic valve.

1 left ventricle
2 aorta
3 coronary arteries
4 right ventricle
5 pulmonary trunk
6 position of native aortic valve
7 catheter

by means of a valved external conduit), and close the VSD (Fig. 16.39). When the truncal valve is incompetent it must be replaced. The most serious late complication is stenosis of the conduit valve. Other complications include dehiscence of the patch used to close the VSD, and obstruction of the left ventricular outflow tract.

SURGICAL REPAIR OF COARCTATION OF THE AORTA

Various operations have been devised to relieve this stenosis, which is located in the upper descending thoracic aorta. The most common operation is resection of the stenotic segment with an end to end anastomosis (Fig. 6.40A). When there is insufficient aortic tissue for an end to end anastomosis, the stenotic aortic segment can be enlarged by interposing the proximal segment of the subclavian artery (Figs. 16.40B and 16.41); many surgeons prefer this approach for young patients. In some instances it is necessary to insert a prosthetic tube between the proximal and distal segments of the aorta, bypassing the stenotic segment (Figs. 16.40C and 16.42).

Coarctation of the aorta is an isolated lesion in 90 percent of patients who present after 6 months of age, who represent the great majority of patients with this malformation. In patients with coarctation and VSD, most surgeons prefer to manage the coarctation first and repair the VSD as a separate lesion. Repair of the coarctation may uncover an unsuspected subaortic stenosis, which must be dealt with separately.

Only 9 percent of patients with aortic coarctation who present under 6 months of age have isolated coarctation; these infants have the same prognosis as older patients with isolated coarctation. In the remainder, aortic coarctation is accompanied by one or more additional anomalies, such as VSD, aortic stenosis, mitral valve abnormalities, or PDA. These infants can be considered to have a form of hypoplastic left heart syndrome, characterized by low flow through the ascending aorta and hypoplasia of the isthmus. They typically present with congestive heart failure and have a high mortality rate, often due to the associated lesions.

Complications of coarctation repair are uncommon. Spinal cord ischemia with paralysis, which may occur even when adequate collaterals are present, is a rare complication of the immediate postoperative period. The postcoarctectomy syndrome, manifested by persistent hypertension and abdominal pain, is an infrequent complication of the early postoperative period. The symptoms are believed to be caused by vasospasm in the target organs (kidneys, adrenals, small intestine) secondary to the sudden increase in perfusion pressure after relief of the aortic obstruction. (The hypertension has been attributed to the release of pressor substances by the kidneys and adrenals.) Plain films of the abdomen and barium studies often reveal bowel edema with "thumb printing." In an exceptional case, the bowel ischemia is severe enough to cause necrotizing enterocolitis and bowel infarction.

The most frequent late complication of coarctation repair is recoarctation, most often seen in patients who underwent sur-

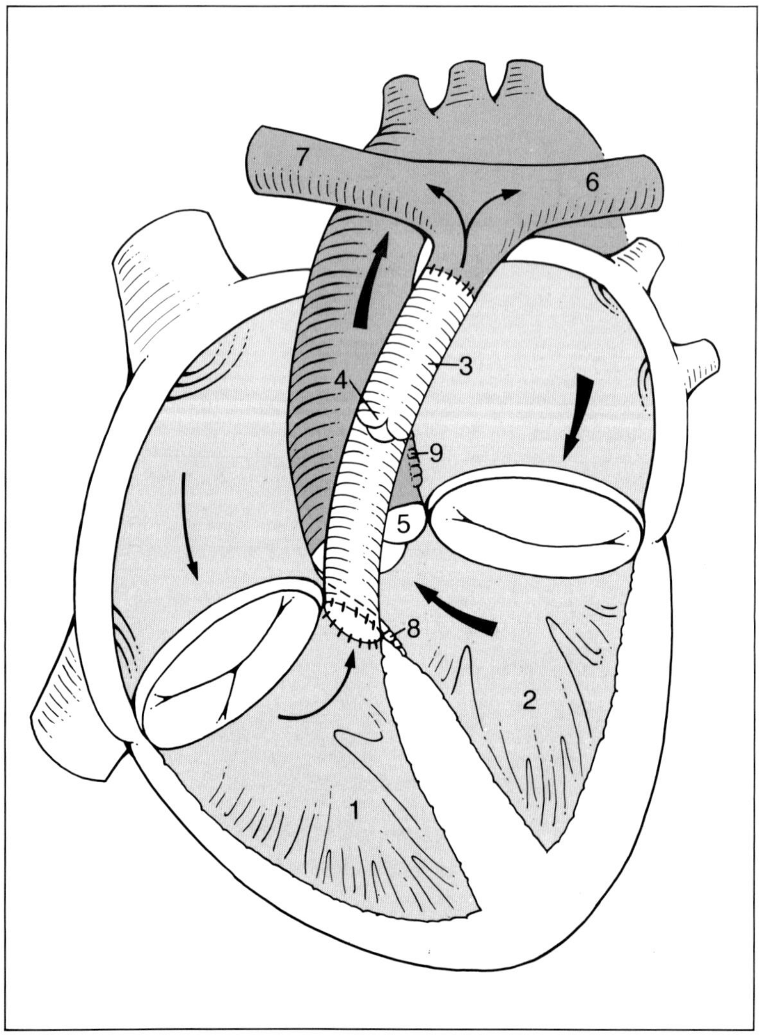

Fig. 16.39 Surgical correction of truncus arteriosus. The truncal valve usually arises from both ventricles, overriding the VSD. To correct this anomaly, the surgeon disconnects the pulmonary trunk and the truncus and inserts a valved external conduit, thus reestablishing the connection between the right ventricle and the pulmonary arteries. The VSD is then closed in such a way that the morphologic left ventricle supports the entire truncal valve.

1 right ventricle
2 left ventricle
3 conduit
4 heterograft valve
5 truncal valve
6 left pulmonary artery
7 right pulmonary artery
8 ventricular septal defect
9 position of native pulmonary trunk

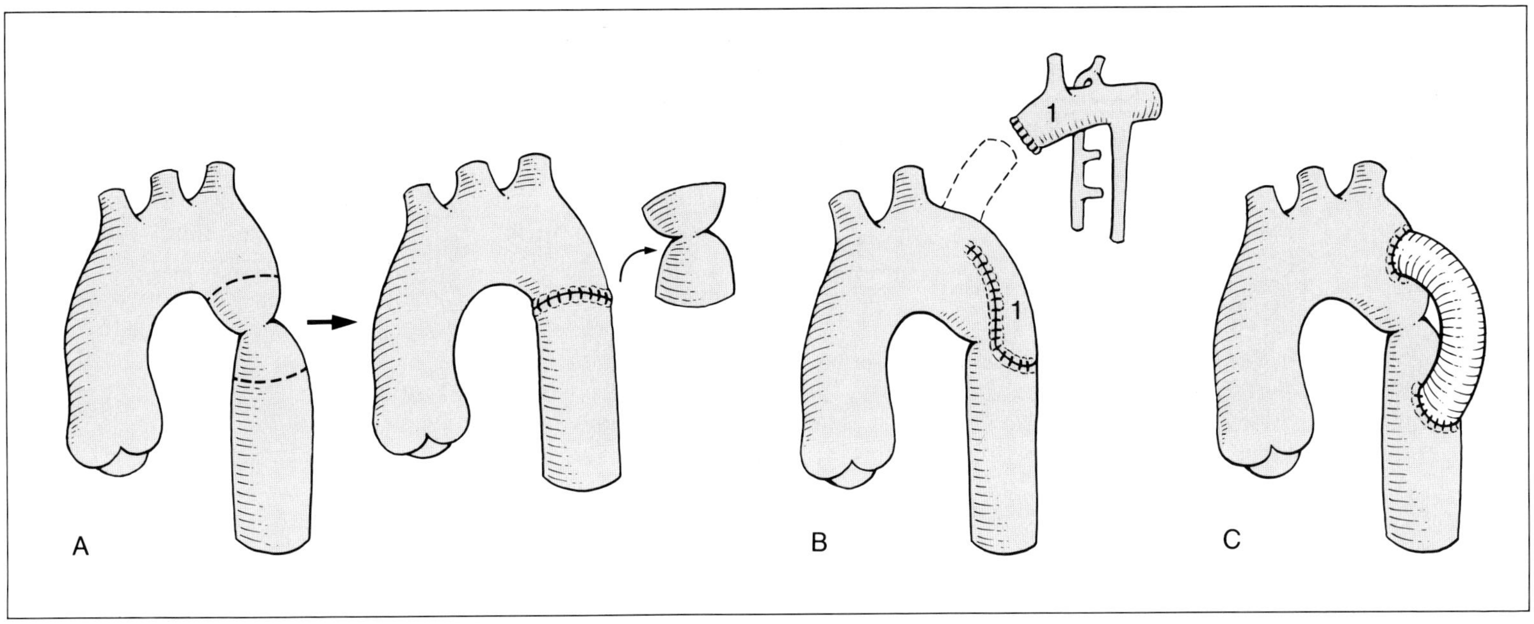

Fig. 16.40 Surgical repair of coarctation of the aorta. (A) Resection of stenotic segment with end to end anastomosis. (B) Left subclavian flap technique. The proximal portion of the left subclavian artery has been used to enlarge the stenotic segment. After the operation, circulation to the territory of the left subclavian artery is provided by collaterals. (C) Bypass technique. An external conduit connects the proximal and distal aorta, bypassing the stenosis.

1 left subclavian artery (used as graft)

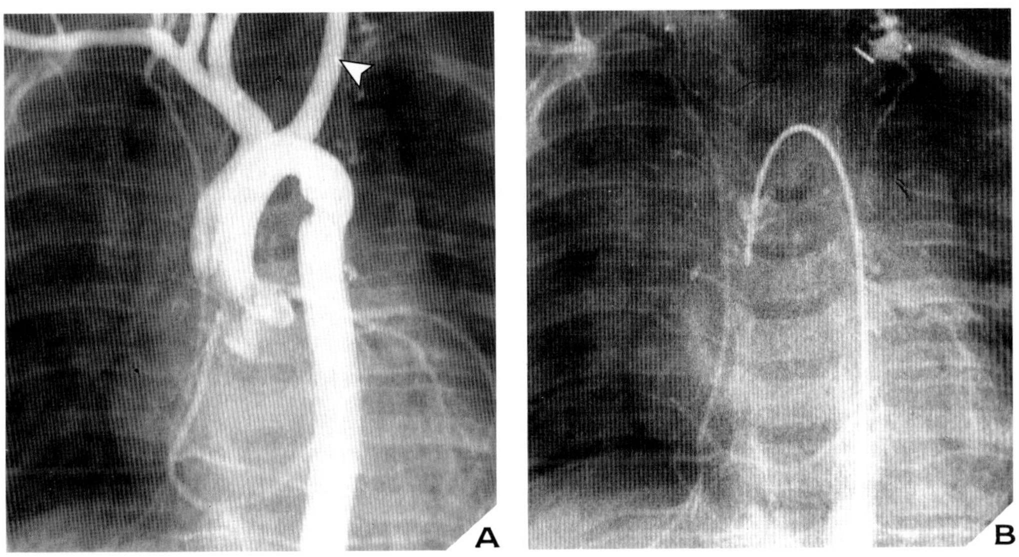

Fig. 16.41 Surgical repair of coarctation of the aorta by the subclavian flap technique. (A, B) Frontal projection of postoperative aortogram. Early phase (A) shows slight narrowing of the lumen at the site of the original coarctation. The metallic clip (*arrow*) indicates where the left subclavian artery has been sectioned. (The proximal portion of the left subclavian artery has been opened, turned down, and sutured to the aorta to enlarge the stenotic segment.) Late phase (B) shows opacification of distal left subclavian artery via collaterals (mainly derived from the vertebral artery).

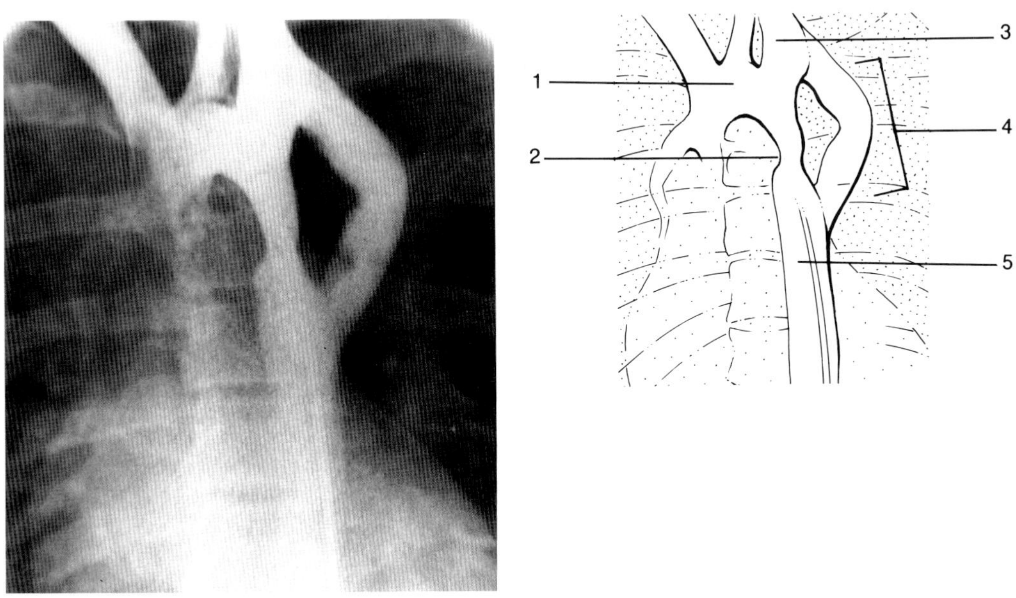

Fig. 16.42 Surgical repair of coarctation of the aorta using a bypass graft. Frontal projection of aortogram after injection of contrast material into the aortic arch shows opacified blood flowing from the left subclavian artery to the descending thoracic aorta via the conduit, bypassing the stenotic segment.

1 aortic arch
2 coarcted segment
3 left subclavian artery
4 conduit
5 descending thoracic aorta

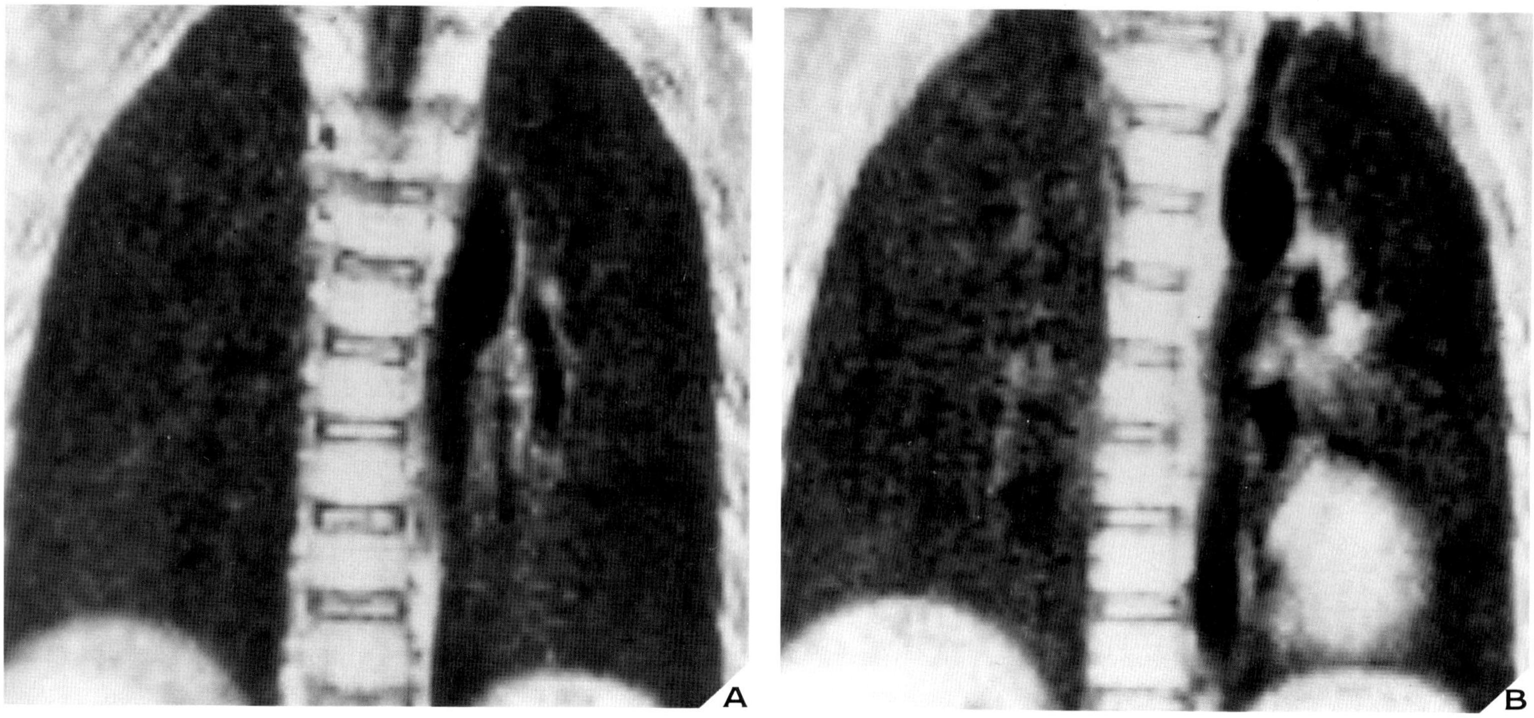

Fig. 16.43 Aneurysmal dilatation after coarctation repair (MRI). (A, B) Coronal ECG-gated spin–echo images obtained 3 years after dacron flap angioplasty demonstrate an area of relatively mild aneurysmal dilatation at the site of the previous repair. Other images demonstrated minimal narrowing of the aortic arch. Cineangiocardiography confirmed the MRI findings. At cardiac catheterization, the peak systolic ejection gradient, measured between the transverse arch and descending aorta, was only 4–5 mm Hg. (Reproduced by permission from Bank et al: Coarctation of the aorta in children undergoing angioplasty: Pretreatment and posttreatment MR imaging. *Radiology* 1987; 162:235).

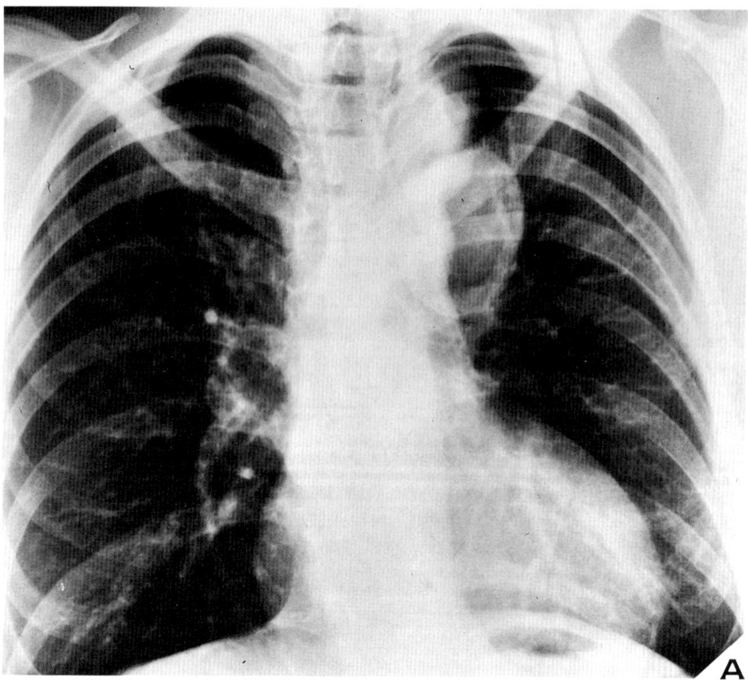

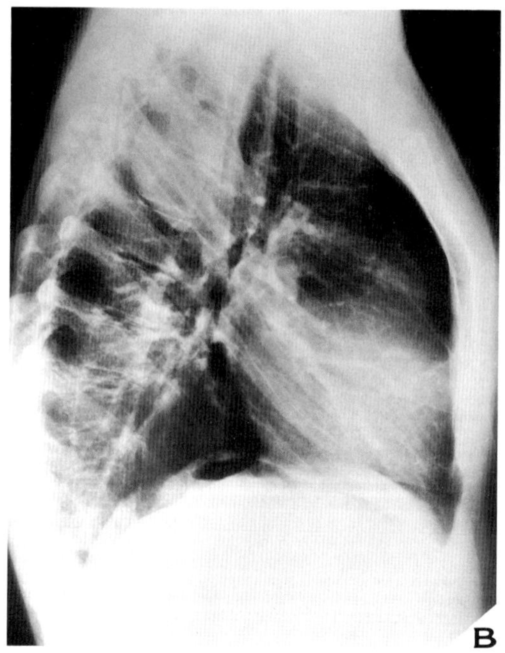

Fig. 16.44 False aneurysm after repair of coarctation of the aorta. (A) Frontal and (B) lateral chest films obtained several years after a coarctation repair show a mediastinal mass contiguous with the aortic arch. Note the deformity of left fourth and fifth posterior ribs at the site of the previous thoracotomy and the absence of rib notching. A false aneurysm of the descending thoracic aorta was found at operation.

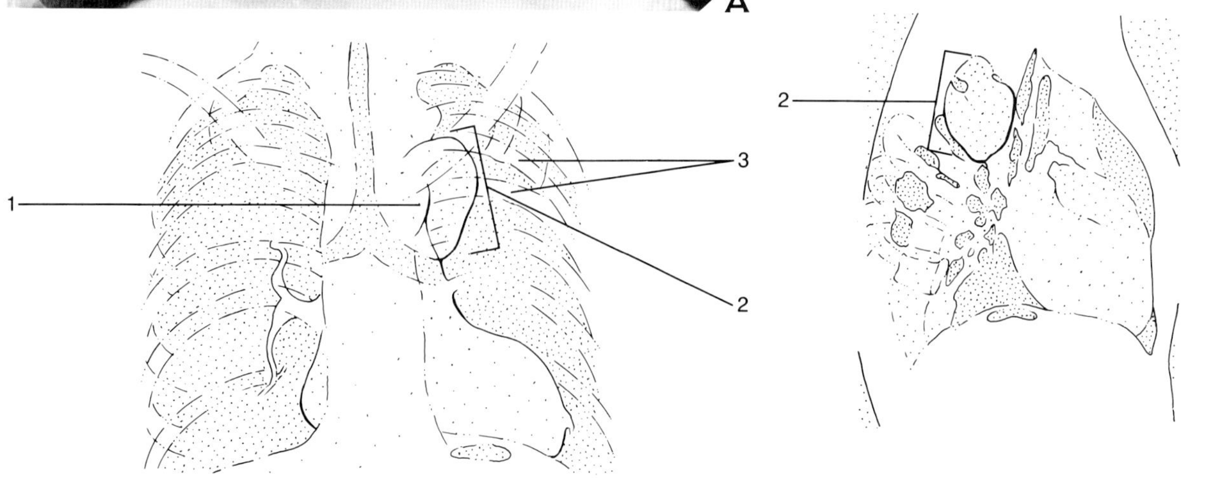

1 left aortic arch
2 pseudoaneurysm
3 deformed ribs (previous thoracotomy)

gery during the first year of life; true or false aneurysm formation is an infrequent late complication (Figs. 16.43 and 16.44).

Delay in diagnosis is not uncommon in patients with isolated coarctation of the aorta, and this undoubtedly contributes to the associated morbidity. For example, it is probable that longstanding hypertension resulting from delay in diagnosis increases the risk of subarachnoid hemorrhage due to a ruptured berry aneurysm of the circle of Willis, a malformation present in about 10 percent of patients with isolated coarctation of the aorta. Persistent postoperative hypertension is more likely to be a problem in patients operated on after 5 years of age; in one series, only 6 percent of patients operated on before 5 years of age had persistent hypertension, whereas 30 percent of those operated on between 6 and 18 years of age and 47 percent of those operated on between 19 and 40 years of age remained hypertensive postoperatively.

SURGICAL TREATMENT OF HYPOPLASTIC LEFT VENTRICLE

In patients with the hypoplastic left ventricle (HLV) complex, the right ventricle supports the entire pulmonary and systemic circulation; the coronary arteries are perfused in retrograde fashion via the ductus arteriosus and the hypoplastic ascending aorta. Without treatment, infants with HLV almost invariably die soon after birth when the ductus arteriosus closes. (Intraductal infusion of prostaglandin E_1 or E_2, which prevents ductus closure, can provide temporary palliation.) The goal of corrective surgery is to decrease the load on the right ventricle while providing an adequate supply of oxygenated blood to the coronary circulation, in retrograde fashion, through the hypoplastic ascending aorta. Some of these critically ill infants have been salvaged by the two-stage Norwood procedure (Figs. 16.45

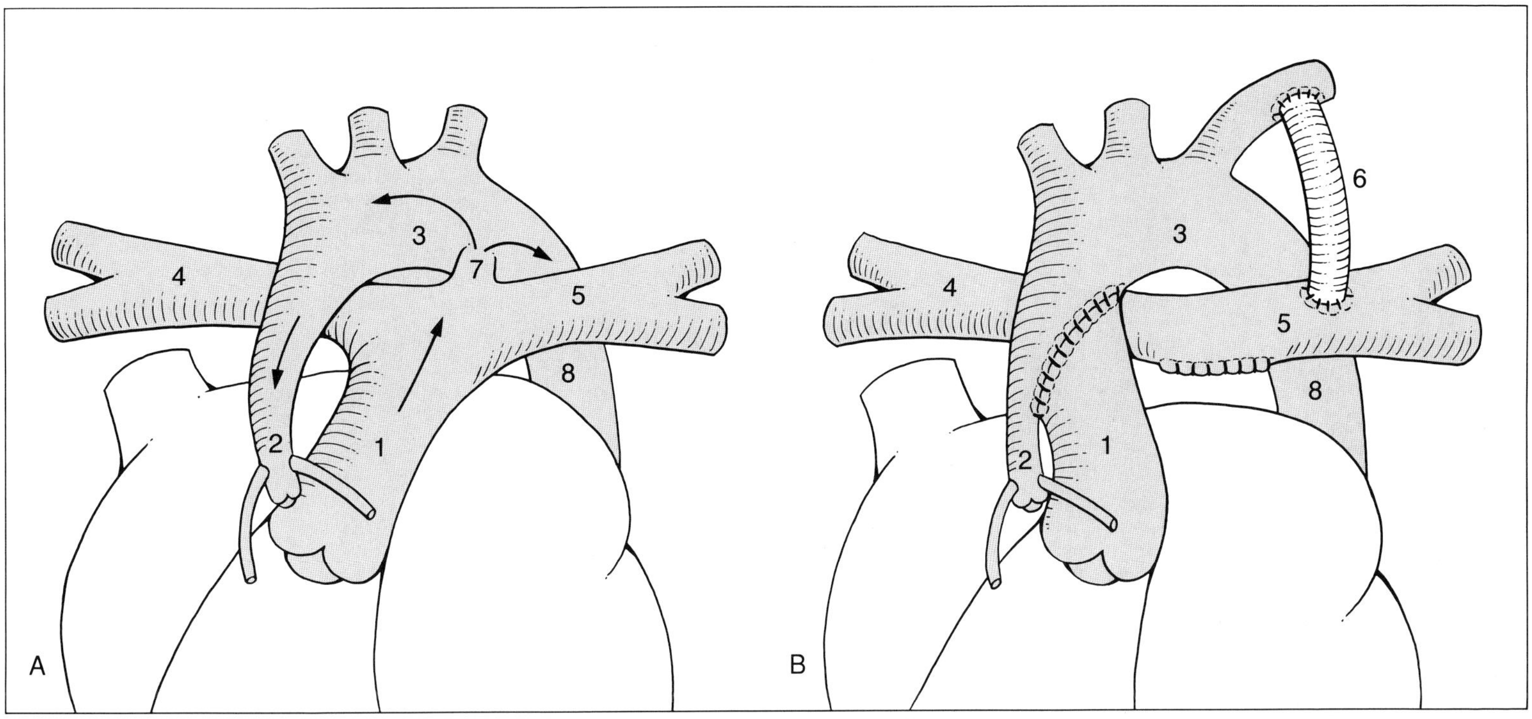

Fig. 16.45 Surgical treatment of hypoplastic left ventricle (Norwood operation). (A) Preoperatively, the hypoplastic ascending aorta supplies the coronary arteries in retrograde fashion. The right ventricle is the only effective pumping chamber: it supplies the pulmonary circulation directly and the systemic circulation via the patent ductus arteriosus. (B) In the first stage of the Norwood operation the pulmonary trunk is disconnected from the right and left pulmonary arteries and connected to the hypoplastic aorta. A Blalock–Taussig anastomosis is then constructed to supply the lungs. In the second stage (not illustrated), the Blalock–Taussig anastomosis is closed and the right atrium is connected to the pulmonary trunk (Fontan operation). Unfortunately, few infants survive long enough to undergo the second stage.

1 pulmonary trunk
2 ascending aorta
3 aortic arch
4 right pulmonary artery
5 left pulmonary artery
6 left Blalock–Taussig anastomosis
7 patent ductus arteriosus
8 descending thoracic aorta

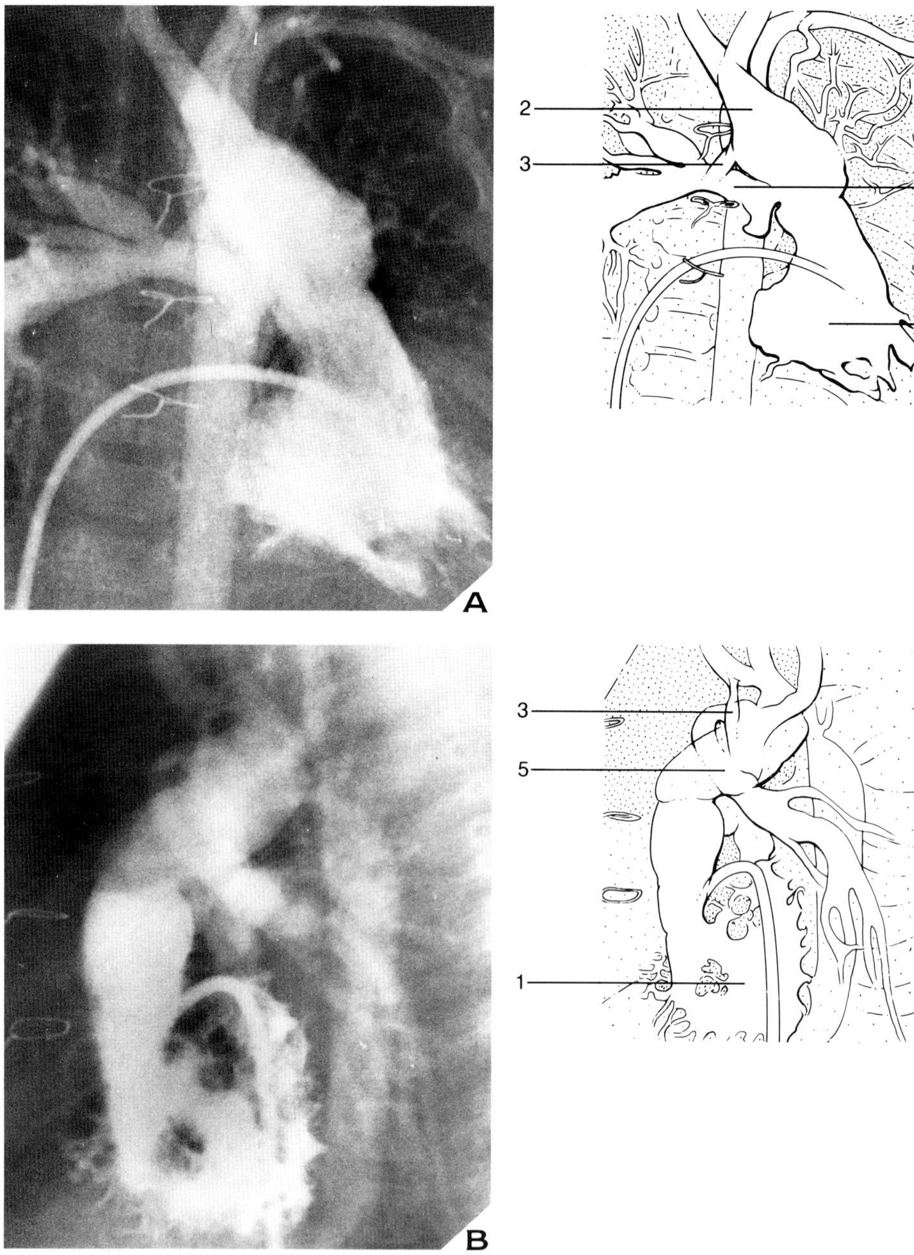

Fig. 16.46 Surgical treatment of hypoplastic left ventricle (Norwood operation). (A) Frontal and (B) lateral projections of left ventriculogram after first stage of the Norwood operation show the surgically created connection between the pulmonary trunk and the hypoplastic ascending aorta. The lungs are perfused via a Blalock–Taussig anastomosis.

1 right ventricle
2 surgical fusion of pulmonary trunk and aorta
3 Blalock–Taussig anastomosis
4 right pulmonary artery
5 hypoplastic ascending aorta

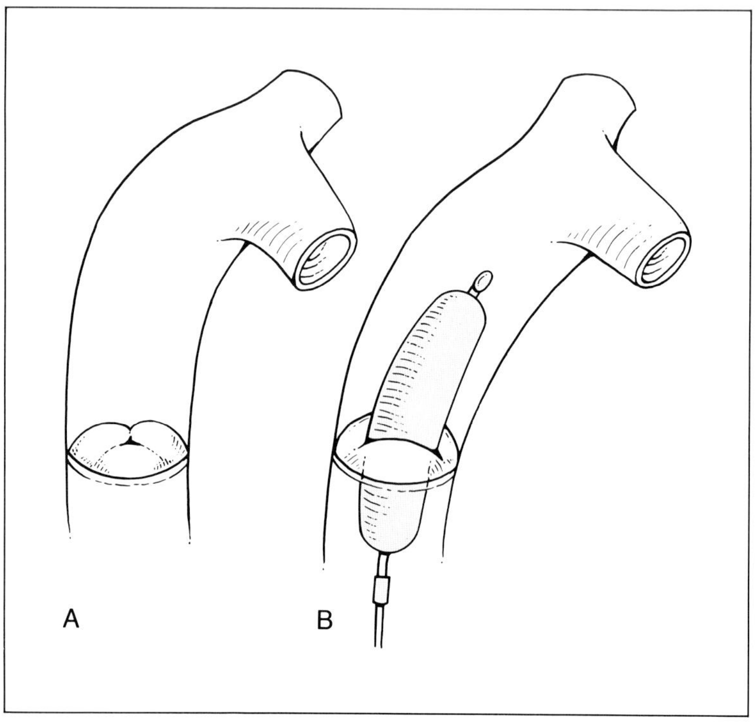

Fig. 16.47 Balloon angioplasty of pulmonic valvular stenosis. (A) Pulmonic valvular stenosis is caused by fusion of the cusps at the commissures. (B) To correct the stenosis, a balloon catheter is introduced via the inferior vena cava, passed across the stenotic valve, and inflated for several seconds.

and 16.46). In the first stage, the pulmonary trunk is disconnected from the right and left pulmonary arteries and is anastomosed to the hypoplastic ascending aorta; a Blalock–Taussig anastomosis is then performed to restore pulmonary blood flow. The first stage is designed to provide adequate circulation to the peripheral and coronary circulation, enabling the infant to survive. In the second stage, an anastomosis is made between the right atrium and the pulmonary trunk (Fontan procedure), and the Blalock–Taussig anastomosis is taken down. Unfortunately, the mortality of the first stage is about 80 percent, and few infants with HLV survive long enough to undergo the second stage.

Some infants with HLV and other lethal cardiac malformations have been salvaged by cardiac transplantation, which some surgeons now consider the operation of choice in such cases.

THERAPEUTIC CATHETER PROCEDURES

The first transcutaneous therapeutic catheter procedure, balloon atrial septostomy, was performed by Rashkind in 1966 (see Fig. 16.12). This palliative procedure has been life-saving in neonates with transposition of the great arteries and tricuspid atresia. Since that time a number of other transcutaneous procedures have been introduced.

As noted above, prostaglandins E_1 and E_2 can be infused directly into the ductus arteriosus (via an indwelling catheter) to maintain ductal patency in infants with ductus-dependent lesions such as hypolastic left ventricle or aortic arch atresia. Balloon catheters have been used with variable success to treat pulmonic valvular stenosis (Figs. 16.47 and 16.48), aortic stenosis, peripheral pulmonic stenosis, and coarctation of the aorta. They have also been used to dilate hypoplastic pulmonary arteries (in patients with tetralogy of Fallot), to enlarge a stenotic Blalock-Taussig anastomosis, to dilate stenotic caval veins, and to treat postoperative re-coarctation of the aorta. Detachable balloons have been used to occlude atrial septal defects, although this technique has not been uniformly successful. Percutaneously introduced clamshell umbrellas, introduced by Mills in the late 1970s, have been used to close ASDs and VSDs with a high initial success rate and few early or late complications. This innovative technique offers an attractive alternative to operative VSD repair in patients in whom a systemic ventriculotomy would be needed to close a muscular VSD, as well as in those with residual defects following corrective surgery and in patients considered poor operative risks.

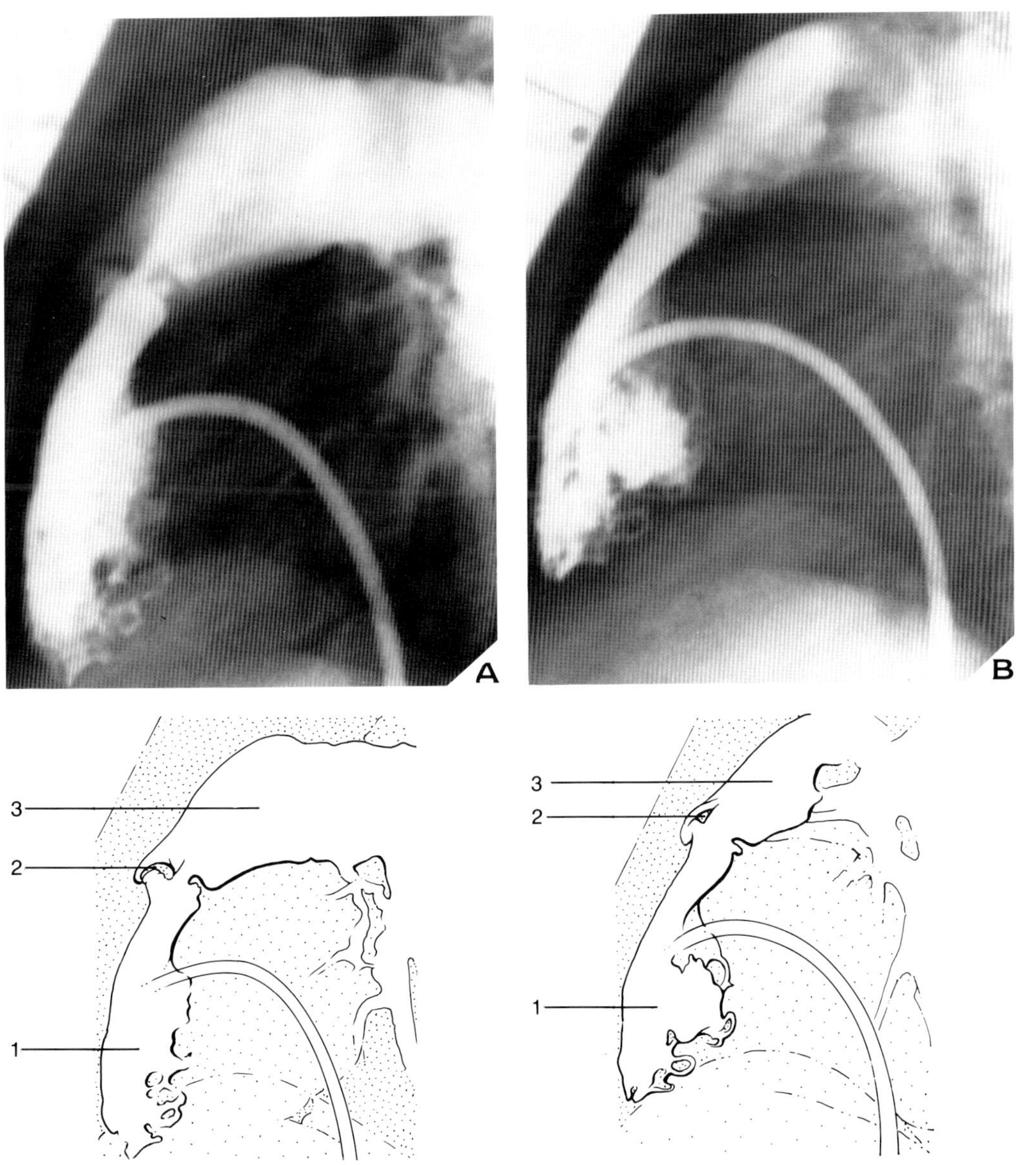

Fig. 16.48 Balloon angioplasty of pulmonic valvular stenosis. Lateral projection of right ventriculogram before (A) and after (B) angioplasty shows marked increase in the diameter of the valve orifice after the procedure. Note poststenotic dilatation of pulmonary trunk.

1 right ventricle
2 pulmonic valve
3 pulmonary trunk

Embolization techniques have been successfully used to occlude large aortopulmonary collaterals, to close a patent ductus arteriosus, or to occlude the arteries supplying an arteriovenous malformation (Figs. 16.49 and 16.50).

THE POSTOPERATIVE PERIOD

NORMAL CONVALESCENCE

After cardiopulmonary bypass is discontinued, the cardiovascular system should be able to maintain adequate (although not necessarily normal) systemic perfusion. During the first few hours, a cardiac index of 1.6 liters per minute per square meter of body surface is acceptable; by the following day, the cardiac index should be 2 or more (2 to 2.2 in infants and small children). When the cardiac index is too low, or when drugs are needed to maintain adequate cardiac output, the convalescence is abnormal. Clinical manifestations of low cardiac output include fluid retention and pulmonary dysfunction.

During the first few postoperative days the patient typically experiences slight pulmonary dysfunction characterized by mild dyspnea, small amounts of mucus and tracheobronchial fluid, and moderate increase of the alveolar–arterial oxygen difference. The pulmonary dysfunction reflects decreased pulmonary and thoracic compliance and localized pulmonary abnormalities (eg, atelectasis). The decreased lung compliance is caused by multiple factors: increased extravascular lung water secondary to increased vascular permeability, perivascular edema, sequestration and breakdown of lymphocytes in the pulmonary capillary bed, and abnormalities of the alveolar lining cells. The decreased pulmonary and thoracic compliance is reflected by mild desaturation (low PaO_2), an increased arterial–venous oxygen difference, and right to left shunting. The latter is the result of a ventilation–perfusion mismatch caused by atelectasis and areas of ventilated but poorly perfused lung. These physiological aberrations usually subside by the third postoperative day and disappear by the fifth postoperative day.

PLAIN FILM FINDINGS DURING THE EARLY POSTOPERATIVE PERIOD

The plain film findings after open heart surgery reflect the operative procedure, the effects of cardiopulmonary bypass and hypothermia, and the postoperative course. The initial postoperative films are a confusing maze of tubes, catheters, sutures, and monitor wires. Because cardiopulmonary bypass and cardiac surgery commonly cause arrhythmias, electrical activity is monitored by atrial and ventricular electrodes. The tips of the electrodes are inserted into the right atrial and right ventricular myocardium and the wires are brought out through an anterior wound. The atrial wire lies to the right of the ventricular wire on the frontal film (Fig. 16.51). Pulmonary wedge pressure reflects

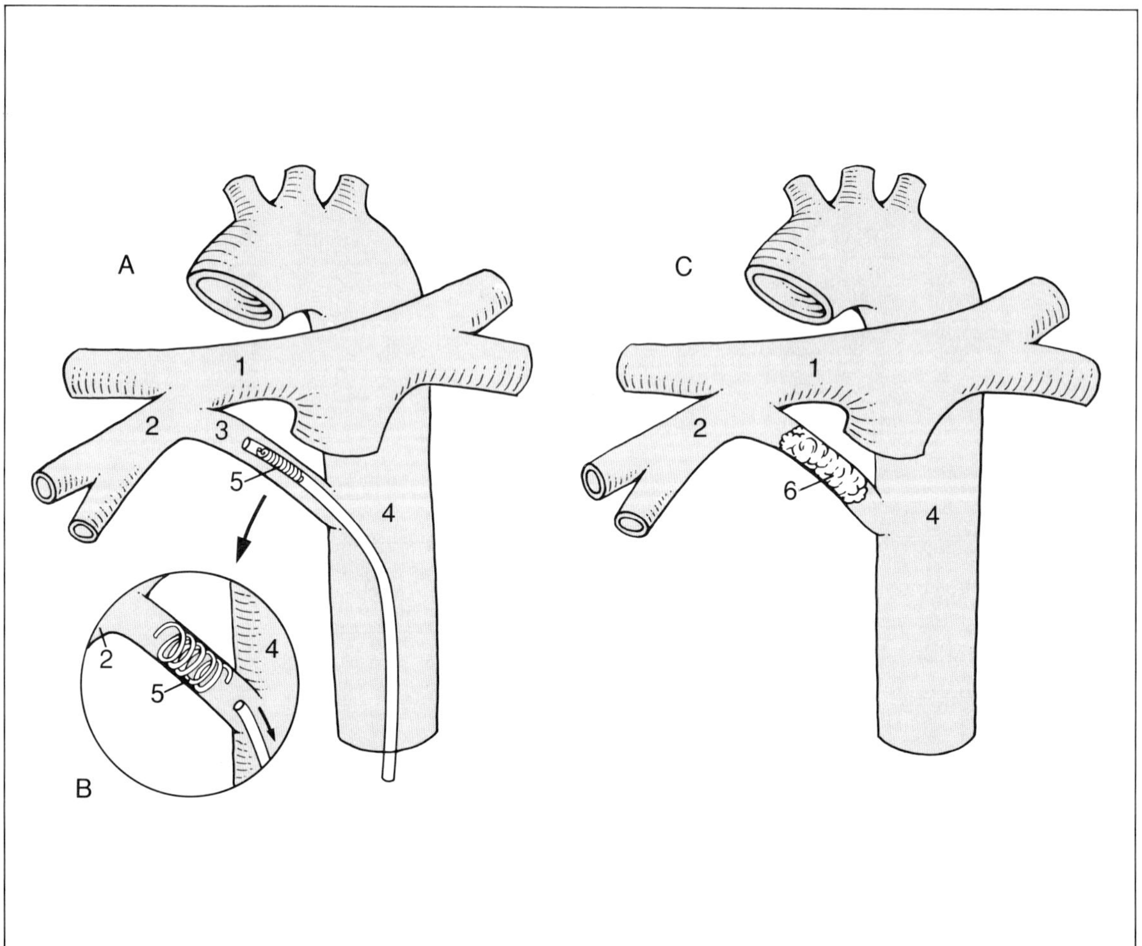

1 right pulmonary artery
2 branch of right pulmonary artery
3 aortopulmonary collateral
4 descending thoracic aorta
5 spring coil
6 thrombus occluding collateral

Fig. 16.49 Percutaneous transvascular embolization. In the example shown, a coiled spring ("coil") is being used to occlude an aortopulmonary collateral connected to a branch of the right pulmonary artery. (A) An end hole catheter with a coil its in its lumen has been advanced into the proximal portion of the collateral artery. (B) When the catheter tip is in proper position, a guidewire is used to dislodge the coil, after which the catheter is removed. Once it is free, the coil expands, partially occluding the arterial lumen. (C) Subsequent platelet aggregation on the coil leads to thrombus formation, completely occluding the collateral artery. Blood from the right pulmonary artery now supplies the territory previously supplied by the collateral.

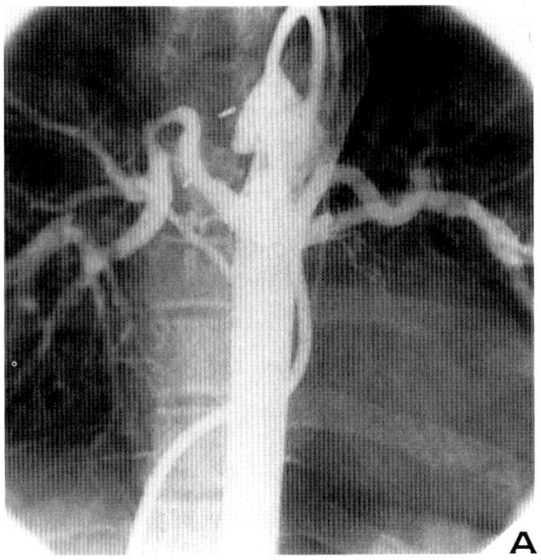

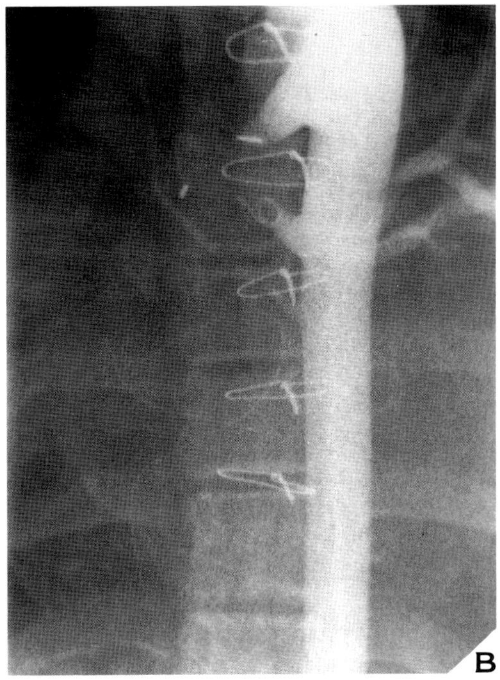

Fig. 16.50 Embolization of aortopulmonary collateral with metal coil. (A) Thoracic aortogram shows a large large collateral supplying the territory of the right pulmonary artery. The stump arising from the upper right border of the descending thoracic aorta is the origin of another large aortopulmonary collateral which had previously been embolized. (B) Repeat aortogram after the second embolization procedure shows the coil occluding the collateral.

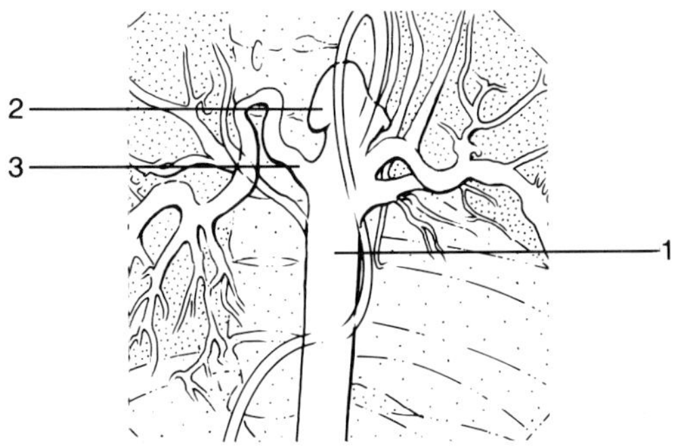

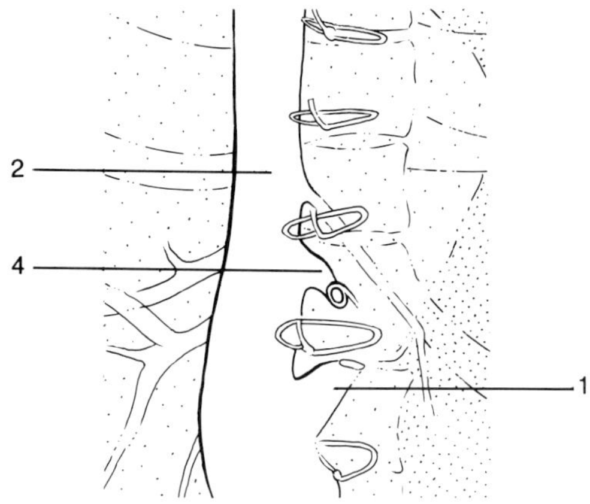

1 descending thoracic aorta
2 site of previously embolized aortopulmonary collateral
3 patent aortopulmonary collateral
4 coil occluding aortopulmonary collateral

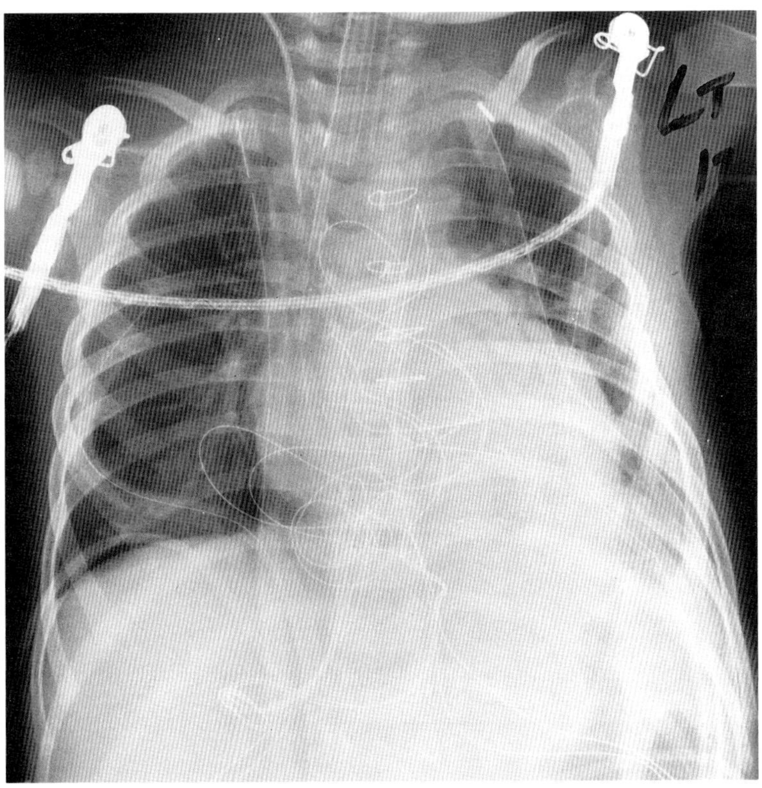

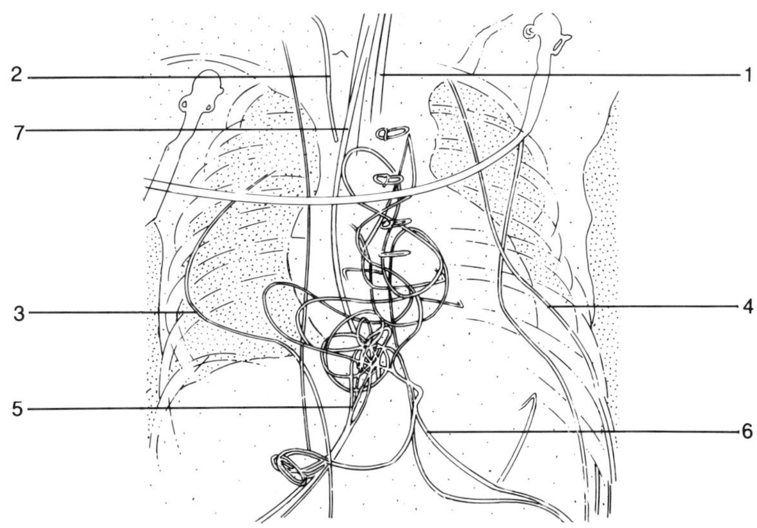

1 endotracheal tube
2 intravenous line
3 right chest tube
4 left chest tube
5 epicardial lead for monitoring right atrial electrical activity
6 epicardial lead for monitoring ventricular electrical activity
7 nasogastric catheter.

Fig. 16.51 Immediate postoperative changes and "hardware." Supine portable chest film immediately after surgery shows a number of tubes, catheters, and monitoring devices. Note mild interstitial edema and left lower lobe atelectasis, common plain film findings in the immediate postoperative period.

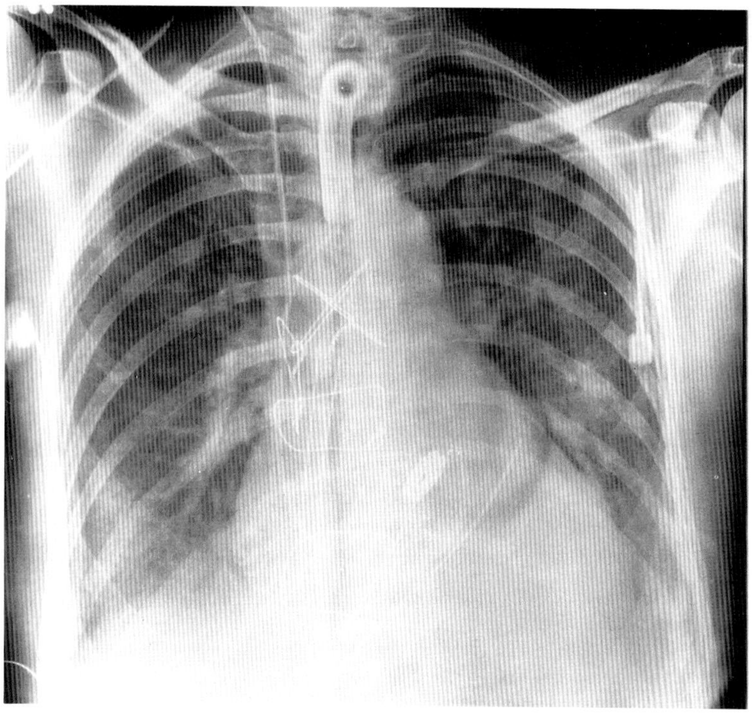

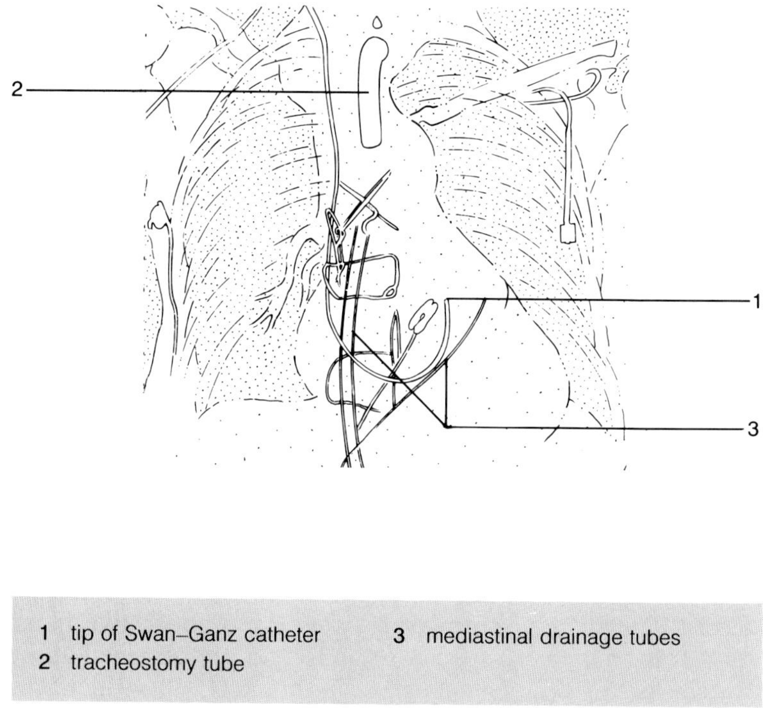

Fig. 16.52 Swan–Ganz catheter. Supine postoperative chest film shows a Swan–Ganz catheter entering the right jugular vein. Its tip is in the right ventricular outflow tract. A tracheostomy tube and mediastinal drainage tubes are also in place.

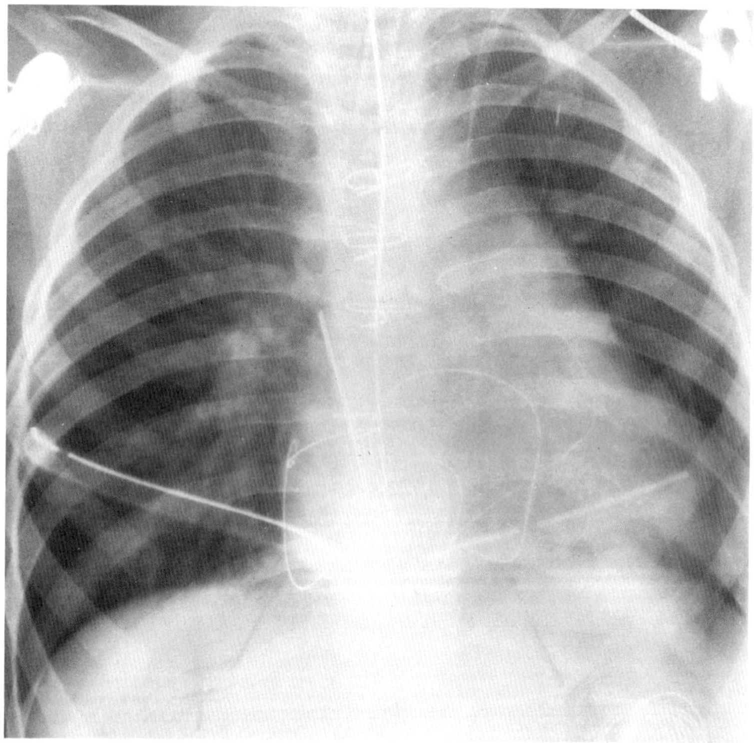

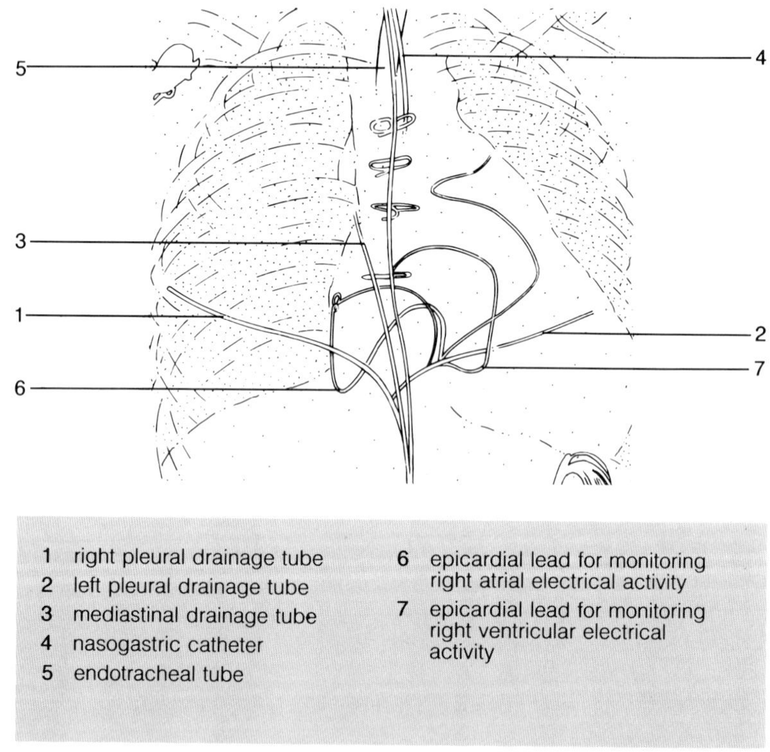

Fig. 16.53 Mediastinal and pleural drainage tubes. A supine portable chest film shows the usual placement of mediastinal and pleural drainage tubes and epicardial monitoring leads. The pleural and mediastinal drains have both been brought out anteriorly.

left atrial pressure cardiac output, provided pulmonary resistance is not markedly elevated. To monitor pulmonary wedge pressure, a pressure-sensing (Swan–Ganz) catheter is passed into the heart via the inferior vena cava, advanced across the tricuspid and pulmonic valves, and allowed to float into a peripheral pulmonary arterial branch (Fig. 16.52). In some patients catheters are also placed in the right and left atrial chambers.

An endotracheal tube is routinely inserted for ventilatory support; its tip should be roughly midway between the carina and the clavicles. Two or three mediastinal drains are left in place. On the frontal film, the pericardial drain is behind and below the heart and anterior mediastinal drains overlie the heart. The mediastinal drainage tubes are brought out through a midline incision. If the pleural space has been opened, one or more pleural drains are left in place and brought out through a midline or a lateral incision (Fig. 16.53). A nasogastric tube is routinely inserted; its tip should be in the stomach.

The heart and mediastinum appear wider on chest films obtained immediately after surgery than on preoperative films. This is not surprising, because the former are obtained at the bedside with the patient supine, using a short (36 to 40 inch) target-film distance (TFD), whereas the latter are usually conventional chest radiographs [ie, posteroanterior projections obtained with the patient erect, using a long (72 inch or greater) TFD]. When the patient's condition permits, a better estimate of heart size can be obtained by portable films obtained in the posterio–anterior projection with a long TFD and the patient erect. Mediastinal structures, such as the descending aorta, are usually obscured as the result of edema or hemorrhage (Fig. 16.54).

Hypoventilation is very common in the early postoperative period. Chest films obtained while the patient is breathing without ventilatory assistance often show slightly decreased lung volume. The lungs tend to be overexpanded on films obtained during the application of positive expiratory pressure.

COMPLICATIONS OF THE EARLY POSTOPERATIVE PERIOD

PULMONARY AND PLEURAL COMPLICATIONS

Atelectasis

Left lower lobe atelectasis is very common during the early postoperative period (Fig. 16.55). Contributory factors include diaphragmatic paresis secondary to intraoperative phrenic nerve trauma, the horizontal course of the left mainstem bronchus (which impedes drainage of secretions), and the inability of the anesthesiologist to suction the left lower lobe bronchus during surgery. Left lower lobe atelectasis usually resolves spontaneously before the end of the first postoperative week. Plate atelectasis, a very common finding, is of no clinical significance and usually clears spontaneously during the second postoperative week.

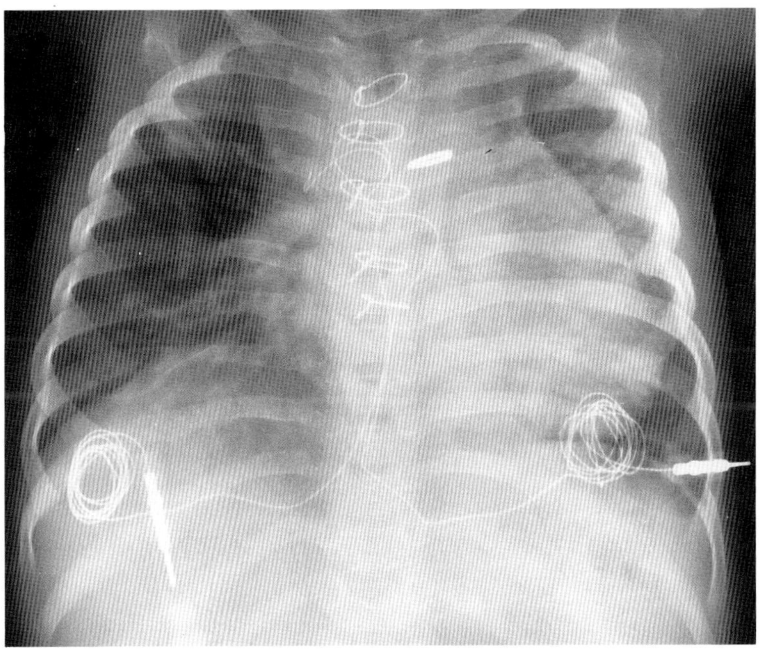

Fig. 16.54 Postoperative mediastinal hemorrhage. Supine portable chest film demonstrates mediastinal widening resulting from mediastinal hemorrhage. There is bilateral pulmonary edema, more severe on the left. Cardiac monitoring leads are in place.

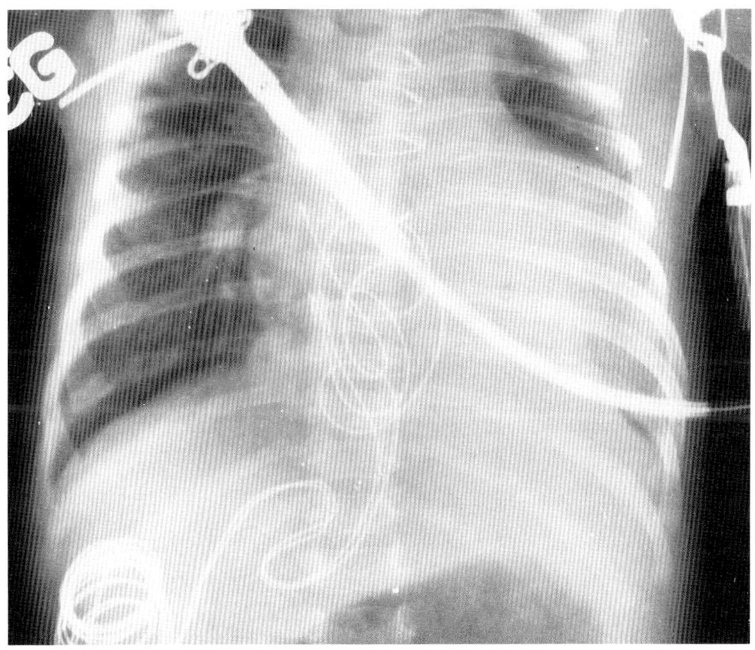

Fig. 16.55 Postoperative left lower lobe atelectasis. A portable chest film obtained immediately after surgery demonstrates a density behind the heart obscuring the diaphragm, which represents the collapsed left lower lobe. There is mild interstitial pulmonary edema. Cardiac monitor leads are in place.

Pulmonary Edema

Postoperative pulmonary edema is very common. Although it may not be evident radiographically, physiologic measurements indicate that pulmonary edema is always present in the first few hours after cardiopulmonary bypass. Postoperative chest films typically show bilateral patchy densities, representing pulmonary edema and/or hemorrhage. When postoperative pulmonary edema persists beyond 48 to 72 hours, the radiographic appearance is typically that of progressive interstitial edema (Fig. 16.56). Postoperative pulmonary edema may be associated with ascites and/or generalized edema.

Several mechanisms are involved in the resolution of postoperative pulmonary edema. Of these, vascular and mechanical factors appear to be the most important. Alveolar and interstitial fluid is cleared by pulmonary capillaries (the rate is driven by a decrease in the oncotic pressure of the interstitial fluid). In addition, interstitial fluid is transported towards the hilum and the pleura through the loose connective tissue that surrounds the blood vessels and bronchi. Edema fluid is also cleared by pulmonary lymphatics and, to a minor extent, by the airways.

Delayed onset interstitial edema, clinically manifested by orthopnea and paradoxical nocturnal dyspnea, may develop during the second postoperative week. It is usually seen in patients who develop pulmonary venous hypertension secondary to ob-

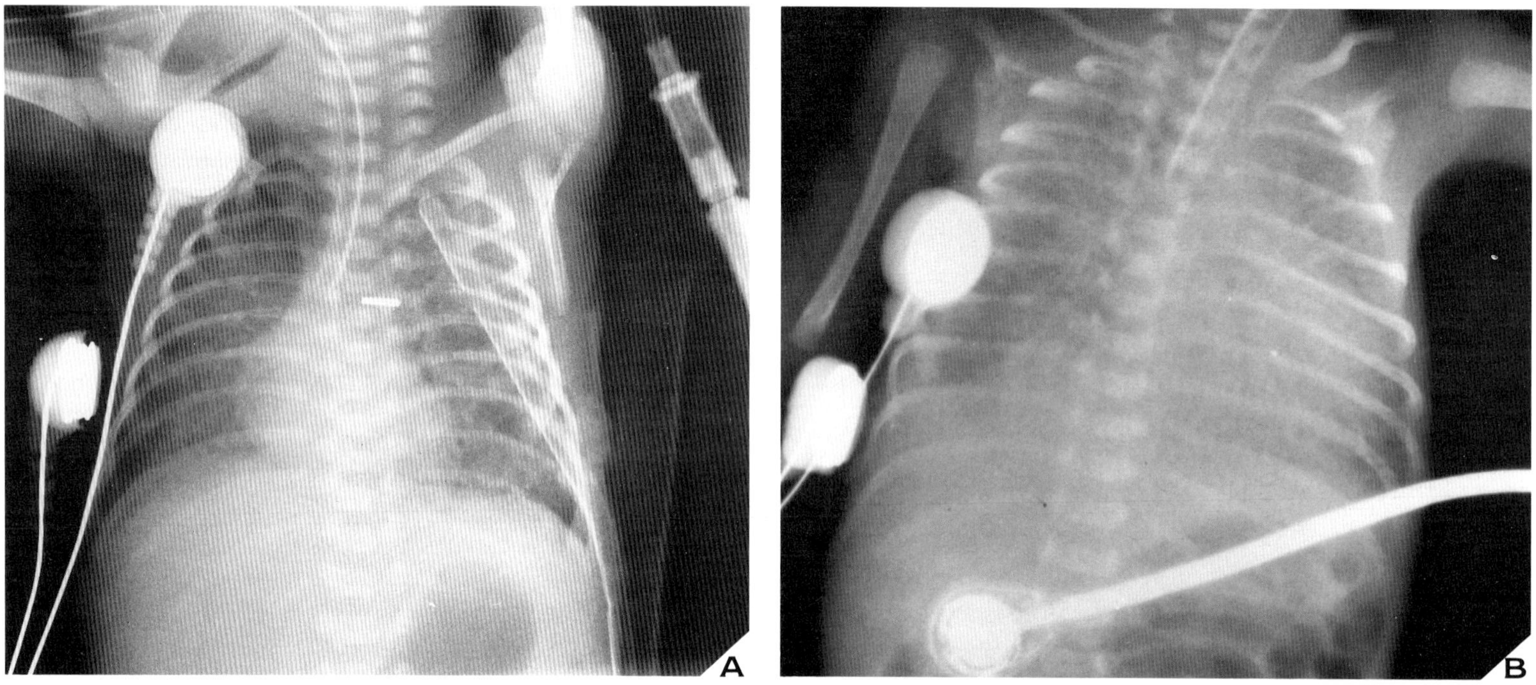

Fig. 16.56 Postoperative pulmonary edema. Early postoperative chest films of two infants demonstrate varying degrees of pulmonary edema. (A) In the first patient, the chest film shows moderate pulmonary edema, manifested by a generalized loss of vascular markings and increased parenchymal density. The endotracheal tube is in the right main bronchus. (B) In the second patient, the chest film shows diffuse opacity of both lungs and loss of the cardiac and diaphragmatic contours, indicating severe pulmonary edema.

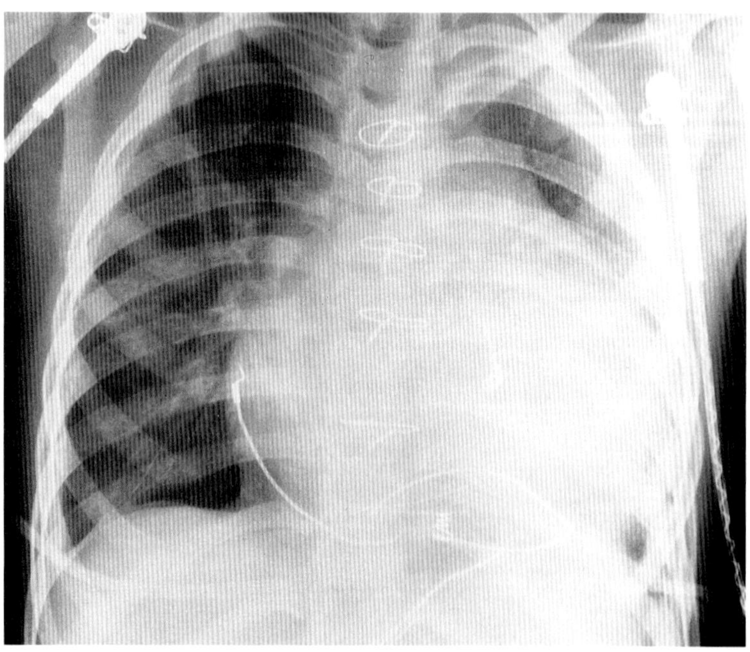

Fig. 16.57 Bilateral hemothorax. Supine film obtained soon after surgery demonstrates a small amount of pleural fluid on the right and a larger amount on the left. When the patient is supine, small amounts of pleural fluid tend to collect in the dependent portion of the thorax and lateral costophrenic angle (as seen at right). Larger effusions tend to collect over the lateral, medial, and apical surfaces of the lung. The latter distribution is seen in the left hemithorax in this patient. A pleural effusion in the immediate postoperative period almost always represents a hemothorax.

struction or to poor left ventricular function. This complication should be suspected when a patient who has been having a normal convalescence begins to cough while lying down or experiences shortness of breath at night. Chest films typically demonstrate interstitial edema, although an occasional patient may exhibit generalized alveolar edema.

Pleural Effusion

Unless the pleural space has been opened, pleural fluid does not accumulate during a normal convalescence. Pleural fluid seen in the immediate postoperative period usually represents blood; a unilateral or bilateral hemothorax is common if the pleura has been violated (Fig. 16.57). A pleural effusion beginning during the first postoperative week usually indicates underlying pulmonary pathology (eg, pneumonia, pulmonary edema). A pleural effusion beginning during or after the third postoperative week is usually due to chylothorax or the postpericardiotomy syndrome (see below).

Pneumothorax

Pneumothorax is an occasional postoperative complication. Although a large pneumothorax is easily detected in an erect patient (Fig. 16.58), a small one may be difficult to appreciate on films obtained on one who is supine. When the patient is supine, intrapleural air tends to collect anteriorly, adjacent to the heart and diaphragm, rather than over the lung apices. Therefore, an unusually deep costophrenic angle, a sharply outlined apical fat pad, or unusual transradiancy of the liver and spleen may be the only radiographic evidence of intrapleural air in a supine patient.

Postoperative Bleeding

Patients who have undergone cardiopulmonary bypass commonly exhibit a bleeding tendency in the immediate postoperative period, manifested by bloody drainage through the pericardial, mediastinal, and pleural drains. A moderate amount of postoperative bleeding is the rule and does not complicate normal convalescence. On the other hand, excessive bleeding or acute cardiac tamponade may necessitate reoperation. A total accumulation of 1500 mL or more in 12 hours should be regarded as excessive in a teenager or adult; a bleeding rate of 300 mL/hr in the first few hours can be considered evidence of acute postoperative hemorrhage. In infants and young children, the bleeding rate must be matched to the patient's size. For example, an accumulation of 100 mL in the first hour is excessive in a 12 kg child.

A marked increase in the width of the cardiac silhouette on a film obtained 8 to 24 hours after surgery is an ominous finding: it usually indicates the presence of a large amount of clot and/or liquid blood within the pericardium. This complication is discussed further in the following section.

CARDIAC AND PERICARDIAL COMPLICATIONS

Acute Complications

Low Cardiac Output. Low cardiac output in the immediate postoperative period can be caused by a decreased preload (eg, low blood volume) or an increased afterload (eg, increased vascular resistance), but the most common causes are related to abnormalities of the heart itself. These include structural defects resulting from an inadequate repair, cardiac tamponade, or depressed myocardial function (with or without myocardial necrosis).

Acute Pericardial Tamponade. Acute pericardial tamponade due to intrapericardial hemorrhage should be considered in patients with a persistently low cardiac output in the early postoperative period. Clinically, there is a rapid hemodynamic deterioration manifested by a rapid rise in right and left atrial pressure, which usually become equal to the end diastolic ventricular pressure. These hemodynamic events can mimic a myocardial infarction.

Chest films usually reveal progressive cardiac enlargement, widening of the superior mediastinum, and clear lung fields. It should be emphasized, however, that the cardiac silhouette may not be enlarged in patients with acute cardiac tamponade. (Delayed tamponade, which is usually

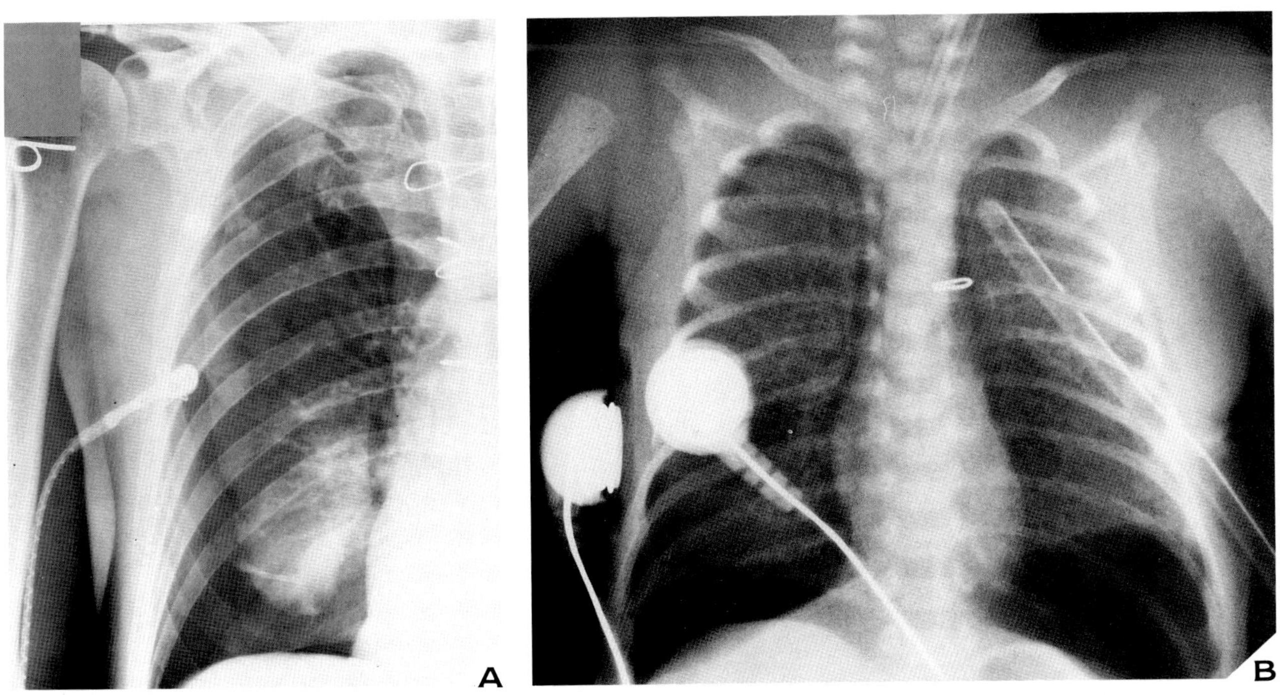

Fig. 16.58 Postoperative pneumothorax. Supine chest films of two patients. (A) Unilateral pneumothorax. The edge of the lung is clearly outlined by air in the pleural space. (B) Bilateral pneumothorax. The severe microcardia and the absence of a mediastinal shift indicate that this is bilateral tension pneumothorax.

more insidious in onset, is almost always associated with an enlarging cardiac silhouette.) The diagnosis is confirmed by echocardiography (Fig. 16.59).

Pneumopericardium is another cause of acute postoperative pericardial tamponade (Fig. 16.60).

Myocardial Depression. Myocardial depression is common in the early postoperative period. It is usually self-limiting, lasting 6 to 18 hours. Acute myocardial infarction is uncommon. The clinical manifestations depend on the extent of the myocardial damage, and the diagnosis is confirmed by typical ECG and enzyme changes. Follow-up studies may reveal abnormal ventricular wall motion or coronary artery occlusion. Acute cardiac failure may also result from excessive loss of functioning myocardium (eg, after an extensive right ventriculotomy).

Subacute and Chronic Complications

Pericardial Effusion. Modest accumulations of pericardial fluid are common after operations in which the pericardium is opened; such collections do not interfere with

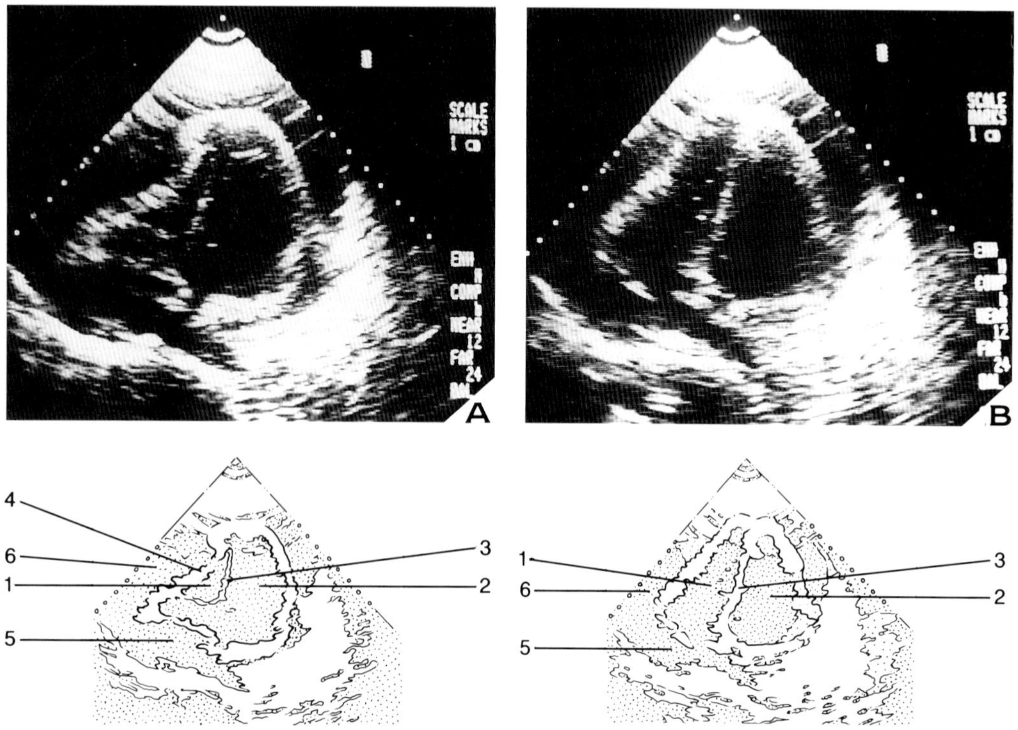

Fig. 16.59 Acute postoperative pericardial tamponade. Echocardiograms (four-chamber view) in diastole (A) and systole (B) demonstrate pericardial fluid. Note medial displacement of the right border of the right ventricle during diastole. This finding reflects decreased right ventricular output, characteristic of acute pericardial tamponade.

1 right ventricle
2 left ventricle
3 ventricular septum
4 displaced right border of right ventricle
5 right atrium
6 pericardial fluid

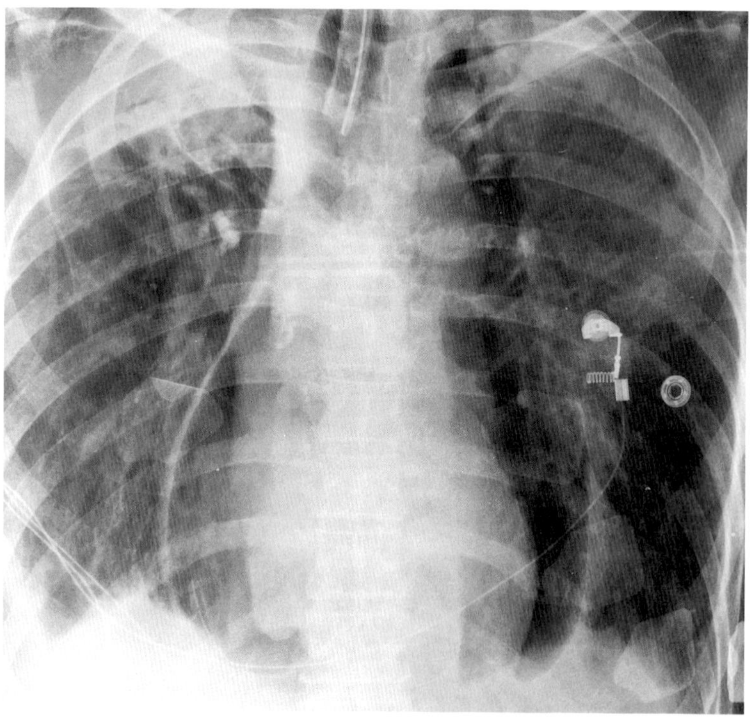

Fig. 16.60 Acute postoperative pericardial tamponade caused by pneumopericardium. The heart is surrounded by air. The pericardium is clearly outlined by air in the pericardial space. A pneumomediastinum is also present (note air outlining structures in upper mediastinum). The small heart and diminished pulmonary vascularity reflect the decreased cardiac output associated with acute pericardial tamponade.

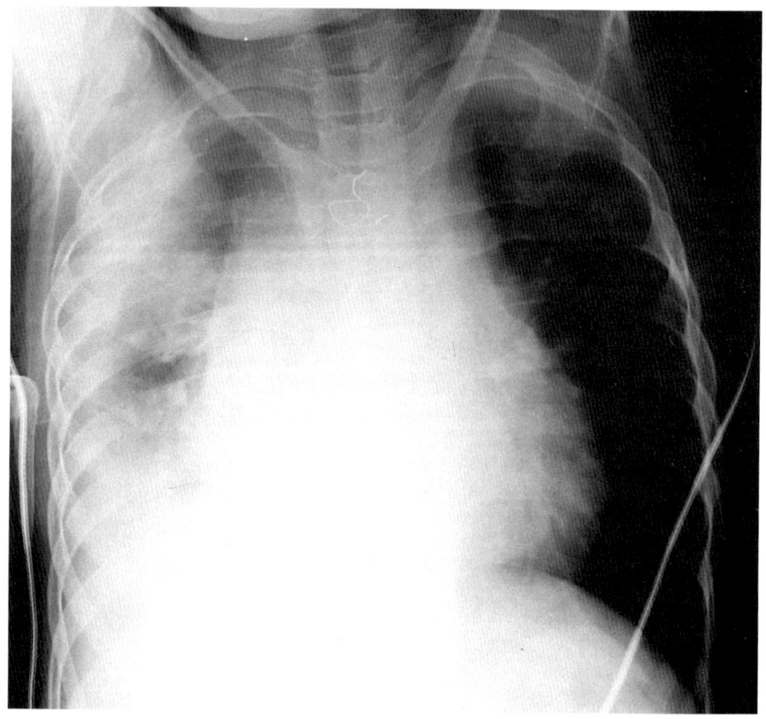

Fig. 16.61 Postpericardiotomy syndrome. This 6-year-old girl had an uneventful postoperative course after an ASD repair until the fourteenth postoperative day, when she began to experience shortness of breath. Right lateral decubitus chest film shows a large right pleural effusion. The fullness of the left upper mediastinal border suggests the presence of a pericardial effusion, which was confirmed by echocardiography.

normal convalescence. Significant pericardial effusions are demonstrated by echocardiography 4 to 10 days after surgery in a small percentage of patients. These effusions, which tend to occur in patients with excessive early postoperative bleeding, typically peak on the tenth postoperative day and regress spontaneously. The affected patients are usually asymptomatic and require no specific therapy; however, tamponade requiring pericardiocentesis occurs in about 1 percent.

Delayed onset pericardial tamponade is manifested clinically by the late onset (days or weeks after surgery) of progressive weakness, lethargy, dyspnea, orthopnea, hepatomegaly, ascites, and peripheral edema. Physical examination reveals pulsus paradoxicus and an elevated jugular venous pressure. Chest films show an enlarged cardiac silhouette, and echocardiography confirms the diagnosis. (Unexplained cardiac enlargement on a chest film obtained just before discharge warrants echocardiography to rule out an unsuspected pericardial effusion, even when the patient is asymptomatic.) Cardiac catheterization reveals equalization of the right atrial and right ventricular end diastolic pressures and elevation of the pulmonary wedge (capillary) pressure.

Postperfusion (Postpericardiotomy) Syndrome. Patients with this uncommon disorder present weeks or months after open heart surgery with fever and unilateral anterior chest pain, simulating pleuritis. Laboratory studies reveal monocytic leukocytosis, an elevated erthrocyte sedimentation rate, and high titers of anticardiac antibodies. Chest films and echocardiograms reveal pericardial and/or pleural effusion (Fig. 16.61). The amount of fluid is usually small and does not correspond to the severity of the symptoms. Constrictive pericarditis is a rare complication.

COMPLICATIONS OF THORACOTOMY

Posterolateral Thoractomy

A posterolateral thoracotomy through the third or fourth intercostal space is the standard approach for many operations used to treat congenital heart disease. Occasionally a rib is resected, although in most instances adequate exposure can be obtained by widening an intercostal space with a rib spreader. Early complications include wound dehiscence, costal chondritis, and intercostal nerve injury. Scoliosis, with the convexity of the curve opposite the side of the thoracotomy, is an infrequent late complication.

Median Sternotomy

Many cardiac defects are best approached through a median sternotomy. Complications of median sternotomy are related to pleural and pericardial trauma, damage to mediastinal structures, and injury to the sternum itself. Edema at the sternotomy site occurs in a small percentage of cases and subsides in a few days. Sternal osteomyelitis or chondritis should be suspected when the sternum becomes unstable or when there is drainage through the sternum, sternal tenderness, or persistent central chest pain. Chest films demonstrate swelling of the pre- and retrosternal soft tissues and/or gas (produced by bacterial activity) in the soft tissues; typical radiographic changes of osteomyelitis may appear after a few weeks (Fig. 16.62). Because sternal separation is usually due to the wires pulling through the bone, any change in the relative position of the wires, or rotation of the axis of a given suture, suggests sternal dehiscence. (The sternotomy defect itself often appears as a radiolucent cleft. The presence of a cleft is of no consequence unless it is very wide or is accompanied by a shift of the sutures to one side.)

CT can be very helpful in evaluating wound complications. Presternal soft tissue infection is characterized by edema of the presternal soft tissues and loss of the normal tissue planes. Localized air collections and minimal sternal separation are seen in some patients. Anterior mediastinitis is characterized by extensive low-density (0 to 15 Hounsfield units) fluid in the anterior mediastinum (sometimes associated with a pericardial effusion), obliteration of all fat planes, formation of large air pockets, and a wide gap (2 to 10 mm) between the sternal segments. Persistence of pre- and retrosternal soft tissue swelling suggests sternal osteomyelitis, and breakdown of the bone confirms the diagnosis.

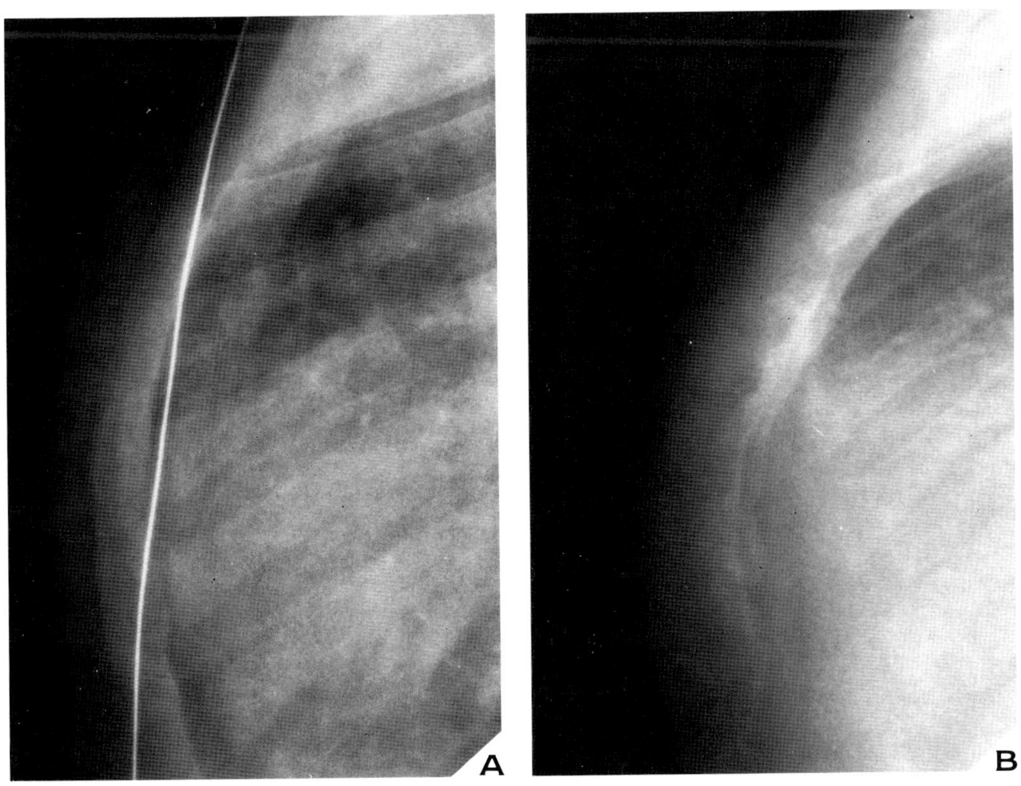

Fig. 16.62 Postoperative sternal osteomyelitis. This 11-month-old girl developed a resistant wound infection after complete repair of an endocardial cushion defect. The wound was explored to the pericardium; the sternum was necrotic and cultures grew out *Pseudomonas* species. Despite continued antibiotic treatment the wound continued to drain and wound cultures were positive for *Staphylococcus aureus*. (A) Initial postoperative radiograph shows soft tissue swelling but the sternum appears intact. (B) Repeat film (three months later) shows marked lysis of the sternal segments. (Courtesy of John C. Leonidas, MD, New Hyde Park, NY.) Reproduced by permission from Kassner EG (ed): *Iatrogenic Disorders of the Fetus, Infant, and Child*. Springer-Verlag, New York, 1985)

Other complications of median sternotomy include rib fracture, which is most readily detected on radionuclide bone scans, and brachial plexus injury. Because mediastinal drains are customarily left in place after median sternotomy, inadvertent injury to abdominal structures (peritoneum, liver, stomach, small intestine, colon, spleen) is another potential hazard. The injury may not become apparent until after the tube is removed and omentum, bile, ascites fluid, gastric juice, or blood appears at the cutaneous end of the drainage tract.

COMPLICATIONS OF THE MEDIASTINAL DISSECTION

Phrenic Nerve Injury

Unilateral diaphragmatic paralysis is a recognized complication of operations that entail dissection in proximity to the phrenic nerve (eg, Blalock–Taussig shunt, Mustard procedure, coarctation repair). Phrenic nerve injury is especially likely to occur during secondary operations, because fibrous adhesions resulting from the initial operation may obscure anatomic relationships. Radiologic diagnosis usually presents no difficulty. In a typical case, serial postoperative films show persistent elevation of the affected hemidiaphragm (Fig. 16.63A). Typical radiographic findings may be absent during the early postoperative period, however, because the paralyzed hemidiaphragm is maintained in normal position while the patient is being mechanically ventilated. Sonography, which can be performed at the bedside, or fluoroscopy will confirm the absence of diaphragmatic movement (Fig. 16.63B).

Unilateral diaphragmatic paralysis is usually well tolerated by patients over 18 months of age. However, it may have serious consequences in young infants, leading to atelectasis, postextubation stridor, CO_2 retention, and respiratory acidosis. Difficulty in weaning the infant from the ventilator may be the first indication of this complication.

The prognosis depends on the severity of the phrenic nerve injury. If the nerve has been transected, permanent paralysis is the rule. However, recovery (usually within 6 months) can be anticipated with most injuries caused by blunt trauma, stretching, or electrocautery.

Chylothorax

Chylothorax is an uncommon postoperative complication. The reported incidence is 0.018 to 0.5 percent in series that include both children and adults, and 0.37 to 1.5 percent in exclusively pediatric series. It is typically seen after operations that entail mobilization of the left subclavian artery and/or aortic arch, such as the Blalock–Taussig shunt, insertion of external conduits, PDA closure, vascular ring repairs, and coarctation repair. In such cases the chylothorax usually results from operative trauma to tributaries of the thoracic duct or, less commonly, from injury to the thoracic duct itself. The latter is most likely to occur during operations in the vicinity of the aortic isthmus (eg, Blalock–Taussig anastomosis, PDA closure, coarctation repair). Chylothorax is not uncommon in patients who have undergone the Fontan, Glenn, or Mustard procedure, in which case it is believed to result from the elevated su-

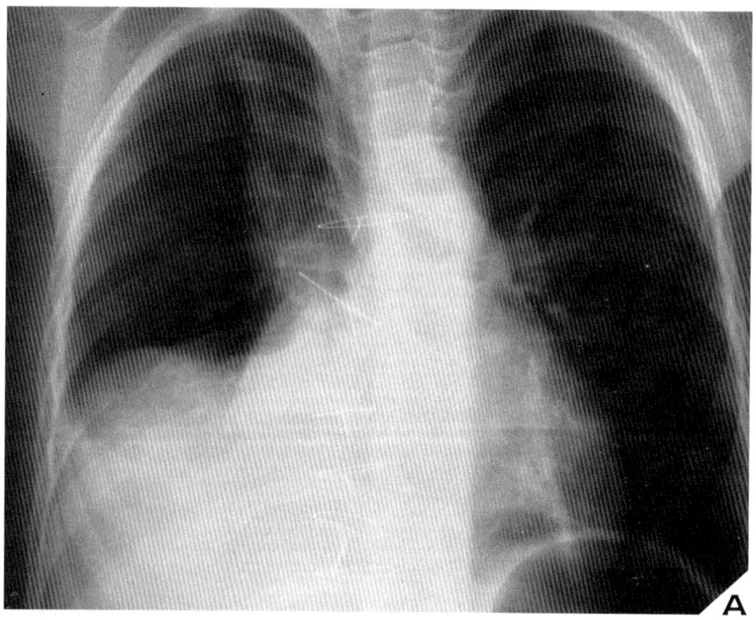

Fig. 16.63 Postoperative diaphragmatic paralysis. This four-year-old girl underwent complete correction of a VSD with pulmonic stenosis through a median sternotomy; a small right atriotomy was made for closure of the foramen ovale. Postoperatively she was tachypneic. Physical examination revealed decreased movements of the right side of the chest and markedly diminished breath sounds over the lower right chest. (A) An erect chest film on the seventh postoperative day shows a density at the right base, which was initially interpreted as a right subpulmonic effusion. (B) Sonogram. Transverse sector scan (transducer at right costal margin and angled cephalad) shows the dome of the liver in a higher position than normal. There is no fluid in the posterior costophrenic sulcus. A follow-up chest film one year later showed persistent elevation of the right hemidiaphragm. Sonography, which can be performed at the bedside, is very helpful in differentiating pleural effusion from diaphragmatic paralysis in the early postoperative period. (Reproduced by permission from Kassner EG (ed): *Iatrogenic Disorders of the Fetus, Infant, and Child.* Springer-Verlag, New York, 1985)

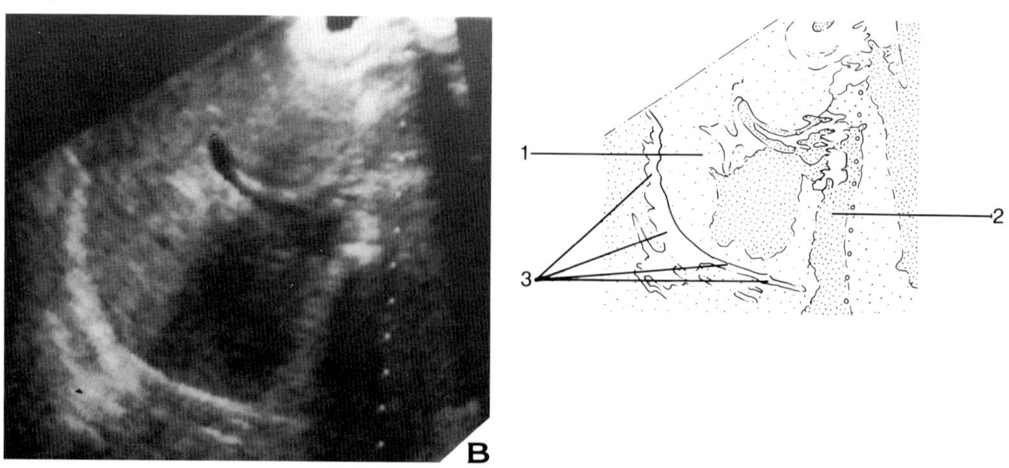

1 liver
2 spine (acoustic shadow)
3 diaphragm

perior vena caval pressure that commonly follows these operations. Because marked elevation of SVC pressure in experimental animals does not result in a chylothorax, it is believed that patients who develop this complication have congenital variations of the thoracic lymphatics that allow thoracic duct chyle to reflux into the lungs (and thence into the pleural space) when SVC pressure is elevated.

Clinical signs (dyspnea, tachypnea, and low-grade fever) usually do not appear for a week or more after surgery; the latent period may be as long as 6 weeks. (Diminished chyle flow secondary to the patient's relative inactivity and restricted oral intake probably account for the frequent failure of chyle to accumulate in clinically significant amounts during the early postoperative period.) Chest radiographs show a pleural effusion, which may be massive (Figs. 16.64 and 16.65). Mediastinal widening resulting from the accumulation of chyle ("chyloma")

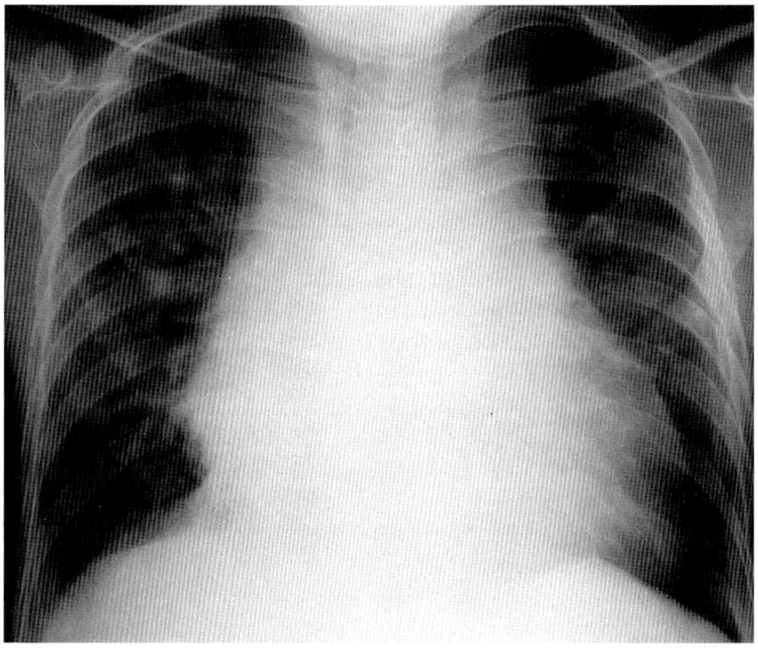

Fig. 16.64 Postoperative chylomediastinum and chylothorax. Supine and right lateral decubitus chest films obtained one week after a VSD repair in a 10-year-old boy show widening of the mediastinum and a large right pleural effusion. Sonography (not illustrated) demonstrated a mediastinal fluid collection. Thoracocentesis revealed a chylous effusion.

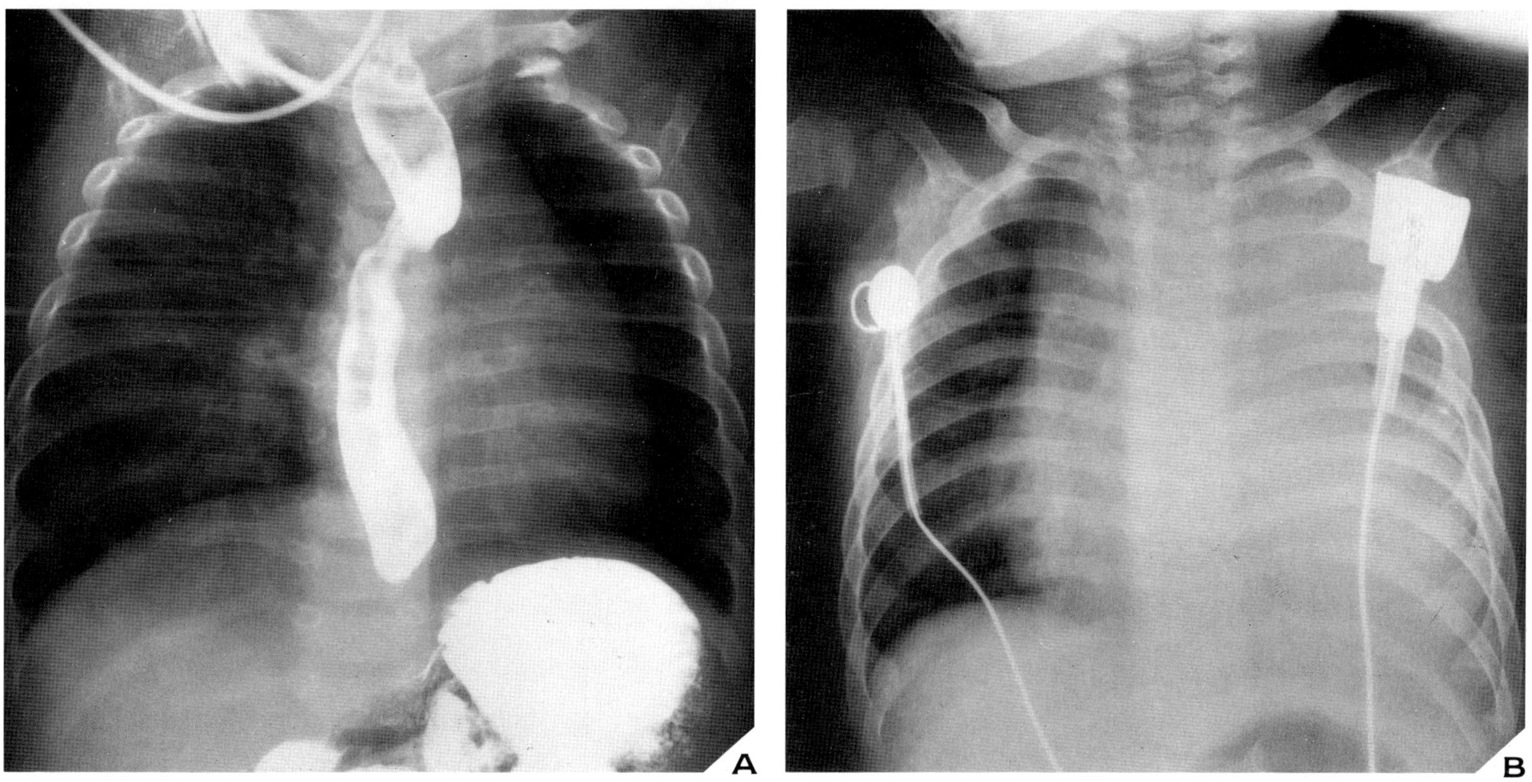

Fig. 16.65 Postoperative chylothorax. This 5-month-old boy had a vascular ring consisting of a right aortic arch, left descending thoracic aorta, and left ligamentum arteriosum. After corrective surgery (left thoracotomy with division of the ligamentum arteriosum), milky drainage from the chest tube was noted on the third postoperative day. (A) Preoperative esophagram shows bilateral indentations on the esophagus caused by the vascular ring. (B) Chest film on the fourth postoperative day shows a massive left pleural effusion with a contralateral mediastinal shift. Despite treatment with a medium-chain triglyceride formula, the chest tube continued to drain as much as 300–400 mL of milky fluid each day. The chyle drainage subsided during the third postoperative week and he was discharged on postoperative day 23. (Reproduced by permission from Kassner EG (Ed); *Iatrogenic Disorders of the Fetus, Infant, and Child.* Springer-Verlag, New York, 1985)

may precede the onset of the pleural effusion, usually becoming less conspicuous or disappearing when the latter appears. Sonography or CT can be used to confirm the cystic nature of the mediastinal mass.

OTHER COMPLICATIONS OF THE EARLY POSTOPERATIVE PERIOD

Renal, gastrointestinal, and neurologic problems may also occur in the early postoperative period (Fig. 16.66). In most instances, these sequelae are the result of decreased cardiac output.

LONG-TERM EFFECTS OF SURGERY FOR CONGENITAL HEART DISEASE

THORACOTOMY

Asymmetry of the soft tissues, deformity of the ribs, and localized pleural thickening indicate a previous left or right posterolateral thoracotomy. The presence of radiopaque sternal wires indicates that the patient has undergone a median sternotomy (nonopaque sutures are occasionally used in infants). Although broken sternal wires can be a source of local chest pain, they are usually of no significance.

A right thoracotomy is commonly employed for palliative shunts [eg, a right Blalock–Taussig (Fig. 16.67) or Waterston anastomosis in patients with a left aortic arch] and for the Glenn procedure (superior vena cava–right pulmonary artery anastomosis); it is seldom if ever employed for intracardiac operations. A left thoracotomy is employed for a left Blalock–Taussig or Pott's anastomosis, ductus ligation, and repair of aortic coarctation. Most intracardiac operations, including the definitive repair of complex malformations, are performed through a median sternotomy, which provides the best access to the ventricular septum, right ventricular outflow tract, and pulmonic valve.

The nature of the thoracotomy can be a helpful clue when the clinical history is unknown. Thus, the presence of a left or right thoracotomy *and* a median sternotomy suggests that the pa-

FIG. 16.66 SYSTEMIC COMPLICATIONS OF THE EARLY POSTOPERATIVE PERIOD

System	Complication
Metabolic	Metabolic acidosis Metabolic alkalosis Hyperthermia Hypoglycemia
Renal	Acute renal insufficiency Acute tubular necrosis Acute cortical necrosis
Neurologic	Seizures (generalized or focal) Flaccid decorticate state (poor prognosis) Choreoathetoid movements
Gastrointestinal	Abdominal distension Massive gastrointestinal bleeding Stress ulcer Gastritis Jaundice Esophagitis Perforation of preexisting peptic ulcer Acute cholecystitis, cholelithiasis

Fig. 16.66 Systemic complications of the early postoperative period.

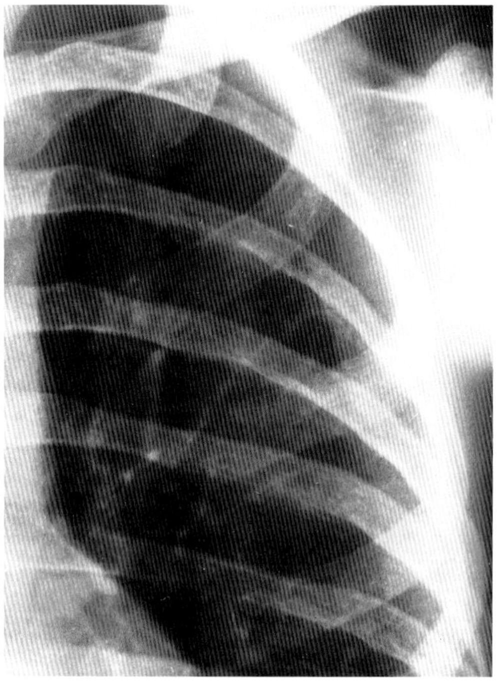

Fig. 16.67 Plain film findings after Blalock–Taussig anastomosis for tetratology of Fallot. The site of the previous thoracotomy, performed during infancy, is indicated by the deformity of the left third, fourth, and fifth posterior ribs. Note notching of the left third and fourth ribs produced by enlarged intercostal arteries providing collateral circulation. The deformity of the left upper mediastinal border is the result of the previous surgery. The heart and pulmonary vasculature are unremarkable.

tient had a congenital defect causing cyanosis (eg, tetralogy of Fallot), that he was initially treated with a palliative shunt, and that he subsequently underwent a definitive repair.

EXTRACARDIAC SHUNTS

After a classical Blalock–Taussig anastomosis, the distal subclavian artery is supplied by collaterals that originate from the upper descending aorta. Large collateral channels cause notching of the second and third ribs, a location different from that usually associated with coarctation of the aorta (Fig. 16.67). Rib notching does not occur when a Goretex tube is used to connect the subclavian and pulmonary arteries, because the distal subclavian artery is not disconnected from the aortic arch.

After a Blalock or Waterston anastomosis, the left atrium increases in size, although this usually cannot be appreciated on chest films. The pulmonary vascularity is usually increased after a palliative shunt; indeed, improved pulmonary perfusion can often be appreciated on immediate postoperative (recovery room) films in patients whose preoperative chest films showed severe pulmonary oligemia. The increased flow across the anastomosis should be distributed equally to both lungs. Symmetrical enlargement of the left and right pulmonary arteries indicates a wide anastomosis and an unobstructed confluence of the pulmonary arteries, whereas asymmetrical enlargement of the pulmonary arteries indicates stenosis of the artery supplying the underperfused lung, a not uncommon postoperative complication in patients with tetralogy of Fallot and pulmonary atresia (Figs. 16.68 and 16.69).

The long-term effects of systemic–pulmonary shunt on the right ventricle are important. After a palliative shunt the stenosis of the right ventricular outflow tract may become tighter,

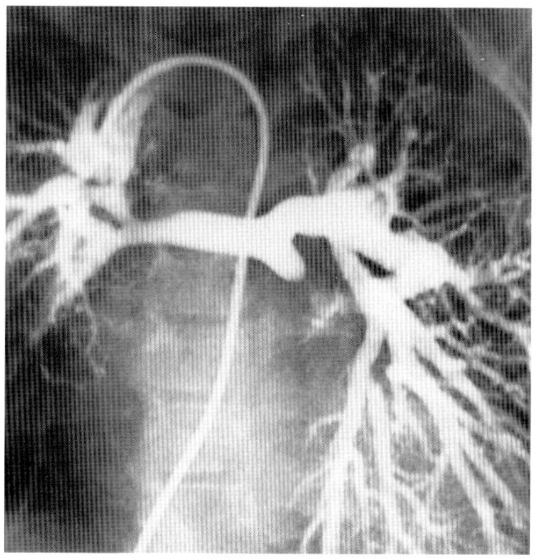

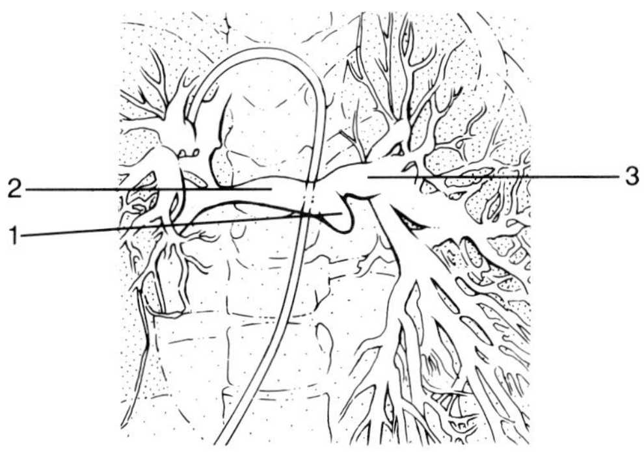

1 pulmonary trunk
2 right pulmonary artery
3 left pulmonary artery

Fig. 16.68 Asymmetrical pulmonary perfusion after palliative shunt. Frontal projection of pulmonary arteriogram in a patient with right Blalock–Taussig anastomosis (obtained after selective injection of the right subclavian artery) demonstrates stenosis of the right pulmonary artery at the level of the hilum. The origin of the artery supplying the right upper lobe is also narrowed. The branches to the right lower lobe are not opacified, presumably owing to the presence of aortopulmonary collaterals. In contrast, the entire left lung is well perfused. The pulmonary branches on the left are much larger than those on the right. Marked asymmetry of the pulmonary vasculature was also evident on frontal chest films (not illustrated).

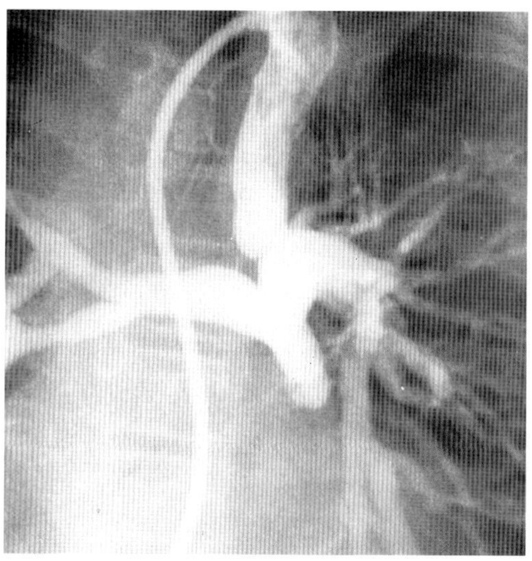

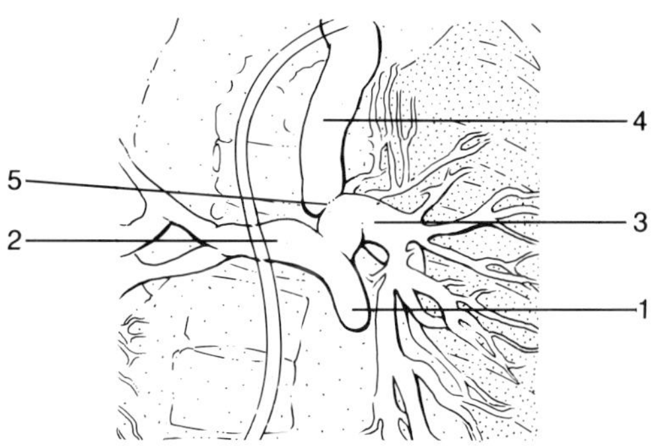

1 pulmonary trunk
2 right pulmonary artery
3 left pulmonary artery
4 left subclavian artery
5 left Blalock–Taussig anastomosis

Fig. 16.69 Asymmetrical pulmonary perfusion after Blalock–Taussig anastomosis. Pulmonary arteriogram in a patient with a left Blalock–Taussig anastomosis, obtained after selective injection of the left subclavian artery, shows opacification of the pulmonary vasculature of both lungs. Arborization of the right lung is abnormal; there are fewer branches than on the left and there are no branches supplying the right upper lobe. The left pulmonary artery is larger than the right and supplies the entire left lung. In this patient the asymmetrical vascularity is due to stenosis of branches of the right pulmonary artery.

causing further right ventricular hypertrophy and eventually leading to complete obliteration of the right ventricle–pulmonary artery connection.

CHEST FILMS AFTER COMPLETE REPAIR OF TETRALOGY OF FALLOT

After operations that employ extracardiac conduits (eg, the Rastelli procedure), chest films show prominence of the left heart border and fullness of the retrosternal space; the mediastinal "mass" represents the conduit (Fig. 16.70). Conduits that incorporate a prosthetic valve have a metallic ring which shows the position of the valve (Fig. 16.70); calcification within the ring indicates significant deterioration of the valve, which may or may not have hemodynamic consequences (Fig. 16.71). Conduits that incorporate a homograft aortic valve do not have a metallic ring.

After a successful total repair, chest films typically show a normal-sized heart with prominence of the right ventricle. The pulmonary arteries are usually of normal size (in an occasional patient they may be smaller than normal). Cardiomegaly with right ventricular and right atrial enlargement, often accompanied by dilatation of the azygos vein, indicates right ventricular failure with tricuspid insufficiency (Fig. 16.71). Significant enlargement of the right ventricular outflow tract on frontal and lateral projections strongly suggests the presence of postoperative pulmonic insufficiency. In patients with this complication, cardiac fluoroscopy reveals massive dilatation of the pulmonary arteries during systole and collapse during diastole. Left ventricular enlargment is uncommon; when present, it is usually a sign of aortic insufficiency.

The presence of a conduit (indicated by a metallic ring) usually indicates a severe malformation, with pulmonary atresia

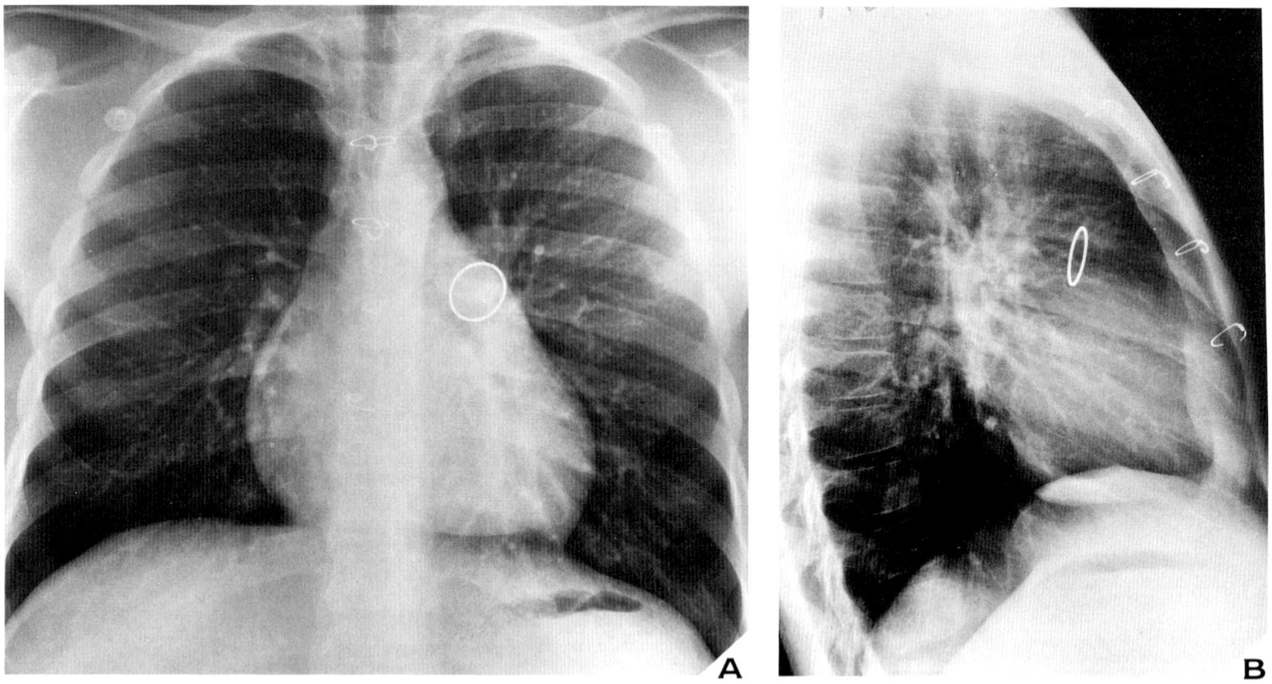

Fig. 16.70 Complete repair of tetralogy of Fallot. (A) Frontal and (B) lateral chest films of a patient with tetralogy of Fallot and pulmonary atresia who had undergone complete repair with insertion of a valved external conduit several years earlier. The site of the conduit is indicated by the slight bulge of the left upper heart border (metallic ring indicates the position of the heterograft valve). The right atrium and right ventricle are slightly enlarged. The pulmonary vasculature is normal.

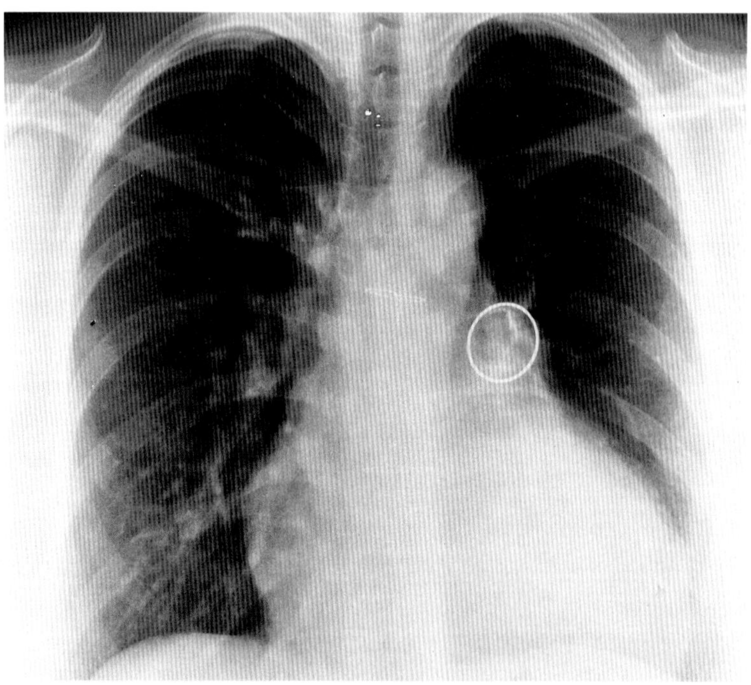

Fig. 16.71 Calcification of heterograft valve and right ventricular failure after complete repair of tetralogy of Fallot. This patient had a complete repair with insertion of a valved external conduit (Rastelli operation) several years earlier. Note extensive calcification within the metallic ring, indicating deterioration of the heterograft valve. Note also the marked right ventricular and right atrial enlargement, which presumably reflects right ventricular failure and tricuspid insufficiency.

and abnormal arborization of the pulmonary arteries. The abnormal pulmonary vascular pattern will persist postoperatively even in patients with a good functional result.

CHEST FILMS AFTER REPAIR OF LEFT TO RIGHT SHUNTS

The plain film findings associated with a large left to right shunt—enlargement of the central pulmonary arteries, plethora, and cardiac enlargement—persist in the early postoperative period. In infants, pulmonary plethora disappears after a period of weeks or months. In adults, especially patients over 50 years of age with ASD, enlargement of the central, lobar, and segmental arteries may persist for months or years. In infants and children with marked right ventricular and right atrial enlargement, films obtained a week after surgery show a decrease in heart size. This is not the case in adults, however, some of whom continue to exhibit marked right ventricular and right atrial enlargement for many years. When preoperative films show only minimal right ventricular and right atrial enlargement, postoperative films are not likely to demonstrate any significant change.

CHEST FILMS AFTER REPAIR OF COARCTATION OF THE AORTA

In patients with a left descending thoracic aorta, the repair is done through a left thoracotomy (in patients with a right descending aorta, it is done on the right). After coarctation repair the appearnace of the aortic arch may change slightly, but the normally rounded appearance of the arch is never restored. Irregularity of the left upper mediastinal border is a common finding. In some patients, rib notching disappears after a successful repair. This is most likely to occur in patients who were 10 to 20 years old at the time of the repair. Rib notching seldom disappears completely in patients who undergo surgery after 30 years of age.

Massive enlargement of the aortic arch, projecting either anteriorly or posteriorly, usually indicates a complication such as pseudoaneurysm of the pre- or postcoarctation segment (see Fig. 16.44). When a prosthetic tube has been used for the repair, the presence of a mediastinal "mass" may indicate detachment of the prosthesis. Postoperative calcification of the post-stenotic segment is quite common.

CHAPTER 17

Plain Film Diagnosis of Congenital Heart Disease in the Adult

Plain films continue to play a central role in the evaluation of adults with known or suspected congenital heart disease. An orderly assessment of the bony thorax, abdominal situs, mediastinal structures, pulmonary vasculature, and cardiac silhouette may be very informative in such patients.

ABNORMALITIES OF THE BONY THORAX

Some cardiac malformations are commonly associated with abnormalities of the ribs, sternum, and/or thoracic spine; conversely, certain abnormalities of the thoracic cage are associated with specific cardiac malformations. Cardiac malformations and abnormalities of the bony thorax coexist in a number of genetic disorders (see Chapter 5). For example, patients with Down syndrome (trisomy 21) commonly have 11 ribs and scoliosis. Females with Turner syndrome, a disorder involving a defective or absent X chromosome, may have coarctation of the aorta, a short neck with fusion of the cervical vertebrae (Klippel–Feil anomaly), and vertebral abnormalities resembling Scheurmann's disease. Abnormalities of the shoulder girdle are not uncommon in patients with the Holt–Oram syndrome, a familial disorder characterized by atrial septal defect, conduction defects, and abnormalities of the upper extremities (see Fig. 5.5).

RIBS

Bilateral rib notching, caused by dilated and tortuous intercostal arteries, is common in patients with coarctation of the aorta (Fig. 17.1; see also Fig. 12.27). In exceptional cases, the coar-

CHAPTER LABELING KEY	
RV right ventricle	Ao aorta
LV left ventricle	PT pulmonary trunk

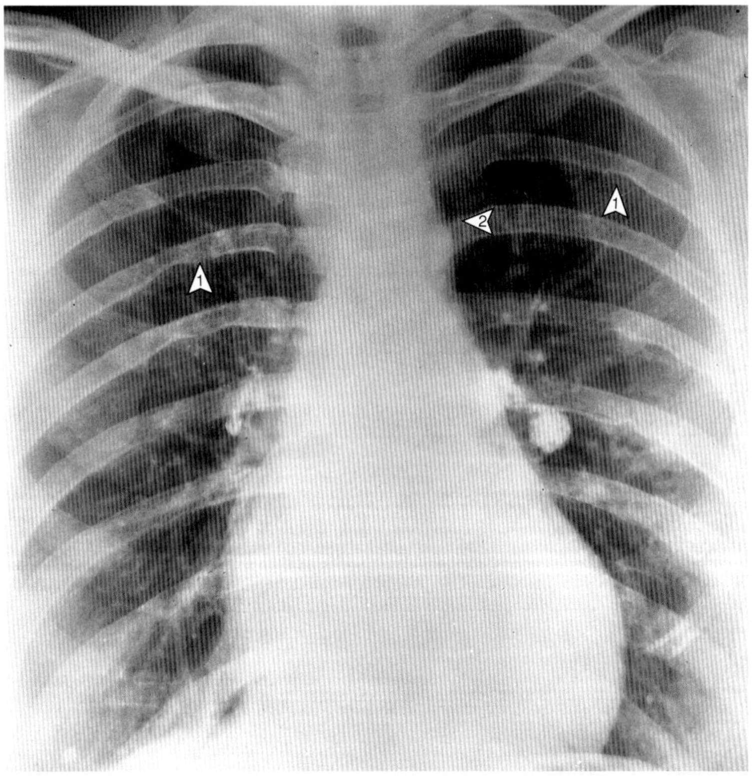

Fig. 17.1 Rib notching. Frontal projection of the chest in a patient with coarctation of the aorta demonstrates bilateral rib notching (*arrows* 1) secondary to dilatation and tortuosity of the intercostal arteries. The diminutive aortic arch (*arrow* 2) is another classic feature of coarctation of the aorta. Incidentally noted are calcified hilar lymph nodes.

cted segment is proximal to the origin of one of the subclavian arteries, in which event unilateral rib notching may occur. Rib notching is common in patients with cyanotic congenital heart disease who have undergone palliative Blalock–Taussig (pulmonary artery to subclavian artery) shunt early in life (Fig. 17.2; see also Fig. 16.67).

STERNUM

Early fusion of sternal segments (manubrial–sternal joint or mesosternum) occurs more often in patients with cyanotic congenital malformations than in the general population, and may be a clue to the presence of congenital heart disease. Delayed fusion of the sternal segments is not uncommon in patients with various cardiac defects (Fig. 17.3).

SPINE

Scoliosis is present in 6 percent of patients with cyanotic disorders and in 0.8 percent of those with acyanotic defects. It is much more common in females with cyanotic defects than in males with acyanotic defects. The spinal curvature usually involves the thoracoabdominal segment, although on occasion only the thoracic spine is affected. A rotatory component is

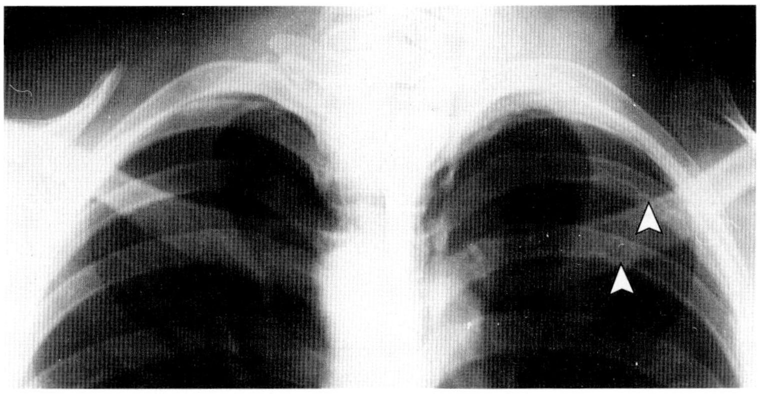

Fig. 17.2 Unilateral rib notching following palliative shunt. Chest film of a 20-year-old patient with tetralogy of Fallot who had previously undergone a left Blalock–Taussig anastomosis shows notching (*arrows*) of the left second and third ribs.

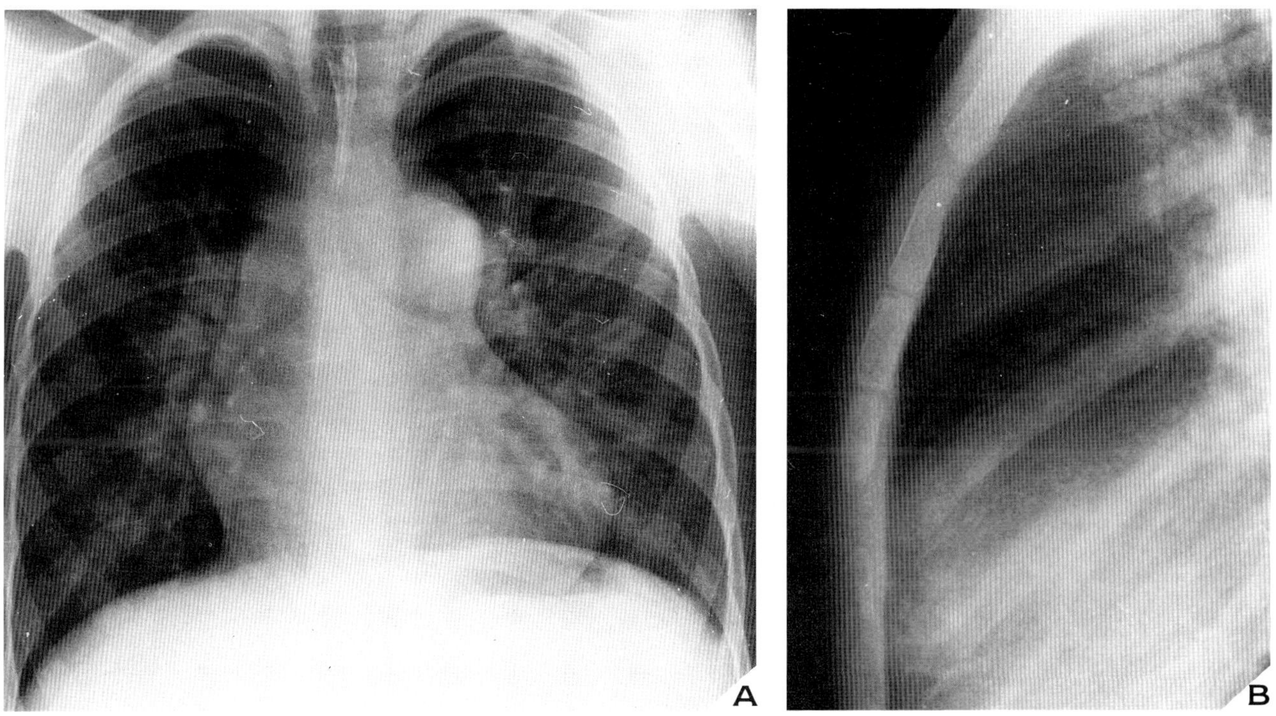

Fig. 17.3 Sternal malformation associated with ventricular septal defect. (A) Frontal and (B) lateral projections show delayed fusion of the sternal segments in an 8-year-old patient with an interventricular septal defect. The enlarged right ventricle, pulmonary plethora, and enlarged pulmonary trunk indicate the presence of a left to right shunt.

usually present (Fig. 17.4). Although an underlying structural malformation (eg, butterfly vertebra or hemivertebrae) is present in a small percentage of cases, a cause for the scoliosis usually cannot be identified.

Kyphoscoliosis and deformities of the anterior chest wall are common in Marfan syndrome, a familial connective tissue disorder associated with aneurysms of the aortic root and mitral insufficiency resulting from prolapse of the mitral valve. Chest films typically show a disproportion between the vertical and the transverse diameter of the thoracic vertebral bodies, as well as an elongated thorax (Fig. 17.5).

ABNORMALITIES OF ABDOMINAL SITUS

Abdominal situs, which does not necessarily correspond to atrial situs, is determined by the position of the stomach and liver. Situs solitus and situs inversus are usually associated with normal visceroatrial relationships, ie, the inferior vena cava drains into the systemic atrium and the normally lateralized liver lies beneath the systemic atrium. Abdominal situs and thoracic situs may not be congruent in patients with atrial isomerism, who often have anomalous patterns of systemic and/or pulmonary venous return (see Chapter 8) (Fig. 17.6).

MEDIASTINAL STRUCTURES

A systematic assessment of the tracheobronchial tree, aortic arch, ascending aorta, descending aorta, pulmonary trunk, and the superior and inferior caval veins may provide important clues in an adult patient with suspected congenital heart disease.

THE AORTIC ARCH

The aortic arch, which gives rise to the brachiocephalic arteries, lies between the ascending and descending segments of the thoracic aorta. A normal (ie, left) arch lies to the left of the trachea, and can be identified on frontal chest films as a round density at the superior margin of the left mediastinal contour. It typically produces a discrete indentation on the left margin of the trachea.

The aortic arch tends to be prominent in conditions associated with excessive blood flow through the systemic circulation. These include certain acyanotic disorders (eg, patent ductus arteriosus) and cyanotic defects in which most of the right ventricular output passes through the aorta (eg, tetralogy of Fallot, pulmonary atresia, severe pulmonary stenosis). The aortic arch is often very conspicuous in nonobstructive coarctation (''pseudocoarctation'') of the aorta, a condition in which

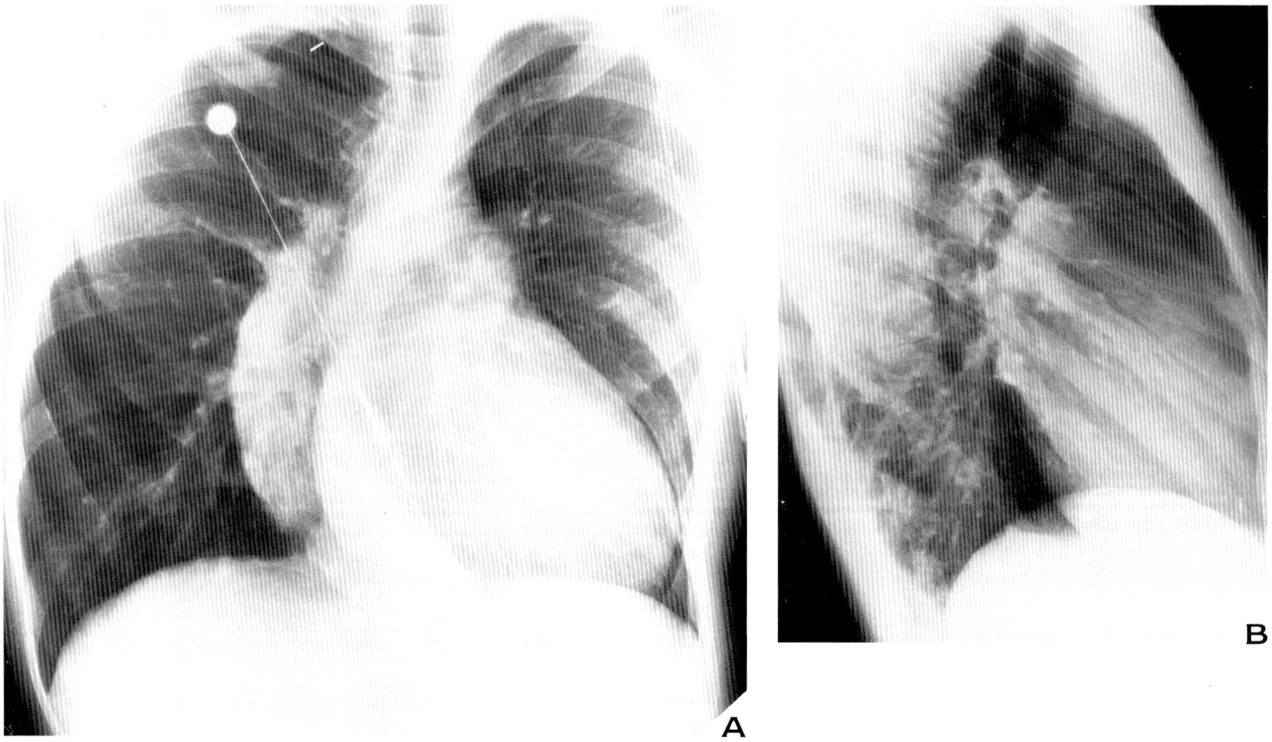

Fig. 17.4 Scoliosis associated with an interatrioventricular septal defect. (A) Frontal and (B) lateral chest radiographs show severe thoracolumbar scoliosis with a rotatory component. The curve is convex to the right in the thoracic segment and convex to the left in the upper lumbar region. Note the enlarged right ventricle and pulmonary plethora, which indicate the presence of a left to right shunt.

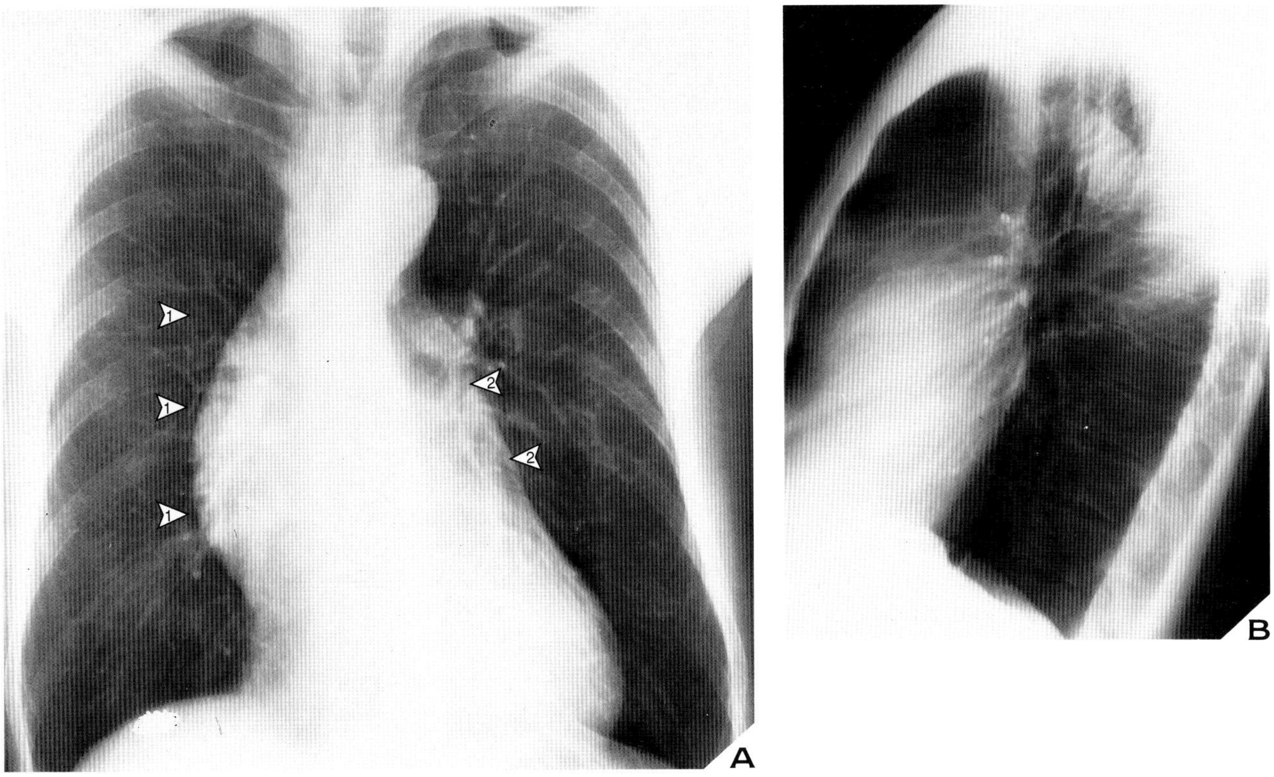

Fig. 17.5 Scoliosis and aortic aneurysm associated with Marfan's syndrome. (A) Frontal and (B) lateral chest radiographs show mild thoracic scoliosis. The thorax is markedly elongated. Note the prominence of the aortic contour on the right (*arrows* 1) and the pulmonary trunk on the left (*arrows* 2) caused by aneurysmal enlargement of the aortic root, a frequent complication of Marfan's syndrome.

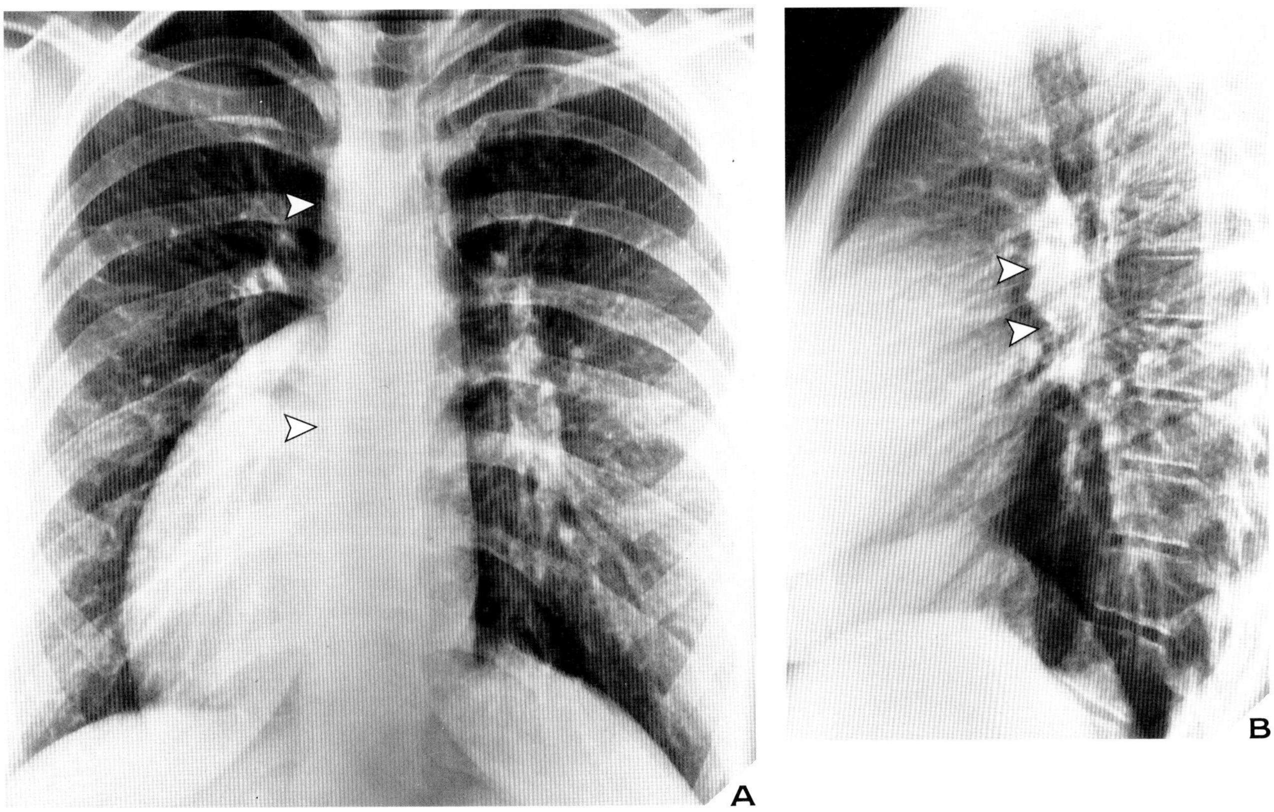

Fig. 17.6 Incongruent thoracic and abdominal situs with thoracic right isomerism. (A) Frontal and (B) lateral chest films in a patient with right atrial isomerism. The cardiac axis is oriented to the right (dextrocardia). The stomach bubble is on the left and the liver on the right, ie, the abdominal (visceral) situs is incongruent with the thoracic situs. The aortic arch and descending thoracic aorta (*arrows* in A) are both on the right. Both frontal and lateral projections demonstrate typical features of right isomerism. On the frontal view, the main bronchi are symmetrical with right-sided morphology; on the lateral, both pulmonary arteries (*arrows* in B) lie anterior to the plane of the trachea. The vascularity of the right lung is diminished, suggesting stenosis of the right pulmonary artery or its branches.

angulation of the distal portion of the arch results in turbulent flow (Fig. 17.7).

The aortic arch tends to be inconspicuous in conditions in which blood flow through the aorta is decreased (eg, atrial or ventricular septal defect) and in those in which the distal aortic arch is malformed (eg, coarctation of the aorta, interruption of the aortic arch). In classical coarctation, the distal part of the aortic arch is displaced medially, so that it appears very small on the frontal chest film (Fig. 17.8).

ABNORMALIES OF THE AORTIC ARCH

In the usual type of left aortic arch the first branch is the right brachiocephalic artery, followed by the left common carotid and left subclavian arteries. Rarely, the right brachiocephalic artery arises distal to the left subclavian artery, an anomaly known as *left arch with aberrant right subclavian artery*.

In *right aortic arch with mirror image branching*, the left brachiocephalic artery arises as the first branch, followed by the right common carotid and right subclavian arteries. This type of right aortic arch is found in approximately 25 percent of patients with tetralogy of Fallot and truncus arteriosus (Fig. 17.9).

The most common anomaly of the aortic arch encountered in individuals without congenital heart disease is *right aortic arch with anomalous left subclavian artery (RAA/ALSA)*. In this condition the left common carotid artery arises as the first branch and the left subclavian artery arises as the fourth branch, distal to the origin of the right subclavian artery. The anomalous left subclavian artery courses posterior to the esophagus to reach the left arm, and is seen on the lateral esophagram to indent the posterior esophageal wall (Fig. 17.10). Although it is usually an isolated malformation, RAA/ALSA is occasionally associated with congenital heart disease, generally of the acyanotic type.

Double aortic arch is an uncommon malformation in which both aortic arches persist, forming a vascular ring which encir-

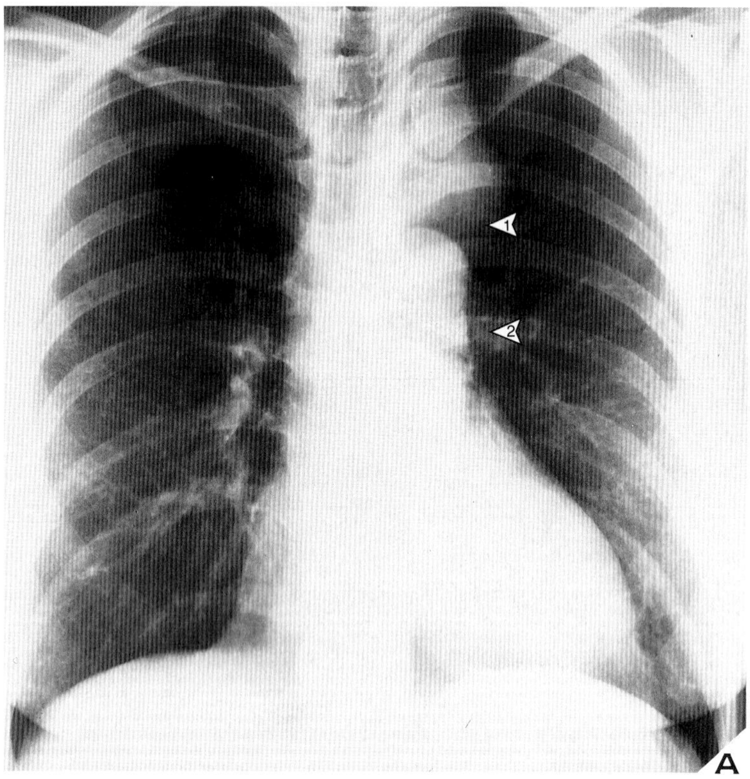

Fig. 17.7 Nonobstructive coarctation of the aorta. (A) Frontal chest radiograph shows a markedly deformed aortic arch, which has the appearance of a numeral "3." The upper part of the "3" is formed by the distal aortic arch and the dilated left subclavian artery (*arrow* 1); the lower part is formed by the dilated descending aorta (*arrow* 2). (B) On the lateral film, the distal aortic arch (*arrow*) is projected behind the trachea (an esophagram would show compression of the esophagus at this level). (C) Frontal and (D) lateral projections of thoracic aortogram (*arrows* indicate coarcted segment).

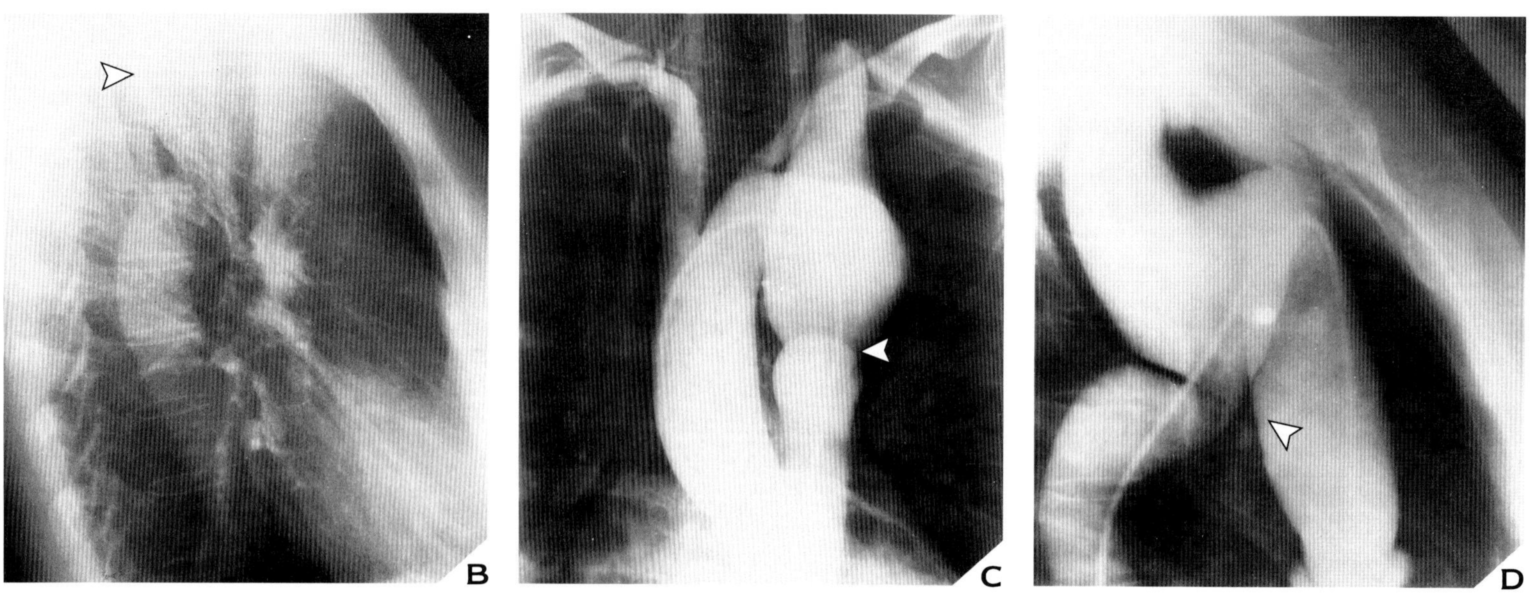

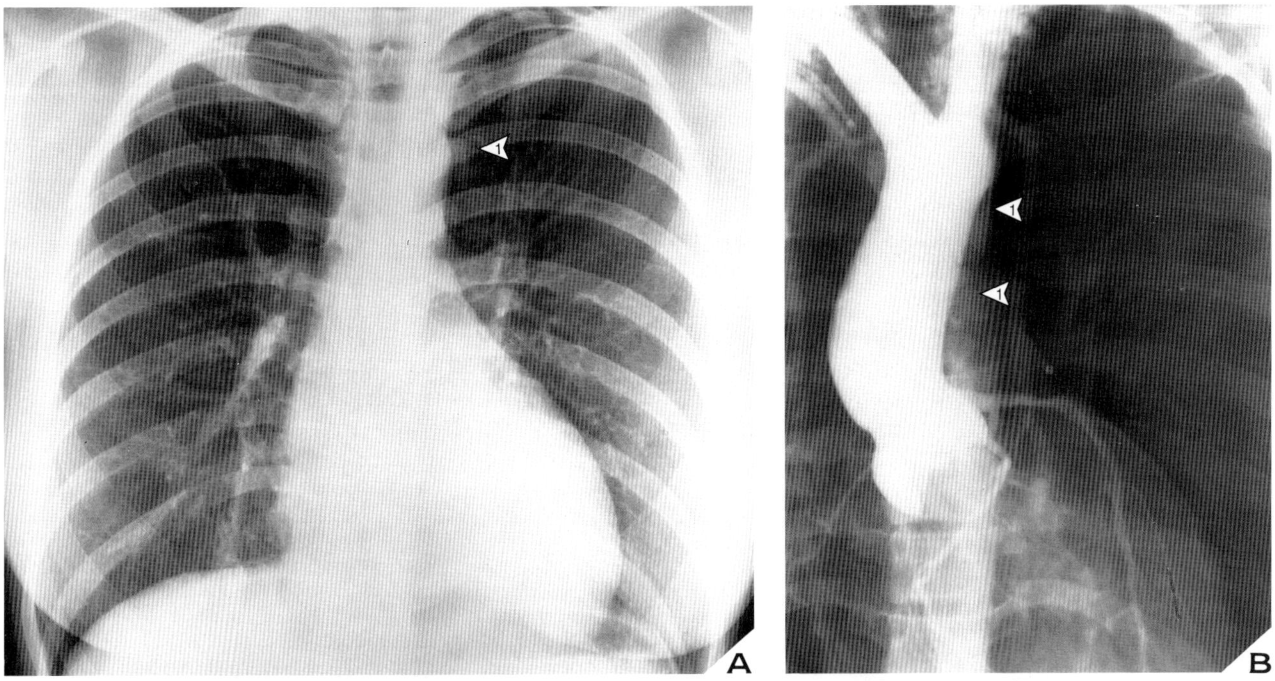

Fig. 17.8 Diminutive left aortic arch associated with coarctation of the aorta. (A) Frontal projection of the chest shows an inconspicuous aortic arch (*arrow* 1) in a 20-year-old woman with hypertension and diminished pulses in the lower extremities. Note left ventricular enlargement and minimal rib notching. (B) Aortogram shows a hypoplastic distal aortic arch and medial displacement of the upper descending thoracic aorta (*arrows* 1).

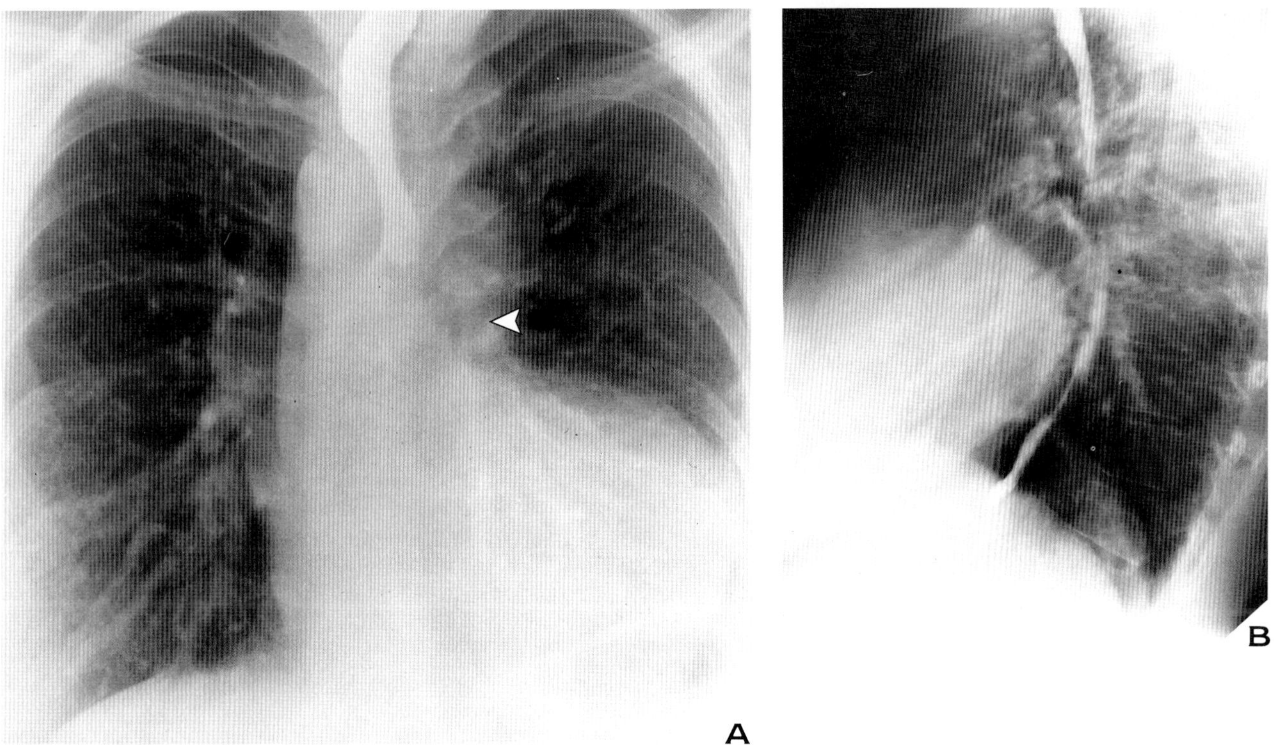

Fig. 17.9 Right aortic arch with mirror-image branching (tetralogy of Fallot). (A) Posteroanterior and (B) lateral chest radiographs. The aortic arch and the proximal portion of the descending thoracic aorta lie to the right of the trachea. The opacified esophagus is displaced to the left. The portion of the left cardiac border normally occupied by the pulmonary trunk (*arrow* in A) is concave; however, the right and left pulmonary arteries appear normal. The cardiac apex is upturned, indicating right ventricular enlargement.

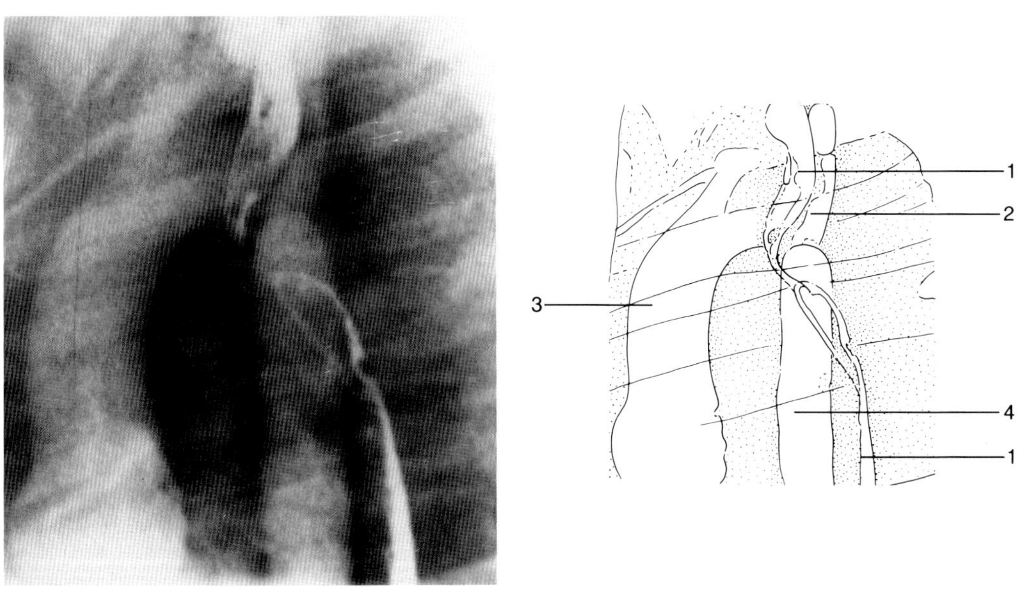

Fig. 17.10 Right aortic arch with anomalous origin of the left subclavian artery. Lateral projection of thoracic aortogram with barium in esophagus. The opacified esophagus is displaced anteriorly by the aberrant left subclavian artery, which arises as the last branch of the aortic arch.

1	esophagus	3	ascending aorta
2	aberrant left subclavian artery	4	descending aorta

cles the trachea and esophagus (see Fig. 15.26). Most patients exhibit symptoms of airway compression and/or dysphagia early in life.

Aortic arch anomalies and their clinical manifestations are discussed further in Chapter 15.

ASCENDING AORTA

The ascending aorta normally forms part of the right superior mediastinal border. The aorta may not be border-forming when the ascending aorta is displaced medially or is hypoplastic. In some cardiac malformations the ascending aorta lies far to the left, in which case it forms part of the left upper mediastinal border (Fig. 17.11). In such patients the right ventricle is commonly displaced to the left (ventricular inversion). A left-sided ascending aorta may also be present in a number of uncommon cardiac malformations associated with atrial situs solitus, eg, congenitally corrected transposition of the great arteries, anatomically corrected malposition of the aorta, double outlet right or left ventricle, or univentricular/atrioventricular connection of the left ventricular type with discordant ventriculoarterial connection (Figs. 17.12 and 17.13).

DISTAL AORTIC ARCH AND DESCENDING THORACIC AORTA

Deformities of the distal aortic arch and the descending thoracic aorta often signal the presence of a cardiovascular malformation. A hypoplastic or inapparent left aortic arch suggests coarctation of the aorta. In classical coarctation, the descending thoracic aorta is dilated immediately beyond the coarcted segment, producing the appearance of a numeral "3" on the frontal chest film. (A portion of the upper part of the "3" represents the dilated left subclavian artery.) The left margin of the opacified esophagus resembles an "E" or an inverted numeral "3" on the barium esophagram (see Fig. 12.29). The distal aortic arch can almost always be identified on the lateral chest film in normal teenagers and adults; its absence favors the diagnosis of coarctation of the aorta (see Fig. 12.28).

Patients with nonobstructive coarctation (pseudocoarctation) of the aorta may have plain film findings resembling those of classic coarctation (ie, a diminutive aortic arch and a dilated descending aorta). In most instances, however, the distal arch and left subclavian artery are markedly dilated, forming a prominent bulge along the left upper mediastinal border (see Fig. 17.7).

In some individuals with a right aortic arch, the thoracic aorta descends on the left. However, this combination of findings usually indicates the presence of a double aortic arch.

THE PULMONARY TRUNK

A prominent pulmonary trunk is a characteristic feature of pulmonic valvular stenosis and conditions associated with increased pulmonary blood flow. A dilated pulmonary trunk appears on the frontal chest radiograph as a smooth bulge of the left upper mediastinal border. In patients with pulmonic valvular stenosis, the right pulmonary artery is of normal size, whereas the pulmonary trunk and left pulmonary artery are en-

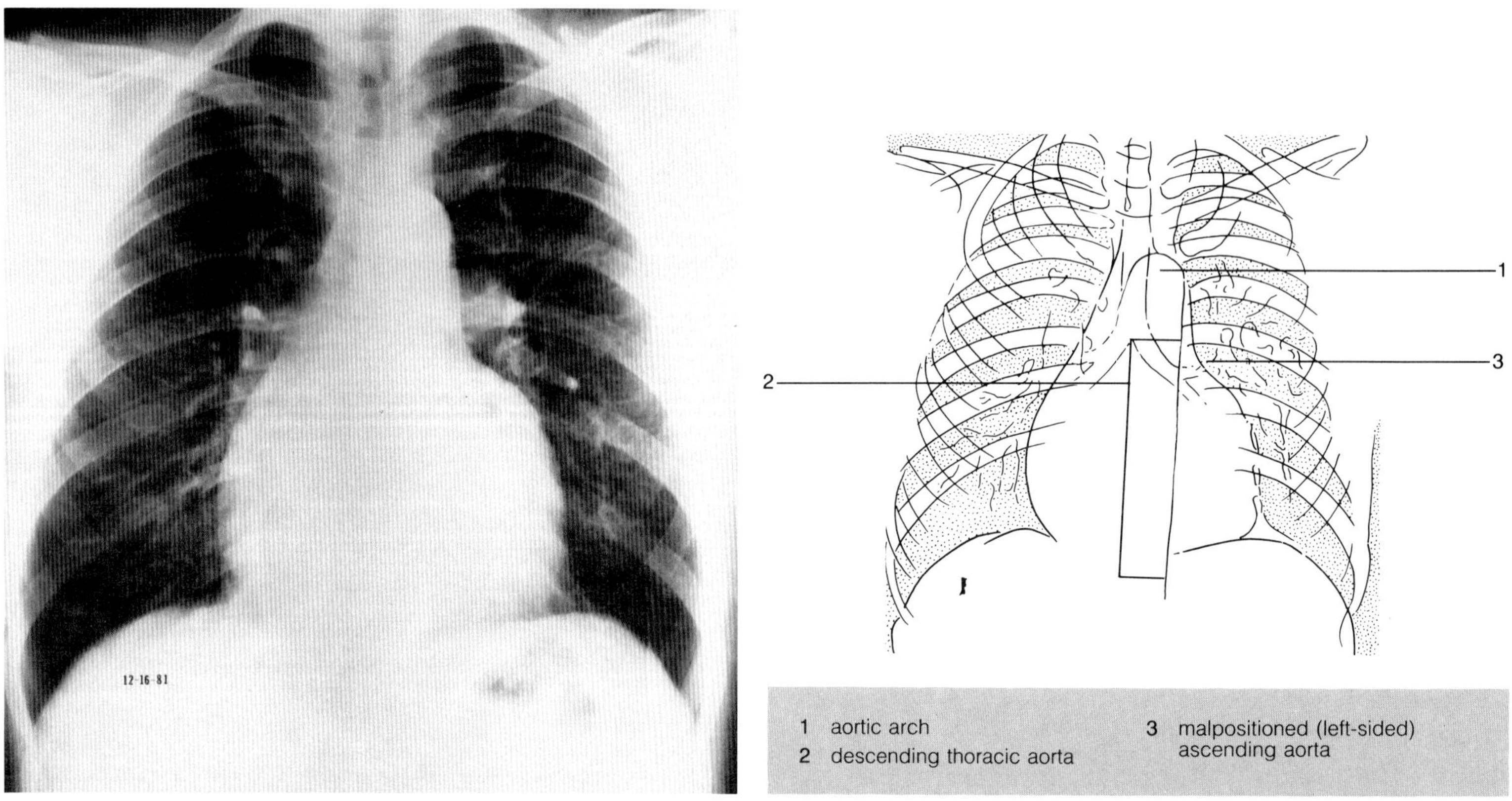

Fig. 17.11 Malposition of the ascending aorta with mesocardia: frontal view in a patient with congenitally corrected transposition of the great arteries. The heart is medially located with its axis oriented anteriorly (ie, parallel to the sagittal plane). There is atrial and visceral situs solitus and the tracheobronchial tree has a left-sided configuration. Both the aortic arch and the descending thoracic aorta are on the left. The straight line forming the superior aspect of the left mediastinal border represents the malpositioned ascending aorta. When associated with situs solitus, the presence of a left-sided ascending aorta indicates ventricular inversion and strongly suggests the disgnosis of congenitally corrected transposition of the great arteries.

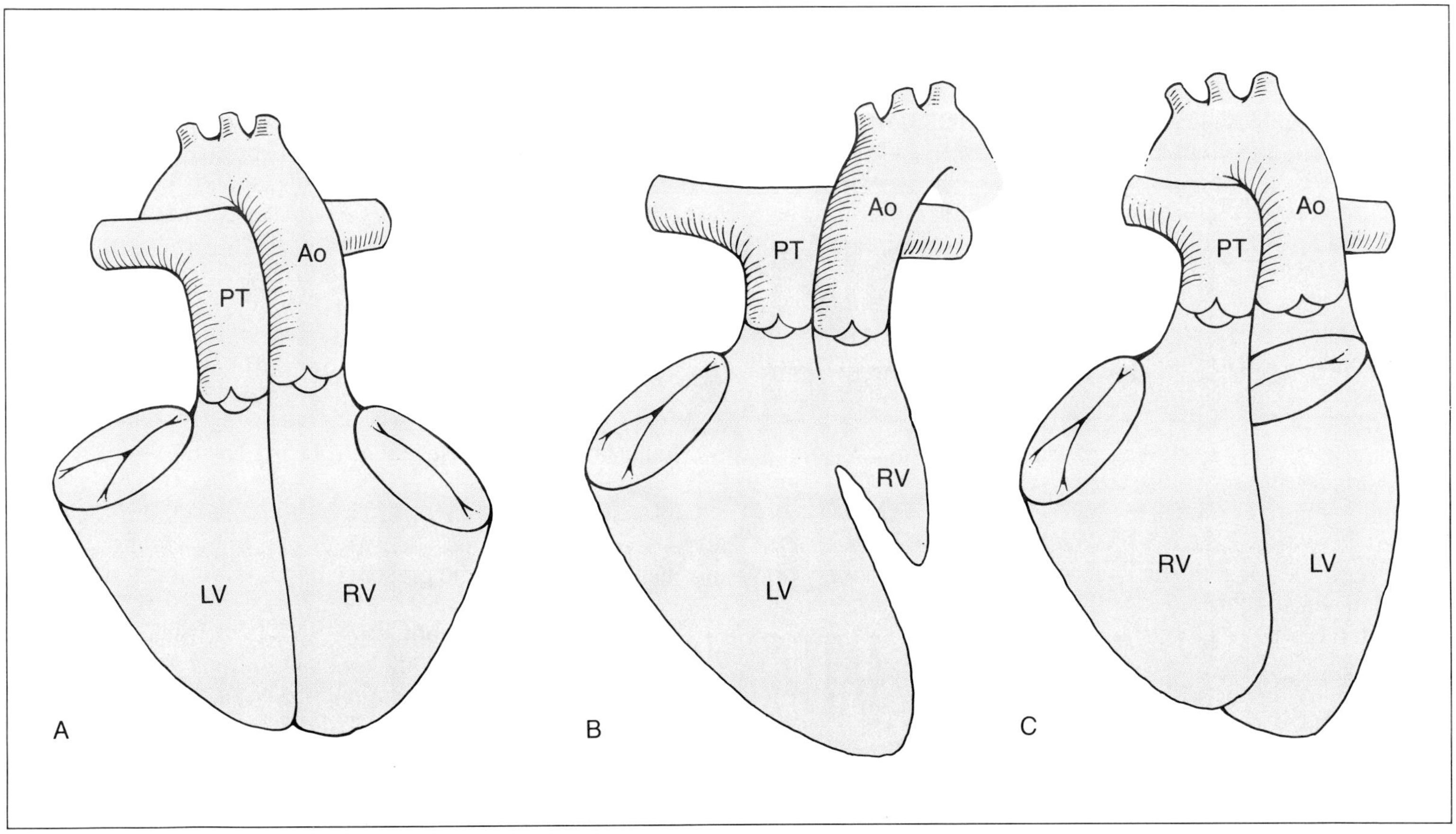

Fig. 17.12 Schematic representation of conditions associated with a left-sided ascending aorta. (A) Corrected transposition of the great arteries. (B) Univentricular atrioventricular connection to the left ventricle with discordant ventricular–arterial connection. (C) Anatomically corrected malposition of the aorta.

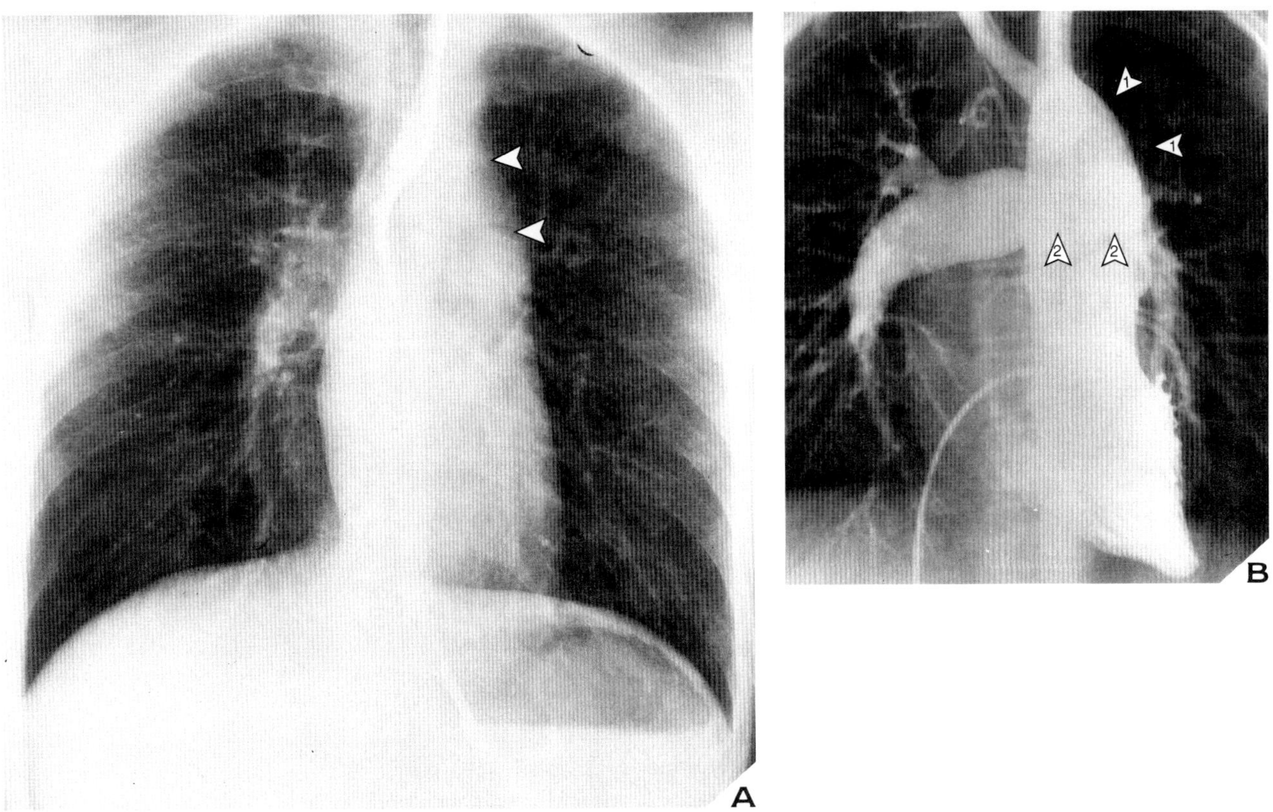

Fig. 17.13 Left-sided ascending aorta. (A) Frontal chest radiograph in a patient with univentricular atrioventricular connection to the left ventricle with discordant ventricular–arterial connection. The left upper mediastinal border to the level of the aortic arch is formed by the ascending aorta (*arrows*). The pulmonary trunk lies in the midline and is inconspicuous on the frontal projection. (B) A left ventricular injection demonstrates the left position of the ascending aorta (*arrows* 1) and its relation to the pulmonary artery. Note the thick, domed pulmonic valve (*arrows* 2), indicating valvular pulmonic stenosis.

larged owing to poststenotic dilatation (Fig. 17.14). Certain congenital cardiac defects (eg, pulmonary hypoplasia associated with tetralogy of Fallot, medial displacement of the ascending aorta associated with double-outlet right ventricle, transposition of the great arteries) are associated with hypoplasia or absence of the pulmonary trunk. The left upper mediastinal border is typically flat or concave in these conditions (see Fig. 17.9A).

THE CAVAL VEINS

The (right) superior vena cava usually forms the right mediastinal border. A patent left superior vena cava should be suspected when the frontal chest film demonstrates a straight line extending from the left border of the heart to the level of the left clavicle (Fig. 17.15). A left superior vena cava is usually associated with an atrioventricular septal defect, in which event atrial isomerism is commonly present as well.

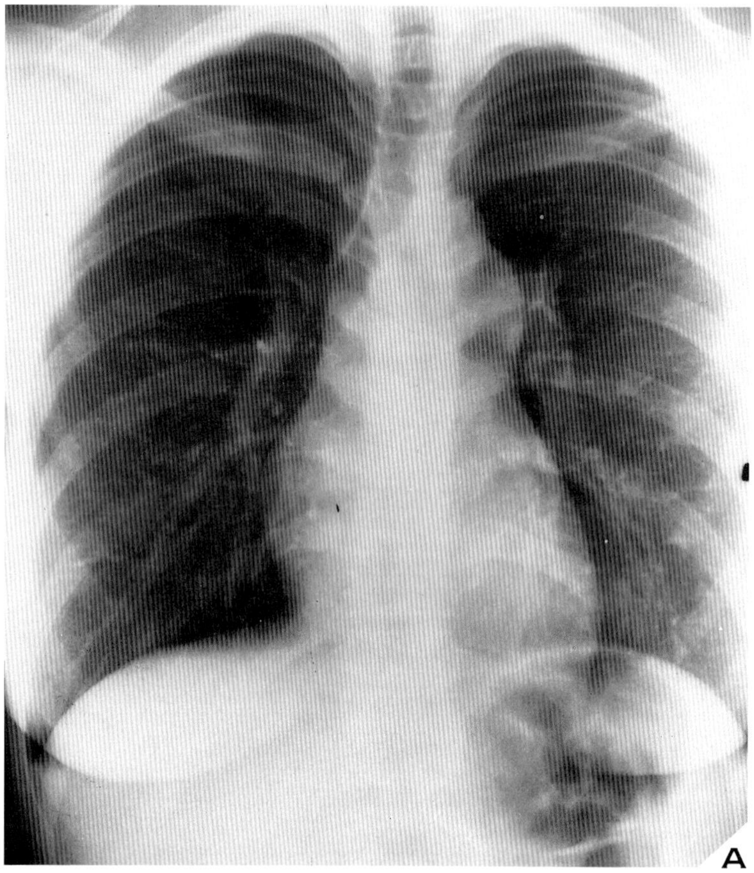

A

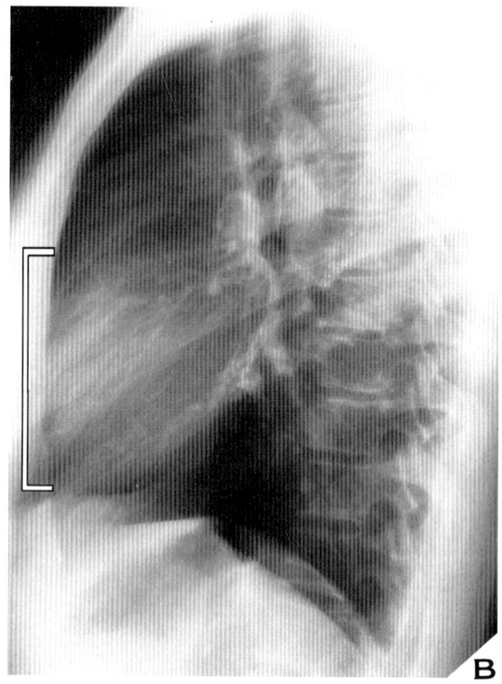

B

Fig. 17.14 Poststenotic dilatation of pulmonary artery (pulmonic valvular stenosis). (A) Posteroanterior and (B) lateral chest films. The main and left pulmonary arteries are dilated, whereas the right pulmonary artery is normal. The peripheral pulmonary vascularity is also normal. On the lateral projection (B) the zone of contact between the right ventricle and the anterior chest wall (*brace*) is greater than normal, indicating right ventricular enlargement.

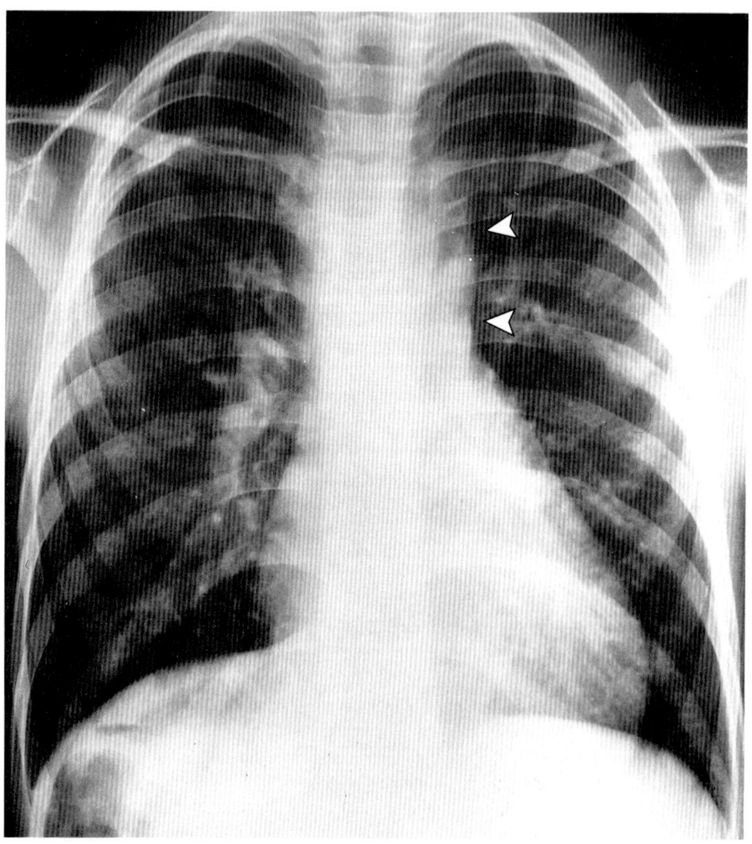

Fig. 17.15 Left superior vena cava; frontal chest film in a patient with right isomerism and stenosis of the left pulmonary artery. The straight line (*arrows*) forming the left upper mediastinal border represents the lateral border of the left superior vena cava. Note that the stomach is on the right, indicating abdominal situs inversus.

Enlargement of the azygos vein suggests absence of the hepatic segment of the inferior vena cava (IVC) with azygos continuation. In this anomaly, the entire venous return from the lower body is carried by the azygos system, which drains into the superior vena cava and thence into the right atrium. Frontal and lateral chest films typically show absence of the inferior vena caval segment (Fig. 17.16). (Its apparent presence does not exclude azgygos continuation of the IVC, because the contour formed by the hepatic veins, which enter the right atrium directly in this anomaly, can simulate a normal inferior vena caval segment on both frontal and lateral projections.) Absence of the hepatic segment of the IVC is frequently associated with atrial isomerism; however, it may also exist as an isolated malformation (see Chapter 8).

THE TRACHEOBRONCHIAL TREE

Thoracic situs, which is closely correlated with atrial situs, is reflected in the anatomy of the tracheobronchial tree (see Chapter 8). In normal thoracic situs *(thoracic situs solitus)*, the

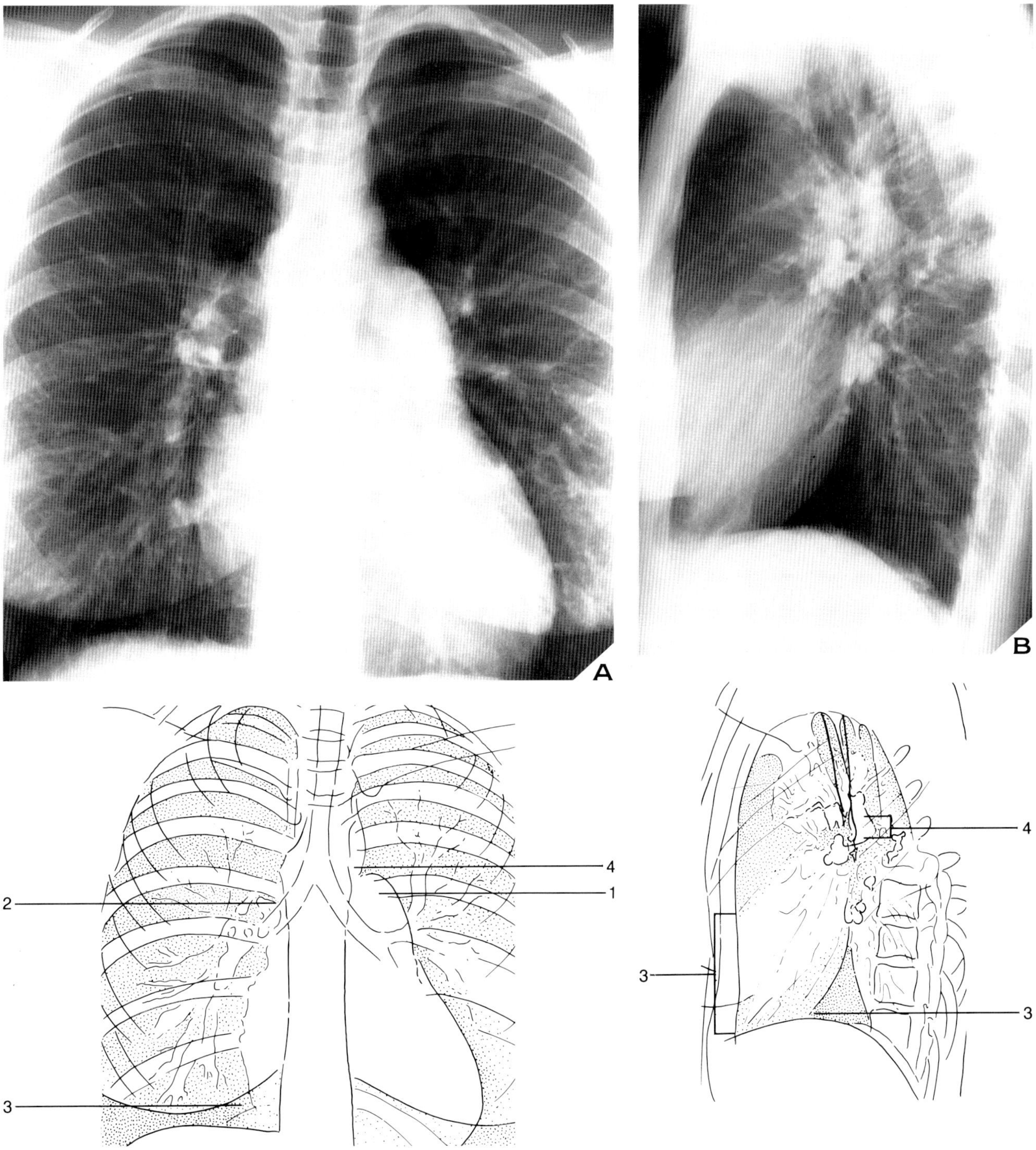

Fig. 17.16 Left atrial isomerism, absence of the hepatic segment of the inferior vena cava with azygos continuation, and atrial septal defect. A frontal chest film demonstrates levocardia and a left aortic arch. The left and right mainstem bronchi are almost equal in length. The enlarged left and right main pulmonary arteries lie superior to their corresponding bronchi and course posteriorly; these are typical features of left isomerism. The azygos vein is prominent. The inferior vena cava cannot be identified on either the frontal or the lateral projection. Note the increased contact between the heart and the anterior chest wall in B, indicating right ventricular enlargement. The pulmonary vascularity is slightly increased.

1 dilated main pulmonary artery
2 epiarterial right pulmonary artery
3 absence of inferior vena caval segment
4 eparterial left pulmonary artery

left mainstem bronchus is longer than the right mainstem bronchus in the ratio of 1.4 to 1 (*see* Fig. 17.14A). The left mainstem bronchus lies immediately inferior to the left pulmonary artery and the right mainstem bronchus lies superior and posterior to the right pulmonary artery. (In thoracic situs inversus, this relationship is reversed.) Thoracic isomerism is considered to be present when the right and left bronchi are relatively equal in length (ie, when the ratio is less than 1.4 to 1). In *left atrial isomerism (left isomerism)*, both pulmonary arteries course superior and posterior to the mainstem bronchi (Fig. 17.16). In *right atrial isomerism (right isomerism)*, both pulmonary arteries course anterior and inferior to the mainstem bronchi (*see* Fig. 17.6).

In atrial isomerism, the atrial chambers are morphologically similar; they may resemble the normal right atrium (right isomerism) or the normal left atrium (left isomerism). Atrial isomerism implies the presence of abnormal connections between the atria and the venous system.

RIGHT ATRIAL ISOMERISM

Because the left atrium is absent, the pulmonic venous return is usually abnormally connected in patients with right atrial isomerism. Most patients with right atrial isomerism have the supracardiac type of anomalous connection; however, the abnormal connection may be infracardiac or even cardiac. Anomalies of systemic venous drainage (eg, left superior vena cava) are commonly present as well (see Fig. 17.15).

LEFT ATRIAL ISOMERISM

Because the right atrium is absent, the systemic venous connection is usually abnormal in patients with left atrial isomerism. The most common pattern is interruption of the inferior vena cava between the renal veins and the atrial chambers; blood from the inferior part of the body flows through the azygos system and drains into the superior vena cava (Fig. 17.16). Other venous systemic anomalies associated with left atrial isomerism include bilateral superior venae cavae and absence of the right superior vena cava with absence of the coronary sinus.

Both left and right isomerism are commonly associated with complex congenital malformations of the atrioventricular valves, ventricles, and great arteries. To sum up, the presence of atrial isomerism implies the existence of associated severe congenital cardiac malformations, mainly at the level of the venoatrial connections.

THE PULMONARY VASCULATURE

The pulmonary vascular markings reflect blood flow and pulmonary vascular pressure. Several patterns of pulmonary vascularity can be identified radiographically: normal; plethoric; pulomonary venous hypertension; oligemic; disordered or systemic arrangement; and asymmetric.

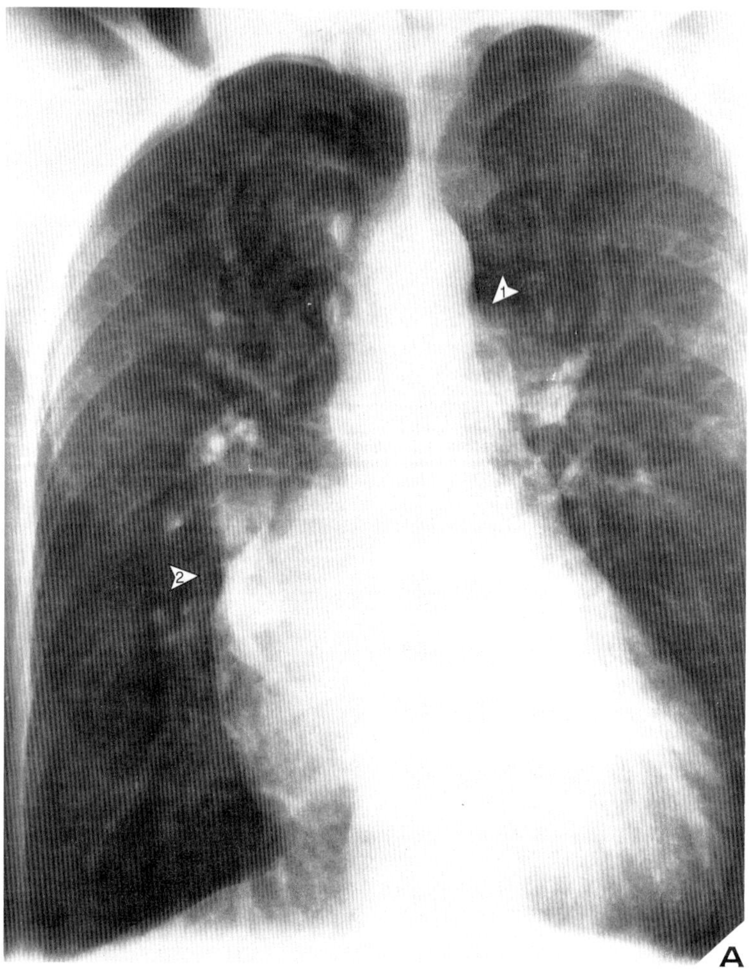

A

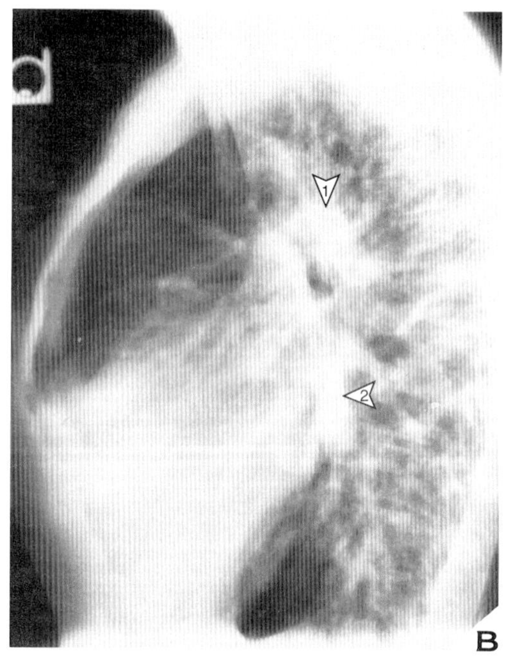

B

Fig. 17.17 Large left to right shunt (truncus arteriosus). (A) Frontal and (B) lateral projections show marked pulmonary plethora. The right and left pulmonary arteries, as well as their lobar and segmental branches, are enlarged. Dilated arteries are equally distributed throughout the superior and inferior zones of the lungs. Enlarged peripheral arterial branches can be followed almost to the margins of the lungs. Note the high take-off of the left pulmonary artery (*arrows* 1 in A and B) and the small aortic arch. There is right atrial, right ventricular, and left atrial enlargement. The markedly enlarged left atrium is border-forming on the right (*arrow* 2 in A) and forms the posterosuperior heart border on the lateral projection (*arrow* 2 in B).

NORMAL

Normal pulmonary vascularity indicates that both lungs are receiving a normal amount of blood per minute and per square meter of body surface area, under normal pressure. Because the right central pulmonary artery divides within the mediastinum, the right hilum includes the truncus anterior and interlobar arteries. On the lateral projection, the right hilum appears as an oval opacity which projects anterior to the tracheobronchial plane (see Fig. 17.14). On the frontal projection, the left pulmonary artery lies superior to the left main bronchus. On the lateral view, it lies superior and posterior to the left main bronchus.

The main pulmonary arteries supply the central, interlobar, and intraparenchymal vascular segment of each lung. The lower lobe branches appear larger than the upper lobe branches on an erect frontal chest film obtained in deep inspiration. This disparity, which is due to gravity, is not seen on chest films obtained with the patient supine. Normally, pulmonary vessels cannot be identified in the upper lung zones on an erect chest film; however, because of the greater flow to the more dependent portions of the lungs, they are normally visible in the lower zones. The main pulmonary veins enter the left atrium below the level of the hila (see Fig. 17.14).

PLETHORA

Pulmonary plethora reflects increased pulmonary blood flow; in patients with congenital heart disease, it usually indicates a systemic to pulmonary shunt. Other conditions associated with increased pulmonary blood flow include volume overload, high cardiac output (eg, thyrotoxicosis), and peripheral arteriovenous shunt. The chest films of well-conditioned athletes sometimes exhibit minimal plethora.

Pulmonary plethora is characterized radiographically by dilatation of pulmonary arteries at the level of the hila as well as peripherally; an increased number of arteries can be identified in any given region of the lung. Dilated vessels are seen close to the lateral margins of the lungs. Pulmonary veins are enlarged to a degree commensurate with the arterial dilatation. Dilated superior and inferior pulmonary veins are easily identified in patients with large shunts (Fig. 17.17; see also Fig. 17.16).

OLIGEMIA

Generalized pulmonary oligemia reflects a reduction in pulmonary blood flow. It is characterized radiographically by a significant reduction in the number and size of the pulmonary vascular markings (Fig. 17.18). With severely decreased pulmonary

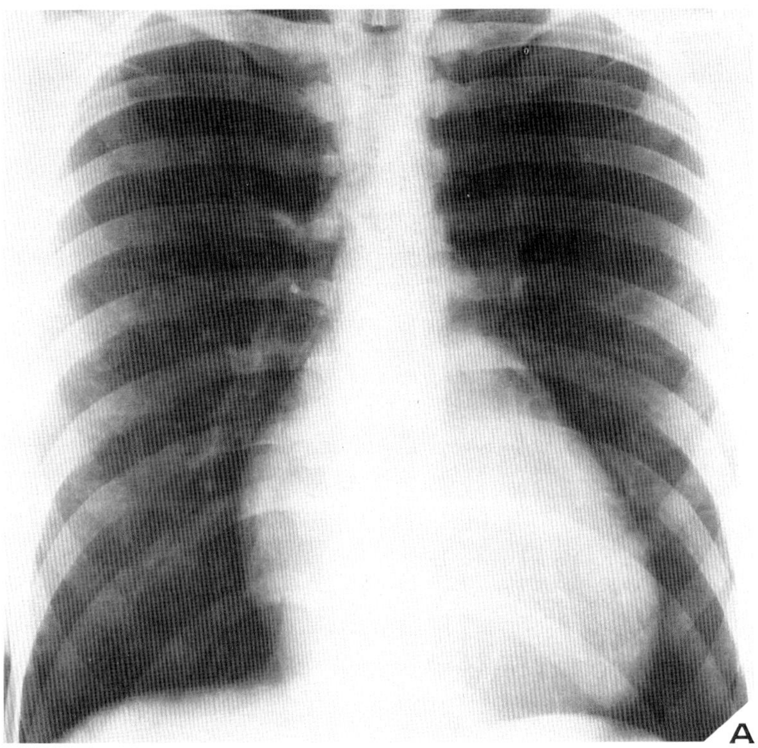

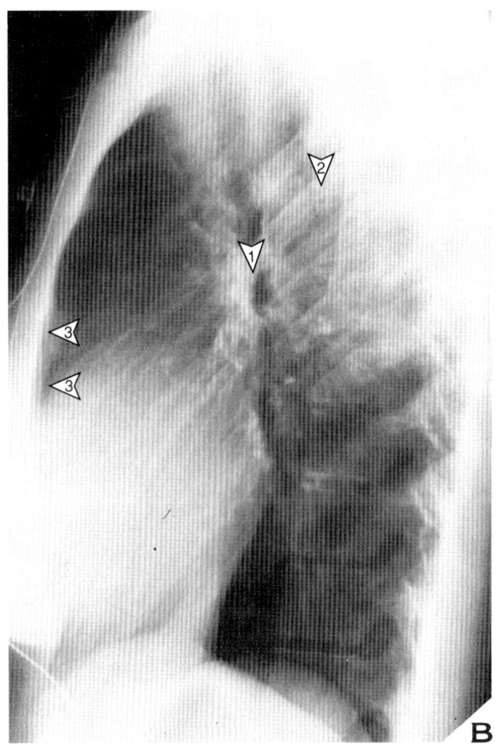

Fig. 17.18 Pulmonary oligemia (Ebstein's anomaly). (A) Frontal and (B) lateral views of a patient with Ebstein's malformation of the tricuspid valve. Note marked narrowing of the mediastinum, which reflects the diminished size of the pulmonary trunk and main pulmonary arteries. The lobar and segmental branches are minute and cannot be traced beyond the inner zone of the lung fields. The lateral projection demonstrates a diminutive right pulmonary artery (*arrow* 1 in B): the left pulmonary artery cannot be identified. Left upper border of the cardiovascular silhouette is formed by the right ventricular outflow tract (*arrow* 2 in B). There is marked right atrial enlargement, manifested by the prominent right lower cardiac border in A and effacement of the retrosternal space (*arrows* 3 in B). Right ventricular enlargement is present as well (note the elevation of the apex in A and increased contact of the heart with the anterior chest wall in B).

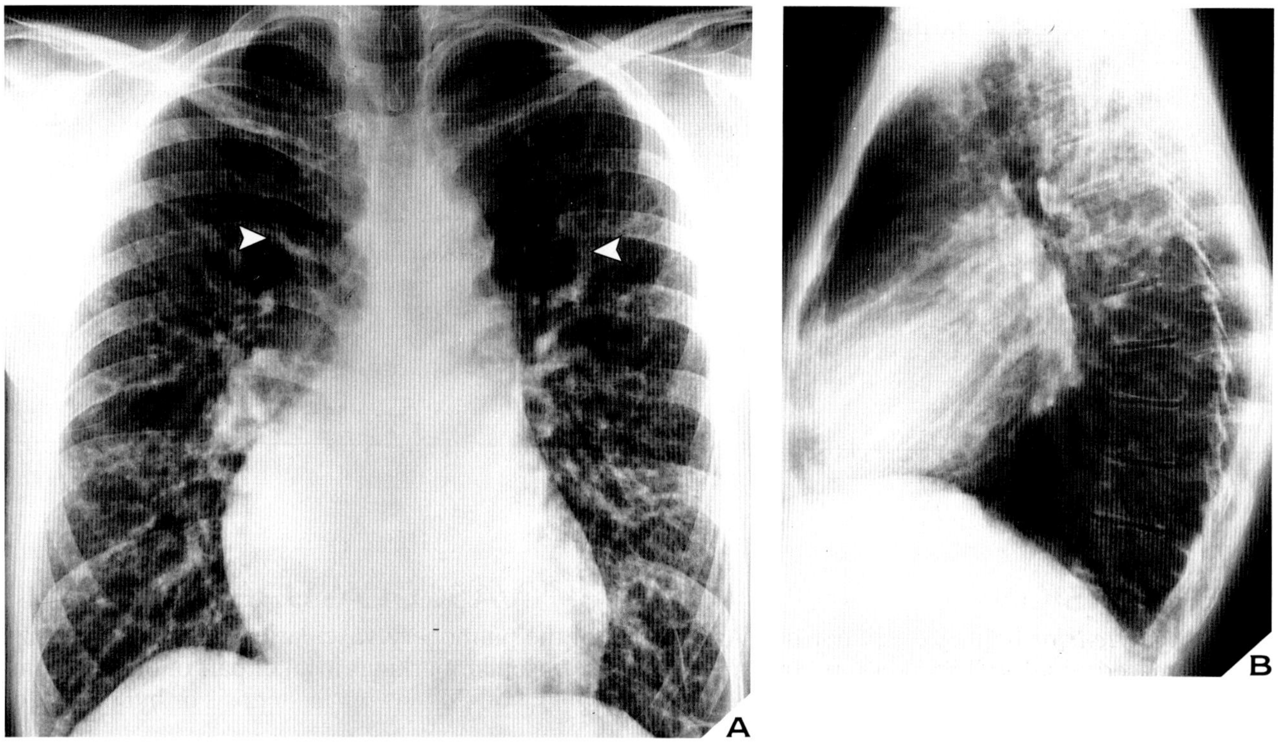

Fig. 17.19 Severe pulmonary venous hypertension. (A) Frontal and (B) lateral chest radiographs in a patient with cor triatriatum. The right and left pulmonary arteries are enlarged. The lobar and segmental arteries in the upper zones are dilated when compared with those in the lower zones. The veins in the upper zones (*arrows*) are also prominent. The interstitial edema reflects the chronically increased pressure in the pulmonary venous system. Left ventricular function was preserved in this patient (note the normal-sized left atrium).

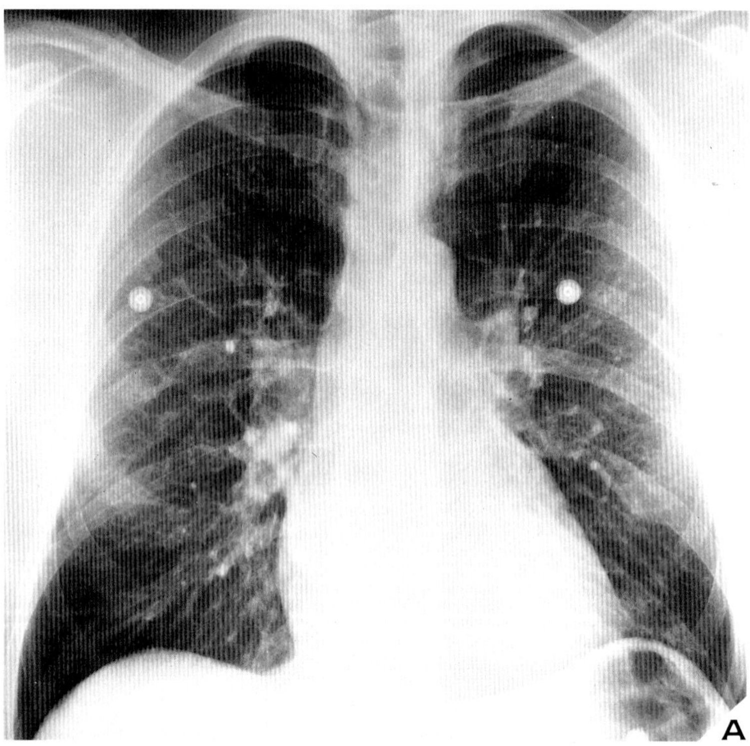

Fig. 17.20 Moderate pulmonary venous hypertension due to cor triatriatum. (A) Frontal chest radiograph shows evidence of moderate pulmonary venous hypertension in a patient with cor triatriatum. The arteries and veins are dilated in the upper zones and constricted in the lower zones. The pulmonary trunk is slightly enlarged. The left atrium is normal. (B) Selective left atriogram (right anterior oblique projection) in another patient. The true left atrium is a small chamber located above the mitral valve. The larger chamber receiving the pulmonary venous blood communicates with the true left atrium via a restricted opening. The left atrial appendage is connected to the atrium.

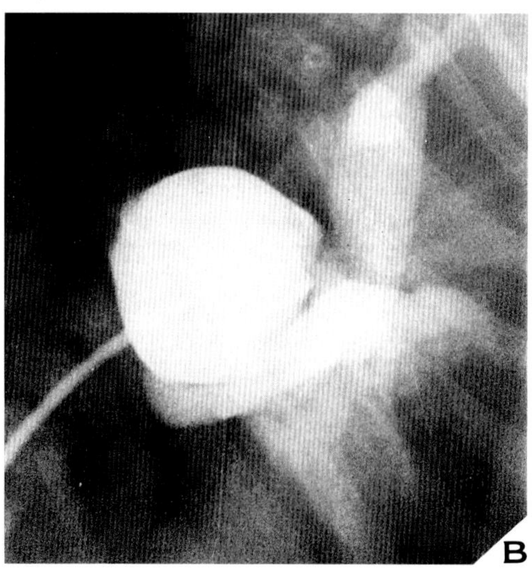

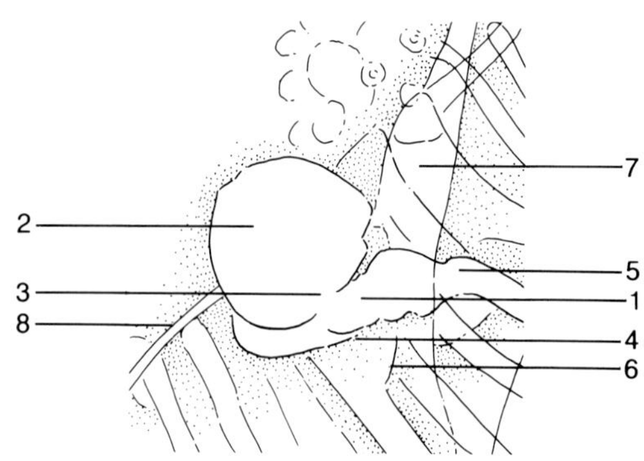

1 true left atrium
2 chamber receiving pulmonary venous blood
3 communication between true left atrium and pulmonary venous chamber
4 mitral valve
5 left atrial appendage
6 left ventricle
7 aorta
8 angiographic catheter (in left atrium)

blood flow, the hilar arteries are diminutive. In the most severely affected individuals, only a few tiny vascular markings can be identified in the perihilar region, and none in the periphery. A number of congenital malformations may be associated with severe pulmonary oligemia (and clinical cyanosis) in the adult. These include tetralogy of Fallot, pulmonary atresia and ventricular septal defect, pulmonary atresia with an intact ventricular septum, tricuspid atresia, tricuspid stenosis or regurgitation, and Ebstein's malformation.

Another cause of pulmonary oligemia is an increase in pulmonary vascular resistance, which can be either primary or secondary. In severe pulmonary arterial hypertension, the pulmonary trunk, as well as the right and left hilar arteries, is dilated, whereas the lobar and segmental branches are small and peripheral branches are diminutive or invisible.

PULMONARY VENOUS HYPERTENSION

The term *pulmonary venous hypertension* implies restriction of venous return resulting in increased venocapillary pressure. In congenital heart disease, pulmonary venous obstruction may occur at the level of the pulmonary veins, left atrium, mitral valve, or left ventricle. The appearance of the pulmonary vasculature reflects the severity of the venous obstruction, ie, the degree to which the pulmonary venous pressure is elevated. Chest films typically show redistribution of pulmonary blood flow to the upper zones ("cephalization") (Fig. 17.19). When pulmonary venous pressure is significantly increased, the upper zone vessels appear as large (or larger than) the lower zone vessels. Interstitial and/or aveolar pulmonary edema is commonly present in patients with pulmonary venous hypertension and may obscure the vascular pattern.

Pulmonary venous hypertension in the adult is usually due to acquired heart disease. Occasionally, however, it is caused by a congenital defect, eg, cor triatriatum (septation of the left atrium) (see Chapter 12) or a congenital malformation of the mitral valve not severe enough to produce symptoms early in life (Fig. 17.20; see also Fig. 17.19). Pulmonary venous hypertension is also seen in patients with atrial septal defects that are associated with moderate to severe right ventricular dysfunction (Fig. 17.21).

ASYMMETRY OF THE PULMONARY VASCULATURE

Asymmetry of the pulmonary vascularity (ie, diminished size and number of vascular markings in all or part of one lung) implies differential blood flow owing to stenosis or hypoplasia of the corresponding pulmonary artery (or its branches), and is not uncommon in adults with congenital heart disease. Stenosis or atresia of either main pulmonary artery is frequently associated with congenital heart disease, although it may exist as an isolated lesion. The latter is usually the case in patients with ste-

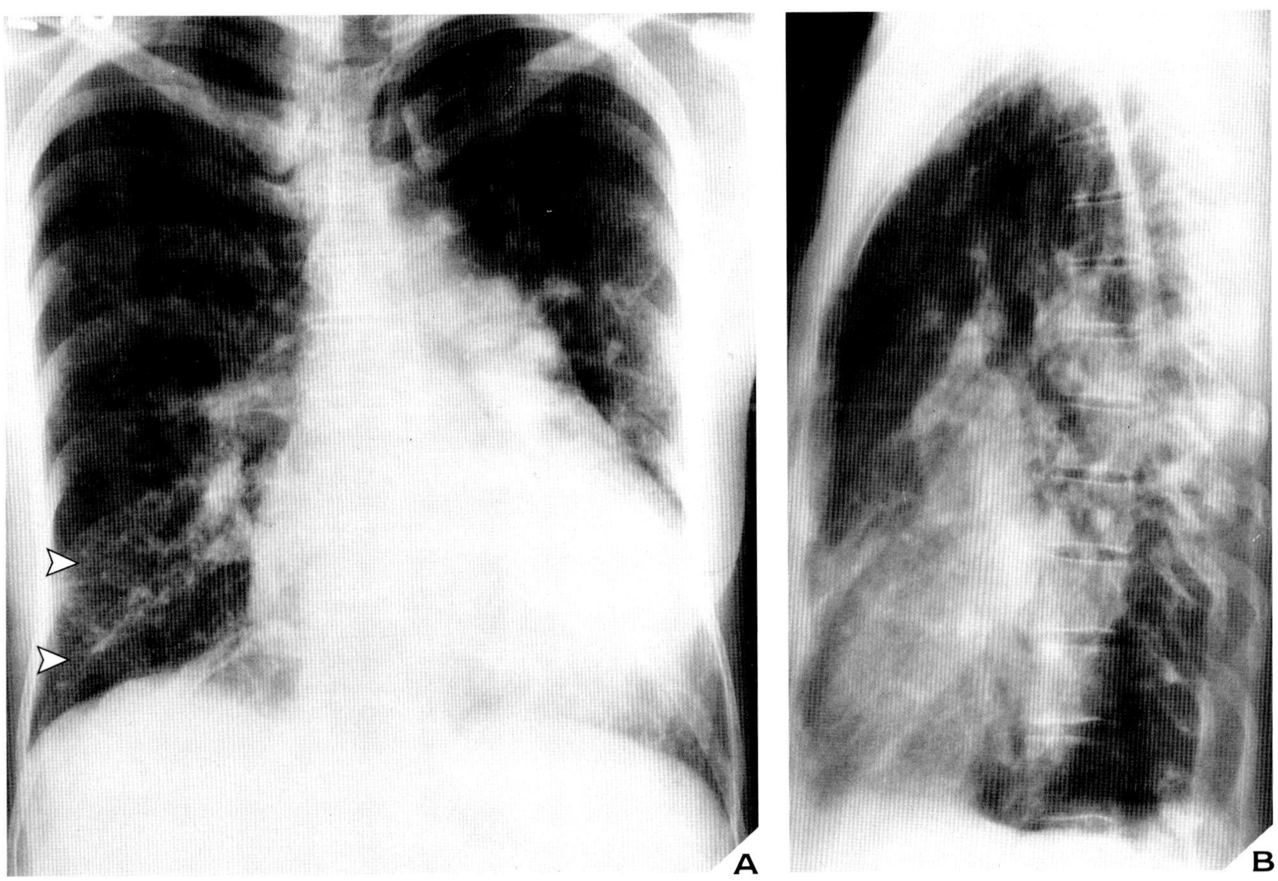

Fig. 17.21 Atrial septal defect (secundum type) with congestive heart failure. (A) Frontal and (B) lateral projections show marked enlargement of the pulmonary trunk and hilar arteries; vessels in the pulmonary parenchyma are also dilated. Note the Kerley B lines (*arrows*), which reflect interstitial pulmonary edema. The right ventricle is enlarged (note elevation of the cardiac apex in A and filling in of the retrosternal space in B). A longstanding left to right shunt at the atrial level has produced right ventricular failure in this patient.

nosis or atresia of the right pulmonary artery (Fig. 17.22). Stenosis or atresia of the left pulmonary artery is generally associated with congenital cardiac malformations, tetralogy of Fallot in particular.

Peripheral pulmonary artery stenosis is not uncommon in tetralogy of Fallot, in which case the left pulmonary artery and its branches are invariably affected. Stenosis may occur at the bifurcation, in the intrapericardial segments of the main arteries, at the hilum, or peripherally (Fig. 17.23). In general, stenosis of the pulmonary artery at the central or hilar level can be detected on the plain film, whereas stenosis of peripheral branches is difficult to appreciate, especially when it is sym-

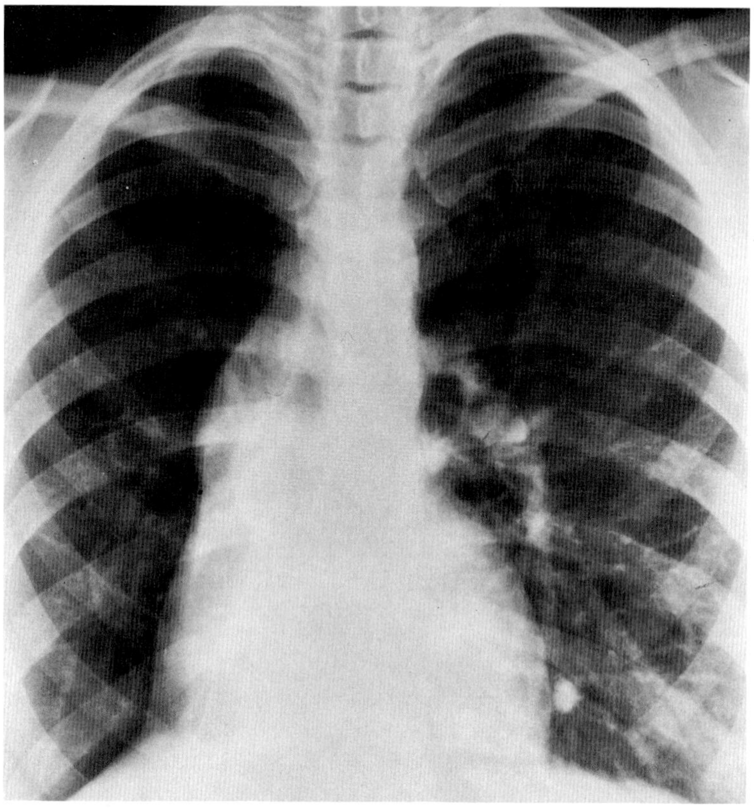

Fig. 17.22 Agenesis of the right pulmonary artery. The right lung is smaller than the left and the heart is displaced. The right pulmonary artery is absent. Note the sparse vascular markings in the inner third of the right lung, which represent systemic collaterals. The left pulmonary artery is slightly larger than normal.

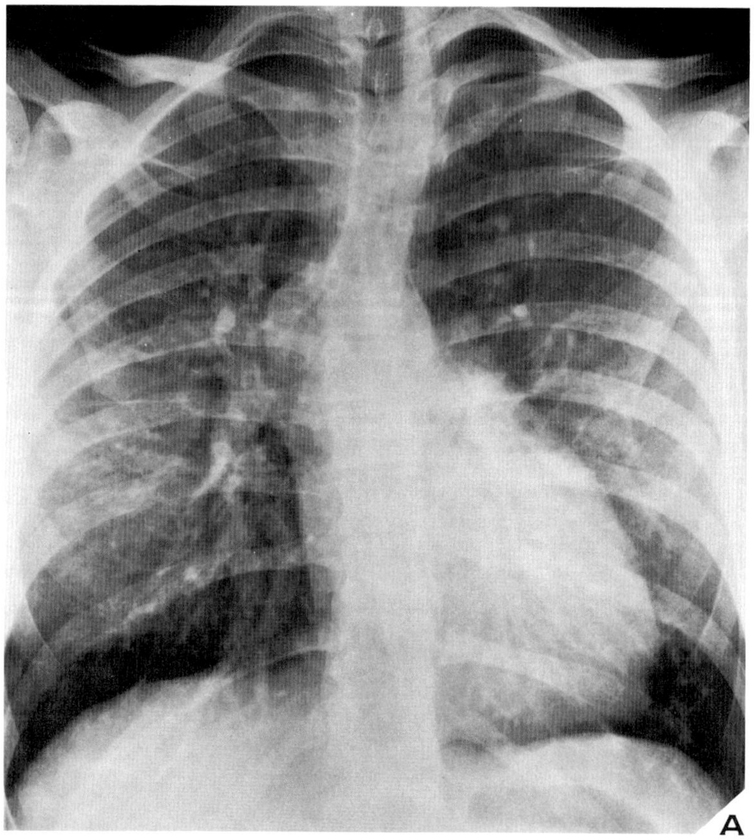

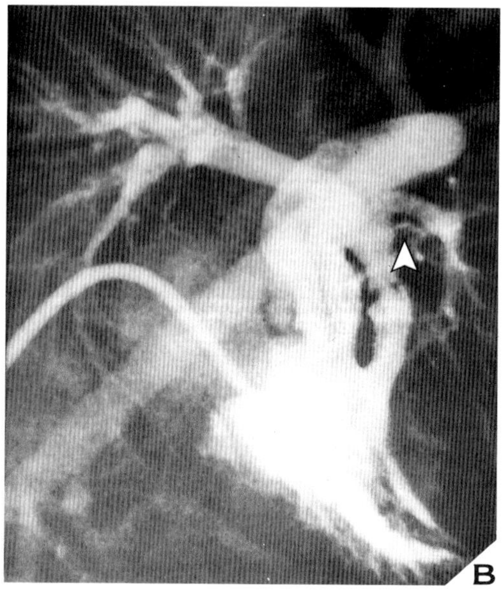

Fig. 17.23 Peripheral pulmonary stenosis. (A) Chest film of a cyanotic patient shows a paucity of vascular markings in the left upper zone. The left pulmonary artery cannot be identified. Angiography demonstrated stenosis of the left upper lobe artery. (B) Right ventricular injection in a patient with tetralogy of Fallot demonstrates severe stenosis (*arrow*) of the left pulmonary artery.

metrical. Unusually small vascular markings at the level of the lobar and segmental branches suggest the presence of bilateral peripheral pulmonary stenosis.

Other causes of asymmetrical pulmonary vascularity include hypoplasia of the pulmonary artery associated with partial anomalous venous connection (scimitar syndrome, hypogenetic lung syndrome) (Fig. 17.24) and pulmonary valvular stenosis with poststenotic dilatation of the left pulmonary artery (see Fig. 17.14A).

CARDIOVASCULAR SILHOUETTE

CHAMBER ENLARGEMENT: GENERAL OBSERVATIONS

The appearance of the cardiac silhouette on frontal and lateral projections in adults with congenital heart disease depends on the size and position of the cardiac chambers.

RIGHT ATRIUM

On the frontal projection, the right atrium forms the right contour of the heart; its inferior (juxtadiaphragmatic) margin is smoothly curved (see Fig. 17.14A). The only part of the right atrium normally visible on the lateral projection is a small portion of the atrial appendage situated above the right ventricular outflow tract (see Fig. 17.14B). Although minimal right atrial enlargement may be difficult to appreciate on chest radiographs, significant right atrial enlargement is easily detected on both frontal and lateral views. On the frontal projection, the right cardiac contour is deviated laterally and inferiorly; on the lateral projection, the retrosternal space may be obscured by the dilated right atrial appendage (see Fig. 17.18).

RIGHT VENTRICLE

The right ventricle lies anterior to the right atrium and left ventricle; it normally forms part of the left heart border on the frontal projection. On the lateral view, the anterior margin of the right ventricle is closely opposed to the inferior third of the anterior chest wall (Figs. 17.14B and 17.16B). When the right ventricle is enlarged, it projects anteriorly and to the left, resulting in elevation of the apex on the frontal projection and increased contact between the superior border of the manubrium and the anterior costophrenic angle. Examples of right ventricular enlargement are shown in Figs. 17.3, 17.4, 17.14, 17.16, and 17.21.

As noted above, right atrial enlargement can also result in increased contact between the heart and the anterior chest wall on the lateral projection. Differentiation from right ventricular enlargement is usually possible on the frontal projection, be-

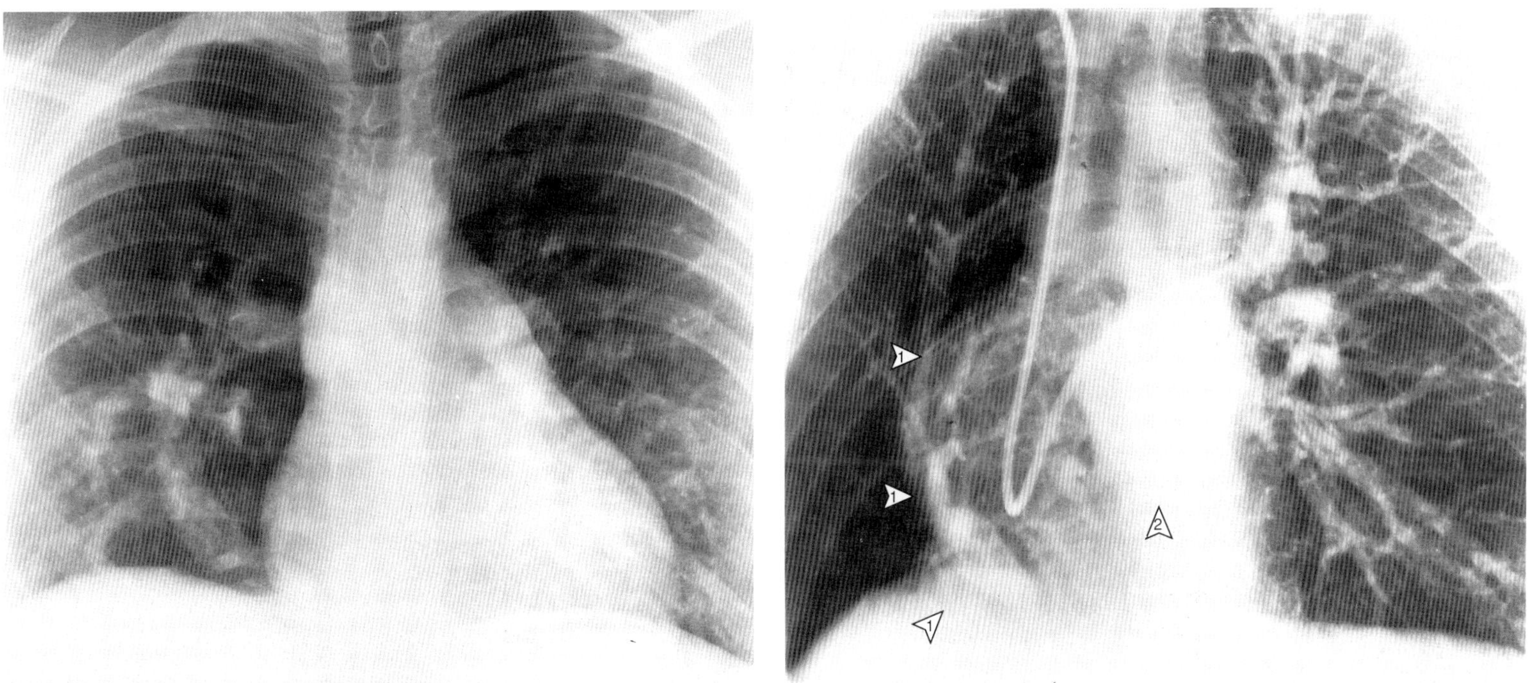

A B

Fig. 17.24 Hypogenetic right lung with partial anomalous pulmonary venous return (scimitar syndrome). (A) Frontal chest radiograph of a patient with partial anomalous pulmonary reveals venous connection of the right pulmonary vein to the inferior vena cava. The right lung is slightly smaller than the left. The only pulmonary vein draining the right lung courses medially and inferiorly towards the right cardiophrenic angle. The pulmonary vasculature is of left to right shunt type in the left lung and is normal to slightly decreased on the right. The pulmonary trunk is dilated. (B) Venous phase of a pulmonary angiogram in another patient. The entire venous return of the right lung is carried by a scimitar-shaped pulmonary vein (*arrows* 1) which drains into inferior vena cava below the diaphragm. The veins draining the left lung are connected to the left atrium (*arrow* 2).

cause the right heart border is displaced to the right and appears more convex than normal in patients with right atrial enlargement (Figs. 17.17 and 17.18).

LEFT ATRIUM

The left atrium forms the posterior and superior contours of the heart. On the frontal projection, the enlarged left atrial appendage forms the contour between the pulmonary artery and the left ventricle (Figs. 17.25A, 17.25C, and 17.26A). Other manifestations of left atrial enlargement include elevation and posterior displacement of the left main bronchus, widening of the carinal angle, and posterior displacement of the barium-filled esophagus (Figs. 17.25B, 17.26B, and 17.27). In extreme instances, the enlarged left atrium projects beyond the right atrium, in which case it forms the right border of the cardiac silhouette (Fig. 17.17A).

LEFT VENTRICLE

On the frontal projection, The left ventricle forms the inferior aspect of the left cardiac contour, curving smoothly downward to the level of the diaphragm. On the lateral projection, it forms the posterior and inferior contours of the cardiac silhouette.

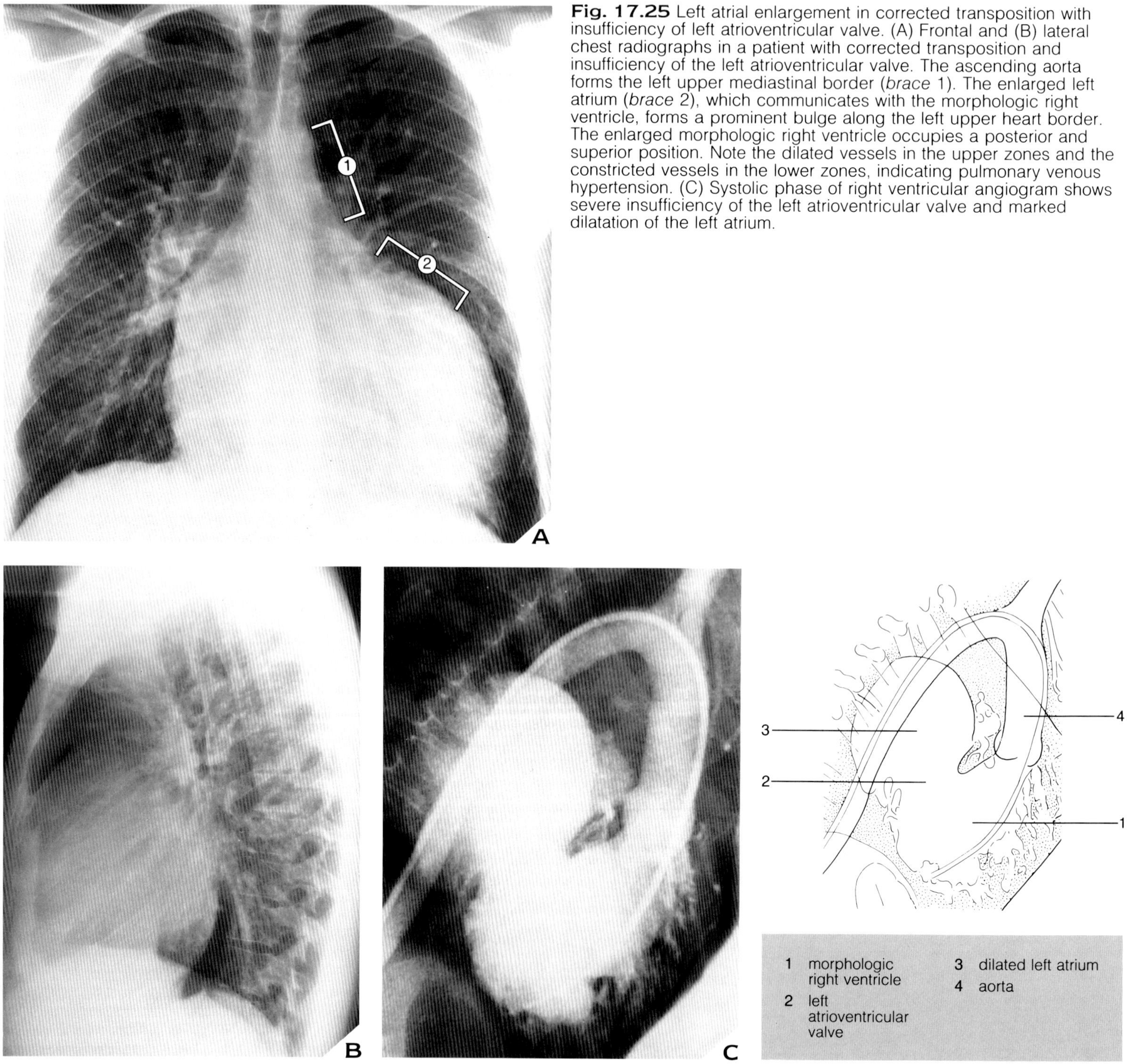

1 morphologic right ventricle
2 left atrioventricular valve
3 dilated left atrium
4 aorta

Fig. 17.25 Left atrial enlargement in corrected transposition with insufficiency of left atrioventricular valve. (A) Frontal and (B) lateral chest radiographs in a patient with corrected transposition and insufficiency of the left atrioventricular valve. The ascending aorta forms the left upper mediastinal border (*brace* 1). The enlarged left atrium (*brace* 2), which communicates with the morphologic right ventricle, forms a prominent bulge along the left upper heart border. The enlarged morphologic right ventricle occupies a posterior and superior position. Note the dilated vessels in the upper zones and the constricted vessels in the lower zones, indicating pulmonary venous hypertension. (C) Systolic phase of right ventricular angiogram shows severe insufficiency of the left atrioventricular valve and marked dilatation of the left atrium.

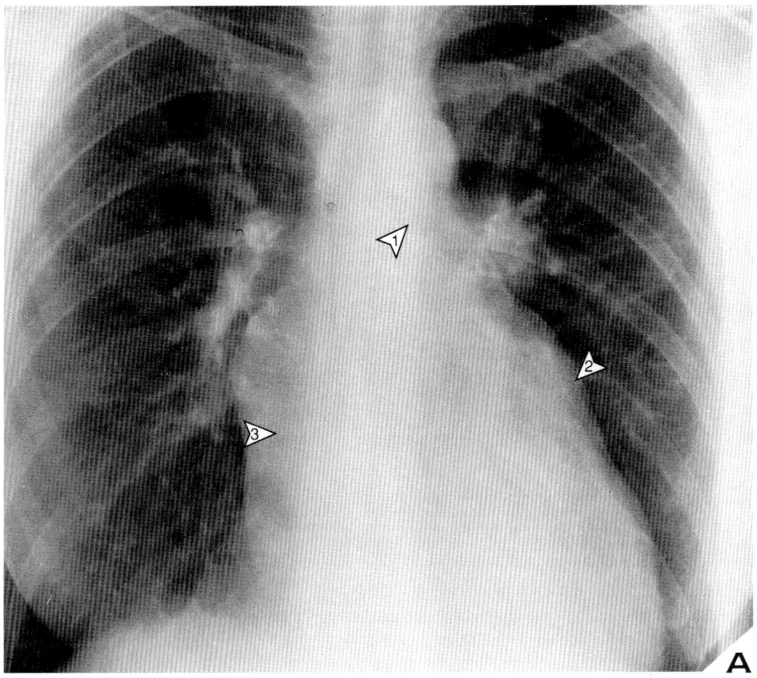

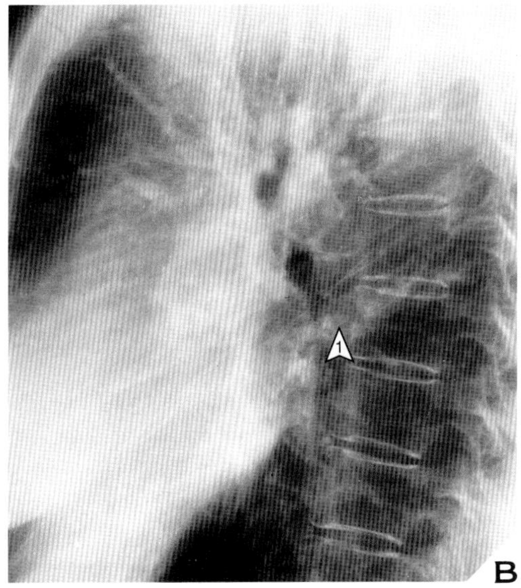

Fig. 17.26 Left atrial enlargement. (A) Frontal and (B) lateral radiographs show moderate left atrial enlargement in a patient with congenital mitral insufficiency. Note elevation of the left mainstem bronchus (*arrow* 1), a double density within the cardiac silhouette, and enlargement of the left atrial appendage (*arrow* 2). The enlarged left atrium forms a portion of the right heart border (*arrow* 3). (B) Lateral projection shows prominence of the upper posterior border of the heart and elevation of the left main bronchus (*arrow* 1).

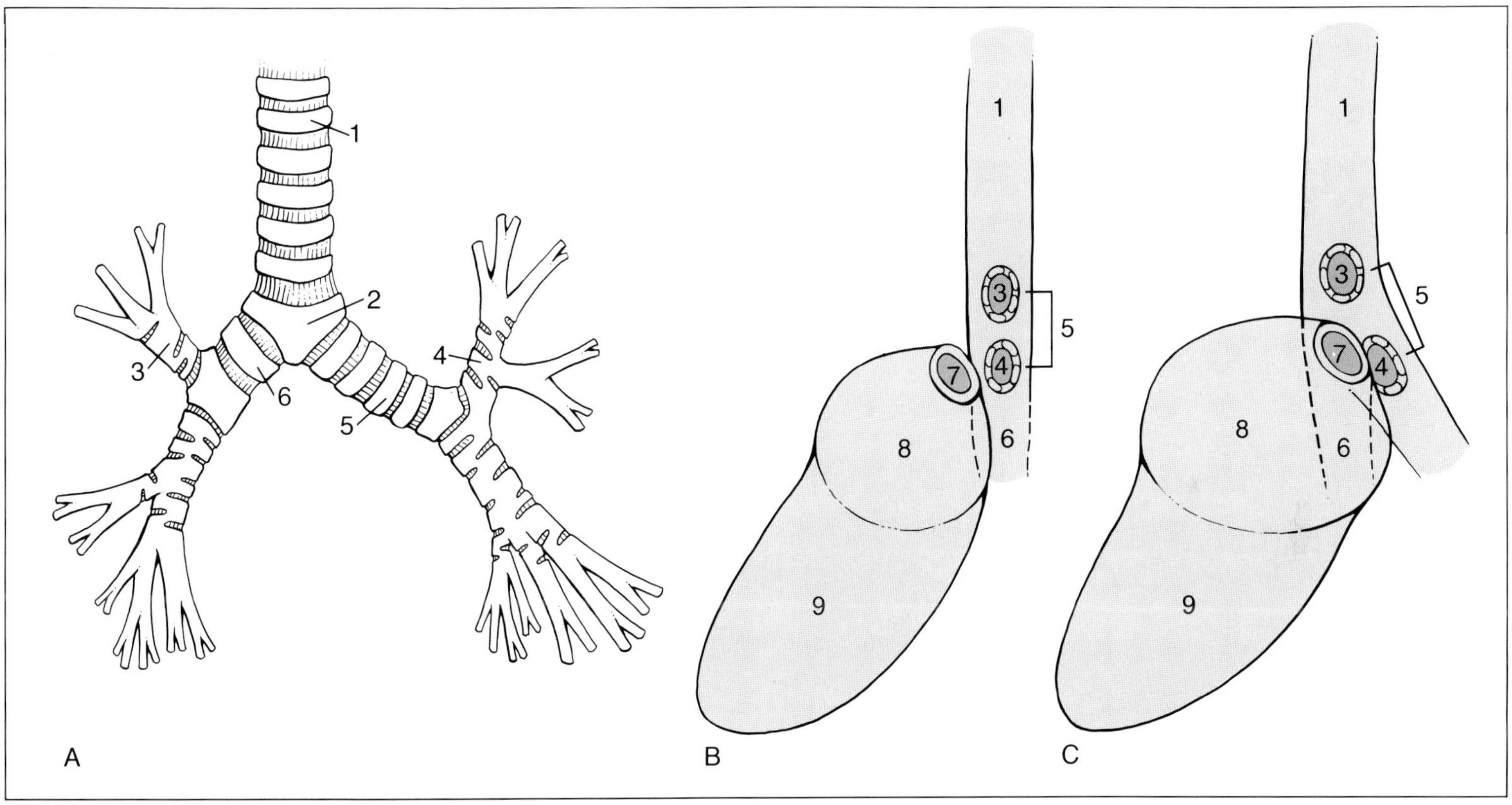

1 trachea	4 left upper lobe bronchus	7 left superior pulmonary vein
2 bifurcation (carina)	5 left main bronchus	8 left atrium
3 right upper lobe bronchus	6 right main bronchus	9 left ventricle

Fig. 17.27 Displacement of left main bronchus by enlarged left atrium as seen on lateral chest film. Diagrammatic representation of normal tracheobronchial tree in frontal (A) and lateral (B) projections. The left main bronchus, which abuts the posterosuperior border of the left atrium, normally merges imperceptably with the tracheal air column. Although the carina cannot be identified on the lateral projection, the left main bronchus roughly corresponds to the portion of the air column between the right and left uper lobe bronchi, which are seen *en face* on this view. Normally, the trachea, left main bronchus, and right main bronchus are in perfect alignment on a well-positioned left lateral film. The superior pulmonary vein and/or left atrium lie immediately anterior to the left main bronchus; with left atrial enlargement, the left main bronchus is displaced posteriorly (C). Posterior displacement of the left upper lobe bronchus on a well-positioned lateral view is reliable evidence of the left atrial enlargement. Because the esophagus is related to the right portion of the left atrium, and the left main bronchus is related to the left portion of the left atrium, asymmetrical enlargement of the left atrium may cause esophageal displacement without displacement of the left main bronchus. Posterior displacement of the left main bronchus is not a valid indicator of left atrial enlargement in patients with other causes of bronchial rearrangement (eg, lobar collapse), mediastinal masses, or marked dilatation of the central pulmonary arteries. (Adapted from Lane EJ Jr, Whalen JP: A new sign of left atrial enlargement: Posterior displacement of the left bronchial tree. *Radiology* 1969; 93:289)

When the left ventricle is enlarged, the cardiac apex is displaced downward on the frontal projection (Figs. 17.8A and 17.28A), and the posteroinferior margin of the heart projects beyond the plane of the inferior vena cava on the lateral (Fig. 17.28B). It must be emphasized, however, that the latter finding is valid only on a true lateral projection obtained in deep inspiration.

CHAMBER ENLARGEMENT ASSOCIATED WITH ABNORMALITIES OF THE ATRIOVENTRICULAR VALVES

Careful assessment of chamber size may provide an important clue to the diagnosis of congenital malformations of the atrioventricular valves.

TRICUSPID INSUFFICIENCY

The prototype of congenital tricuspid insufficiency is Ebstein's malformation. In this anomaly, the tricuspid valve leaflets are plastered to the right ventricular wall, resulting in severe tricuspid insufficiency. The classical radiographic findings are enlargement of the right atrium and right ventricle, associated with diminished pulmonary vascularity (see Fig. 17.18). Tricuspid insufficiency may also be associated with corrected transposition. In such patients the tricuspid valve leaflets are short and have rolled margins.

MITRAL INSUFFICIENCY

Prolapse of the mitral valve is a common cause of mitral insufficiency in adults; chest films typically show left atrial and left ventricular enlargement (see Chapter 18). A cleft mitral valve associated with an atrioventricular septal defect (atrioventricular canal) is an uncommon cause of mitral insufficiency in adults. In the great majority of cases the left atrium is decompressed via the atrial septal defect, and the plain film findings are those of an atrial septal defect (ie, pulmonary plethora and right atrial enlargement). However, patients with an intact atrial septum or a restricted atrial septal defect exhibit left atrial enlargement. Mitral insufficiency may also be associated with corrected transposition (see Fig. 17.25).

MITRAL STENOSIS

Congenital stenosis of the mitral valve is occasionally found in adults, and is usually due to a malformed parachute valve that was not stenotic enough to produce severe symptoms in early life. Chest films typically show severe dilatation of the left atrium and signs of pulmonary venous hypertension, findings indistinguishable from those seen in mitral stenosis secondary to rheumatic heart disease (see Chapter 18).

DEFORMITY OF THE LEFT BORDER OF THE CARDIOVASCULAR SILHOUETTE

Patients with certain cardiac malformations commonly exhibit a prominent bulge in the midportion of the left cardiovascular silhouette, between the main pulmonary artery and the left ventricular contour, on the frontal projection (Fig. 17.29). Malformations associated with this appearance include hypoplastic right ventricle in an inverted position, juxtaposition of the atrial appendages, dilatation of the left atrial appendage secondary to left atrial enlargement, and partial absence of the pericardium with herniation of a cardiac or vascular structure (Fig. 17.30). In a cyanotic patient with this finding, the diagnostic possibilities include univentricular atrioventricular connection to the left ventricle with the aorta arising from the hypoplastic left-sided right ventricle (see Fig. 17.29), juxtaposition of the atrial appendages associated with tricuspid atresia, and transposition of the great arteries.

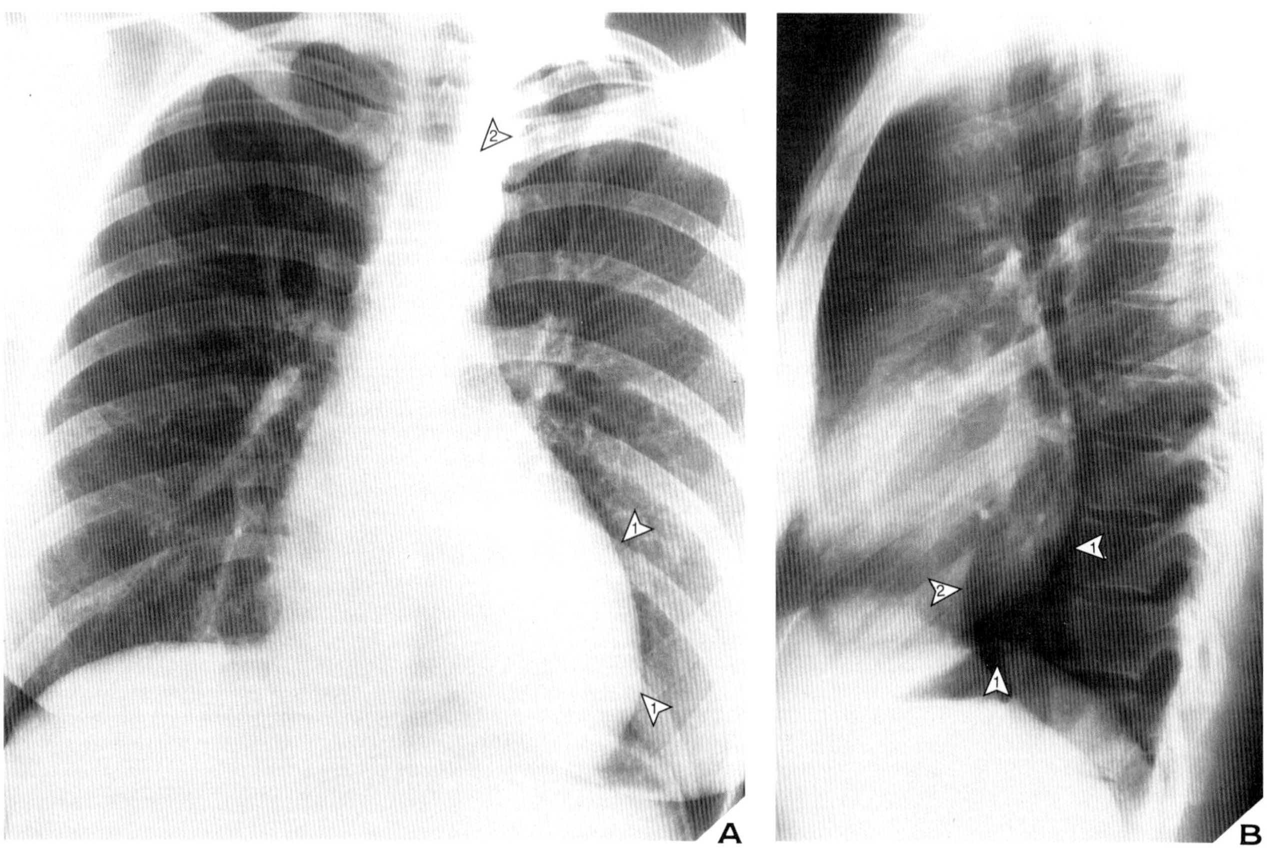

Fig. 17.28 Left ventricular hypertrophy (coarctation of the aorta). (A) Frontal and (B) lateral projections show bulging of the inferior portion of the left cardiac border (*arrows* 1 in A) and the posteroinferior margin of the heart (*arrows* 1 in B) margins. Note that the posteroinferior margin of the heart, which represents the left ventricle, projects well beyond the plane of the inferior vena cava (*arrow* 2 in B). The aortic arch is hypoplastic and the left subclavian artery is prominent (*arrow* 2 in A). These findings strongly suggest aortic coarctation even when rib notching is absent.

CARDIAC AXIS

The cardiac axis is normally directed anteriorly, inferiorly, and to the left; this arrangement is known as *levocardia* (see Fig. 17.1). In some instances the cardiac axis is directed to the right (*dextrocardia;* see Fig. 17.6A) or lies parallel to the diaphragm (*mesocardia;* see Fig. 17.11). It should be emphasized that the orientation of the cardiac axis does not provide an indication of the anatomy of the cardiac chambers and great arteries; however, certain arrangements do suggest specific congenital malformations. For example, a patient with atrial situs solitus and dextrocardia is likely to have a severe congenital heart malformation (usually congenitally corrected transposition of the great arteries). Similarly, congenital heart disease is very common in patients with atrial situs inversus and levocardia (Fig. 17.6).

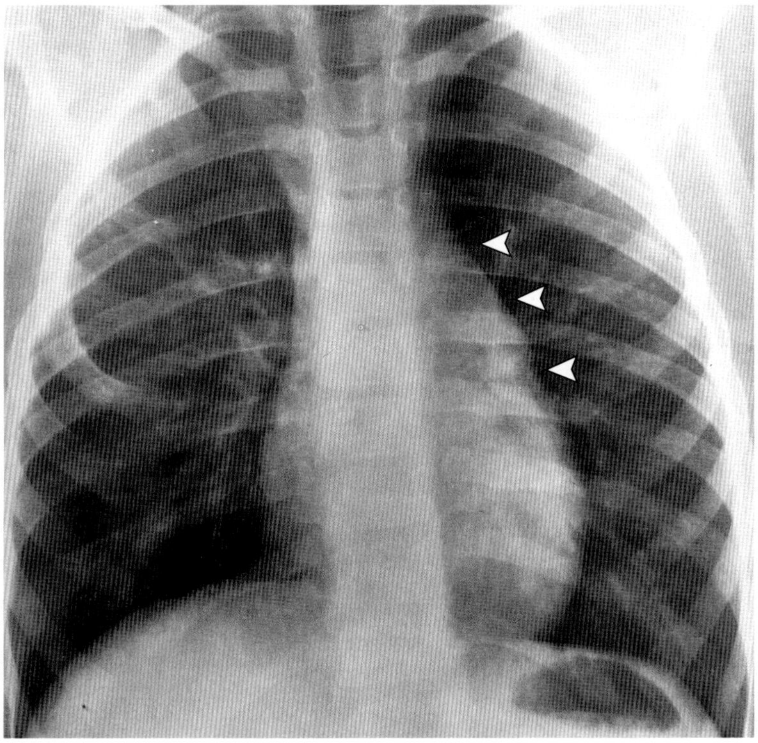

Fig. 17.29 Abnormal convexity of left heart border due to left-sided right ventricle (univentricular atrioventricular connection to a morphologic left ventricle). Posteroanterior chest film shows abnormal convexity of the left heart border (*arrows*), which represents the ascending aorta; it merges superiorly with the aortic arch and inferiorly with the small left-sided right ventricle. (In some individuals with this malformation the right ventricle forms an additional convexity along the left heart border.) The descending thoracic aorta and the aortic arch are right sided. The tracheobronchial tree is normal, indicating atrial situs solitus. Angiocardiography demonstrated ventricular inversion; the right ventricular outlet chamber was hypoplastic and displaced to the left. The presence of a left-sided ascending aorta, in conjunction with the deformity of the middle portion of the left cardiac border, strongly suggests the diagnosis of univentricular atrioventricular connection to the left ventricle with discordant ventriculoarterioal connection ("single ventricle" or "double-inlet left ventricle with transposition of the great arteries"). It should be emphasized that a similar deformity of the left heart border can be produced by juxtaposition of the atrial appendages or by a prominent left atrial appendage caused by left atrial enlargement.

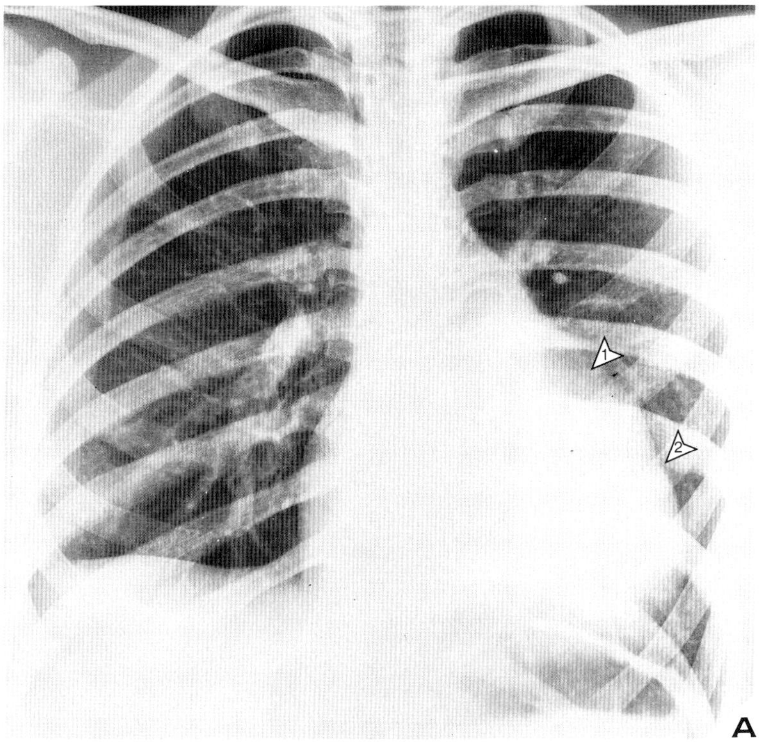

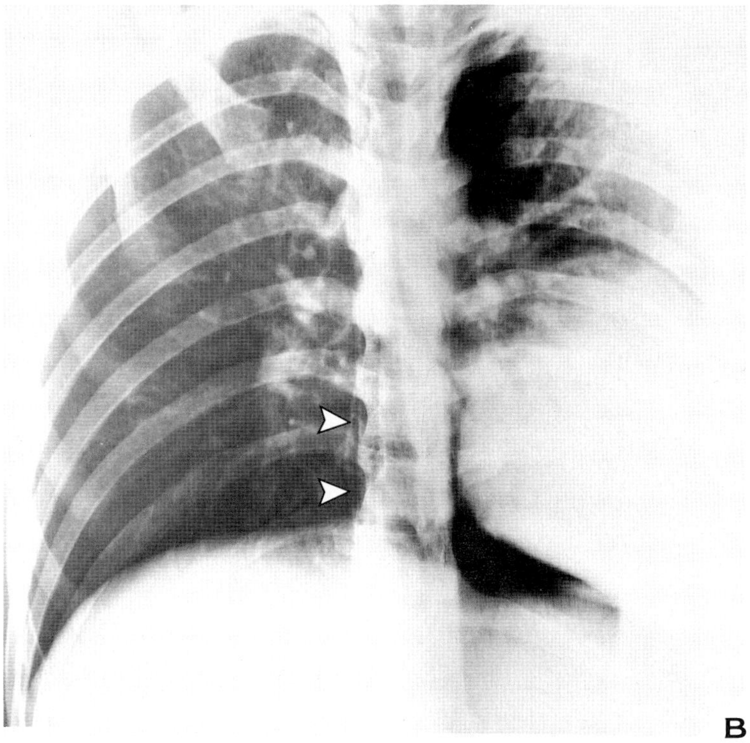

Fig. 17.30 Congenital absence of left pericardium. (A) Frontal projection of the chest. The heart is displaced to the left and the left heart border is close to the lateral chest wall. The left atrial appendage (*arrow* 1) and left ventricle (*arrow* 2) are sharply outlined. The cardiac apex is slightly elevated. (B) Left lateral decubitus projection obtained after injection of air into the left pleural space. Air has entered the pericardial space through the defect in the left pericardium and outlines the intact right pericardium (*arrows*).

A GENERAL APPROACH TO CONGENITAL CARDIAC MALFORMATIONS IN ADULTS

The plain film findings, taken together with the arterial oxygen saturation, allow one to suggest an appropriate differential diagnosis in an adult patient with known or suspected congenital heart disease, as follows.

1. Acyanotic conditions
   A. Pulmonary plethora
      i. Aortopulmonary shunt, such as aortopulmonary window or patent ductus arteriosis
      ii. Cardiac level shunts, such as atrial or atrioventricular septal defect
      iii. Peripheral arteriovenous fistula
   B. Normal-sized peripheral pulmonary vessels with right ventricular enlargement.
      i. Pulmonary valvular stenosis
      ii. Peripheral pulmonary arterial stenosis
   C. Normal pulmonary vasculature and left ventricular enlargement
      i. Aortic stenosis
      ii. Coarctation of the aorta
2. Cyanotic conditions
   A. Pulmonary plethora
      i. Transposition of the great arteries
      ii. Truncus arteriosus
      iii. Total anomalous pulmonary venous connection
      iv. Other admixture lesions, including single ventricle, isolated atrioventricular discordance, double outlet ventricle, etc.
   B. Normal or decreased pulmonary vasculature
      i. Tetralogy of Fallot
      ii. Pulmonary atresia with ventricular septal defect
      iii. Tricuspid atresia with normally related great arteries
3. Admixture syndromes
   A. Ascending aorta forming the left upper mediastinal contour
      i. Cyanotic conditions
         a. Univentricular, atrioventricular connection with inverted ventricles.
         b. Double outlet right ventricle
         c. Double outlet left ventricle
         d. Isolated atrioventricular discordance
      ii. Noncyanotic conditions
         a. Congenitally corrected transposition of the great arteries
         b. Anatomically corrected malposition of the aorta
   B. Cardiac silhouette with a hump in its left mid contour
      i. Cyanotic conditions
         a. Juxtaposition of the atrial appendages (associated with transposition of the great arteries or tricuspid atresia)
         b. Hypoplastic right ventricle and inverted position in the setting of univentricular atrioventricular connection
      ii. Noncyanotic conditions
         a. Partial pericardial defect
         b. Enlarged left atrial appendage associated with a stenotic mitral valve or isolated left atrial appendage aneurysm

References

GENERAL REFERENCES

Amplatz K, Moller JH, Castaneda WR: *Radiology of Congenital Heart Disease.* New York: Thieme Medical Publishers, Inc, 1986.

Braunwald E: *Heart Disease. A Textbook of Cardiovascular Medicine.* 3rd ed. Philadelphia: WB Saunders Co., 1988.

Gillette PC: Cardiac dysrhythmias in infants and children. In Allen Engle MA, ed. *Pediatric Cardiovascular Disease.* Philadelphia: FA Davis, 1981:79.

Doyle EF, Engle MA, Gersony WM, Rashkind WJ, Talner NS, Eds: *Pediatric Cardiology.* New York: Springer-Verlag, 1985.

Jefferson K, Rees S: *Clinical Cardiac Radiology.* 2nd ed. London: Butterworths, 1980.

Kassner EG, ed: *Iatrogenic Disorders of the Fetus, Infant, and Child.* New York: Springer-Verlag, 1985.

Kirklin JW, Barratt–Boyes B: *Cardiac Surgery.* New York: John Wiley & Son, 1986.

Moss AF, Adams FM, Emmanoulides GS, eds: *Heart Disease in Infants, Children and Adolescents.* Baltimore: Williams & Wilkins, 1977.

Rowe RD, Freedom RM, Mehrizi A, eds: *The Neonate with Congenital Heart Disease.* 2nd ed. Philadelphia: WB Saunders, 1981.

Soto B, Pacifico AD: *Angiocardiography in Congenital Heart Malformations.* New York: Futura Publishing, 1990.

Spindola–Franco H, Fish BG: *Radiology of the Heart: Cardiac Imaging in Infants, Children and Adults.* New York: Springer-Verlag, 1985.

CHAPTER REFERENCES

CHAPTER 1: NONINVASIVE RADIOLOGIC TECHNIQUES AND ELECTROCARDIOGRAPHY

CHEST RADIOGRAPHY, FLUOROSCOPY, COMPUTED TOMOGRAPHY

Eldredge WJ, Flicker S: Evaluation of congenital heart disease using cine-CT. *Am J Cardiac Imag* 1987; 1:38.

Jefferson K: *Clinical Cardiac Radiology.* London: Butterworths, 1970.

Joseph PM, Berdon WE, Baker DH, et al: Upper airway obstruction in infants and small children. *Radiology* 1976; 121:143.

Lipton MJ: Quantitation of cardiac function. *Radiol Clin No Am* 1985; 23:613.

Sethna DH, Bateman TM, Whiting JS, Forrester JS: Comprehensive and quantitative cardiac assessment using cine-CT: Description of a new clinical diagnostic modality. *Am J Cardiac Imag* 1987; 1:18.

ELECTROCARDIOGRAPHY

Anderson RH, Ho SY, Becker AE: The clinical anatomy of cardiac conduction system. In Rowlands DJ, ed. *Recent Advances in Cardiology.* New York: Churchill Livingstone, 1984: 1.

Bigger JT: Mechanisms and diagnosis of arrhythmias. In Brunwald E, ed. *Heart Disease.* Philadelphia: WB Saunders, 1980: 630.

Chou TC: *Electrocardiolography in Clinical Practice.* 2nd ed. Baltimore: Williams & Wilkins, 1983.

Fisch CH: Electrocardiography and vectorcardiography. In Brunwald E, ed. *Heart Diseases.* 3rd ed. Philadelphia: WB Saunders, 1988:180.

Gillette PC: Cardiac dysrhythmia in infants and children. In Allen Engle MA, ed. *Pediatric Cardiovascular Disease.* Philadelphia: FA Davis, 1981: 79.

Marriott H: *Practical Electrocardiography.* 8th ed. Baltimore: Williams & Wilkins, 1988.

Myerburg R, Castellanos A: Cardiac arrest and sudden cardiac death. In Brunwald E, ed. *Heart Disease.* 3rd ed. Philadelphia: WB Saunders, 1988:742.

Zipes DP, Jalife J: *Cardiac Electrophysiology from Cell to Bedside.* Philadelphia: WB Saunders, 1990.

CHAPTER 2: ECHOCARDIOGRAPHY

Anderson RH, Macartney FJ, Shinebourne EA, et al: *Pediatric Cardiology.* New York: Churchill Livingstone, 1987: 65.

Feigenbaum H: *Echocardiography.* 4th ed. Philadelphia: Lea & Febiger, 1986.

Hatle L, Angelsen B: *Doppler Ultrasound in Cardiology.* Philadelphia: Lea & Febiger, 1985.

Helmcke F, Nanda NC, Hsiung MC, et al: Color Doppler assessment of mitral regurgitation with orthogonal planes. *Circulation* 1987; 75:175.

Nanda NC: *Atlas of Color Doppler Echocardiography.* Philadelphia: Lea & Febiger, 1989.

Nanda NC: Congenital heart disease. In Nanda NC, ed.: *Atlas of Color Doppler Echocardiography.* Philadelphia: Lea & Febiger, 1989.

Nanda NC: *Textbook of Color Doppler Echocardiography.* Philadelphia: Lea & Febiger, 1989.

Nishimura RA, Miller FA, Callahan MJ, et al: Doppler echocardiography: Theory, instrumentation, technique, and application. *Mayo Clin Proc* 1985; 60:321.

Omoto R: *Color Atlas of Real Time Two-dimensional Doppler Echocardiography.* Tokyo: Shindan-To-Chiryo, 1984.

Perry GJ, Helmcke F, Nanda NC, et al: Evaluation of aortic insufficiency by Doppler color flow mapping. *J Am Coll Cardiol* 1987; 9:952.

Ritter SB: Transesophageal echocardiography in children. New peephole to the heart. Editorial Comments. *J Am Coll Cardiol* 1990; 16:447.

Sciller NB, Shah PM, Crawford M, et al: Recommendations for quantitation of the left ventricle by two-dimensional echocardiography. *J Am Soc Echo* 1989; 2:358.

Tajik AJ, Seward JB, Hagler DJ, et al: Two-dimensional real-time ultrasonic imaging of the heart and great vessels: Technique, image orientation, structure identification, and validation. *Mayo Clin Proc* 1978; 53:271.

CHAPTER 3: INVASIVE DIAGNOSTIC PROCEDURES

Balter S, Sones M, Brancato R: Radiation exposure to the operator performing cardiac angiography with U-arm system. *Circulation* 1979; 58:925.

Baxley WA, Soto B: Hemodynamic evaluation of patients with mechanical prosthesis in both mitral and aortic position. *Am J Cardiol* 1980; 45:542.

Braunwald E, Ross J, Sonnenblick EH: *Mechanism of Contraction of the Normal and Failing Heart.* 2nd ed. Boston: Little, Brown, and Co, 1976.

Gertz EW, Wisneski JA, Gould RG, et al: Improved radiation protection for physicians performing cardiac catheterization. *Am J Cardiol* 1982; 50:1283.

Gomes AS, Baker JD, Paredero VM, et al: Acute renal dysfunction after major arteriography. *AJR* 1985; 145:1249.

Lassen EC, Berry CC, Talner LB, et al: Pretreatment with corticoids to alleviate reactions to intravenous contrast material: A randomized multi-institutional study. *N Engl J Med* 1987; 317:845.

Lister G, Talner NS: Oxygen transport in congenital heart disease. In Engle MA, ed. *Pediatric Cardiovascular Disease.* Philadelphia: FA Davis, 1981:129.

Parfrey PS, Griffiths SA, Barrett BJ: Contrast material induced renal failure in patients with diabetes mellitus, renal insufficiency, or both. *N Engl J Med* 1989; 320:143.

Reagan K, Bettman MA, Finkelstein BA, et al: Double-blind study of a new nonionic contrast agent for cardiac angiography. *Radiology* 1988; 167:409.

Rudolph A: *Congenital Disease of the Heart.* Chicago: Year Book Medical Publishers, 1974.

Rueter FG: Physician and patient exposure during cardiac catheterization. *Circulation* 1978; 58:134.

Schwab SJ, Hlatky MA, Pieper KS: Contrast nephrotoxicity: A randomized controlled trial of a nonionic and an ionic radiographic contrast agent. *N Engl J Med* 1989; 320:149.

Stacul F, Carraro M, Magnaldi S, et al: Contrast agent nephrotoxicity: Comparison of ionic and nonionic contrast agents. *AJR* 1987; 149:1287.

Weber KT, Janicki JS, Shroff SG, et al: The mechanics of ventricular function. *Hosp Prac* May 1983; 113.

CHAPTER 4: MAGNETIC RESONANCE IMAGING

Aisen AM, Chenevert TL: MR spectroscopy: Clinical perspective. *Radiology* 1989; 173:593.

Bittner V, Cranney GB, Lotan CS, et al: Overview of cardiovascular nuclear magnetic resonance imaging. *Cardiol Clin* 1989; 7:631.

Council on Scientific Affairs of the American Medical Association: Report of the Magnetic Resonance Imaging Panel. Fundamentals of magnetic resonance imaging. *JAMA* 1987; 258:3417.

Council on Scientific Affairs of the American Medical Association: Report of the Magnetic Resonance Imaging Panel. Present state of the art and future potential. *JAMA* 1988; 259:253.

Cranney GB, Lotan CS, Pohost GM: Evaluation of aortic regurgitation by magnetic resonance imaging. *Curr Prob Cardiol* 1990; 15:87.

Gangarosa RE, Minnis JE, Nobbe J, et al: Operational safety issues in MRI. *Magn Reson Imaging* 1987; 5:287.

Klipstein RH, Firmin DN, Underwood SR, et al: Blood flow patterns in the human aorta studied by magnetic resonance. *Br Heart J* 1987; 58:316.

Lim TH, Saloner D, Anderson CM: Current applications of magnetic resonance vascular imaging. *Cardiol Clin* 1989; 7:661.

Lotan CS, Cranney GB, Bouchard A, et al: The value of cine nuclear magnetic resonance imaging for assessing regional ventricular function. *J Am Coll Cardiol* 1989; 14:1721.

Nazarian GK, Julsrud PR, Elman RL, et al: Correlation between magnetic resonance imaging of the heart and cardiac anatomy. *Mayo Clin Proc* 1987; 62:573.

Pettigrew RI: Dynamic cardiac MR imaging. Technique and applications. *Radiol Clin No Am* 1989; 27:1183.

Schaefer S, Massie B, Weiner MW: Magnetic resonance spectroscopy of the heart. *Cardiol Clin* 1989; 7:697.

Stehling MJ, Howseman AM, Ordidge RJ, et al: Whole-body echo-planar MR imaging at 0.5 T. *Radiology* 1989; 170:257.

CHAPTER 4A: NUCLEAR CARDIOLOGY

Berman DS, ed: A symposium: Technetium-99m myocardial perfusion imaging agents and their relation to thallium-201. *Am J Cardiol* 1990; 66:1E.

Callahan RF, Froelich JW, McKusick KA, et al: A modified method for in vivo labelling of red blood cells with Tc99-m: Concise communication. *J Nucl Med* 1982; 23:315.

Dilsizian V, Rocco TP, Freedman NMT, et al: Enhanced detection of ischemic but viable myocardium by the reinjection of thallium after stress-redistribution imaging. *N Engl J Med* 1990; 323:141.

Gould KI, Westcott RJ, Albro PC, et al: Noninvasive assessment of coronary stenoses by myocardial imaging during pharmacologic coronary vasodilation: II. Clinical methodology and feasibility. *Am J Cardiol* 1978; 41:279.

Hendel RC, McSherry B, Karimeddini M, et al: Diagnostic value of a new myocardial perfusion, agent, Teboroxime (SQ 30,217), utilizing a rapid planar imaging protocol: Preliminary results. *J Am Coll Cardiol* 1990; 16:855.

Johnson LL, Seldin DW, Becker LC, et al: Antimyosin imaging in acute transmural myocardial infarctions: Results of a multicenter clinical trial. *J Am Coll Cardiol* 1989; 13:27.

Kiat H, Berman DS, Maddahi J, Yang LDL, et al: Late reversibility of tomographic myocardial thallium-201 defects: An accurate marker of myocardial viability. *J Am Coll Cardiol* 1988; 12:1456.

Leppo JA, O'Brien J, Rothendler JA, et al: Dipyridamolel-thallium-201 scintigraphy in the prediction of future cardiac events after acute myocardial infarction. *N Engl J Med* 1984; 310:1014.

Passamani E, Davis KB, Gillespie MJ, et al: A randomized trial of coronary artery bypass surgery: Survival in patients with low ejection fraction. *N Engl J Med* 1985; 312:1665.

Pohost GM, Zir LM, Moore RH, et al: Differentiation of transiently ischemic from infarcted myocardium by serial imaging after a single dose of thallium-201. *Circulation* 1977; 55:294.

Schelbert HR, Phelps ME, Hoffman E, et al: Regional myocardial blood flow, metabolism, and function assessed noninvasively with positron emission tomography. *Am J Cardiol* 1980; 80:1269.

Verani MS, Mahmarian JJ, Hixson JB, et al: Diagnosis of coronary artery disease by controlled coronary vasodilation with adenosine and thallium-201 scintigraphy in patients unable to exercise. *Circulation* 1990; 82:80.

CHAPTER 5: THE CHILD WITH CONGENITAL HEART DISEASE

de la Cruz MV, Gomez CS, Arteaga MM, et al: Experimental study of the development of the truncus and the conus in the chick embryo. *J Anat* 1977; 123:661.

Martin EC: Heritable syndromes and skeletal abnormalities and congenital heart disease. *NY State J Med* 1977; 77:944.

Nora JJ, Nora AH: The evolutions of specific genetic and environmental counseling in congenital heart diseases. *Circulation* 1978; 57:205.

Rudolph AM: Development consideration in neonatal failure. *Hosp Prac* January 15, 1985; 53.

Van Mierop LHS, Alley RD, Kausel HW, et al: Pathogenesis of transposition complexes. I. Embryology of the ventricles and great arteries. *Am J Cardiol* 1963; 12:216.

Van Mierop LHS, Wiglesworth FW: Pathogenesis of transposition complexes. II. Anomalies due to faulty transfer of the posterior great artery. *Am J Cardiol* 1963; 12:226.

Van Mierop LHS, Wiglesworth FW: Pathogenesis of transposition of the great vessels: III. True transposition of the great vessels. *Am J Cardiol* 1963; 12:233.

Van Praagh R, Van Praagh S: Embryology and anatomy: Keys to the understanding of complex congenital heart disease. *Coeur* 1982; 13:315.

CHAPTER 6: CARDIAC ANATOMY RELEVANT TO CONGENITAL HEART DISEASE

Anderson RH, Becker AE, Lucchese FE, et al: *Morphology of Congenital Heart Disease. Angiographic, Echocardiographic and Surgical Correlates.* Kent, UK: Castle House Publications, 1983.

Anderson RM, Baker AE: *Cardiac Anatomy.* New York: Gower Medical Publishing, 1980.

Becker AE, Anderson RH: *Pathology of Congenital Heart Disease.* London: Butterworths, 1981.

Ceballos R, Soto B, Bargeron LM: Angiographic anatomy of the normal heart through axial angiography. *Circulation* 1981; 64:351.

Hurst JW: *Atlas of the Heart.* New York: Gower Medical Publishing, 1988.

Van Mierop LHS: Diagnostic code for congenital heart disease. *Pediatr Cardiol* 1984; 5:331.

CHAPTER 7: PLAIN FILM EVALUATION OF CONGENITAL HEART DISEASE

Amplatz K, Moller JH, Zuniga WR: *Radiology of Congenital Heart Disease.* New York: Thieme Medical Publishing, 1986.

Elliott LP: Radiological differentiation of the common congenital malformations of the heart and great vessels. In Robert WC, ed. *Congenital Heart Disease in Adults.* Philadelphia: FA Davis, 1979: 91.

Jefferson K: *Clinical Cardiac Cardiology.* 2nd ed. London: Butterworths, 1973.

Kirklin JW, Pacifico AD, Bargeron LM, et al: Cardiac repair in anatomically corrected malposition of great arteries. *Circulation* 1973; 68:153.

Shinebourne EA, Macartney FJ, Anderson RH: Sequential chamber localization—logical approach to diagnosis in congenital heart disease. *Br Heart J.* 1976; 38:327.

White RI, Jordan CHE, Fisher KC, et al: Skeletal changes associated with adolescent congenital heart disease. *AJR* 1972; 110:531.

CHAPTER 8: ABNORMALITIES OF THE ATRIAL SEGMENT

De Tommasi SM, Daliento L, Ho SY, et al: Analysis of atrioventricular junction, ventricular mass and ventriculoarterial junction in 43 specimens with atrial isomerism. *Br Heart J* 1981; 45:236.

Diethelm L, Dery R, Lipton MJ: Atrial level shunts: Sensitivity and specificity of MR in diagnosis. *Radiology* 1987; 162:181.

Ettedgui JA, Siewers R, Anderson RH, et al: Diagnostic echocardiographic features of the sinus venous defect. *Br Heart J* 1990; 64:329.

Gutgesell HP, Cheatham J, Latson LA, et al: Atrioventricular valve abnormalities in infancy. Two-dimensional echocardiographic and angiographic comparison. *J Am Coll Cardiol* 1983; 2:531.

Gutgesell HP, Huhta JC, Latson LA, et al: Accuracy of two-dimensional echocardiography in the diagnosis of congenital heart disease. *Am J Cardiol* 1985; 55:514.

Hernanz–Schulman M, Ambrosino MM, Geneiser NB, et al: Current evaluation of the patient with abnormal visceroatrial situs. *AJR* 1990; 154:797.

Jacobstein MD, Fletcher BD, Goldstein S: Evaluation of atrioventricular septal defect by magnetic resonance imaging. *Am J Cardiol* 1985; 55:1158.

Macartney FJ, Patridge JB, Shinebourne EA, et al: Identification of atrial situs. In Anderson RH, Shinebourne EA, eds. *Pediatric Cardiology.* London: Churchill Livingstone, 1978: 16.

Parsons JM, Baker EJ, Anderson RH, et al: Morphological evaluation of atrioventricular septal defects by magnetic resonance imaging. *Br Heart J* 1990; 64:138.

Sanders C, Bittner V, Nath PH, et al: Atrial septal defect in older adults: Atypical radiographic appearance. *Radiology* 1988; 167:123.

Sanders SP: Echocardiography and related techniques in the diagnosis of congenital heart defects. Part II. Atrioventricular valves and ventricle. *Echocardiography* 1984; 1:333.

Soto B, Banuelos C, Ceballos R: Angiographic recognition of atrial septal defect. *Rev Latinoam Cardiol* 1986; 1:181.

Soto B, Pacifico AD, Souze AS, et al: Identification of thoracic isomerism from the plain chest film roentgenogram. *AJR* 1978; 131:995.

Stanger P, Rudolph AM, Edwards JE: Cardiac malpositions. An overview based on study of sixty-five necropsy specimens. *Circulation* 1977; 56:159.

Stumper OFW, Sreeram N, Elzenga NJ, et al: Diagnosis of atrial situs by transesophageal echocardiography. *J Am Coll Cardiol* 1990; 16:442.

Winer–Muran HT, Tonkin ILD: The spectrum of heterotaxic syndromes. *Radiol Clin No Am* 1989; 27:1147.

CHAPTER 9: VENTRICULAR AND ATRIOVENTRICULAR SEPTAL DEFECTS

Bittner V, Colvin EF, Soto B, et al: Diagnosis of atrioventricular septal defects. *Rev Latina de Card Inf* 1987; 3:177.

Gutgesell HP, Cheatham J, Latson LA, et al: Atrioventricular valve abnormalities in infancy. Two-dimensional echocardiographic and angiographic comparison. *J Am Coll Cardiol* 1983; 2:531.

Gutgesell HP, Huhta JC, Latson LA, et al: Accuracy of two-dimensional echocardiography in the diagnosis of congenital heart disease. *Am J Cardiol* 1985; 55:514.

Jacobstein MD, Fletcher BD, Goldstein S: Evaluation of atrioventricular septal defect by magnetic resonance imaging. *Am J Cardiol* 1985; 55:1158.

Parsons JM, Baker EJ, Anderson RH, et al: Morphological evaluation of atrioventricular septal defects by magnetic resonance imaging. *Br Heart J* 1990; 64:138.

Piccoli GP, Gerlis LM, Wilkinson JL, et al: Morphology and classification of atrioventricular defects. *Br Heart J* 1979; 42:621.

Sanders SP: Echocardiography and related techniques in the diagnosis of congenital heart defects. Part II. Atrioventricular valves and ventricles. *Echocardiography* 1984; 1:333.

Santamaria H, Soto B, Ceballos R, et al: Angiographic differentiation of types of ventricular septal defects. *AJR* 1983; 141:273.

Silverman NH, Ho SY, Anderson RH, et al: Atrioventricular septal defect with intact atrial and ventricular septal structures. *Int J Cardiol* 1984; 5:567.

Soto B, Bargeron LM, Pacifico AD, et al: Angiography of atrioventricular canal defects. *Am J Cardiol* 1981; 48:492.

Soto B, Becker AE, Moulaert AJ, et al: Classification of ventricular septal defects. *Br Heart J* 1980; 43:332.

Soto B, Ceballos R, Kirklin JW: Ventricular septal defects: A surgical viewpoint. *J Am Coll Cardiol* 1989; 14:1291.

CHAPTER 10: ABNORMAL ATRIOVENTRICULAR CONNECTIONS

Allwork S, Bentall HH, Becker AE, et al: Congenitally corrected transposition of the great arteries: Morphological study of 32 cases. *Am J Cardiol* 1976; 38:910.

Anderson RH, Becker AE, Macartney FJ, et al: Is "tricuspid atresia" a univentricular heart? A question of definition. *Pediatr Cardiol* 1979; 1:51.

Anderson RH, Lenox C, Zuberbuhler JR, et al: Double inlet left ventricle with rudimentary right ventricle and ventriculoarterial concordance. *Am J Cardiol* 1983; 52:573.

Anderson RH, Wilkinson JL, Gerlis LM, et al: Atresia of the right atrioventricular orifice. *Br Heart J* 1977; 39:414.

Fletcher BD, Jacobstein MD, Abramowsky CR, et al: Right atrioventricular valve atresia: Anatomic evaluation with MR imaging. *AJR* 1987; 148:671.

Girod DA, Lima RL, Anderson RH, et al: Double inlet ventricle: Morphological analysis and surgical implications in 32 cases. *J Thor Cardiovasc Surg* 1984; 88:590.

Gittenberger–de-Groot A, Wenick ACG: Mitral atresia. *Br Heart J* 1984; 51:522.

Hagler D, Tajik A, Seward JB, et al: Atrioventricular and ventriculo arterial discordance (corrected transposition of the great arteries). *Mayo Clin Proc* 1981; 56:591.

Losekoot TG, Anderson RH, Becker AE, et al: *Congenitally Corrected Transposition.* New York: Churchill Livingstone, 1983.

Ottenkamp J, Wenink CG, Rohmer J, et al: Tricuspid atresia with overriding imperforate tricuspid membrane, an anatomical variant. *Int J Cardiol* 1984; 6:599.

Rigby ML, Anderson RM, Gibson D, et al: Two-dimensional echocardiographic categorization of the univentricular heart. *Br Heart J* 1981; 46:603.

Rossi MB, Ho SY, Anderson RH: Double inlet ventricle and its relationship to heart with straddling and overriding atrioventricular valves. *Rev Latina de Card Inf* 1989; 3:171.

Soto B, Ceballos R, Nath PH, et al: Overriding atrioventricular valves. An angiographic-anatomical correlate. *Int J Cardiol* 1985; 9:327.

Soto B, Pacifico AD, DiSciascio G: "Univentricular heart: An angiographic study. *Am J Cardiol* 1982; 49:787.

Tenorio A, Rigby ML, Anderson RH, et al: The spectrum of atrioventricular discordance: A clinical study. *Br Heart J* 1984; 51:498.

Van Praagh K, Plett JA, Van Praagh S: Single ventricle. *Herz* 1979; 4:113.

Wilkinson JL, Becker AE, Tynan M, et al: Nomenclature of univentricular heart. *Herz* 1979; 4:107.

CHAPTER 11: ABNORMAL VENTRICULOARTERIAL CONNECTIONS

TETRALOGY OF FALLOT

Becker AE, Connor M, Anderson RH: Tetralogy of Fallot: A morphometric and geometric study. *Am J Cardiol* 1975; 35:402.

Gomes AS, Lois JF, Williams RG: Pulmonary arteries: MR imaging in patients with congenital obstruction of the right ventricular outflow tract. *Radiology* 1990; 174:51.

Kirklin JW, Bargeron LM, Pacifico AD, et al: Management of Tetralogy of Fallot with large aortopulmonary collateral arteries. In Burakosky VI, Bockeria LA, eds. Fourth Joint Symposium on Congenital Heart Disease. Moscow: MIR Publishers, 1981: 569.

Mirowitz SA, Gutierrez FR, Canter CE, et al: Tetralogy of Fallot: MR findings. *Radiology* 1989; 171:207.

Rosenquist GG, Sweeney LJ, Stemple AR, et al: Ventricular septal defect in tetralogy of Fallot. *Am J Cardiol* 1973; 31:749.

Soto B, Pacifico AD, Ceballos R, et al: Tetralogy of Fallot: Angiographic–pathological correlative study. *Circulation* 1981; 64:558.

Van Praagh R, Van Praagh S, Nebesar RA, et al: Tetralogy of Fallot. Underdevelopment of the pulmonary infundibulum and its sequela. *Am J Cardiol* 1970; 26:25.

PULMONARY ATRESIA

Bharati S, Paul M, Idriss FS: The surgical anatomy of pulmonary atresia with ventricular septal defect. *J Thorac Cardiovasc Surg* 1975; 69:713.

Blackston EH, Kirklin JW, Bertranou EG, et al: Preoperative prediction from cineangiograms of post repair right ventricular pressure in tetralogy of Fallot. *J Thorac Cardiovasc Surg* 1979; 78:542.

Burrows PE, Freedom RM, Benson LN, et al: Coronary angiography of pulmonary atresia, hypoplastic right ventricle, and ventriculocoronary communications. *AJR* 1990; 154:789.

Haworth SG: Collateral arteries in pulmonary atresia with ventricular septal defect. *Br Heart J* 1980; 44:5.

DOUBLE OUTLET RIGHT VENTRICLE

Akins EW, Martin TD, Alexander JA: MR imaging of double outlet right ventricle. *AJR* 1989; 152:128.

Anderson RH, Becker AE, Wilcox B, et al. Surgical anatomy of double outlet right ventricle. A reappraisal. *Am J Cardiol* 1983; 52:555.

Battistessa S, Soto B: Double outlet right ventricle with discordant atrio-ventricular connection: An angiographic analysis of 19 cases. *Int J Cardiol* 1990; 27:253.

Brandt PW, Calder L, Barratt–Boyes B, et al: Double outlet left ventricle. Morphology. Cineangiographic diagnosis and surgical treatment. *Am J Cardiol* 1976; 38:897.

de la Cruz MV, Espino–Vela J, Vizcaino A, et al: Double outlet right ventricle. Anatomo-embryological classification with angiographic and surgical considerations. *Il Cuore* 1986; 3:25.

Lev M, Bharati S, Meng CC, et al: A concept of double outlet right ventricle. *J Thorac Cardiovasc Surg* 1972; 64:271.

Piccoli G, Pacifico AD, Kirklin JW, et al: Changing results and concepts in surgical treatment of double outlet right ventricle: Analysis of 137 operations in 126 patients. *Am J Cardiol* 1983; 52:549.

Robertson D, Silverman NH: Malalignment outlet septum with subpulmonary ventricular septal defect and abnormal ventriculoarterial connection: A morphologic spectrum defined echocardiographically. *J Am Coll Cardiol* 1990; 16:459.

TRANSPOSITION OF THE GREAT ARTERIES

de la Cruz MV, Arteaga M, Espino–Vela J, et al: Complete transposition of the great arteries: Types and morphogenesis of ventriculoarterial discordance. *Am Heart J* 1981; 102:271.

Kirklin JW, Barratt–Boyes B. Complete transposition of the great arteries. In Kirklin JW, Barratt–Boyes B, eds. *Cardiac Surgery*. New York: John Wiley & Sons, 1986: 1129.

Tynan M: Transposition of the great arteries. Changes in the circulation after birth. *Circulation* 1972; 46:809.

Tynan M, Anderson RH: Terminology of transposition of the great arteries. In Goodman M, Marquis R, eds. *Pediatric Cardiology*. Vol 2. Edinburgh: Churchill Livingstone, 1978: 341.

Van Praagh R: Transposition of the great arteries II. Transposition clarified. *Am J Cardiol* 1971; 28:739.

Van Praagh R, Perez–Trevino C, Lopez C, et al: Transposition of the great arteries with posterior aorta, anterior pulmonary artery, subpulmonary conus and fibrous continuity between aortic and atrioventricular valves. *Am J Cardiol* 1971; 28:621.

CORRECTED TRANSPOSITION OF THE GREAT ARTERIES

Anderson RH: Criss-cross atrioventricular relationship producing paradoxical atrioventricular concordance or discordance. Their significance to nomenclature of congenital heart disease. *Circulation* 1974; 50:176.

Kirklin JW, Pacifico AD, Bargeron LM, et al: Cardiac repairs in anatomically corrected malposition of the great arteries. *Circulation* 1973; 48:153.

Van Praagh R, Weinberg PM. Double outlet left ventricle. In Moss AJ, Adams FH, eds. *Heart Disease in Infants, Children and Adolescents*. Baltimore: Williams & Wilkins, 1977: 367.

PULMONARY ATRESIA WITH INTACT VENTRICULAR SEPTUM

Bull C, DeLeval M, Mercanti C, et al. Pulmonary Atresia and Intact Ventricular Septum: A Revised Classification. *Circulation* 1982; 66:266.

Freedom RM: *Pulmonary Atresia with Intact Ventricular Septum*. New York: Futura Publishing, 1989.

TRUNCUS ARTERIOSUS

Calder L, Van Praagh R, Van Praagh S, et al: Truncus arteriosus communis. *Am Heart J* 1976; 92:23.

Ceballos R, Soto B, Kirklin JW, et al: Truncus arteriosus. An anatomical–angiographic study. *Br Heart J* 1983; 49:589.

Crupi G, Maccartney F, Anderson RH: Persistent truncus arteriosus. *Am J Cardiol* 1977; 40:569.

Van Praagh R: Classification of truncus arteriosus communis. *Am Heart J* 1976; 92:129.

CHAPTER 12: OBSTRUCTING LESIONS
OBSTRUCTIONS ON THE LEFT SIDE OF THE HEART

Allan LD, Chita SK, Anderson RH: Coarctation of the aorta in prenatal life: An echocardiographic, anatomical and functional study. *Br Heart J* 1980; 59:356.

Beuren AJ, Schulze C, Eberke P, et al: The syndrome of supravalvular aortic stenosis, peripheral pulmonary stenosis, mental retardation and similar facial appearance. *Am J Cardiol* 1964; 13:471.

Carpenter A, Brauchini B, Cour JC, et al: Congenital malformation of the mitral valve in children: Pathology and surgical treatment. *J Thorac Cardiovasc Surg* 1976; 72:854.

Chen JTT, Khoury M, Kirks DR, et al: Obscured aortic arch on the lateral view as a sign of coarctation. *Radiology* 1984; 153:595.

Collins–Nakai RL, Dick M, Parisi–Buckley L, et al: Interrupted aortic arch in infancy. *J Pediatr* 1976; 88:959.

Edwards IE, Clagett OT, Drake RL, et al: The collateral circulation in coarctation of the aorta. *Proc Staff Meet Mayo Clin* 1948; 23:324.

Freedom RM, Culham JAC, Rowe RD: Angiocardiography of subaortic obstruction in infancy. *AJR* 1977; 129:813.

Gupta TC, Wiggens CJ: Basic hemodynamic changes produced by aortic coarctation of different degrees. *Circulation* 1951; 3:17.

Higgins CB, French JW, Silverman JF, et al: Interruption of the aortic arch. Preoperative and postoperative clinical, hemodynamic and angiographic features. *Am J Cardiol* 1977; 39:563.

Ho SY, Anderson RH: Coarctation, tubular hypoplasia and the ductus arteriosus. Histological study of 35 specimens. *Br Heart J* 1979; 41:268.

Hoeffel JC, Gengler L, Henry M, et al: Angiocardiography in congenital subvalvular aortic stenosis: Prognosis and operative indications. *Ann Thorac Surg* 1977; 23:122.

Julsrud PR, Ehman RL: Magnetic resonance imaging of vascular rings. *Mayo Clin Proc* 1986; 61:181.

Moller JH, Nakib A, Eliot RS, et al: Symptomatic congenital aortic stenosis in the first year of life. *J Pediatr* 1966; 69:728.

Nanda NC: *Atlas of Color Doppler Echocardiography*. Philadelphia: Lea & Febiger, 1989.480.

Neufeld HN, Wagenvoort CA, Onley PA, et al: Hypoplasia of ascending aorta. An unusual form of supravalvular stenosis with reference to localized coronary arterial hypertension. *Am J Cardiol* 1962; 10:746.

Ostman–Smith I, Silverman NH, Oldershaw P, et al: Cor triatriatum sinistrum. Diagnostic features on cross section echocardiography. *Br Heart J* 1984; 51:211.

Richardson JR, Doty DB, Siewers RD, et al: Cor triatriatum (subdivided left atrium). *J Thorac Cardiovasc Surg* 1981; 81:232.

Roberts WC: The structure of the aortic valve in clinically isolated aortic stenosis. An autopsy study of 162 patients over 15 years of age. *Circulation* 1970; 42:72.

Shone JD, Sellers RD, Anderson RC, et al: The developmental complex of "parachute mitral valve" supravalvular ring of left atrium, subaortic stenosis and coarctation of the aorta. *Am J Cardiol* 1963; 11:714.

Smallhorn J, Tommasini G, Deanfield J, et al: Congenital mitral stenosis: Anatomical and functional assessment by echocardiography. *Br Heart J* 1981; 45:527.
Snider AR, Roge CL, Schiller NB, et al: Congenital left ventricular inflow obstruction evaluated by two dimensional echocardiography. *Circulation* 1980; 61:848.
Soto B, Shin MS, Papapietro SF: Non-obstructive coarctation. *Cardiovasc Radiol* 1979; 2:231.
Starr A, Dotter C, Griswold H: Supravalvular aortic stenosis. Diagnosis and treatment. *J Thorac Cardiovasc Surg* 1961; 41:134.
Van Praagh R, Corsini I: Cortriatriatum pathologic anatomy and a consideration of morphogenesis based on 13 post mortem cases and a study of normal development of the pulmonary vein and atrial septum in 83 human embryos. *Am Heart J* 1969; 78:379.
Van Schulthess GK, Hagishino SM, Higgins SS, et al: Coarctation of the aorta: MR imaging. *Radiology* 1986; 158:469.
Williams JCP, Barratt–Boyes BC, Lowe JB: Supravalvular aortic stenosis. *Circulation* 1961; 24:1311.

OBSTRUCTIONS ON THE RIGHT SIDE OF THE HEART

Adey CK, Soto B, Shin MS: Congenital pulmonary vein stenosis: A radiographic study. *Radiology* 1986; 161:113.
Geggel RL, Ruthellen F, Tuuri DT, et al: Congenital pulmonary vein stenosis. *J Am Coll Cardiol* 1984; 3:193.
Glancy DL, Roberts WC: Congenital obstructive lesions involving the major pulmonary veins, left atrium or mitral valve: A clinical, laboratory and morphologic survey. *Cathet Cardiovasc Diagn* 1976; 2:215.
Johnson LW, Grossman W, Dalen JE, et al: Pulmonic stenosis in the adult. Long-term follow-up results. *N Eng J Med* 1972; 287:1159.
McDonald AH, Gerlis LM, Somerville J: Familial arteriopathy associated pulmonary and systemic arterial stenosis. *Br Heart J* 1969; 31:375.
Rudhe U: Angiocardiography in pulmonary stenosis. *Radiol Clin No Am* 1964; 2:395.
Sullivan ID, Robinson PJ, Macartney FJ, et al: Percutaneous balloon valvuloplasty for pulmonary valve stenosis in infants and children. *Br Heart J* 1985; 54:435.

CHAPTER 13: VALVULAR INSUFFICIENCY

VALVULAR INSUFFICIENCY ON THE RIGHT SIDE OF THE HEART

Anderson KR, Zuberbuhler JR, Anderson RH, et al: Morphological spectrum of Ebstein's anomaly of the heart. *Mayo Clin Proc* 1979; 54:174.
Calder AL, Brandt PWT, Barratt–Boyes BG, et al: Variant of tetralogy of Fallot with absence of pulmonary valve leaflets and origin of one pulmonary artery from the ascending aorta. *Am J Cardiol* 1980; 46:106.
Clink KM, Herrera MA, D'Souza VJ, Formanek AG: MR imaging of Ebstein's anomaly. Results in four cases. *AJR* 1988; 150:363.
Giuliani ER, Foster V, Brandenburg RO, et al: Ebstein's anomaly. The clinical feature and natural history of Ebstein's anomaly of the tricuspid valve. *Mayo Clin Proc* 1979; 54:163.
Lokier JB, Stanger P, Heymann MA, et al: Tetralogy of Fallot with absent pulmonary valve. Natural history and hemodynamic considerations. *Circulation* 1974; 30:167.
Ports TA, Silverman NH, Schiller MB: Two-dimensional echocardiographic assessment of Ebstein's anomaly. *Circulation* 1987; 58:336.
Rabinovitch M, Grady S, David I, et al: Compression of intrapulmonary bronchi by abnormally branching pulmonary arteries associated with absent pulmonary valves. *Am J Cardiol* 1982; 50:804.
Zuberbuhler JR, Allwork SP, Anderson RH: The spectrum of Ebstein's anomaly of the tricuspid valve. *J Thorac Cardiovasc Surg* 1979; 77:202.

VALVULAR INSUFFICIENCY ON THE LEFT SIDE OF THE HEART

Edwards JE, Burchell HB: Specimen exhibiting the essential lesion in aneurysm of the aortic sinus. *Proc Staff Meet Mayo Clin* 1956; 31:407.
Fishbein MC, Obma R, Roberts WC: Unruptured sinus of Valsalva aneurysm. *Am J Cardiol* 1975; 35:918.
Humes RA, Hagler DJ, Julsrud PR, et al: Aorto-left ventricular tunnel: Diagnosis based on two dimensional echocardiography, color-flow Doppler imaging and magnetic resonance imaging. *Mayo Clinic Proc* 1986; 61:901.
Jain SP, Mahan EF, Nanda NC, et al: Doppler color flow mapping in the diagnosis of sinus of Valsalva aneurysm. *Echocardiography* 1989; 6:533.
Kieffer SA, Winchell P: Congenital aneurysms of the aortic sinuses with cardioaortic fistula. *Chest* 1960; 38:79.
March JE, Greenwood WF: Rupture of the sinus of Valsalva: A study of eight cases with discussion on the different diagnosis of continuous murmurs. *Am J Cardiol* 1966; 18:827.
Sakakibara S, Konno S: Congenital aneurysm of the sinus of Valsalva: Anatomy and classification. *Am Heart J* 1962; 63:405.
Tonkin ILD, Garcia JM, Paul RN, et al: Ruptured sinus of Valsalva aneurysm in children. *Cardiovasc Intervent Radiol* 1984; 7:78.

CHAPTER 14: EXTRACARDIAC SHUNTS

Blieden LC, Moller JH: Aortopulmonary septal defect. An experience with 17 patients. *BR Heart J* 1974; 36:630.
Campbell CD, Wernly JA, Koltip PC, et al: Aberrant left pulmonary artery (pulmonary artery sling): Successful repair and 24 year follow-up report. *Am J Cardiol* 1980; 45:316.
Cumming GR, Ferguson C, Sanchez J: Aortic origin of the right pulmonary artery. *Am J Cardiol* 1972; 30:674.
Dines DE, Sewart JB, Bernatz PE: Pulmonary arteriovenous fistula. *Mayo Clin Proc* 1983; 58:176.
Doty DB, Richardson JB, Falkovsky GE, et al: Aorto pulmonary septal defect. Hemodynamic angiographic and operation. *Ann Thorac Surg* 1981; 32:244.
Duncan WJ, Freedom RM, Olley PM, et al: Two-dimensional echocardiographic identification of hemitruncus: Anomalous origin of the pulmonary artery from ascending aorta with the other pulmonary artery arising normally from the right ventricle. *Am Heart J* 1981; 102:892.
Fan PH, Philpot E, Nanda NC: Color Doppler echocardiography in congenital heart disease. *Diagn Imag* 1987; 9:288.
Fisher RG, Moodie DS, Sterva R, et al: Patent ductus arteriosus in adults—long term follow up. Nonsurgical versus surgical treatment. *J Am Coll Cardiol* 1986; 8:280.
Fong LV, Anderson RH, Siewers RD, et al: Anomalous origin of one pulmonary artery from the ascending aorta: A review of echocardiographic, catheter and morphological features. *Br Heart J* 1989; 62:389.
Gittenberger de Groot AC: Persistent ductus arteriosus most probably a primary congenital malformation. *Br Heart J* 1977; 39:610.
Hoffman JI, Hayman MA, Claiman RI: Patent ductus arteriosus in premature infants. *Rev Latina de Card Inf* 1986; 4:293.
Hyo S, Shime H, Omoto R, et al: Evaluation of intracardiac shunt flow in premature infants by color flow mapping real-time two-dimensional Doppler echocardiography. *Circulation* 1984; 70:456.
Jureidini S, Nouri S, Goel DP: Similarity of anomalous origin of right pulmonary artery from ascending aorta to d-transposition of the great arteries: 2-D echographic and Doppler study. *Am Heart J* 1986; 112:175.
Kirks DR, McCook, TA, Serwer GA, et al: Aneurysm of the ductus arteriosus in neonate. *AJR* 1980; 134:573.
Lundell C, Finck E: Arteriovenous fistulas originating from Rasmussen aneurysms. *AJR* 1983; 140:687.

Pool PE, Vogel AK, Blount G: Congenital unilateral absence of a pulmonary artery. *Am J Cardiol* 1962; 11:706.

Sahn DJ, Allen HD: Real time cross-sectional echocardiographic imaging of the patent ductus arteriosus in infants and children. *Circulation* 1987; 58:343.

Sapire DW, Casta A, Donner RM, et al: Dilatation of the descending aorta: A radiologic and echocardiographic diagnostic sign in arteriovenous malformation in neonates and young infants. *Am J Cardiol* 1979; 44:493.

CHAPTER 15: ANOMALIES OF THE AORTIC ARCH AND PULMONARY ARTERIES

Berdon WE, Baker DH, Wung J-T, et al: Complete cartilage-ring tracheal stenosis associated with anomalous left pulmonary artery: The ring-sling complex. *Radiology* 1984; 152:57.

Bisset GS III, Strife JL, Kirks DR, et al: Vascular rings: MR imaging. *AJR* 1987; 159:251.

Capitanio MA, Ramos R, Kirkpatrick JA: Pulmonary sling: Roentgen observations. *AJR* 1971; 112:28.

Cohen SR, Landing BH: Tracheostenosis and bronchial abnormalities associated with pulmonary artery sling. *Ann Otol Rhinol Laryngol* 1976; 85:582.

Contro S, Miller RA, White H, et al: Bronchial obstruction due to pulmonary artery anomalies: I. Vascular sling. *Circulation* 1958; 17:418.

Edwards JE: Anomalies of the derivatives of the aortic arch system. *Med Clin No Am* 1948; 32:925.

Ekstrom G, Sandblom P: Double aortic arch. *Acta Chir Scand* 1951; 102:183.

Ericsson ND, Saderland S: Compression of the trachea by an anomalous innominate artery. *J Pediatr Surg* 1969; 4:424.

Fletcher BD, Cohn RC: Tracheal compression and the innominate artery in infants and children. *Radiology* 1989; 170:103.

Fletcher BD, Jacobstein MD: MRI of congenital abnormalities of the great arteries. *AJR* 1986; 146:941.

Frey EE, Sato Y, Smith WI, Franken EA Jr: Cine CT of the mediastinum in pediatric patients. *Radiology* 1987; 165:19.

Gomes AS: MR Imaging of congenital anomalies of the thoracic aorta and pulmonary arteries. *Radiol Clin No Am* 1989; 27:1171.

Gomes AS, Lois JF, George B, et al: Congenital abnormalities of the aortic arch: MR imaging. *Radiology* 1987; 165:191.

Hiller MG, Maclear AD: Pulmonary artery ring. *Acta Radiol* 1957; 48:434.

Joseph PM, Berdon WE, Baker DH, et al: Upper airway obstruction in infants and small children. *Radiology* 1976; 121:143.

Moncada R, Shannon M, Miller R, et al: The cervical aortic arch. *AJR* 1975; 125:591.

Murdison K, Andrews BA, Chin AJ: Ultrasonographic display of complex vascular ring. *J Am Coll Cardiol* 1990; 15:1645.

Proto AV, Cuthbert NW, Raider L: Aberrant right subclavian artery: Further observations. *AJR* 1987; 148:253.

Shuford WH, Sybers RG. *The Aortic Arch and Its Malformations with Emphasis on the Angiographic Features.* Springfield, IL: Charles C. Thomas, 1974.

Smith RJH, Smith MCF, Glossup LP, et al: Congenital vascular anomalies causing tracheoesophageal compression. *Arch Otolaryngol* 1984; 110:82.

Soulen RL, Donner RM: Advances in noninvasive evaluation of congenital abnormalities of the thoracic aorta. *Radiol Clin No Am* 1985; 23:727.

Stewart JR, Kincaid OW, Edwards JE: *An Atlas of Vascular Rights and Related Malformations of the Aortic Arch System.* Springfield, IL: Charles C. Thomas, 1964.

Strife JL, Baumel AS, Dunbar JS: Tracheal compression by the innominate artery in infancy and childhood. *Radiology* 1981; 139:73.

Strife JL, Matsumoto J, Bissett GS III, Martin R: The position of the trachea in infants and children with right aortic arch. *Pediatr Radiol* 1989; 19:226.

Tonkin ILD, Elliott LP, Bargeron LM Jr: Combined axial cineangiography and barium esophagography in the evaluation of vascular rings. *Radiology* 1980; 135:69.

Tonkin ILD, Gold RE, Moser D, Laster RE Jr: Evaluation of vascular rings with digital subtraction angiography. *AJR* 1984; 142:1287.

Whitman G, Stephenson LW, Weinberg P: Vascular ring: Left cervical aortic arch, right descending aorta, and right ligamentum arteriosum. *J Thorac Cardiovasc Surg* 1982; 83:31.

Wittenburg MH, Tahtimongse T, Rosenburg BF: Anomalous course of the left pulmonary artery with respiratory obstruction. *Radiology* 1956; 67:339.

Wychulis AR, Kincaid OW, Danielson GS: Congenital vascular ring: Surgical considerations and results of operation. *Mayo Clin Proc* 1971; 46:182.

CHAPTER 15A: IMAGING THE FETAL HEART

INTRODUCTION: FETAL CIRCULATION

Allan LD, Tynan MJ, Campbell S, et al: Echocardiographic and anatomical correlates in the fetus. *Br Heart J* 1980; 44:444.

Egeblad H, Bang J, Northeved A: Ultrasonic identification and examination of fetal heart structures. *J Clin Ultrasound* 1975; 3:95.

Garrett WJ, Robinson DE: Fetal heart size measured in vivo by ultrasound. *Pediatrics* 1970; 46:25.

Kleinman CS, Donnerstein RL, DeVore GR: Fetal echocardiography for evaluation of in utero congestive cardiac failure: A technique for study of non-immune hydrops. *N Engl J Med* 1982; 306:568.

Kleinman CS, Hobbins JC, Jaffee CC: Echocardiographic studies of the human fetus: Prenatal diagnosis of congenital heart disease and cardiac dysrhythmias. *Pediatrics* 1980; 60:1059.

Rudolph AM, Heymann MA: The circulation of the fetus in utero, methods for studying distribution of blood flow, cardiac output, and organ blood flow. *Circ Res* 1967; 21:163.

FETAL TWO-DIMENSIONAL ECHOCARDIOGRAPHY

Allan LD, Crawford DC, Anderson RH, et al: Spectrum of congenital heart disease detected echocardiographically in prenatal life. *Br Heart J* 1985; 54:523.

Allan LD, Tynan M, Campbell S, et al: Identification of congenital cardiac malformations by echocardiography in the midtrimester fetus. *Br Heart J* 1981; 46:358.

Anzacot A: Analysis of ventricular shape by echocardiography in normal fetuses. Circulation 1983, 68:1201.

Axel L: Real-time sonography of fetal cardiac anatomy (pictorial essay). *AJR* 1983; 141:283.

Bennacerraf BR, Galman R, Frigoletto FD: Sonographic identification of second trimester fetuses with Down syndrome. *N Engl J Med* 1987; 317:1371.

Bennacerraf BR, Miller WA, Frigoletto FD: Sonographic detection of fetuses with trisomy 13 and 18: Accuracy and limitations. *Am J Obstet Gynecol* 1988; 158:404.

Brown DL, Emerson DS, Cartier MS, et al: Congenital cardiac anomalies: Prenatal sonographic diagnosis (pictorial essay). *AJR* 1989; 153:109.

Copel JA, Pilu G, Green J: Fetal echocardiographic screening for congenital heart disease: The importance of the four-chamber view. *Am J Obstet Gynecol* 1987; 157:648.

Devore GR: The prenatal diagnosis of congenital heart disease. A practical approach for the fetal sonographer. *J Clin Ultrasound* 1985: 13:229.

Devore GR, Siassi B, Platt LD: Fetal echocardiography: IV. M-mode assessment of ventricular size and contractility during the second and third trimesters of pregnancy in the normal fetus. *Am J Obstet Gynecol* 1984; 150:981.

Huhta JC, Smallhorn JF, Macartney FJ: Two dimensional echocardiographic diagnosis of situs. *Br Heart J* 1982; 48:97.

Kleinman CS, Donnerstein RL: Ultrasonic assessment of cardiac function in the intact human fetus. *J Am Coll Cardiol* 1985; 5:84S.

Sahn DJ, Lange LW, Allen HD: Quantitative cross-sectional echocardiography in the developing normal human fetus and newborn. *Circulation* 1980; 62:588.

St John Sutton MB, Gewitz MH, Shah B: Quantitative assessment of growth and function of the cardiac chambers in the normal human fetus: A prospective longitudinal echocardiographic study. *Circulation* 1984; 69:645.

Schmidt KG, Silverman NH, Harrison MR, et al: High-output cardiac failure in fetuses with large sacrococcygeal teratoma: Diagnosis by echocardiography and Doppler ultrasound. *J Pediatr* 1989; 144:1023.

Wladimiroff JW, Vosters R, Vletter W: Ultrasonic measurement of fetal and neonatal ventricular dimensions. *Contrib Gynecol Obstet* 1979; 6:109.

FETAL HEART RATE AND RHYTHM

Devore GR, Siassi B, Platt LD: Fetal echocardiography: III The diagnosis of cardiac arrhythmias using real-time directed M-mode ultrasound. *Am J Obstet Gynecol* 1983; 146:792.

Klein CS, Donnerstein RL, Jaffee CC: Fetal echocardiography: A tool for evaluation of in utero cardiac arrhythmias and monitoring of in utero therapy. Analysis of 71 patients. *Am J Cardiol* 1983; 51:237.

Silverman NH, Enderlein BS, Stanger P, et al: Recognition of fetal arrhythmias by echocardiography. *J Clin Ultrasound* 1985; 13:255.

Strasburger JF, Huhta JC, Carpenter RJ, et al: Doppler echocardiography in the diagnosis and management of persistent fetal arrhythmias. *J Am Coll Cardiol* 1986; 7:1386.

FETAL CIRCULATORY FUNCTION

Allan LD, Joseph MC, Boyd EGCA: M-mode echocardiography in the developing human fetus. *Br Heart J* 1982; 47:573.

Beisher NA, Fortune DW, MacAfee J: Nonimmunologic hydrops fetalis and congenital abnormalities. *Obstet Gynecol* 1971; 38:86.

De Smedt MCH, Visser GHA, Meijboom EJ: Fetal cardiac output estimated by Doppler echocardiography during mid- and late gestation. *Am J Cardiol* 1987; 60:338.

Devore GR, Donnerstein RL, Kleinman CS, et al: Real-time M-mode echocardiography: A new technique for accurate and rapid quantitation of the fetal pre-ejection period and ventricular ejection time of the right and left ventricles. *Am J Obstet Gynecol* 1981; 15:470.

Huhta JC: Fetal examination. In Ludomirsky A, Huhta JC, eds. *Color Doppler in Congenital Heart Disease in the Child and Adult.* Mount Kisco, NY: Futura, 1987.

Huhta JC, Strasburger JF, Carpenter RJ: Pulsed Doppler fetal echocardiography. *J Clin Ultrasound* 1985; 13:247.

Hutchinson AA, Drew JH, Uyu VYH: Nonimmunologic hydrops fetalis: A review of 61 cases. *Obstet Gynecol* 1982; 59:347.

Maulik M, Nanda NC, Saini VD: Fetal Doppler echocardiography: Methods and characterization of normal and abnormal hemodynamics. *Am J Cardiol* 1984; 53:572.

Reed KL, Meijboom EJ, Sahn D: Cardiac Doppler flow velocities in human fetuses. *Circulation* 1986; 73:41.

Silverman NH, Kleinman CS, Rudolph AM: Fetal atrioventricular valve insufficiency associated with nonimmune hydrops: A two dimensional echocardiographic and pulsed Doppler ultrasound study. *Circulation* 1985; 78:825.

Wladimiroff JW, McGhin JS: M-mode ultrasonic assessment of fetal cardiovascular dynamics. *Br J Obstet Gynecol* 1981; 88:1241.

Wladimiroff JW, Vosters R, McGhie JS: Normal cardiac ventricular geometry and function during the last trimester of pregnancy and early neonatal period. *Br J Obstet Gynecol* 1982; 89:839.

RISKS AND BENEFITS

Mole R: Possible hazards of imaging and Doppler ultrasound in obstetrics. *Birth* 1986; 13:29.

National Council on Radiation Protection and Measurement (NCRPM): Biological effects of ultrasound: mechanisms and clinical implications. Report No. 74. Bethesda, 1984.

National Institutes of Health: Diagnostic ultrasound imaging in pregnancy. National Institutes of Health Consensus Development Conference Consensus Statement 5:1, 1984.

CHAPTER 16: TREATMENT OF CONGENITAL HEART DISEASE BY SURGERY AND CATHETER TECHNIQUES

GENERAL

Kirklin JW, Barratt–Boyes B: *Cardiac Surgery.* New York: John Wiley & Sons, 1986.

Martin EC: Cardiac surgery: Residual problems and complications. In Kassner EG, ed. *Iatrogenic Disorders of the Fetus, Infant, and Child.* New York: Springer-Verlag, 1985.

Stark J, de Leval M: *Surgery for Congenital Heart Defects.* London: Grune & Stratton, 1983.

PALLIATIVE SURGERY

Albert HM, Fohler RL, Craighead CC, et al: Pulmonary artery banding. A treatment for infants with intractable cardiac failure due to interventricular septal defect. *Circulation* 1961; 23:16.

Parenzan L, Alfieri O, Vanini V, et al: Waterston anastomosis for initial palliation of tetralogy of Fallot. *J Thorac Cardiovasc Surg* 1981; 82:176.

Parks WJ, Smith S, Gibson S: An anastomosis of aorta to pulmonary artery: Certain types in congenital heart disease. *JAMA* 1946; 132:627.

Redo S, Ecker R: Intrapericardial aortopulmonary artery shunt. *Circulation* 1963; 28:520.

Turley K, Tucker WY, Ebert PA: The changing role of palliative procedures in the treatment of infants with congenital heart disease. *J Thorac Cardiovasc Surg* 1980; 79:194.

CORRECTION OF TOTAL ANOMALOUS VENOUS CONNECTION

Katz NM, Kirklin JW, Pacifico AD: Concepts and practice in surgery for total anomalous venous connection. *Ann Thorac Surg* 1978; 25:479.

Trusler GA, Kazenelson G, Freedom RM, et al: Late result following repair of partial anomalous venous connection with sinus versus atrial septal defect. *J Thorac Cardiovasc Surg* 1980; 79:776.

Whight WM, Barratt–Boyes BG, Calder AL, et al: Total anomalous venous connection. Long-term results following repair in infancy. *J Thorac Cardiovasc Surg* 1978; 75:52.

CORRECTION OF SEPTAL DEFECTS

Blackstone DH, Kirklin JW, Bradley EL, et al: Optimal age and results in repair of large ventricular septal defect. *J Thorac Cardiovasc Surg* 1976; 72:661.

Bulle C, Deanfield J, de Laval M, et al: Correction of isolated secundum atrial septal defect in infancy. *Arch Dis Child* 1981; 56:184.

Carpenter A: Surgical anatomy and management of the mitral component of atrioventricular canal defect. In Anderson RH, Chamber EA, Shinebourne EA, eds. *Pediatric Cardiology.* Edinburgh: Churchill Livingstone, 1977: 477.

Kirklin JW, Harshbarger HG, Donald TE, et al: Surgical correction of ventricular septal defect. Anatomic and technical considerations. *J Thorac Surg* 1957; 33:45.

Pacifico AD: Atrioventricular septal defect. In Stark J, de Laval M, eds. *Surgery for Congenital Heart Defects.* London: Grune & Stratton, 1983: 285.

Rastelli GC, Weidman WH, Kirklin JW: Surgical repair of the partial form of persisting atrioventricular canal with special reference to the problem of mitral valve incompetence. *Circulation* 1965; 81(suppl 1):31.

REPAIR OF EBSTEIN'S MALFORMATION

Danielson JK, Maloni JD, Devloo RA: Surgical repair of Ebstein's anomaly. *Mayo Clin Proc* 1979; 54:185.

Westaby S, Carp RB, Kirklin JW, et al: Surgical treatment in Ebstein's malformation. *Ann Thorac Surg* 34; 388.

REPAIR OF HEARTS WITH ABSENCE OF ONE ATRIOVENTRICULAR CONNECTION OR UNIVENTRICULAR ATRIOVENTRICULAR CONNECTION

Fontan F, Baudet E: Surgical repair of tricuspid atresia. *Thorax* 1971; 240.

Kirklin JW, Blackstone EH, Kirklin JW, et al: The Fontan's operation: Ventricular hypertrophy, age, and date of operation as risk factors. *J Thorac Cardiovasc Surg* 1986; 92:1149.

Kreutzer GO, Vargas FJ, Schlichter AJ, et al: Atriopulmonary anastomosis. *J Thorac Cardiovasc Surg* 1982; 83:427.

Puga FJ, Chiavarelli, Hagler DJ: Modification of the Fontan operation applicable to patients with left atrioventricular valve atresia or single atrioventricular valve. *Circulation* 1987; 76(suppl 1): 111.

COMPLETE CORRECTION OF TETRALOGY OF FALLOT

Alferi O, Blackstone EH, Kirklin JW, et al: Surgical treatment of tetralogy of Fallot with pulmonary atresia. *J Thorac Cardiovasc Surg* 1978; 76:321.

Blalock A, Taussig HB: The surgical treatment of malformation on the heart in which there is pulmonary stenosis or pulmonary atresia. *JAMA* 1945; 128:189.

Castaneda AR, Freed MD, Williams RG: Repair of tetralogy of Fallot in infancy. Early and late results. *J Thorac Cardiovasc Surg* 1977; 74:372.

Fujino M, Kozuka T, Yokata K, et al: Angiography after total correction of tetralogy of Fallot using large homograft arteries. *AJR* 1977; 128:243.

Ferencz C: The pulmonary vascular bed in tetralogy of Fallot II. Changes following a systemic-pulmonary artery anastomosis. *Bull Johns Hopkins Hosp* 1960; 106:100.

Kirklin JW, Blackstone EH, Pacifico AD, et al: Routine primary repair versus two stage repair of tetralogy of Fallot. *Circulation* 1979; 60:373.

Kirklin JW, Karp R: *Tetralogy of Fallot—From a Surgical Viewpoint.* Philadelphia: WB Saunders, 1970.

McGoon DC, Baird DK, Davis GD: Surgical management of large bronchial collateral arteries with pulmonary stenosis or atresia. *Circulation* 1975; 52:109.

SURGICAL CORRECTION OF TRANSPOSITION OF THE GREAT ARTERIES

Blalock A, Hanlon CR: The surgical treatment of complete transposition of the aorta and the pulmonary artery. *Surg Gynecol Obstet* 1950; 90:1.

Eber PA, Turley K, Stanger P, et al: Surgical treatment of truncus arteriosus in the first six months of life. *Ann Surg* 1984; 200:451.

Egloff LP, Freed MD, Dick M: Early and late results with the Mustard operation in infancy. *Ann Thorac Surg* 1978; 26:474.

Jatene AD, Fontes VF, Paulista PP, et al: Anatomical corrections of transposition of the great vessels. *J Thorac Cardiovasc Surg* 1976; 72:364.

Kirklin JW, DeVloo RA, Weidman WH: Open intracardiac repair of transposition of the great arteries. *Surgery* 1961; 50:58.

Ochsner JL, Cooley DA, Harris LC, et al: Treatment of complete transposition of the great vessels with the Blalock-Hanlon operation. *Circulation* 1961; 24:51.

Quaegebeur JM, Romhmer J, Ottenkamp J, et al: The arterial switch operation. *J Thorac Cardiovasc Surg* 1986; 92:361.

Rastelli GC: A new approach to anatomic repair of transposition of the great arteries. *Mayo Clin Proc* 1969; 44:1.

Rastelli GC, McGoon DC, Wallace RB: Anatomic correction of transposition of the great arteries with ventricular septal defect and subpulmonary stenosis. *J Thorac Cardiovasc Surg* 1969; 58:545.

Parenson L, Alfieri O: Surgical repair of persistent truncus arteriosus in infancy. In Anderson RH, Shinebourne EA, eds. *Pediatric Cardiology.* Edinburgh: Churchill Livingstone, 1978: 551.

Poirier RN, Berman MA, Stansle HC: Current status of the surgical treatment of truncus arteriosus. *J Thorac Cardiovasc Surg* 1975; 69:169.

SURGICAL REPAIR OF COARCTATION OF THE AORTA

Korfer R, Meyer H, Kleikamp G, et al: Early and late results after resection in end-to-end anastomosis of coarctation of the thoracic aorta in early infancy. *J Thorac Cardiovasc Surg* 1985; 89:616.

Meier M, Lucchese FA, Jazbik W, et al: A new technique for repair of aortic coarctation. Subclavian flap aortoplasty with preservation of arterial blood flow to the left arm. *J Thorac Cardiovasc Surg* 1986; 92:1005.

Metzdorff MT, Cobanoglu A, Grunkemeir GL: Influence of age at operation and late results with subclavian flap aortoplasty. *J Thorac Cardiovasc Surg* 1985; 89:235.

Reul GJ, Kabbani SS, Sandefor FM: Repair of coarctation of the thoracic aorta by patch craft aortoplasty. *J Thorac Cardiovasc Surg* 1974; 68:696.

THERAPEUTIC CATHETER PROCEDURES

Bank ER, Aisen AM, Rocchini AP, et al: Coarctation of the aorta in children undergoing angioplasty: Pretreatment and posttreatment MR imaging. *Radiology* 1987; 162:235.

Barth KH, White RI, Kaufman S, et al: Embolotherapy of pulmonary arterio-venous malformation with detachable balloon. *Radiology* 1982; 142:599.

Fellows KE: Therapeutic catheter procedures in congenital heart disease: Current status and future prospect. *Cardiovasc Intervent Radiol* 1984; 7:170.

Keller FS, Rosch J, Baker AF, et al: Pulmonary arterio-venous fistula occluded by percutaneous introduction of coiled spring. *Radiology* 1984; 192:373.

Lasjaunias P, Rodesch G, Pruvost P, et al: Treatment of vein of Galen aneurysmal malformation. *J Neurosurg* 1989; 70:746.

Locke JE, Neimi BA, Burke B: Transcutaneous angioplasty of experimental aortic coarctation. *Circulation* 1982; 66:1280.

Medellin GJ, Di Sessa TG, Tonkin ILD: Interventional catheterization in congenital heart disease. *Radiol Clin No Am* 1989; 27:1223.

Mills NL: Nonoperative closure of atrial septal defect. *Surgery* 1974; 75:383.

Mills NL, King TD: Nonoperative closure of left-to-right shunt. *J Thorac Cardiovasc Surg* 1976; 72:371.

O'Neill WW: Predictors of long-term survival after percutaneous aortic valvuloplasty: Report of the Manfield Scientific Balloon Aortic Valvuloplasty Registry. *J Am Coll Cardiol* 1991; 17:193.

Park JH, Tynan MJ, Finley JP, et al: Balloon angioplasty for the treatment of native coarctation. Results of valvuloplasty and angioplasty of congenital anomalies. Congenital Anomalies Registry. *Am J Cardiol* 1990; 65:790.

Park SC, Neches WH, Zuberbuhler JR, et al: Clinical use of blade atrial septostomy. *Circulation* 1977; (suppl III):172.

Rashkind WJ: Palliative procedures for transposition of the great arteries. *Br Heart J* 1971; (suppl)33:69.

Redington AN, Booth P, Shore DF, et al: Primary balloon dilatation of coarctation of the aorta in neonates. *Br Heart J* 1990; 64:277.

Robicsek F, Harbold NB, Scotten LN, et al: Balloon dilatation of the stenosed aortic valve: How does it work? Interrogation. Why does it fail? Interrogation. *Am J Cardiol* 1990; 65:761.

Stanger P, Cassidy SC, Girod DA, et al: Balloon pulmonary valvuloplasty. Results of the valvuloplasty and angioplasty of congenital anomalies. Anomalies Registry. *Am J Cardiol* 1990; 65:775.

PHARMACOTHERAPY OF PATENT DUCTUS ARTERIOSUS IN PRETERM INFANT

Huhta JC: Patent ductus arteriosus in the preterm neonate. In Long WA, ed. *Fetal and Neonatal Cardiology.* Philadelphia: WB Saunders, 1990: 389.

Olley PM, Coceani F, Freedom RM, et al: Pharmalogical manipulation of the ductus arteriosus. In Godman MC, ed. *Pediatric Cardiology. Vol 4.* Edinburgh: Churchill Livingstone, 1981: 259.

THE POSTOPERATIVE PERIOD

Amplatz K, Formanek A, Knight, et al: Radiographic changes in the post operative patient. *Prog Cardiovasc Dis* 1975; 17:403.

Bream PR, Elliott LP, Sousa AS, et al: Postoperative findings common to acquired and congenital heart disease. In Teplic JG, Haskin ME, eds. *Surgical Radiology.* Philadelphia: WB Saunders, 1981.

Carter AR, Sostman HB, Curtis AM, et al: Thoracic alteration after cardiac surgery. *AJR* 1983; 140:475.

Goodman LR, Kay HR, Teplick SK, et al: Complications of median sternotomy: Computed tomographic evaluation. *AJR* 1983; 141:225.

Henry TA, Jolles H, Berberich JJ, et al: The post cardiac surgery chest radiography: A clinically integrated approach. *J Thorac Imag* 1989; 4:20.

Kassner EG, Kottmeier PK: Surgery of the airway, thorax, and diaphragm. In Kassner EG, ed. *Iatrogenic Disorders of the Fetus, Infant, and Child.* New York: Springer-Verlag, 1985.

Kay HR, Cuttman LR, Teplick SK, et al: Use of computed tomography to assess mediastinal complication after medial sternotomy. *Ann Thorac Surg* 1983; 36:706.

Landay MJ, Mootz AR, Estrera AS, et al: Apparatus seen on chest radiographs after cardiac surgery in adults. *Radiology* 1990; 174:477.

Thorsen MK, Goodman LR, Sagel SS, et al: Ascending aorta complication of cardiac surgery: CT evaluation. *J Comput Assist Tomogr* 1986; 10:219.

CHAPTER 17: CONGENITAL HEART DISEASE IN THE ADULT

Danielson JK, McGoon DC: Surgical consideration in treatment of adults with congenital heart disease. In Roberts WC, ed. *Congenital Heart Disease in Adults*. Philadelphia: FA Davis, 1979: 543.

Garson A, McNamara DG, Cooley DA: Tetralogy of Fallot in adults. In Roberts WC, ed. *Congenital Heart Disease in Adults*. Philadelphia: FA Davis, 1979: 341.

Kidd L, O'Neil J: Transposition of the great Arteries in the adult. In Roberts WC, ed. *Congenital Heart Disease in Adults*. Philadelphia: FA Davis, 1979: 543.

Murphy ML, Lieu LR, Thenabatu PN, et al: The reliability of the routine chest roentgenogram for determination of heart size based on a specific chamber evaluation at post mortem. *Invest Radiol* 1985; 20:21.

Sanders C, Bittner V, Nath PH, et al: Atrial septal defect in older adults: A typical radiographic appearance. *Radiology* 1988; 167:123.

Index

A

Note: Numbers in **boldface** refer to Figure numbers.

B

C

D

E

F

G

H

I

J

K

L

M

N

O

P

Q

R

S

T

U

V

W

COLOR APPENDIX

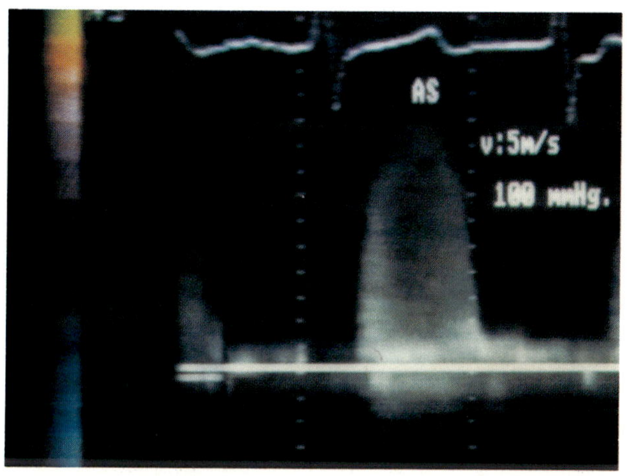

Fig. 2.12 Spectral wave form by continuous Doppler in aortic stenosis from suprasternal approach. The vertical axis measures the velocity of the blood through the aortic orifice during systole (5 meters per second). The calculated gradient through the aortic valve is 100 mm Hg. (AS = aortic stenosis; V = velocity of blood through the aortic valve; mm Hg = pressure.measured in millimeters of Hg)

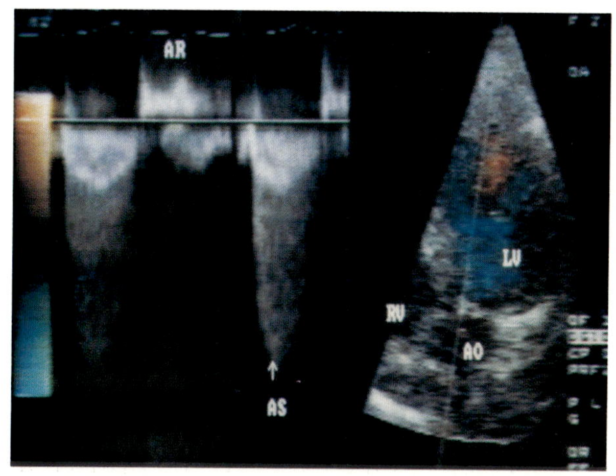

Fig. 2.13 Spectral wave form of Doppler, demonstrating high velocity through the aortic valve. (left) From an apical window, aortic insufficiency is demonstrated on top of the baseline and the stenosis is towards the lower part in the opposite direction. (right) Continuous-wave Doppler beam directed through the area of the aortic valve. The blue color signals indicate laminar velocity during systole, located before the site of obstruction. (AR = aortic regurgitation; AS = aortic stenosis; CD = continuous Doppler)

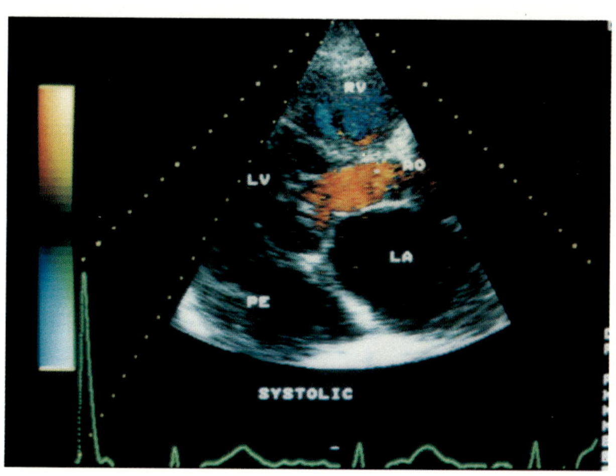

Fig. 2.14 Long-axis view of the heart from the parasternal window. Systolic frame. Red signal in LV represents the laminar blood flow towards the aorta. The red and blue signals to the right of the septum represent the turbulent jet produced by blood passing through the ventricular septal defect.

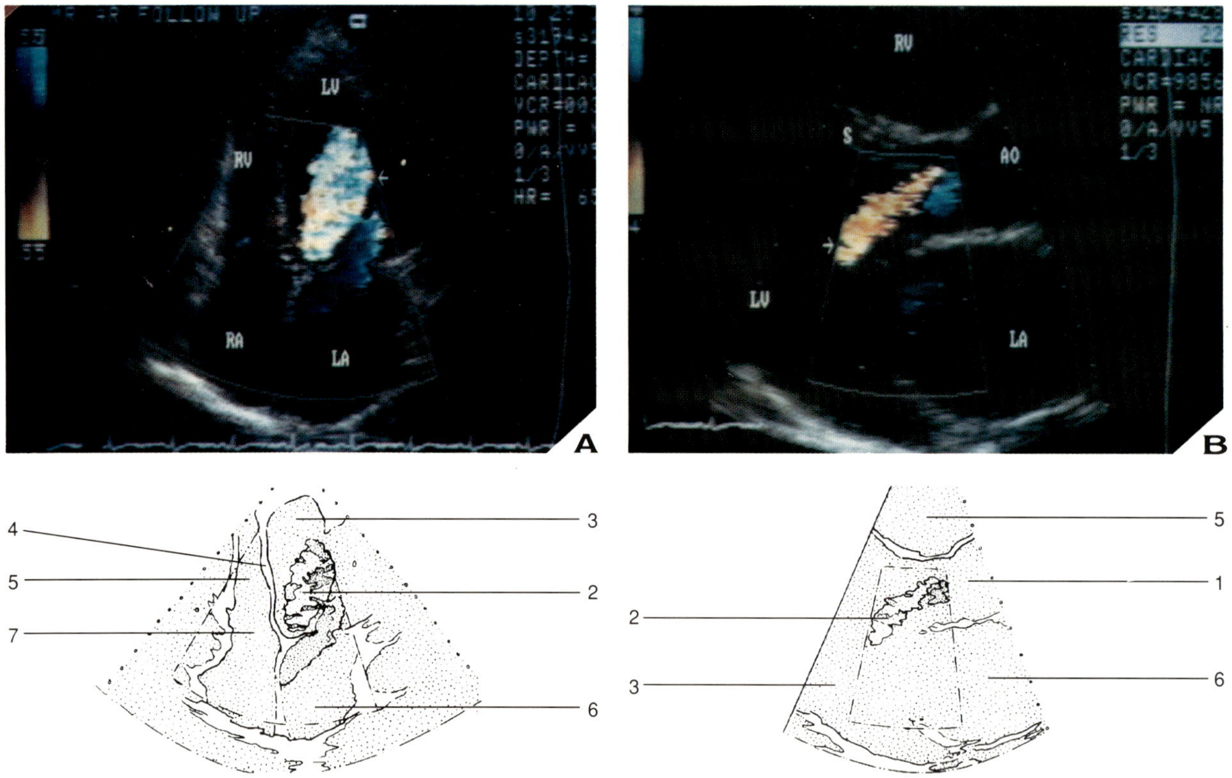

Fig. 18.22 Aortic insufficiency demonstrated by color flow Doppler echocardiography. (A) Apical five-chamber view (diastole) in a patient with severe (Grade 5) aortic insufficiency demonstrates a mosaic color-flow jet in the left ventricular outflow tract, originating at the aortic valve. (B) Parasternal long axis view (diastole) in a patient with mild (Grade 2) aortic insufficiency demonstrates a mosaic color-flow jet in the left ventricular outflow tract, originating at the aortic valve. The jet is smaller than the one shown in A.

1 aorta
2 regurgitant jet in left ventricular outflow tract
3 left ventricle
4 ventricular septum
5 right ventricle
6 left atrium
7 right atrium

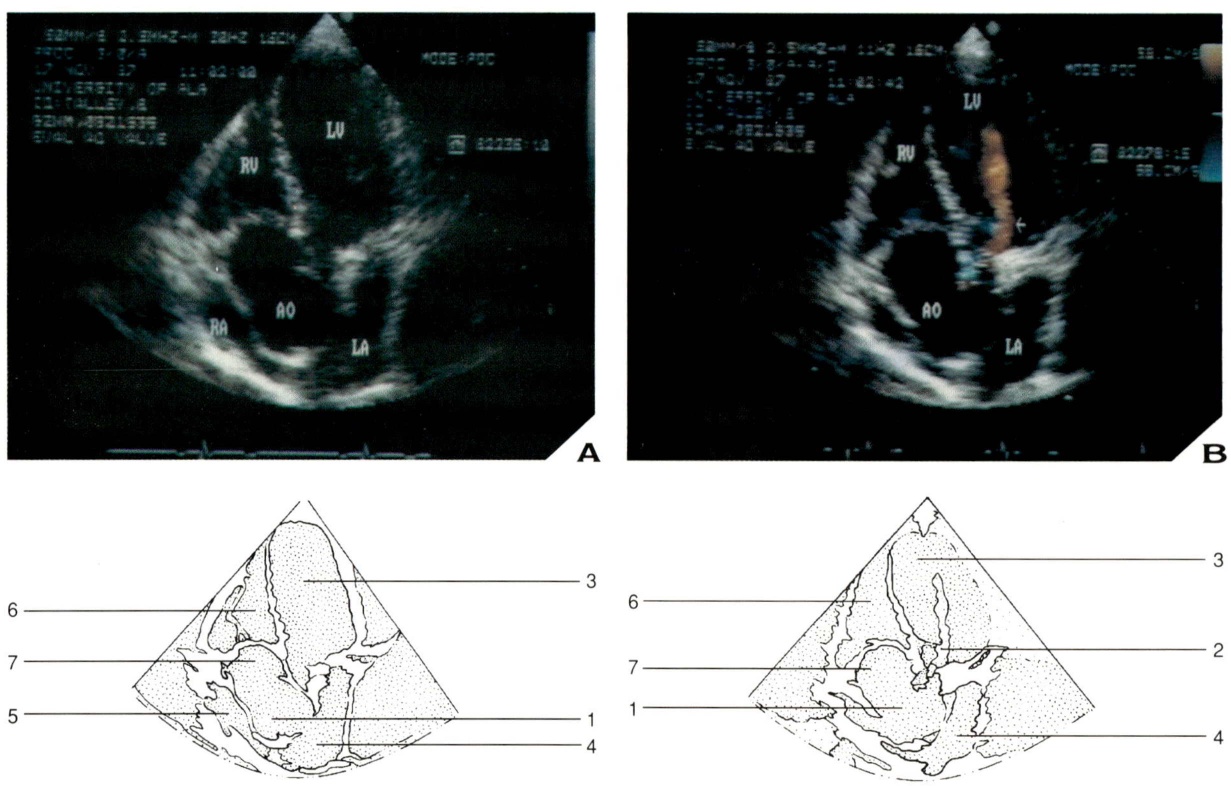

Fig. 18.28 Acute aortic insufficiency secondary to ruptured sinus of Valsalva aneurysm. Two-dimensional echocardiogram (apical five-chamber view) without (A) and with (B) color Doppler imaging. Note the regurgitant jet into the left ventricular outflow tract in B. The aortic root is markedly dilated. The aneurysmally enlarged right coronary sinus protrudes into the right ventricle.

1 dilated aortic root
2 regurgitant jet in left ventricular outflow tract
3 left ventricle
4 left atrium
5 right atrium
6 right ventricle
7 aneurysm of right coronary sinus of Valsalva

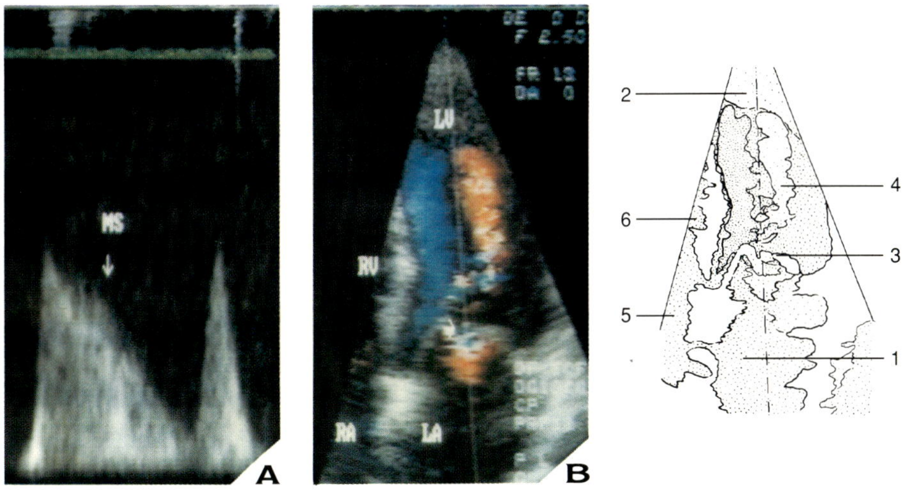

1 left atrium
2 left ventricle
3 domed, stenotic mitral valve
4 turbulent flow
5 right atrium
6 right ventricle

Fig. 18.40 Mitral stenosis. (A) Color Doppler guided continuous wave echocardiography shows findings typical of mitral stenosis. Left atrial emptying is prolonged (100 milliseconds; normal, 20 to 60 milliseconds) and the slope of the run-off curve is abnormally flat. The time needed to decrease the left atrium–left ventricle gradient by 50 percent from its baseline value at the beginning of diastole ($T_{1/2}$) is abnormally long. (B) Two-dimensional color Doppler echocardiogram during diastole (four-chamber view) shows restricted opening of the leaflets with doming of the mitral valve and turbulent flow in the left ventricle.

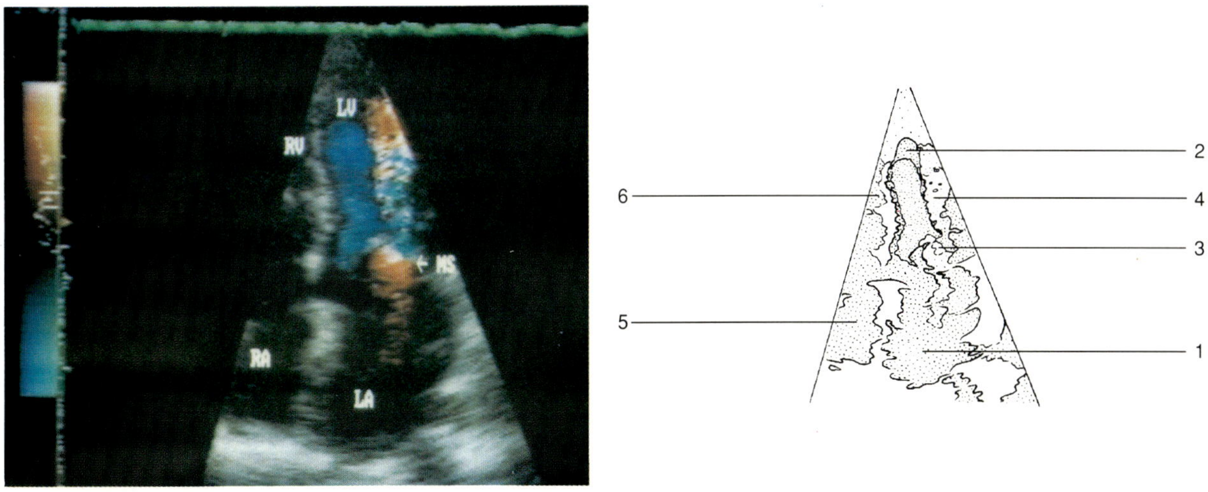

Fig. 18.41 Mitral stenosis. Transthoracic two-dimensional echocardiogram with color Doppler imaging, during diastole (apical four-chamber view). Note the mosaic pattern of the jet originating at the level of the mitral valve. The turbulent jet is directed towards the apex of the left ventricle.

1 left atrium
2 left ventricle
3 stenotic mitral valve
4 jet (turbulent flow)
5 right atrium
6 right ventricle

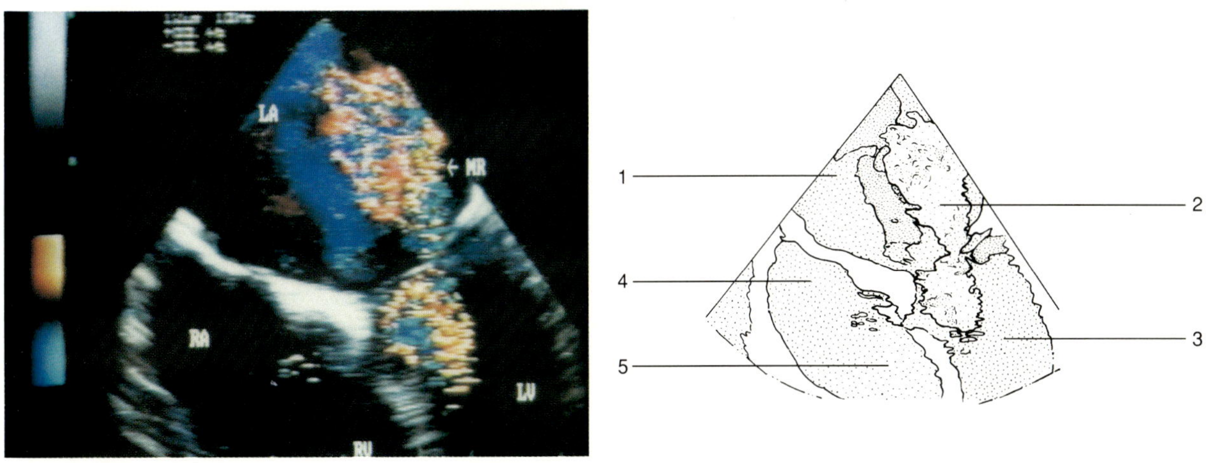

Fig. 18.52 Severe mitral insufficiency demonstrated by color Doppler. Transesophageal echocardiogram (long-axial four-chamber view, in systole) demonstrates a mosaic pattern color-flow jet extending from the mitral valve into the left atrium. The large area occupied by the turbulent jet indicates severe mitral insufficiency.

1 left atrium
2 regurgitant jet
3 left ventricle
4 right atrium
5 right ventricle

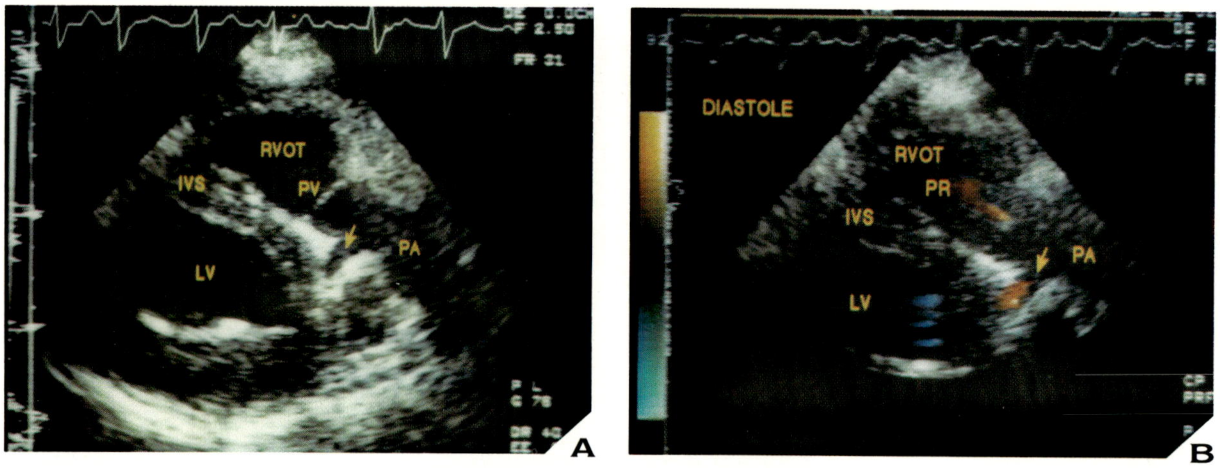

Fig. 20.39 Anomalous origin of the left coronary artery from the pulmonary trunk (echocardiographic findings). (A and B) Short-axis views obtained via a parasternal window. One wall of the pulmonary trunk (PA) is interrupted (*arrow*) at the origin of the anomalous left coronary artery. Diastolic flow (red) from the left coronary artery into the pulmonary trunk can be seen on the color Doppler image (B). (LV = left ventricle; IVS = ventricular septum; RVOT = right ventricular outflow tract)

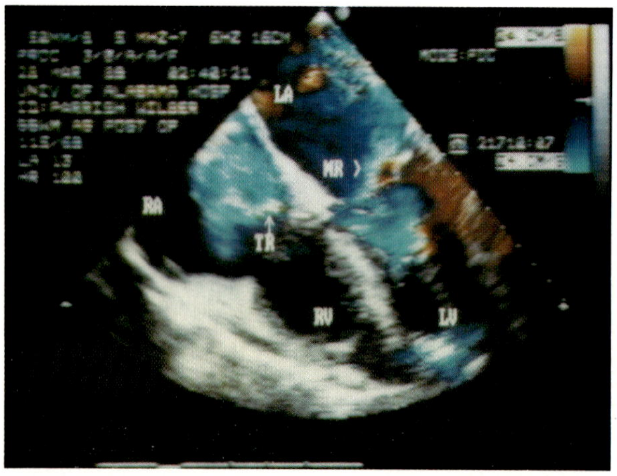

Fig. 23.10 Bacterial endocarditis involving mitral and tricuspid valves. Four-chamber view of color Doppler image at the level of atrioventricular valves (in systole). The blue color in the right atrium (RA) indicates turbulent flow produced by the regurgitant jet (TR) through the incompetent tricuspid valve during systole. The smaller area of blue color (MR) in the left atrium indicates the regurgitant jet through the incompetent mitral valve. (RV = right ventricle; LV = left ventricle)

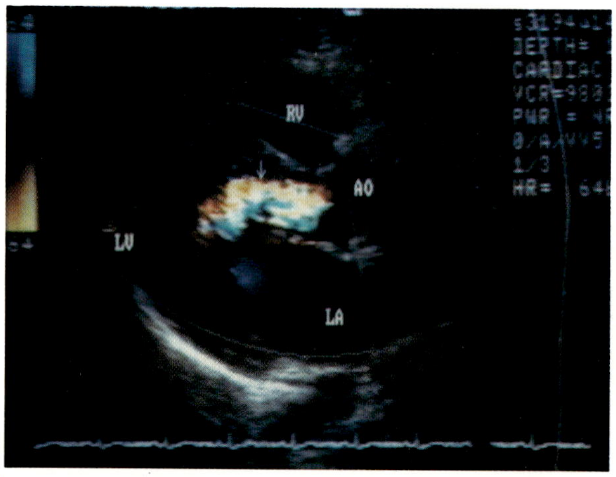

Fig. 23.11 Bacterial endocarditis with aortic insufficiency. Color Doppler echocardiogram. Long axial view (via parasternal window) in diastole demonstrates moderate enlargement of the left atrium (LA). The mosaic color (*arrow*) in the left ventricular outflow tract indicates regurgitant flow through the incompetent aortic valve during diastole. (AO = aorta; LV = left ventricle; RV = right ventricle)

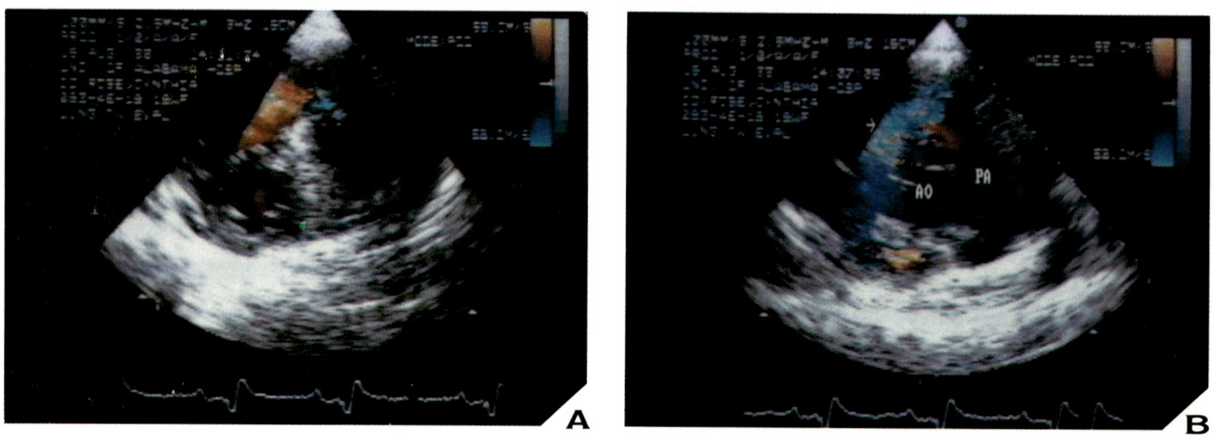

Fig. 24.7 Echocardiographic findings in chronic cor pulmonale. (A and B) Color Doppler images in short axis projection (diastole) show marked dilatation of the pulmonary trunk. Note turbulent flow in the right ventricular outflow tract indicating pulmonic valvular insufficiency.

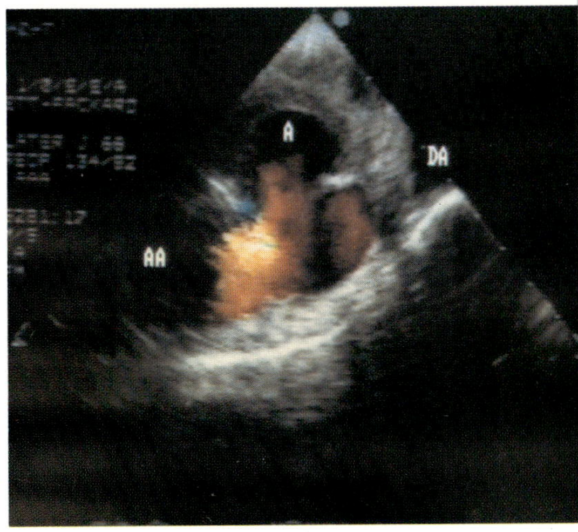

Fig. 27.40 Aortic arch aneurysm (echocardiographi
findings). Transesophageal scan of aortic arch demonst
a large aneurysm arising from the inferior wall of the aor

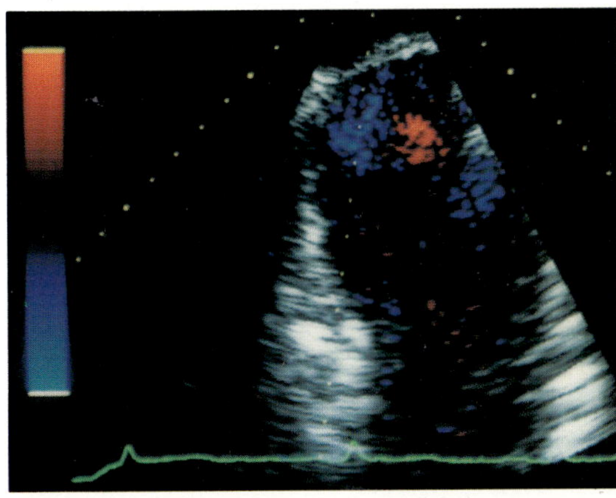

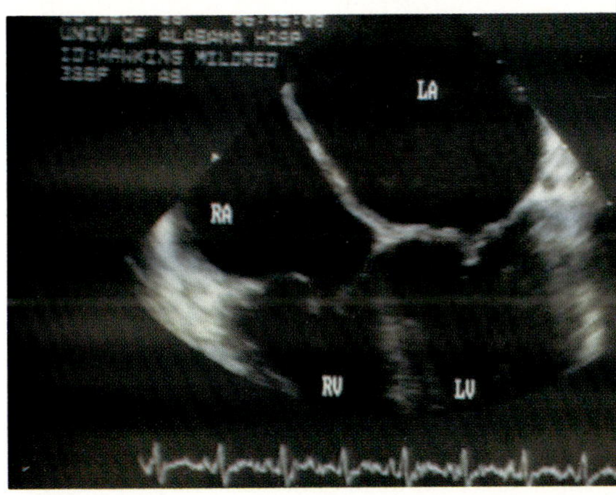

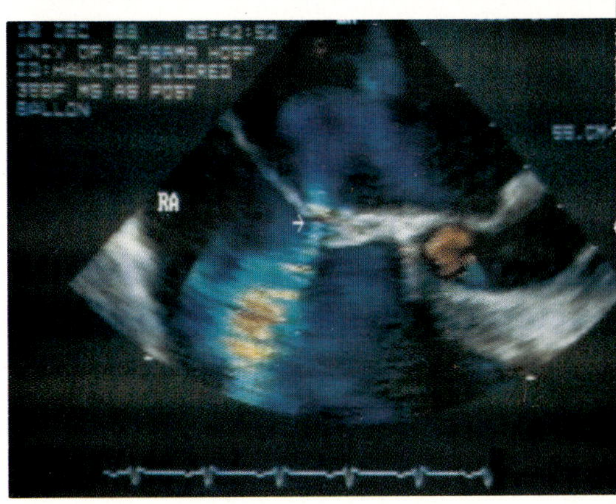

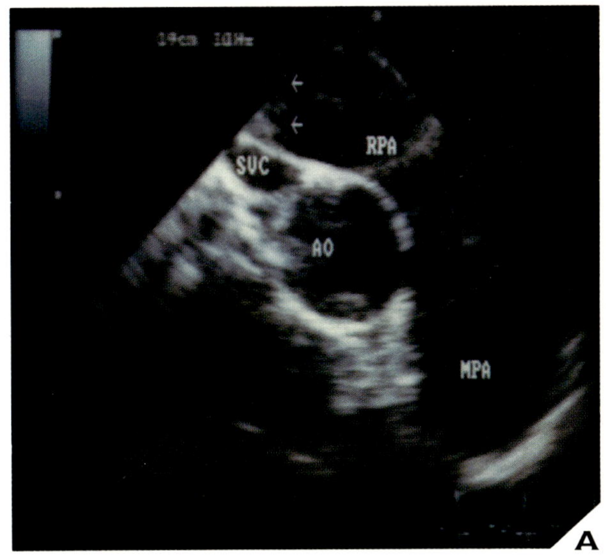

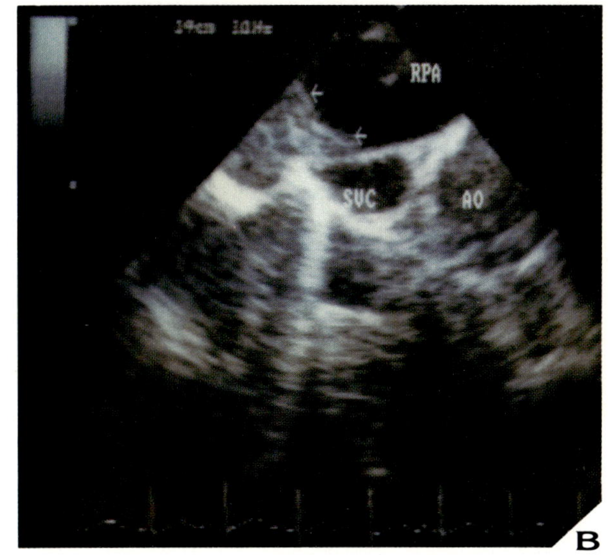

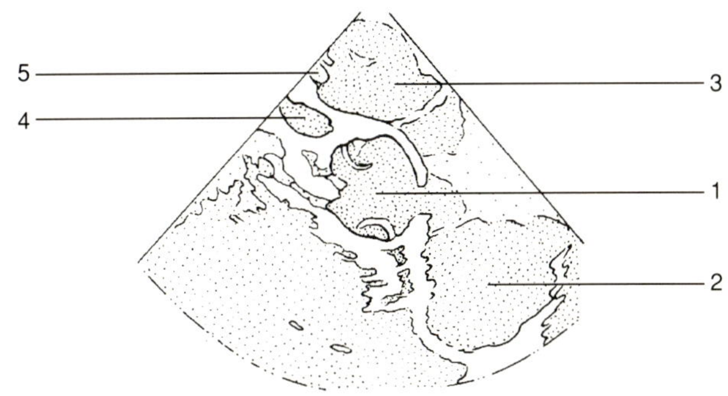

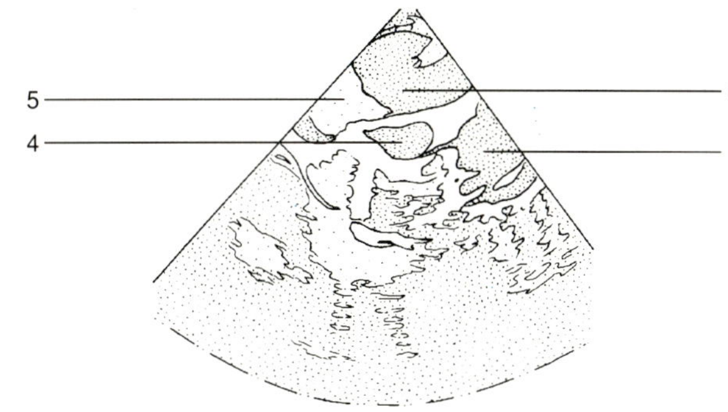

Fig. 24.17 Echocardiographic demonstration of pulmonary embolism. (A and B) Basal short axis images of transesophageal echocardiogram demonstrate dilatation of the pulmonary trunk and right pulmonary artery. The filling defect in the distal portion of the right pulmonary artery represents a thromboembolus.

1 aorta	4 superior vena cava
2 pulmonary trunk	5 intraluminal embolus
3 right pulmonary artery	

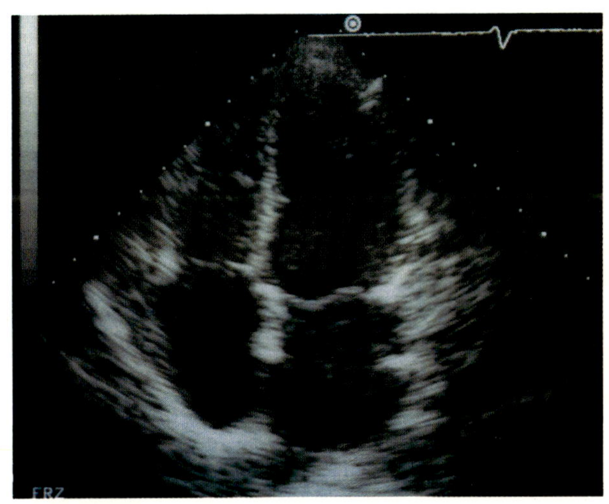

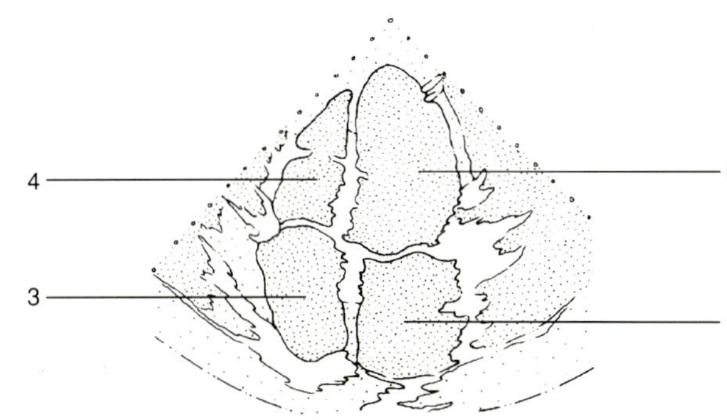

1 left atrium	3 right atrium
2 left ventricle	4 right ventricle

Fig. 24.28 Echocardiographic findings in primary pulmonary hypertension. Apical four-chamber view demonstrates enlargement of the right atrium. The tricuspid and mitral valves are within normal limits. The filling defect in the right atrium represents a mural thrombus, a common finding in patients with primary pulmonary hypertension.

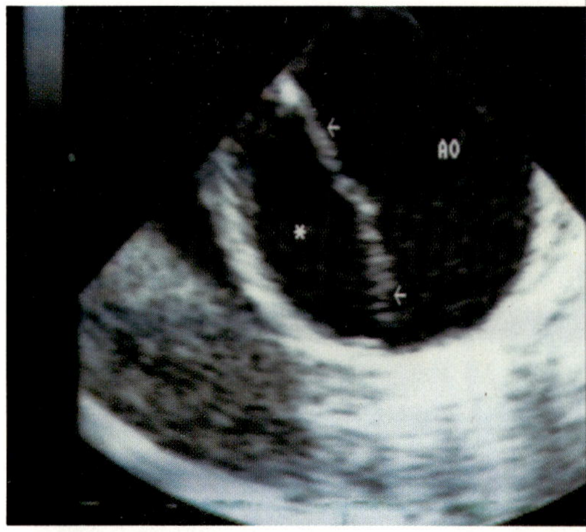

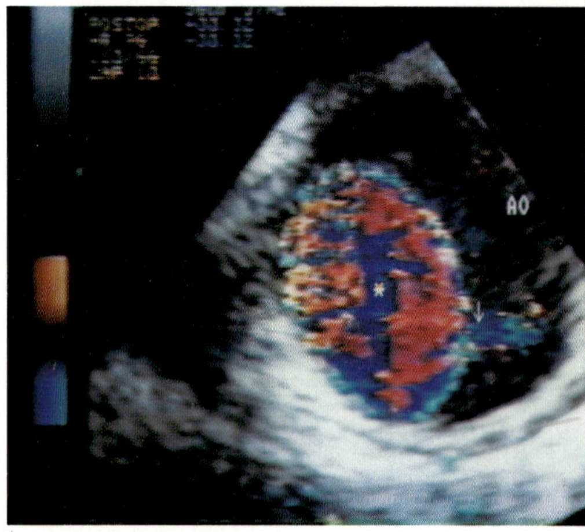

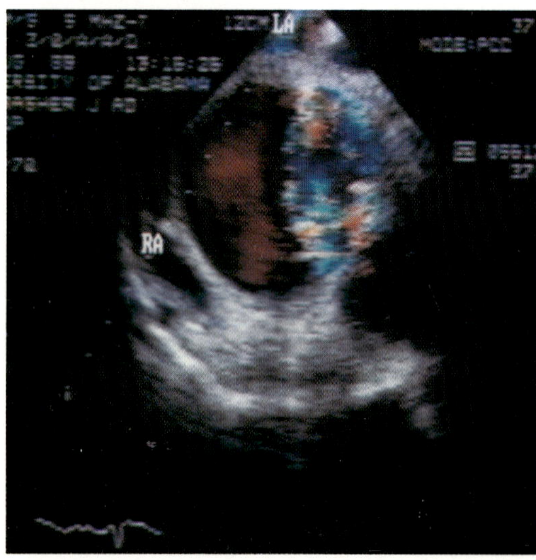

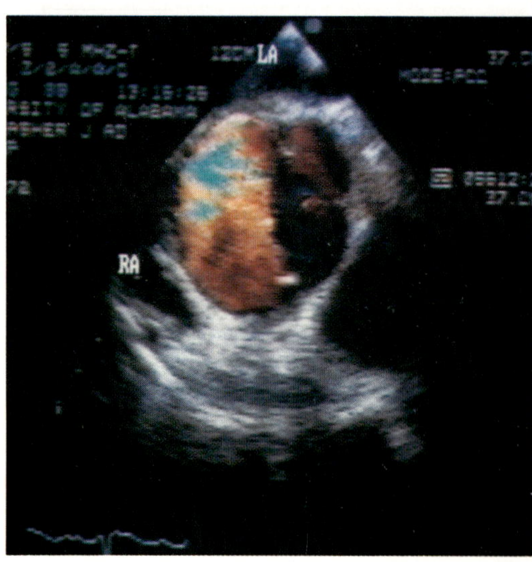

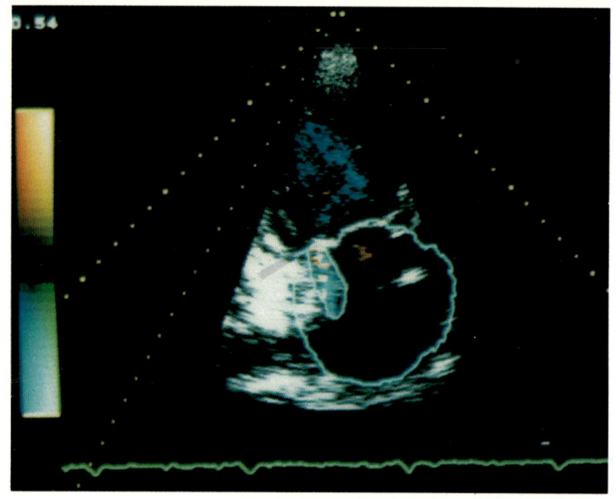

Fig. 32.10 Acute rejection. Color Doppler echocardiogram (apical four-chamber view) demonstrates dilatation of the left atrium and left ventricle. Note moderate mitral insufficiency, which was not evident on previous postoperative studies. Left ventricular systolic function was normal. Endocardial biopsy revealed acute rejection.

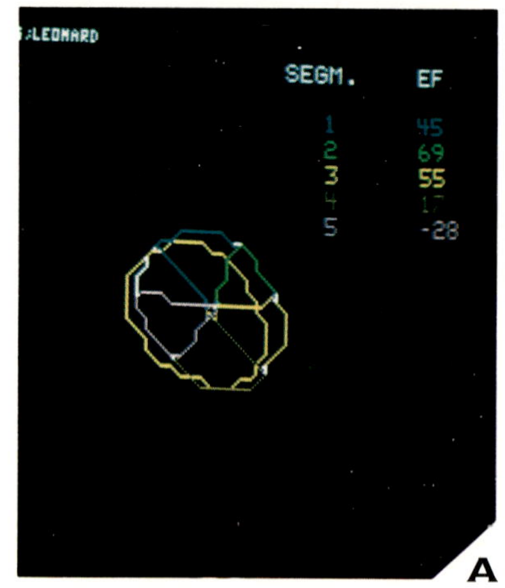

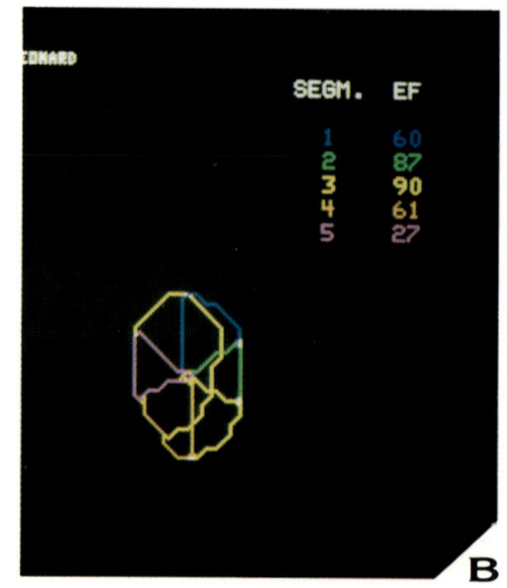

Fig. 32.14 Ischemic cardiomyopathy secondary to accelerated arteriosclerosis (demonstrated by nuclear ventriculography). (A and B) Computer-generated diagrams of left ventriculogram in LAO projection (^{99}Tc-labeled RBCs, 24 mCi). (A) Study obtained 3 years after cardiac transplantation demonstrates dilatation of the left ventricle with poor contraction of all segments and akinesis of the ventricular septum. The measured ejection fraction was 40 percent. Coronary arteriography revealed diffuse stenosis of the left anterior descending artery and stenosis of the middle and distal segments of the right coronary artery (see Figs. 32.15 and 32.16). Re-transplantation was performed several months later. (B) Study obtained several months after the second cardiac transplant demonstrates hypokinesis of the septum; however, the other left ventricular segments contract normally. The measured ejection fraction was 60 percent.